1994
MEDICAL AND HEALTH ANNUAL

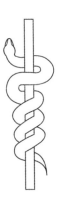

Encyclopædia Britannica, Inc.

CHICAGO

AUCKLAND·LONDON·MADRID·MANILA·PARIS·ROME·SEOUL·SYDNEY·TOKYO·TORONTO

1994 Medical and Health Annual

Editor	Ellen Bernstein
Senior Editor	Linda Tomchuck
Contributing Editors	Charles Cegielski, Daphne Daume, Melinda C. Shepherd

Creative Director, Art	Cynthia Peterson
Operations Manager, Art	Marsha Mackenzie
Senior Picture Editor	Holly Harrington
Picture Editors	Karen Wollins, Amy Zweig
Art Production Supervisor	Stephanie Motz
Illustrators/Layout Artists	Kay Diffley, John L. Draves, Steven N. Kapusta, James I. Montes
Art Staff	Patricia A. Henle, Diana M. Pitstick, Rebecca L. Porter

Manager, Cartography	Barbra A. Vogel
Cartography Staff	Steven Bogdan, Robert G. Kowalski, Michael D. Nutter, Kathryn A. Piffl

Manager, Copy Department	Sylvia Wallace
Copy Supervisor	Barbara Whitney
Copy Staff	Philip Colvin, Madolynn Cronk, Anthony L. Green, John Mathews, Deirdre McAllister

Manager, Production Control	Mary C. Srodon
Production Control Staff	Marilyn L. Barton, Stephanie A. Green

Manager, Composition/Page Makeup	Melvin Stagner
Supervisor, Composition/Page Makeup	Michael Born, Jr.
Coordinator, Composition/Page Makeup	Danette Wetterer
Composition/Page Makeup Staff	Griselda Cháidez, Carol A. Gaines, John Krom, Jr., Thomas J. Mulligan, Arnell Reed, Gwen E. Rosenberg, Tammy Yu-chu Wang

Director, Management Information Systems	Michelle J. Brandhorst
Management Information Systems Staff	Steven Bosco, Philip Rehmer, Vincent Star

Manager, Index Department	Carmen-Maria Hetrea
Index Supervisor	Edward Paul Moragne
Index Staff	Stephen S. Seddon, Gayl E. Williams

Librarian	Terry Passaro
Associate Librarian	Shantha Uddin
Curator/Geography	David W. Foster
Assistant Librarian	Robert M. Lewis

Yearbook Secretarial Staff	Dorothy Hagen, Catherine E. Johnson

Editorial Advisers

Stephen Lock, M.D.	Drummond Rennie, M.D.
Research Associate,	Professor of Medicine,
Section of History of 20th Century Medicine,	Institute for Health Policy Studies,
Wellcome Institute for the History of Medicine, London;	University of California at San Francisco;
Editor Emeritus,	Deputy Editor (West),
British Medical Journal	*Journal of the American Medical Association*

Editorial Administration

Robert McHenry, Editor in Chief
Robert F. Rauch, Director of Yearbooks
Elizabeth P. O'Connor, Director, Finance and Operations

Encyclopædia Britannica Publishing Group
Joseph J. Esposito, President
Karen M. Barch, Executive Vice President, Associate Publisher

Encyclopædia Britannica, Inc.
Robert P. Gwinn, Chairman of the Board
Peter B. Norton, President

Library of Congress Catalog Card Number: 77-649875
International Standard Book Number: 0-85229-590-1
International Standard Serial Number: 0363-0366
Copyright © 1993 by Encyclopædia Britannica, Inc.
All rights reserved for all countries.
Printed in U.S.A.

Foreword

The editors of the 1994 *Medical and Health Annual* have endeavored to prepare a volume that is informative, up-to-date, stimulating, and attractive—an authoritative resource that addresses subjects of interest and concern to our readers.

In this volume we are pleased to introduce a new section, **Newsmakers** (pages 6–23), in which are highlighted notable achievements and contributions of individuals—some well known, some not—who, for a wide assortment of reasons, have lately made medical news. Although most are human, they are joined by several animals, a robot that recently made its debut in the operating room, a cartoon character, a doll, and a beloved character from fiction.

In-depth **Feature** articles, appearing on pages 24–192, are meant to convey the challenge and excitement in the very broad areas of medicine and health. All are lavishly illustrated; the subjects range from world hunger to American Indian health to the behind-the-scenes work of pathologists to mental breakdown in travelers to the Holy City of Jerusalem.

Certainly it is no easy task for the layperson to keep up with the rapidly evolving developments in medicine and health today. Indeed, each day brings reports of new treatments and new ways to diagnose and prevent disease, as well as new causes for anxiety and alarm—environmental threats to health, dangers posed by drugs, foods that are unsafe to eat or suspected of causing cancer or heart disease—not to mention frequent and often conflicting admonitions about what constitutes a healthy lifestyle. To sort it all out, the *Annual* turns to experts. In the alphabetically organized **World of Medicine** (pages 222–406), these authorities—medical scientists and health specialists who are well recognized in their respective fields—evaluate so-called breakthroughs and put health risks in perspective.

As always, this edition of the *Annual* has not restricted its focus to medicine and health in the United States. Rather, it offers an international perspective. Accordingly, this year's **World of Medicine** includes the following **Special Reports**:

● "Health Care Reform in Eurasia: The Next Revolution" (pages 292–299)
● "John Snow Gets His Monument: London's Tribute to a Medical Pioneer" (pages 344–348)
● "Health for All: A Dream Realized in Cuba" (pages 357–362)
● "Work: Dying for It in Japan" (pages 373–375)
● "France: Fuming over a New Law?" (pages 386–391)

The section of the *Annual* that we call **HealthWise** (pages 417–482) was conceived in response to an evident and timely need for sound medical information for laypeople who wish to take a measure of responsibility for their own health. Here readers will find instructive articles that provide basic understanding of common and not-so-common diseases; articles that focus on women's, men's, and children's health concerns; articles about diet, nutrition, and physical fitness; and articles that are concerned with psychological health and emotional well-being.

We emphasize that the intention of the *Medical and Health Annual* is to *inform,* not to prescribe. We hope the **HealthWise** articles will help readers become more knowledgeable about how and when to seek professional help; however, this book should never serve as a substitute for the advice and care of a physician.

Three selections in this volume are designated **Editors' Choice**:

● "America's Children: Our Vision of the Future" (pages 212–221) is an adaptation of a lecture given by M. Joycelyn Elders at the time she received the prestigious Joseph W. Mountin Award from the Centers for Disease Control and Prevention in Atlanta, Georgia. We think readers will find her message an especially compelling one. At the time the *Annual* went to press, Elders was Pres. Bill Clinton's nominee for the nation's top health post, surgeon general; her confirmation by the U.S. Senate was expected shortly.

● Of course, as a yearbook of medicine and health, the *Annual,* to quite a large extent, focuses on subjects that are very serious in nature—*e.g.,* illness, disability, and death. However, as most physicians would be quick to point out, laughter is excellent medicine. Therefore, the editors offer a selection of pertinent humor, which we call "A Cartoon a Day . . ." (pages 245–249).

● The editors wonder how much the *Annual*'s readers know about the foods they eat—or *should be* eating. They can find out by taking the quiz "What's Your Nutrition IQ?" (pages 407–416). We suspect that many will find they know less than they thought they did.

*   *   *

Finally, the editors are indebted to our many contributors, without whose considerable cooperation this volume would not be possible. We also wish to express our gratitude to our two medical advisers, Drummond Rennie in San Francisco and Stephen Lock in London, for their continuing good counsel.

Ellen Bernstein

—Editor

Contents

Features

World of Medicine

Editors' Choice

HealthWise

NEWSMAKERS

Both mice and men and not a few women were in the news as medicine and health care moved to the top of the agenda with the inauguration of William Jefferson (Bill) Clinton as president of the United States in January 1993. The White House acted quickly to reverse restrictive abortion policies of the administrations of George Bush and Ronald Reagan, including lifting a five-year ban on fetal tissue research. Clinton also proposed bold initiatives to ensure that all U.S. children are fully immunized and created a commission, headed by his wife, lawyer Hillary Rodham Clinton, to develop a national health plan that would, among other things, provide coverage for the estimated 37 million Americans who have no medical insurance.

While the spotlight was on Washington, AIDS continued its relentless course worldwide, claiming the lives of numerous public figures and, often unnoted except in statistics, thousands of others. At the same time, the politics surrounding the pandemic drew researchers, political activists, and others into the news. In a controversial film, actors portraying the struggle of a real-life family brought attention to a rare inherited disorder and its treatment. There were, in addition, many sung and unsung heroes and heroines who made an impact in one way or another on matters of health and sadly, quite a few medical pioneers died.

It was not just bipedal mammals that took front and center in health and medicine, however. They were joined by a menagerie of quadrupedal kin, ranging from mice to baboons, as well as such inanimates as a doll, a robot, and a cartoon character who promotes carrots to kids on television.

Capital health

While Clinton was still a candidate, his health became the focus of controversy when he declined to make public his doctors' reports. Critics argued that the public was entitled to information about the health of a presidential candidate, citing previous cover-ups of the seriousness of the medical conditions of such presidents as Franklin D. Roosevelt and John F. Kennedy.

During the campaign for the presidential nomination, controversy arose over the medical status of candidate Paul E. Tsongas, a former Democratic senator from Massachusetts. Tsongas had been treated with a bone marrow transplant for lymphoma in 1986. During the primaries Tsongas said that he was cancer free. However, his doctors subsequently acknowledged that lymphoma had been found in 1987 in a lymph node in his armpit. He withdrew from the race after faring poorly in early primaries, and later he was hospitalized for treatment of a recurrence of cancer. Tsongas acknowledged that he had erred in not providing full disclosure, and his doctors at the Dana-Farber Cancer Institute in Boston also conceded that they had made mistakes in describing the candidate's health as being better than it was.

Once Clinton's doctors were permitted to disclose his medical history, they told rather more than many voters might want to know, including the fact that the 46-year-old president had suffered from hemorrhoids in 1984 but on subsequent examination showed no significant rectal pathology. One of his doctors described

The 42nd U.S. president, like several of his predecessors, jogs to keep fit. Soon after Bill Clinton moved to the capital, private donors paid for a jogging track to be built on the grounds of the presidential abode.

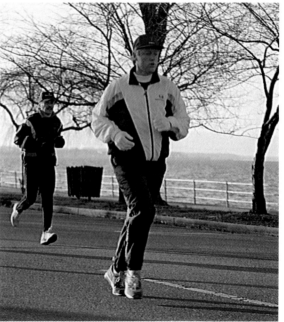

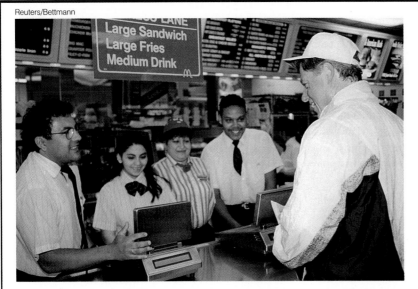

President-elect Clinton chats with employees at a McDonald's restaurant after an early-morning run. Despite his efforts to keep fit and stick to a heart-healthy diet, Clinton makes no secret of the fact that he has trouble resisting an occasional Big Mac and fries.

him as being "a well-developed, well-nourished white male" with blood pressure and pulse in the normal range. Although he is an avid jogger, the president also has an affinity for fast food—greasy french fries and hamburgers—which undoubtedly contributed to his being a tad overweight (102.5 kilograms [226 pounds]) and to his mildly elevated blood cholesterol. He showed no cardiovascular problems, however, and was found to have a normal prostate and no traces of blood in his stool. Because of a gastric reflux problem, Clinton had switched from regular coffee, which he formerly consumed in large quantities, to decaffeinated. He also consumes alcohol moderately and, though a nonsmoker, sometimes chews on a fat unlit cigar.

During the campaign Clinton suffered from laryngitis resulting from excessive use of his voice and from allergies, which also have contributed to his sinusitis. Tests have shown that he is allergic to house dust, mold spores, weed pollen, grass pollen, beef, milk, and—yes—cat dander, even though daughter Chelsea's feline friend, Socks, lived with the family in the Governor's Mansion in Little Rock, Arkansas, and now has free run of the White House. He also reacts to Christmas trees, presumably from mold spores, but endures the discomfort caused by the family tree for the sake of the season. He is treated for his allergies with decongestants and a prescription antihistamine and receives periodic desensitization shots. During the last stretch of the campaign and on election day, he used an inhaled corticosteroid, beclomethasone, for his swollen vocal cords, a medication that could have systemic side effects with extended use.

A few months into his administration, the president was reported to be working long days and late nights and keeping a feverish pace. Some staff and friends noted he was "puffy-eyed" and expressed concern that he was overdoing it—getting by on less than five hours of sleep on an average night.

With national security less of a campaign issue than in previous years, voters chose Clinton to deal with pressing domestic problems—among the top ones being health care. Once elected, he hit the ground running, literally and figuratively. (His penchant for jogging in the unsecured streets of the capital raised concerns about Clinton's safety, and so private donors paid to have a jogging track built on White House grounds.) It was his high-profile appointments and other actions related to health care, however, that created excitement—and some criticism.

Clinton had pledged during the campaign to create an administration more representative of the nation's diversity, and the elections themselves created a Congress that included more women and minorities than anytime in history. Making good on his pledge, Clinton named as one of his first appointments Donna E. Shalala, chancellor of the University of Wisconsin since 1988 and former president of Hunter College in New York City, to be secretary of health and human services. Shalala, who holds a doctorate in political science from Syracuse (New York) University, had experience primarily in education. Though not a physician, she had served for 20 months on the institutional advisory panel of the National Institutes of Health (NIH), and she had succeeded Hillary Clinton as head of the Children's

Defense Fund. Shalala also pointed out that at Wisconsin she oversaw the university's teaching hospital, which gave her insight into the financing of health care.

As surgeon general, Clinton appointed an outspoken legend in Arkansas politics, M. Joycelyn Elders, a pediatric endocrinologist who had been president of the Association of State and Territorial Health Officials. Elders, an African-American, had headed Governor Clinton's state health department, where she was both colorful in her language and controversial in her policies. She worked to reduce adolescent pregnancy and was an advocate of school-based family-planning clinics. When she was once asked if such clinics would dispense contraceptives, she replied, "We're not going to put them on the lunch trays. But yes." She also advocated sex education beginning in kindergarten. "I really feel we must put our children first, and I'm willing to do whatever we have to do to save the children," she has said. (*See* Editors' Choice: "America's Children: Our Vision of the Future," page 213.)

To deal with the problems of the nation's network of veterans hospitals, Clinton appointed Jesse Brown, also an African-American, who had been executive director of the Disabled Veterans of America, to head the Department of Veterans Affairs. Brown, who has a partially paralyzed arm, was awarded a Purple Heart for service in the Marine Corps during the Vietnam war. Although his appointment was greeted with widespread approval from leaders of veterans organizations, his diplomatic skills were expected to be challenged as he sought to deal with the largest health-care-delivery system in the free world—employing 200,000 people; comprising 172 hospitals, 229 outpatient clinics, 117 nursing homes, and other facilities; and costing taxpayers $13.8 billion a year. Numerous VA hospitals have been under fire for delivering poor-quality care and for being underutilized at a time when the nation's health care resources are severely strained.

From the Bush administration Clinton retained David A. Kessler as commissioner of the Food and Drug Administration (FDA). Kessler, a physician, lawyer, and former congressional aide, has been widely admired for his technical expertise and nonpolitical approach to carrying out the business of an agency that is frequently criticized for inefficiency and for delaying the approval of drugs. He has been credited with reorganizing what had become a beleaguered bureaucracy and making the FDA both aggressive and innovative.

Clinton asked for the resignation, however, of Bernadine P. Healy, the controversial director of the NIH. The physician had been accused of being abrasive in her dealings with top government officials and many university-based researchers. Shortly after taking charge of the institute, she openly clashed with the powerful Rep. John Dingell (Dem., Mich.), who chaired a key committee with extensive power over NIH affairs. In a statement following her dismissal, Healy said that her primary achievements at the NIH had been the creation of a strategic plan for biomedical research, the advancement of a major women's health initiative, and expansion of the Human Genome Project. Critics contested her assertions.

Donna E. Shalala visits with youngsters at a day-care center. Expanding the Head Start preschool program and ensuring that all American children are fully immunized before their sixth birthday were among the top orders of business of the new secretary of the Department of Health and Human Services during her first year. Though not a physician, Shalala came to her post with vast administrative experience—most recently as chancellor of the University of Wisconsin. At her confirmation hearings she told senators that she had "no problem switching hats" from education to health.

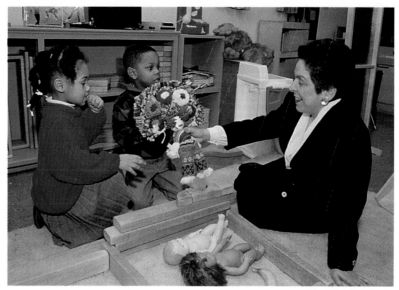

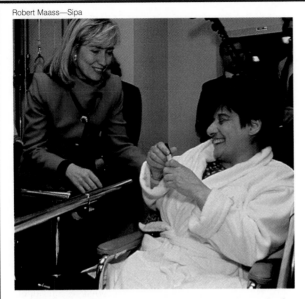

Hillary Rodham Clinton visits a patient at St. Agnes Medical Center in Philadephia. As the president's choice to head a task force on health policy reform, the first lady has traveled nationwide to learn firsthand how Americans feel about the health care that is available to them.

Also dismissed was Burton J. Lee, a political appointee who served as Bush's personal physician, reportedly because he refused to give the president an allergy shot in January. Lawrence C. Mohr, a military doctor, remained on at the White House; he and his staff now provide the medical care for the Clintons.

When Clinton appointed his wife as head of the President's Task Force on National Health Care Reform, he said that he had chosen her because "she's better at organizing and leading people from a complex beginning to a certain end than anybody I've ever worked with in my life." While it is not unusual for wives to play a role in their husbands' administrations, Hillary Clinton was the first to be assigned such an important policy-making position. Although unpaid, she was given an office in the West Wing of the White House. Prior to her husband's election to the presidency, she was a highly successful lawyer in Little Rock, earning more than her husband did as governor. Her first Washington assignment was to head a committee appointed to prepare legislation to overhaul the nation's costly health care system, one that delivers the highest-quality care in the world to those who can afford it but leaves millions without adequate care—or with no care at all.

The first lady drew attention to personal health matters straightaway by saying that she and the president wished to ban smoking throughout the White House,

just as she and her husband had done in the Governor's Mansion in Little Rock. She reinstated broccoli on the White House menu, restoring it to a place of proper nutritional esteem after President Bush had banished the vegetable from his plate. "We are big broccoli eaters.... We do a lot of vegetables and a lot of fiber and a lot of fruit," she remarked, in announcing that the White House would emphasize American rather than French-style food.

AIDS: the unrelenting toll

Just as the rain falls on the just and the unjust, so does AIDS wipe out the bright, the brilliant, and the beautiful as well as the ordinary. While scientists worked to develop a cure for AIDS and a vaccine against human immunodeficiency virus (HIV), the virus that causes it, the disease continued its relentless decade-long decimation throughout the world, especially in poverty-ridden less developed countries. In the industrialized Western world, AIDS continued to take a phenomenal toll on a generation of creative artists and performers, and many other high-profile personalities, thus making the disease real for some to whom it might otherwise represent nothing more than cold statistics.

Few disclosures of HIV infection have had such an electrifying effect as that of Earvin ("Magic") Johnson, the world-famous Los Angeles Lakers basketball star. Although asymptomatic for AIDS, Johnson announced in November 1991 that he was retiring from professional basketball. He soon began playing again, however. But because players on competing teams made public their concerns about contracting HIV from contact with Johnson on the ball court—a possibility that remains unlikely and controversial—he quit the game again a year later. Controversy did not end there. Johnson had been appointed by President Bush to the National Commission on AIDS in 1991 but resigned on Sept. 25, 1992, telling the president in a letter that he and his fellow commission members had "been increasingly frustrated by the lack of support, and even opposition, of your administration to our recommendations— recommendations that have an urgent priority and for which there is broad consensus in the medical and AIDS communities." He was replaced on the commission by Mary Fisher, an artist and heiress from Florida, who is HIV positive. Fisher had earlier made a passionate speech before the 1992 Republican national convention in Houston, Texas, talking about the prejudice she and other victims of the epidemic face.

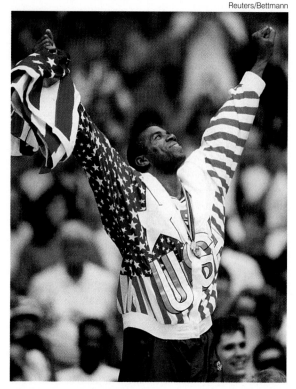

Johnson's announcement has had major repercussions nationally and internationally. Other infected celebrities have also disclosed their illness; condom use among some groups has increased; and there are reportedly fewer individuals having one-time sexual encounters and multiple sexual partners.

Another distinguished athlete, tennis champion Arthur Ashe, died of complications of AIDS on Feb. 6, 1993, at age 49. Ashe was the first African-American to win the Wimbledon and U.S. Open titles and to play for the U.S. Davis Cup team, for which he later served as captain. During his career he won 33 titles. After retiring from active competition, he wrote *A Hard Road to Glory,* a three-volume history of the black athlete in America. Throughout his life he fought diligently in defense of civil rights and other causes. Just weeks before his death, he visited the State University of New York Health Science Center at Brooklyn to announce the creation of the Arthur Ashe Institute for Urban Health. Ashe was believed to have contracted HIV from a blood transfusion he received during heart surgery in 1983, 18 months before blood supplies started being routinely tested for the virus. He revealed his condition

A jubilant Magic Johnson, a player for the U.S. "Dream Team," displays his gold medal at the 1992 summer Olympic Games. Nine months earlier Johnson shocked the sporting world when he announced he was HIV positive. The basketball star served on the National Commission on AIDS but quit in September 1992, claiming former president George Bush "dropped the ball" on AIDS. He was replaced by Mary Fisher, an artist from Florida who contracted HIV from her former husband. Fisher gained recognition when she pleaded with Republicans at their national convention to have compassion toward people with AIDS.

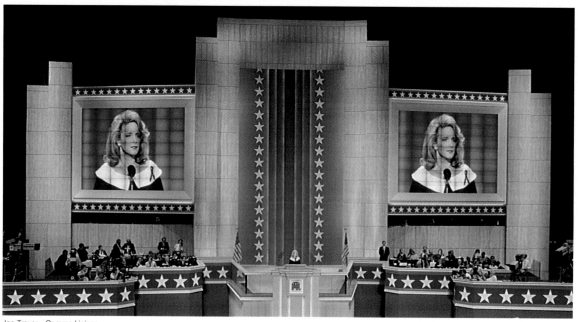

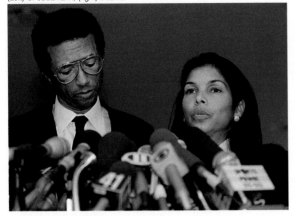

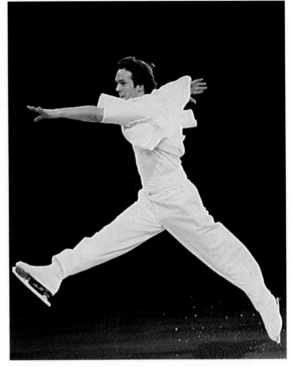

A tearful Arthur Ashe, one of professional tennis' finest players ever and a longtime champion of human rights, reveals publicly in April 1992 that he has AIDS; his wife, Jeanne, helps him through the painful disclosure. Ten months after his announcement, Ashe died of AIDS-related pneumonia. (Right) AIDS has taken an especially grim toll on the professional skating world; the British gold medalist John Curry is just one of dozens of skaters to have contracted the disease.

publicly less than a year before his death after the information was leaked to a national newspaper, which threatened to publicize it. In *Days of Grace: A Memoir,* published posthumously, he reflected on his illness and approaching death: "Did I feel a sense of shame, however subdued, about having AIDS, although I was guilty of nothing in contracting it? Very little. I could not shake off completely that irrational sense of guilt, but I did my best to keep it in check."

The dancer credited with popularizing ballet in the U.S., Rudolf Nureyev, who had defected from the U.S.S.R. in 1961, died in Paris on Jan. 6, 1993, at age 54, from complications of AIDS. Unlike Johnson and Ashe, Nureyev never publicly revealed that he had the disease, and his physician, Michel Canési, announced the cause of death as "a cardiac complication following a grievous illness." After much criticism Canési acknowledged that Nureyev had indeed died of AIDS after contracting the virus 13 or 14 years earlier. His was but the most notable of deaths that have devastated the ballet world, wiping out not only many of today's stars but also several of tomorrow's.

Figure skating, sometimes called ballet on ice, likewise has lost stellar performers to AIDS, with more than 40 top North American skaters having died from complications of the disease, including the Canadian champions Rob McCall, Shaun McGill, Dennis Coi, and Brian Pockar. Another world-class skater to acknowledge publicly that he was infected was British champion John Curry, a 1976 Olympic gold medal winner.

In April 1993, Rubén Palacio of Colombia, holder of the World Boxing Organization's featherweight crown, tested positive for HIV, the first boxing champion to do so. Subsequent to the revelation of his infection, Palacio was stripped of his title and barred from further competition in the sport.

The AIDS epidemic is also diminishing the ranks of another group of performers, gospel singers. Racism is being blamed for the lack of notice that has been given to the many deaths that are depriving African-American churches of many a glorious singer.

One of the most prominent journalists regularly writing about AIDS, *New York Times* reporter Jeffrey Schmalz revealed his own illness in a first-person report in 1992 in that newspaper: "Now I see the world through the prism of AIDS. I feel an obligation to those with AIDS to write about it and an obligation to the newspaper to write what just about no other reporter in America can cover in quite the same way." Among many things, he disclosed his feelings about reporting on three brothers with hemophilia, Randy, Robert, and Ricky Ray, sons of Louise and Clifford Ray, who had been barred from school in Arcadia, Florida, after it became known that they were infected with HIV. When a federal court ordered that the boys be readmitted to class, the family's home was destroyed by arson, and they were forced to move to another town. The oldest, Ricky, 15, died of AIDS in December 1992.

Another prominent writer, Randy Shilts of San Francisco, developed full-blown AIDS in the summer of 1992. He had been diagnosed with HIV in 1987 on the day he finished his book on the disease, *And the Band Played On.* In April 1993 his book *Conduct Unbecoming,* a portrait of gays in the military, was published.

The highly acclaimed young playwright and actor Scott McPherson died of AIDS Nov. 7, 1992. He received critical praise for his two plays, *'Til the Fat Lady Sings* and *Marvin's Room,* both of which focused on illness. Another loss to the theatrical world was Anthony Perkins. Best known for his role in Alfred Hitchcock's *Psycho,* the actor died of complications from AIDS on Sept. 12, 1992.

Baritone William Parker, acclaimed for his performances of American music, died on March 29, 1993. He was 49. Parker had commissioned works about the illness (including songs by Ned Rorem and William Bolcom) for a cycle called *The AIDS Quilt Songbook.* In June 1992 he participated in the first performance of the work at Lincoln Center's Alice Tully Hall in New York City.

Among other young AIDS-stricken artists whose illness became publicly known in 1992 are Kevin Oldham of New York City, a highly regarded composer, and Robert Farber, an artist whose exhibition in a Manhattan gallery linked the AIDS crisis with the bubonic plague in 1348. Both received support from the Estate Project for Artists with AIDS, an organization that encourages artists in all disciplines to catalog their works and prepare their estates in order to ensure their artistic posterity.

Peter Jepson-Young, a physician who had appeared on Canadian television in frank discussions about his own illness in an effort to help fight stereotypes and misunderstandings about AIDS, died in Vancouver, British Columbia, on Nov. 15, 1992, of AIDS-related complications. Over a period of two years, more than 100 segments of his "AIDS Diaries" were viewed by millions of Canadians.

Melvin L. Rosen, a social worker who for three years was chairman of Beth Simchat Torah synagogue in New York City, died of AIDS-related lung cancer on Aug. 31, 1992. Rosen had been the first executive director of the Gay Men's Health Crisis/AIDS Fund and the first director of the New York State AIDS Institute, a division of the state's Department of Health. Louis Grant of New York City died on May 22, 1993. An African-American who had lived with the symptoms of AIDS for more than 11 years, he had been vice president of the board of the Gay Men's Health Crisis.

On the West Coast, Daniel P. Warner, founder and executive director of the Los Angeles-based Shanti Foundation, which trains volunteers to care for AIDS patients, succumbed to AIDS complications on June 14, 1993, his 38th birthday. The list of young people in their prime who became AIDS and HIV victims grew daily.

On the research front, a nearly decade-old dispute over who should get credit—and royalties—for discovering the virus that causes AIDS seemed to be closer to resolution when the U.S. Department of Health and Human Services (HHS) issued a report censuring

Peter Jepson-Young delivered frank messages about AIDS on Canadian television. The physician from Vancouver lived with the disease for six years, during which time he lost his sight to the virus and developed AIDS-related skin cancer.

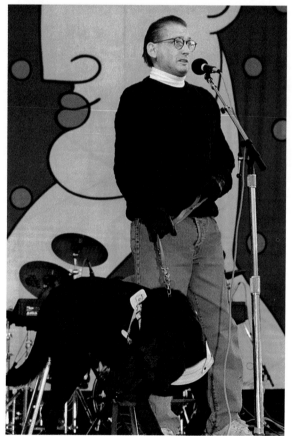

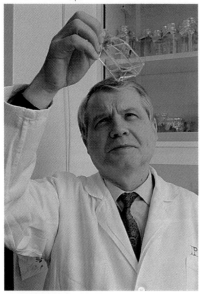

Florence Durand—Sipa

Luc Montagnier investigates the AIDS virus in his lab at the Pasteur Institute in Paris. He and fellow researchers received the 1993 King Faisal International Prize for identifying the virus and elucidating how it attacks the immune system.

Robert C. Gallo, an eminent researcher. The report said that Gallo, director of the National Cancer Institute's Laboratory of Tumor Cell Biology, had committed scientific misconduct in connection with his codiscovery in 1984, with French scientists, of the virus that causes AIDS, then called lymphadenopathy-associated virus (LAV). At stake, in addition to Gallo's position and reputation, were lucrative patent rights to blood tests for AIDS in which pieces of the virus are used to detect antiviral antibodies in infected persons. The HHS report accused Gallo and his colleagues of claiming in a published paper that the virus discovered in their laboratory differed from LAV, which had been isolated by Luc Montagnier and co-workers at the Pasteur Institute in Paris. Evidence showed that the researchers had in fact transferred LAV to a permanent cell line, a crucial step in the production of sufficient viral proteins for development of AIDS-virus antibodies. In June 1993 the government announced it was looking into still further misconduct regarding Gallo's work with the AIDS virus. New charges focused on his withholding of information from competitors and keeping secret data that were "of critical public health importance." By not sharing scientific findings, Gallo is said to have prevented other countries from adopting crucial blood-screening practices.

Meanwhile, three French AIDS researchers from the Pasteur Institute garnered further acclaim for their work when in February 1993 they received the King Faisal International Prize in medicine. The honors went to Montagnier, Jean-Claude Chermann, and Françoise Barré-Sinoussi for their work in identifying the virus subsequently shown to cause AIDS and delineating how it damages the human immune system.

Crusading against cigarettes

Even before the Clintons' insistence on a ban on smoking in the White House, the antismoking campaign was gaining international momentum. The death in July 1992 of "Marlboro Man" Wayne McLaren at age 51 helped diminish the macho image of cigarette smoking. McLaren, who died of lung cancer, had appeared in the 1970s and '80s in billboard and magazine advertisements depicting a rough-riding, cigarette-smoking cowboy in "Marlboro Country." A rodeo rider, actor, and Hollywood stuntman, McLaren had smoked a pack and a half of cigarettes a day for more than 25 years. After he developed his fatal disease, he became an ardent campaigner against smoking. In one of his last acts, McLaren appeared at a meeting of Philip Morris shareholders, urging them to call upon the company to investigate its advertising practices—in particular, the ways in which the ads influence children. McLaren said that tobacco companies had a moral obligation to "end this war to gain young smokers." The resolution was defeated.

After his death McLaren's wife, Ellen, appealed to members of the European Community (EC) to ban tobacco advertising and promotion except at the point of sale. Five EC nations were resisting a ban on tobacco advertising. "There is nothing macho or glamorous about smoking," she said. Joining McLaren in the European lobbying efforts was the "Lucky Strike Girl," 61-year-old Janet Sackman, who modeled for ads in the 1950s. She, too, subsequently developed cancer and had to have her larynx and part of a lung removed. "Children must never learn to smoke and ruin their healthy bodies," she told the Europeans, who only recently had to adapt to the kind of restrictions on smoking in public areas that have become the rule in the United States.

A popular athlete also joined the public health campaign against smoking. Kirby Puckett, star batter for the Minnesota Twins, volunteered to work with the Minnesota Department of Health in an effort to discourage school-age children from taking up the habit. Puckett, wielding a baseball bat, is featured on posters

In 1954 Daniel E. Horn (left) and E. Cuyler Hammond sort through a veritable mountain of statistics in their office at the national headquarters of the American Cancer Society. They were among the first to establish a link between cigarette smoking and lung cancer, and their statistical studies provided the impetus for the government to adopt an aggressive antismoking stance. Horn continued to conduct smoking-related research throughout his professional career and was a committed health advocate until his death in late 1992.

and billboards saying, "I can handle smoking fastballs. It's smoking cigarettes I've got a problem with."

Meanwhile, a cigarette called Death, with a skull and crossbones on its package, widened its distribution in the U.S. and the U.K. The brand's chief promoter is entrepreneur Charles Southwood of Venice, California, who believes that people have the right to smoke (he does so himself occasionally) but that they should also know the consequences of what they are doing.

One of the scientists whose pioneering research first demonstrated scientifically the harm induced by cigarette smoking died of a heart attack in October 1992 at age 76. Psychologist Daniel Horn was assistant director of statistical research at the American Cancer Society in the 1950s, when he and statistician E. Cuyler Hammond published studies establishing a statistical link between cigarette smoking and the subsequent development of lung cancer. The studies helped turn public opinion against smoking and prod the government to act more aggressively against it. Horn later worked at the Centers for Disease Control in Atlanta, Georgia, where he continued his research on the impact of smoking on health and on the most effective ways to persuade people to stop smoking.

Doing it their way

Alternative, unproven therapies for the treatment of disease were debated anew after the movie *Lorenzo's*

Oil opened in late 1992. The film personalizes the story of a young boy afflicted with the rare, fatal hereditary disease adrenoleukodystrophy (ALD). The film portrays how loving parents, played by Nick Nolte and Susan Sarandon, fought against the seeming indifference of the medical establishment to the lack of available treatments and, using published scientific research, came up with what they claimed would be a cure for their dying son (played by Zack O'Malley Greenburg). The film was based on the true-life story of Lorenzo, the son of Augusto and Michaela Odone of Fairfax, Virginia. The parents were told by doctors in 1984 that their six-year-old boy suffered from ALD. The disease, which is passed from symptomless mothers to their sons, destroys the myelin sheath around nerve fibers, and soon after onset those who are afflicted generally lose the ability to walk or talk, and they become deaf, blind, and demented. Although the symptoms vary widely among those who have the disease, children usually die within two years of its onset.

Neither of the Odones is medically trained—the mother, an editor, and the father, a native of Italy, an economist with the World Bank in Washington, D.C. In their private research the parents discovered in obscure medical journals that two naturally occurring oils, erucic and oleic acids, could be used to lower certain very long-chain saturated fatty acids (VLCFAs) in the blood; ALD is marked by abnormal levels of such compounds. The parents deduced that giving their son a mixture of the oils would alleviate the symptoms. The underlying principle of such a treatment had been discovered by William B. Rizzo, a researcher at the Medical College of Virginia, but it was the Odones who found companies to produce the oils, which they have used to treat Lorenzo.

Rizzo and other scientists, however, say there is no proof that the treatment changes or improves the course of the disease, even though the oil does reduce the level of VLCFAs in the blood. Hugo Moser of the Johns Hopkins University School of Medicine, Baltimore, Maryland, used the oil to treat 70 children with rapidly progressing disease from the time of onset until they went blind and lost the ability to move. He concluded that the oil made no difference.

At the time the film was released, the real-life Lorenzo was 14 years old. He could communicate only by wiggling the fingers of his right hand to answer yes and closing his eyes to say no. He is fed by nurses, who must suction the mucus from his mouth that he cannot bring up himself. The Odones insist that they have found a way to remedy this hopeless disease and that scientists are trying to discredit them.

Many scientists and ethicists were deeply troubled because the movie powerfully conveys the failure of traditional science to offer any treatment and may create distrust of scientific methodology. They are also concerned about the overly dramatic depiction of the disease in the film. In fact, subsequent to the release of the movie, a team of scientists from France, Germany, and the U.S. identified the gene involved in ALD—a discovery that may lead to a cure.

Fuss over food

Benjamin Spock, the renowned child-rearing specialist, became involved in a widely publicized controversy when he appeared at a press conference with members of the Physicians Committee for Responsible Medicine to warn parents about the dangers of milk, which had long been for children the nutritional equivalent of nectar of the gods. The committee urged that cow's milk be eliminated from the diets of adults as well as those of children because, they said, it contributes to diabetes, ovarian cancer, cataracts, iron deficiency, and allergies. None of these assertions has been proved. For adults the committee also advocates a strict vegetarian diet, without eggs or dairy products.

Spock, not infrequently in the eye of the storm, did not endorse the committee's position entirely, although he became ensnared in disputes among pediatricians that followed. In fact, he agrees with the widely held position of the pediatric community that breast-feeding is the preferred method of infant feeding. But for bottle-fed babies, he now believes that cow's milk should not be the choice because it is low in iron and can lead to iron deficiency anemia; rather, soy-based infant formula should be given to infants under one year.

What older kids consume was the target of a new campaign sponsored jointly by *Consumer Reports* magazine and the Home Box Office cable TV channel. Comedian Jim Fyfe went on the air and, in a kid-friendly manner, ridiculed many of the junk foods that are widely pitched, often with celebrity endorsements, during children's TV programs. Among others, he lam-

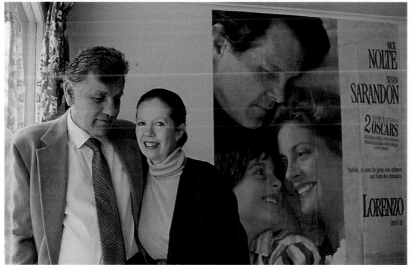

Augusto and Michaela Odone, whose son, Lorenzo, suffers from adrenoleukodystrophy, were unwilling to accept the failure of medical science to find a treatment for the rare hereditary disorder. They believe that a special combination of oils, discovered through their own research, has kept Lorenzo alive. The Odones' dramatic story was portrayed on-screen by actors Nick Nolte, Susan Sarandon, and Zack O'Malley Greenfield in the movie Lorenzo's Oil.

basted sugarcoated cereals, calling them "candy for breakfast." Willie Munchright began delivering a similar message on the CBS network on Saturday mornings. In public service announcements aimed at the three million kids aged 2 to 11 who are then glued to their television sets, Willie, an animated clay cartoon character, is host for the "What's on Your Plate" series. The 55-second nutrition messages produced by McDonald's and the Society for Nutrition Education encourage children to eat at least three servings of vegetables a day and to snack on apples, carrots, low-fat yogurt, bananas, unbuttered popcorn, and pretzels.

Phil Sokolof, who has been called an amateur cardiologist, has been waging a one-person national campaign against saturated fat and cholesterol since 1985. A septuagenarian from Omaha, Nebraska, Sokolof founded the National Heart Savers Association to spread the word that high cholesterol kills. Through self-financed national newspaper advertising, radio announcements, and brochures, Sokolof has brought pressure on manufacturers of commercially processed foods to substitute polyunsaturated oils for tropical oils in their products and on fast-food restaurants to reduce the saturated fat content in their offerings. His latest campaign was a personal lobbying effort for better nutritional labeling so that Americans know what they are getting from their food. In full-page newspaper ads in September

Carrots beat candy and "dudes with brains eat foods with grains" are among the healthy-eating messages that Willie Munchright delivers to kids on Saturday-morning television in the "What's on Your Plate" nutrition-education series.

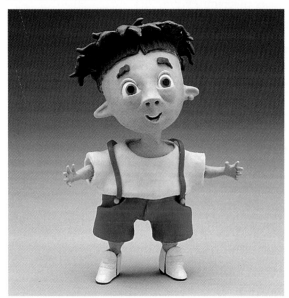

1992, he claimed that "The Food Processors and the Meat Industry are at it again" and that the American public could be the losers. At the 11th hour, he said, "tremendous pressure is being exerted . . . to dramatically weaken the implementation of a new nutrition labeling law that the American public demanded." Sokolof became interested in heart-healthy diets after he suffered a massive heart attack in 1966. He did not smoke and he exercised regularly. Examining his personal lifestyle, he decided that his regular fare of "tamales, hot dogs, and hamburgers" had to go when he learned that his cholesterol level was 300. It went. Today his cholesterol is at a healthy low of around 150.

Mavericks of another ilk

John M. Smith of Colorado Springs, Colorado, broke ranks with his profession in writing a book in which he argued that men should not be obstetrician-gynecologists. Smith had trained and practiced for a decade as an OB/GYN before he quit the discipline to work in administrative medicine. In *Women and Doctors* he asserts that many male doctors do physical and psychological harm to their female patients. "Ingrained male prejudices" are the reason men make bad gynecologists, he says. Many gynecologic surgeries, especially hysterectomies, are done, he claims, solely so the doctors and hospitals can make money. While female patients may hail Smith's candid position, a male gynecologist, reviewing the book in the *Journal of the American Medical Association,* called Smith's contentions "more bombastic than enlightening."

Another career-switching physician, Eddie Joe Reddick of Nashville, Tennessee, had been a pioneer in the development of the minimally invasive technique for removing the gallbladder, known as laparoscopic cholecystectomy (which was the subject of an article he wrote for the 1992 *Medical and Health Annual*). The approach, which involves suctioning out the intestinal organ through a tiny "belly-button" incision, has now largely replaced major surgery for gallbladder disease. Exchanging scalpel for guitar pick, Reddick has temporarily given up his lucrative surgical practice and teaching activities to pursue a lifelong love, country-music songwriting. He has no idea whether he will achieve stardom in his new venture, but at least he will not be a starving artist.

Another physician, Raymond O. West of Belfair, Washington, may have patients beating a path to his office door. West has invented something many have

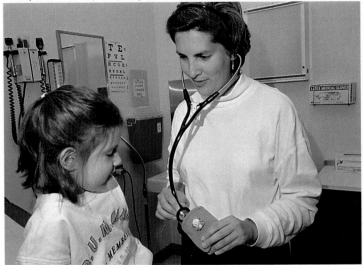

A pediatrician tries out a patient-friendly stethoscope warmer—the invention of Raymond O. West, who received a patent for his device in December 1992. Marketed under the name Nice Touch, the simple-to-use, inexpensive scope-warming method is aimed at eliminating the shock of cold metal on bare skin.

long yearned for: a warm stethoscope. No longer will patients have to dread the shock of frosty metal on their bare chests or backs once other doctors adopt West's ingenious device—a chemical heat reactor kept in a small pouch that activates once it has been punctured and keeps a stethoscope warm for up to 12 hours. Recently patented by West, the patient-friendly invention can be worn on a belt and will sell for about $8.

Medical technology was advanced in a major way when "Robodoc" made its debut in the operating room in November 1992. The first of its kind, Robodoc is a multifunctional, computer-guided robotic system, whose first surgical undertaking was assisting in the hip-replacement surgery on a 64-year-old man at Sutter General Hospital in Sacramento, California. The robot-surgeon, which has a 1.5-meter (5-foot) arm and relies on complex imaging technology, drilled a precise shaft in the patient's femur (thigh bone) so that a pin could be implanted to hold the ball that fits into the artificial hip socket. The patient got out of bed the day after his new hip was implanted and on the second day was able to walk.

Conceived and developed by Howard Paul, a veterinarian, and William Bargar, an orthopedic surgeon, both at the University of California at Davis, Robodoc provides far greater surgical accuracy than is possible with human hands. Robodoc has since assisted in at least a dozen orthopedic operations. Surgeons now envision robots assisting in surgery on the brain, eye, ear, and perhaps other organs as well. Sadly, Paul will not be able to follow the blossoming of his invention's career. He died of leukemia at age 59 in February 1993.

Trials, tribulations, and triumphs

When the pop music idol Michael Jackson disclosed in a television interview with the talk show host Oprah Winfrey that his light skin was not the result of bleaching but resulted from a skin disorder—probably vitiligo—he brought public attention to a little-known but not uncommon disease. Vitiligo is not contagious but leaves discolored areas, often quite pronounced, on the face and body. Jackson said he uses makeup to give his skin an even tone. Vitiligo is thought to be a genetic disorder; it often begins in childhood, although it can start at any age. It can be limited to a few spots, or the depigmented areas can spread; in severe cases the person loses all pigment cells. Treatment generally involves a drug called 8-methoxypsoralen, which patients take before being exposed to ultraviolet A radiation in a special tanning booth. The process is lengthy and expensive, and some patients become nauseated and dizzy from the treatment; it is said to be successful in about 65% of cases. For many people with vitiligo, the social effects can cause more hardship than the physical aspects. Studies of vitiligo patients have shown that about 7% are severely depressed by the disease, 32% suffer acute embarrassment, and 27% claim to experience some embarrassment, while about 34% are well adjusted to their disease.

Beat Richner, a Swiss pediatrician, might be called a contemporary Albert Schweitzer. Richner had been caring for ailing children in Phnom Penh, Cambodia, where he established a modern hospital in a country whose medical services were almost nonexistent. He

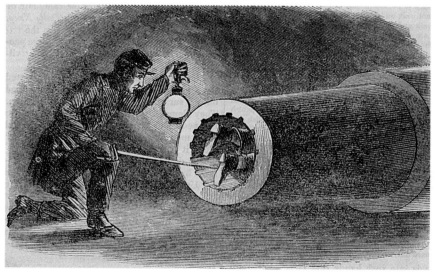

Pop music superstar Michael Jackson discloses to talk show hostess Oprah Winfrey that his light skin is not from bleaching, as the popular media had alleged, but the result of a skin disease, presumably vitiligo. Vitiligo causes discoloration of the face and body owing to a loss of the skin's pigment-producing cells; it is difficult to treat and often causes its sufferers considerable emotional distress.

was forced to flee in 1975 when the Khmer Rouge were victorious in that country's civil war, returning home to Zürich. But his heart was still in Cambodia, and in 1991 he returned to rebuild his hospital, which had been demolished. In 1993 the restoration was completed, thanks to his efforts, which included raising $4.6 million from private sources. His "mission" includes teaching in the country's only medical school and training Cambodians to provide pediatric care.

Justice finally was served, if only informally, when a moot court in February 1993 cleared the name of Samuel A. Mudd, who was convicted as a conspirator in the assassination of Pres. Abraham Lincoln. Mudd

had set the broken leg of John Wilkes Booth, Lincoln's assassin, when he arrived at the physician's Maryland home after committing the deed at Ford's Theatre in nearby Washington, D.C. Mudd was sentenced to life in prison. But a three-member panel of moot-court judges at the T.C. Williams School of Law at the University of Richmond, Virginia, held that the military commission that convicted Mudd had no right to try him in the first place. Mudd served four years of his sentence before he was pardoned by Pres. Andrew Johnson, but the conviction remained. The moot court's verdict did not do much good for Mudd, but it pleased his descendants, who wanted their family name cleared and had

Physician Samuel Mudd tries to escape imprisonment in the cannon of a steamer ship. Mudd was convicted in 1865 as a conspirator in the murder of Abraham Lincoln because he set the broken leg of John Wilkes Booth just after the assassin shot the president. The doctor contended that he did not know of Booth's act. In 1993 a moot court cleared Mudd's name—much to the relief of his descendants, who insist that the conviction was unjust.

18

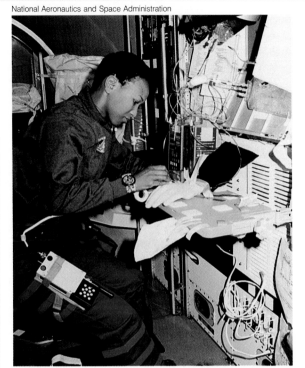

Mae C. Jemison conducts a medical experiment on board the space shuttle Endeavour *on its September 1992 flight. The first black woman physician astronaut in space, Jemison now teaches science at Dartmouth College.*

sought restoration—unsuccessfully—through the legal justice system.

Mae C. Jemison, the first African-American woman in space, decided to abandon her career with the National Aeronautics and Space Administration (NASA) for earthbound pursuits. A medical doctor and chemical engineer, Jemison, prior to becoming an astronaut, was a medical officer for the Peace Corps in Sierra Leone and Liberia. At age 36 she decided to pursue interests in "teaching, mentoring, health care issues and increasing participation in science and technology of those who have traditionally been left out." She began teaching at Dartmouth College, Hanover, New Hampshire, in 1993. She has been an especially inspiring instructor to minority students, whom she tells, "Don't be limited by others' limited imaginations."

Chiaki Mukai became the first Japanese female physician-astronaut to be chosen to travel on a NASA space shuttle flight, scheduled for 1994. She will participate in medical experiments on the effects of low levels of gravity on the body.

Another female physician who scored a first was Carrie Lee Davis, who was chosen Miss South Caro-

lina to represent her state in the 1992 Miss America pageant. A 1991 graduate of the Medical University of South Carolina College of Medicine, she took a year off before doing her radiology residency to promote preventive medicine and mandatory public service work by medical students. Other pageant contestants have gone on to become physicians, but Davis was the first physician to compete.

Miss America 1993, Leanza Cornett, made AIDS awareness the focus of her yearlong reign. Talking about her activities, she told an interviewer: "I've gotten letters from people saying we don't want Miss America talking about sex, and that's fine. But hopefully the perception of most people about Miss America is changing."

Rebecca Cole of Jacksonville, North Carolina, was recognized by the FDA in 1992 for her efforts to improve labeling for corticosteroids (drugs that function as immunosuppressants). Her 12-year-old son, who was being treated for asthma with corticosteroid medication, died in 1988 when he contracted chicken pox, a disease that is generally mild for a child with a normally functioning immune system. Cole's work led the FDA to ask the makers of such drugs to include a warning that long-term or high-dose use may put a patient exposed to chicken pox or measles at risk of serious illness or even death.

Of mice, pigs, baboons, and men

After a moratorium of nearly three years, the U.S. government again began approving patents for genetically engineered animals. Early bioengineering research was designed to produce cows that would give more milk and pigs that would provide leaner bacon. More recent research involves manipulation of animal genes to benefit human health.

The first patent had been awarded in April 1988 to Harvard University for a genetically altered mouse that was predisposed to cancer. The world's second animal patent was awarded in December 1992 to Ohio University for a strain of mice carrying a human gene that makes them resistant to viral infections. The animal was genetically altered to continuously produce a low level of interferon, a protein used by the human body to attack invading viruses.

Geneticists at the University of Cambridge announced in March 1993 that they had bred the first two pigs with genetically modified hearts developed from human genes. While transgenic heart transplants into humans are still years away, the success of this experiment is

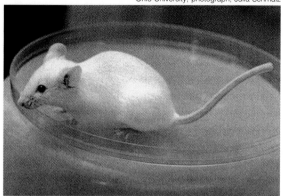

On Dec. 29, 1992, Ohio University received a U.S. patent for a transgenic mouse developed by two of its scientists. The furry research animal carries a human gene that makes it resistant to viral infections and useful for immunity studies.

a first step. The demand for hearts for transplant far exceeds supply. Pig hearts that have genes from human hearts are less likely to be rejected, and so they might eventually provide the needed supply.

Indeed, unsuccessful efforts to transplant baboon organs into dying humans already have stimulated demands that such experimentation cease. The second human to receive a baboon liver transplant—a 62-year-old man—died in February 1993, 26 days after the operation to replace his diseased liver. At the time of the transplant, done at the University of Pittsburgh, Pennsylvania, the man was near death from hepatitis B infection. The first patient to undergo the surgery also was infected with hepatitis B as well as HIV. His

transplant, done at the same institution, kept him alive 70 days. He died in September 1992 after an overdose of an antirejection drug hastened a fatal infection. The experimental transplants were done under the direction of Thomas E. Starzl, the world-renowned liver transplant pioneer, who performed the first human liver transplantation in 1963. Starzl, who published his autobiography, *The Puzzle People: Memoirs of a Transplant Surgeon,* in 1992, believes that the future of transplants lies in using animal parts. "We've got to turn to animals," he said, "or we'll never advance."

Small but special

Dolly Downs made her debut in 1992 to serve as an identifiable companion for people with Down syndrome, a congenital disorder resulting in mental retardation that occurs in about one in 800 live births. Manufactured at Camp Venture, Inc., Stony Point, Long Island, New York, the doll was the idea of John Lukens, a child psychologist, and Kathleen Lukens, executive director of the camp, who have a son with autism. The doll has the broad face and slanting eyes of a child with Down syndrome. Children with the syndrome have warmly welcomed her. The Lukenses have also used Dolly to help teach children who do not have the condition to be more tolerant of those who do. The doll is assembled by retarded people in a workshop at the camp and sells for about $25.

Donald Lewis, a pediatric neurologist, has concluded that Tiny Tim, the invalid boy in Charles Dickens'

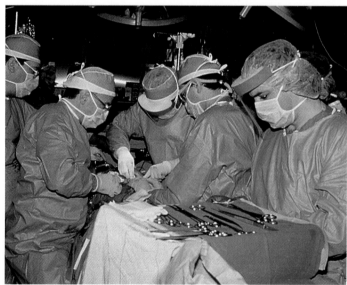

Surgeons at the University of Pittsburgh (Pennsylvania) Medical Center perform the first baboon-to-human liver transplant. The historic operation was carried out under the direction of transplant pioneer Thomas E. Starzl. The patient was a 35-year-old man dying from liver disease caused by the hepatitis B virus; he was ineligible for a human liver because that organ too would be attacked by the virus. A second patient—male, aged 62, and also a victim of hepatitis B—subsequently received a baboon's liver from the same surgical team. Though neither patient survived, Starzl remains committed to the use of animal parts in human transplantation, particularly because of the continuing shortage of human organs.

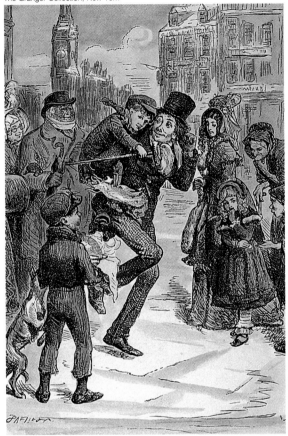

Charles Dickens' beloved Tiny Tim Cratchit suffered from a kidney ailment according to physician Donald Lewis, whose study of the fictional boy's condition was published in the December 1992 American Journal of Diseases of Children.

popular *A Christmas Carol,* suffered from distal renal tubular acidosis—a kidney disease that makes the blood too acidic. Dickens never told his teary audiences what the fragile lad who rode on his father's shoulders was suffering from, but Lewis, who practices at the U.S. Naval Hospital in Portsmouth, Virginia, believes he has ended the suspense. Lewis came up with his diagnosis by examining the literature on Timmy Cratchit. In Dickens' 19th-century story, Tiny Tim survives his illness to enjoy Christmases Yet to Come. But that might be expected, given that doctors of the day, even with their limited armamentarium of palliatives, had an effective treatment: an antacid.

Many sad losses to medicine

Among the many heroes and heroines of medicine who died in late 1992 and early 1993 were:

● Barbara McClintock, 90, winner of the 1983 Nobel Prize for Physiology or Medicine for her work in genetics, in Huntington, New York, on Sept. 2, 1992. Considered one of the most influential geneticists of the century, she did research for more than 50 years at Cold Spring Harbor Laboratory, Long Island. McClintock is best remembered for delineating how "jumping" genes work—that is, how transposable DNA fragments can modify the ways in which genes are expressed.

● Leon J. Davis, 85, founder of the nation's largest labor organization of health care workers, in New York City on Sept. 14, 1992. He was leader for many years of Local 1199 of the Hospital and Health Care Employees Union, which transformed the workplace for thousands of workers.

● Clara M. Hale, 87, a self-taught New York City social worker who cared for hundreds of abandoned and orphaned babies, including victims of drug-abusing mothers and AIDS, on Dec. 18, 1992. Mother Hale, as she was known, opened her Harlem home to the babies in 1969. Soon afterward she moved into a five-story brownstone where she was able to care for even more children. Her methods were unorthodox by official government standards, and she had to battle the bureaucracy to continue her work. She herself reared 40 foster children in addition to three of her own.

● Jean Mayer, 72, nutritionist and university administrator, on Jan. 1, 1993. Born in France and decorated for service in the Free French and Allied forces, he became a U.S. citizen after World War II. He conducted pioneering research on malnutrition and obesity and was one of the first to show the relationship between coronary heart disease and risk factors such as smoking, high cholesterol, hypertension, and lack of exercise. As an adviser to the U.S. government, he influenced policy and programs to combat hunger, including expansion of the federal school-lunch program for needy children. He also served on missions to Africa and India to assess starvation problems. In 1976 he became president of Tufts University, Medford, Massachusetts, transforming it into a major research institution.

● Leonard A. Scheele, 85, U.S. surgeon general under Presidents Harry S. Truman and Dwight D. Eisenhower, on Jan. 8, 1993. Scheele led the 1955 effort to ensure the safe distribution of the Salk polio vaccine to millions of children and adults.

● Audrey Hepburn, 63, actress and advocate for children, on Jan. 20, 1993, several weeks after surgery for colon cancer in Switzerland, where she lived. She had been a special ambassador for the United Nations

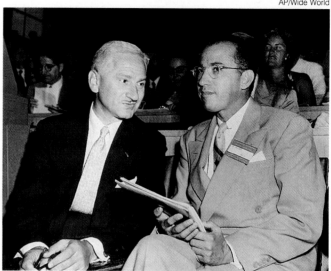

Albert B. Sabin (left), seated next to Jonas Salk, attends the third International Polio Congress in Rome in September 1954. Both medical scientists developed immunizations against poliomyelitis. Though Salk's killed-virus vaccine was widely used at first, Sabin's rival live-virus oral vaccine became the immunization of choice in most parts of the world. Sabin, who was known for his brilliance and his diligent commitment to research, spent the latter part of his career investigating the relationship between human cancer and viruses. His death on March 3, 1993, at age 86, marked the loss of a true medical pioneer.

Children's Fund (UNICEF) since 1988. She traveled to Latin America, Africa, and Asia on behalf of UNICEF. To call attention to the plight of starving children, the actress visited Ethiopia at the time that country was suffering a devastating drought.

• Albert B. Sabin, 86, the pioneering researcher who developed the live-virus oral polio vaccine, on March 3, 1993. Sabin's vaccine generally supplanted the killed-virus injected vaccine developed by Jonas Salk. Sabin, a native of Poland, was on the staff at the University of Cincinnati, Ohio, and its Children's Hospital Research

Foundation when he and his co-workers developed the vaccine that helped virtually eliminate polio in developed countries and is making inroads toward ending the crippling disease in the rest of the world. Sabin once said, "A scientist who is also a human being cannot rest while knowledge which might be used to reduce suffering rests on the shelf."

• Denis Burkitt, 82, a renowned missionary doctor and epidemiologist, in England on March 23, 1993. While working as a surgeon in Africa, he helped map the incidence of a cancer of the immune system (now called

Barbara McClintock enjoys an early-morning walk along Long Island Sound near her home and workplace for over 50 years, the Cold Spring Harbor Laboratory. McClintock carried out interbreeding experiments with maize (corn) to determine that genes "jump" around on chromosomes. Thus, transposable DNA fragments modify how genes are expressed, which is noted in the color variations of corn kernels. This crucial genetics discovery won her the 1983 Nobel Prize for Physiology or Medicine.

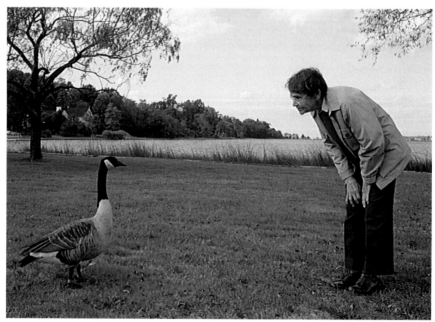

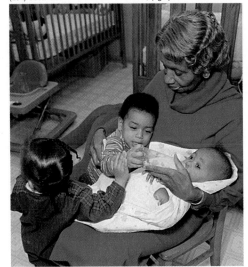 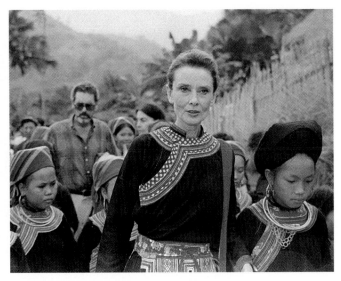

*Great losses for the world's less fortunate children were the deaths of Clara M. Hale and Audrey Hepburn.
Hale took in and cared for hundreds of abandoned and orphaned babies in her Harlem, New York, home.
Actress Hepburn served for many years as a "goodwill ambassador" for UNICEF. (Above) In 1990 she brought
attention to the plight of Vietnam's poorest children living in the country's remote northern mountains.*

Burkitt's lymphoma), showing that it occurred in areas where yellow fever and malaria also were found. His theory that the cancer might be caused by a virus (now known as the Epstein-Barr virus) and his development of effective drug treatments were major contributions to cancer research. In a later study of the differences between diseases affecting poor Africans and affluent Westerners, Burkitt suggested a connection between colon cancer and the consumption of refined carbohydrates, which led to an awareness of the importance of dietary fiber in the prevention of disease.

● John M. Morris, 78, who made important contributions in the field of gynecology, in Woodbridge, Connecticut, on April 8, 1993. A missionaries' son, he grew up in China, where he observed the harsh treatment of women, which led to his interest in women's health. In the late 1930s he identified the rare disorder testicular feminization (now known as Morris' syndrome), in which persons born with normal male chromosomes develop as females because they are insensitive to testosterone. Later, with Gertrude Van Wagenen, he developed the "morning after" birth-control pill, which worked by preventing implantation of the egg in the womb. Morris also helped develop radiation therapy as a treatment for cancer.

● Daniel X. Freedman, 71, a psychiatrist and pharmacologist who was a pioneer in the use of drugs to treat mental illness, in Los Angeles on June 2, 1993. In the 1950s he established a link between the psychedelic drug LSD and serotonin, a brain hormone that plays a role in depression and other illnesses. Among his many other contributions were studies on the effects of stress on the brain and the biology of diseases such as schizophrenia, anxiety, and sleep disturbances. The psychiatrist had a distinguished academic career at Yale University, the University of Chicago, and the University of California at Los Angeles. He was also a prolific author and had been a contributor to Encyclopædia Britannica's *Medical and Health Annual*. One of his UCLA colleagues called Freedman "the most pivotal thinker in psychiatry in the second half of the 20th century."

● Binay Ranjan Sen, 94, in Calcutta on June 10, 1993. His lifelong concern was "that huge portion of the human race that lives one drought, one flood, one crop failure away from starvation." He first became involved in combating hunger as a government official in his native India. Later, as director general of the UN Food and Agriculture Organization, he promoted the development of food reserves and of distribution systems to relieve famine and hunger throughout the world and organized the Freedom from Hunger campaign (1960) and the World Food Congress (1963).

*—prepared by Charles-Gene McDaniel, M.S.J.,
Professor and Chair, Department of Journalism,
Roosevelt University, Chicago*

Can One Shot Do It All?

by Scott B. Halstead, M.D., and Bruce G. Gellin, M.D., M.P.H.

The year is 2010. The place: the village of Manpura-Upazila, Bangladesh, one of thousands of small farming settlements along the deltaic branches of the Ganges and Brahmaputra rivers. The annual floods and the fierce cyclones that roar off the Bay of Bengal, only 80 kilometers (50 miles) distant, serve as a reminder that life here, in one of the most densely populated lands on Earth, is precarious. Despite efforts over the years to improve living standards, the persistence of severe overcrowding, an unreliable source of clean water, an inadequate food supply, and primitive sanitation methods still create extremely poor health conditions; the organisms that cause contagious respiratory and diarrheal infections are ubiquitous.

On this day a young Bangladeshi mother has just given birth to her first child. She is attended at home by a nurse-midwife, who, after assisting with a long and tiring but uncomplicated delivery, administers to the newborn a few drops of a white liquid. Over the next three months the infant will develop strong and lasting immunity to some two dozen infectious diseases—infections that had been the most important childhood killers during the 20th century. Six months earlier the mother-to-be had done her part by swallowing a single pill—a vaccine capsule designed to stimulate high levels of protective antibodies that would be carried through her placenta into her unborn baby's blood. After the birth other antibodies that developed in response to the same capsule will be secreted in her breast milk; these secretory antibodies will play a further role in protecting her infant by creating a barrier to infections caused by organisms that are carried in food and water and against respiratory infections transmitted easily from person to person in crowded living conditions.

Is the above scenario an impossible dream? Not if a global effort, conceived in 1990, succeeds. The plan, known as the Children's Vaccine Initiative (CVI), is to bring into existence an ideal vaccine for children—an inexpensive, single-dose, oral immunization that will provide children everywhere with lifelong immunity against a host of infectious diseases. This vaccine will be designed to maintain its potency without refrigeration and to be easily administered at or shortly after birth. Such a vaccine would protect all the world's children against at least nine common childhood

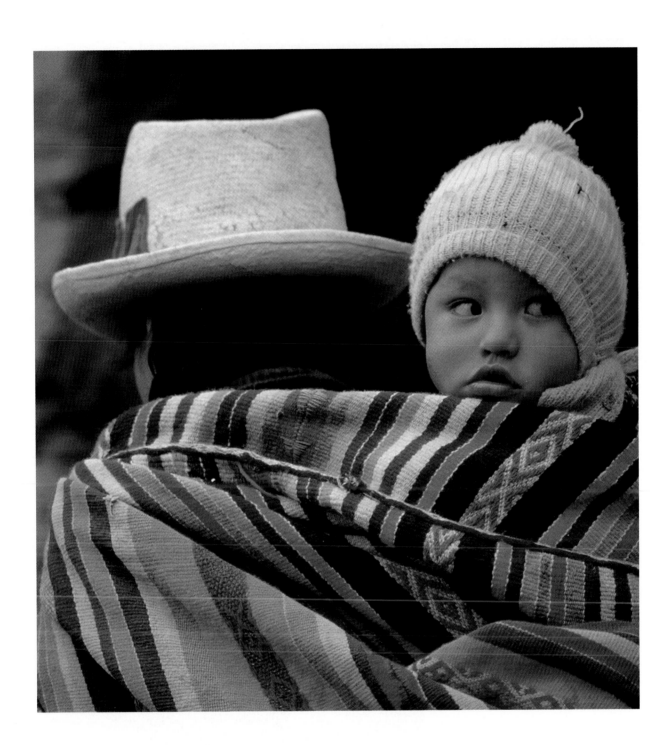

Scott B. Halstead, M.D., is Deputy Director, Health Sciences Division, the Rockefeller Foundation, New York City.
Bruce G. Gellin, M.D., M.P.H., is Assistant Professor, Department of International Health, Johns Hopkins University School of Hygiene and Public Health, Baltimore, Maryland.

(Overleaf) Peruvian mother and child; photograph, Jerry Alexander—Tony Stone Images

diseases—diphtheria, polio, pertussis (whooping cough), measles, mumps, rubella (German measles), tetanus (lockjaw), tuberculosis, and hepatitis B. Where required, special additional components would offer protection against the local or regional infectious diseases, such as the most severe forms of meningitis, diarrhea, pneumonia, malaria, and other diseases that afflict so many children in less developed countries.

Vaccines evolve

Vaccination, or immunization, is one of the safest, most cost-effective, and most powerful tools that medicine has for preventing disease, disability, and death. Indeed, no other intervention has had so profound an impact on the health and well-being of the world's children as the introduction and widespread use of vaccines.

In ancient times it was observed that people who survived an infectious disease rarely were stricken again with the same disease. This led to the centuries-old practice of variolation, injecting pus from smallpox pustules of a sick person directly into the skin of a person not previously affected by smallpox—with the goal of producing a milder form of this disease. Although those who had been so inoculated often developed severe symptoms from this hazardous procedure, fatalities from variolation were a far less common occurrence than from smallpox infection itself.

While variolation has been documented to have been practiced as early as the 10th century in China, vaccines as a *safe,* practical preventive tool are only about 200 years old. Credit for the first modern vaccine goes to the English country doctor Edward Jenner, who made the astute observation that milkmaids who contracted cowpox (a disease of cows that caused only mild illness in humans) rarely became victims of the devastating human illness smallpox. In 1796 Jenner took the fluid from the pustule of a cowpox lesion on the hand of milkmaid Sarah Nelmes and inoculated it into the skin of an eight-year-old boy, James Phipps, who then was protected against smallpox despite exposure to the virus. By the beginning of the

On May 14, 1796, Edward Jenner gives James Phipps, a boy of eight, the first vaccination against smallpox. The inoculation contained matter taken from cowpox lesions on the hand of a young dairymaid, Sarah Nelmes. On July 1 of that year, Jenner inoculated the boy again, this time with infectious material containing live smallpox; no disease developed and protection was complete. Jenner then predicted that "the annihilation of the smallpox—the most dreadful scourge of the human species—must be the final result of this practice."

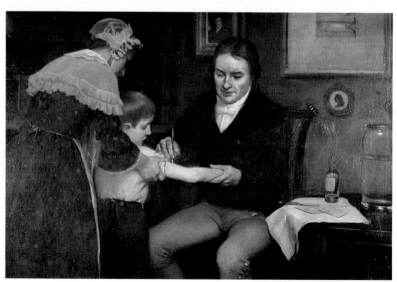

Painting by E. Board; the Wellcome Institute Library, London

19th century, more than 100,000 people had been protected with Jenner's vaccine, and he predicted that "the annihilation of the smallpox—the most dreadful scourge of the human species—must be the final result of this practice" (an accomplishment that would actually take about another 180 years). Appropriately enough, this weakened form of smallpox was called a "vaccine," from *vacca*, the Latin word for "cow."

It took nearly another 100 years for the second useful vaccine to appear—the famous treatment developed by the French chemist Louis Pasteur in 1885 for rabies ("hydrophobia"), an inevitably fatal disease that developed from the bite of a rabid animal. It was Pasteur who suggested that, in Jenner's honor, all inoculations be called "vaccinations" even though, properly speaking, they have nothing to do with cows. Today most scientists prefer the more accurate term *immunization*. However, the two terms continue to be used interchangeably.

In the latter years of the 19th century, as the germ theory of disease was advanced and the science of bacteriology emerged, the identification and laboratory growth of infectious organisms fostered the development of the first generation of vaccines—against diphtheria, tetanus, cholera, typhoid, and plague—some of which were only of limited effectiveness. While the total number of available immunizations is *still* surprisingly small, their impact has been extraordinary. In the United States in 1992, vaccine-preventable diseases were reduced by nearly 99% from their peak levels just a few decades earlier. The World Health Organization (WHO) estimates that in 1990, 80% of the world's children were immunized against measles, diphtheria, pertussis, tetanus, tuberculosis, and polio. In Latin America, a region that has set the goal of polio elimination by the year 2000, the last reported case of paralytic poliomyelitis occurred in Peru on Aug. 23, 1991. Most of these vaccines have appeared in a steady progression over the course of 20th century.

Principles of immunization

The process of immunization represents the creation of a state of protection against an infectious disease. A person can be protected by receiving preformed antibodies, as is the situation when a fetus receives a portion of its mother's antibodies through the placenta or when antibodies are removed from donated blood and administered to people (gamma globulin). These antibodies are used in special circumstances—to prevent a disease from occurring in an exposed individual or in travelers who may encounter a disease such as hepatitis A. These *passively* acquired or administered antibodies, though immediate and effective, are often short-lived in the recipient, usually conferring protection only until the time that the antibodies are degraded as they circulate in the recipient's bloodstream—usually about three to six months.

In contrast, vaccines work by actively eliciting the production of antibodies that seek out and destroy infectious microorganisms or their toxic products once they have entered the body. Antibodies are specific protein molecules (immunoglobulins) produced by white blood cells called B lymphocytes. After being administered orally or by injection, proteins called

Vaccine development*	
1796	smallpox
1885	rabies
1890	diphtheria antitoxin
1892	tetanus antitoxin
1896	cholera
1896	typhoid
1897	plague
1906	pertussis
1909	BCG (tuberculosis)
1914	typhoid (licensed)
1924	tetanus toxoid
1927	diphtheria toxoid (licensed)
1933	tetanus toxoid (licensed)
1935	yellow fever–attenuated live
1945	pneumococcal
1945	influenza (licensed)
1948	pertussis–whole cell (licensed)
1949	DPT (diphtheria/pertussis/tetanus)
1950	cholera (licensed)
1950	BCG (licensed)
1950	polio–attenuated live
1953	polio–inactivated
1955	polio–inactivated (licensed)
1959	measles–attenuated live
1960	polio–attenuated live (licensed)
1963	measles (licensed)
1965	rubella–attenuated live
1967	mumps–attenuated live (licensed)
1969	rubella–attenuated live (licensed)
1969	meningococcus–polysaccharide
1971	MMR (measles/mumps/rubella)
1974	*H. influenzae* type B–polysaccharide
1975	hepatitis B
1977	pneumococcal–14-valent (licensed)
1980	adenovirus (licensed)
1980	*H. influenzae* type B conjugate
1980	rabies–human diploid cell (licensed)
1981	acellular pertussis
1981	hepatitis B–plasma derived (licensed)
1983	pneumococcal–23-valent (licensed)
1985	*H. influenzae* type B polysaccharide (licensed)
1987	polio–enhanced potency inactivated (licensed)
1987	hepatitis B–recombinant (licensed)
1987	*H. influenzae* type B conjugate (licensed)
1991	acellular pertussis (licensed)
1992	Japanese encephalitis (licensed)
1993	DPT/*H. influenzae* type B conjugate (licensed)

*selected vaccines

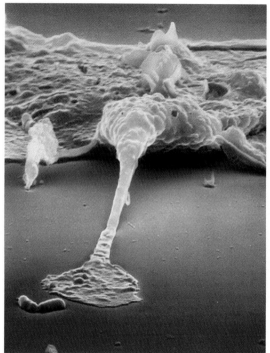

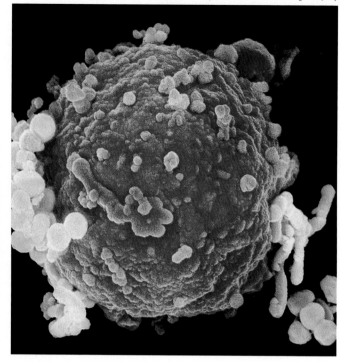

(Above) A macrophage (a type of white blood cell) extends toward bacteria, which it will engulf and break into small molecular bits that will then be delivered to white blood cells called B lymphocytes (above right) to stimulate antibody production. Antibodies fight off invading foreign bacteria and produce "memory cells" that in the future will react swiftly and vigorously to resist infections. To produce vaccines, molecular biologists prepare antigens (components of bacteria or viruses) that will trigger an immune response. Advances in understanding of immunity and novel technologies made possible by the genetic engineering revolution are enabling scientists to create new and better vaccines.

antigens (foreign molecules) are taken up by macrophages, another type of white blood cell. Macrophages digest the antigens into small molecular bits that are delivered to B lymphocytes to stimulate antibody production. For some viral and bacterial infections caused by microbes living inside the body's cells, antigen-containing macrophages induce specific T lymphocytes (yet another white blood cell type) to attack and kill the infected cells, producing cellular immunity. Both cellular and antibody-mediated immune responses are forms of *active* immunization that result in the production of so-called memory cells. Memory cells will react swiftly and vigorously to future encounters with the antigen in question.

There are three kinds of vaccines. They include those based on (1) genetically altered (weakened, or "attenuated") living organisms (viruses or bacteria) that are able to grow in the body after being administered and stimulate an immune response but do not produce disease; (2) inactivated (killed) whole organisms or pieces or organisms; and (3) inactivated toxic products of microorganisms ("toxoid").

The first type includes smallpox, yellow fever, oral polio, measles, mumps, and rubella vaccines—all viral vaccines. In the process of attenuation, the vaccine viruses are modified from the naturally infecting "wild" viruses such that they do not cause disease, yet they stimulate an immune response that is subsequently protective against the natural infection. In general, viral vaccines produce very long-lasting immunity, often for a lifetime. Many bacterial vaccines are also derived from attenuated organisms. Examples of these include bacillus Calmette-Guérin (BCG), developed in 1909 by the French scientists Albert Calmette and Camille Guérin from a form of bovine tuberculosis, and an oral vaccine against typhoid fever.

28

Vaccines made from killed organisms or antigenic components of organisms include whooping cough, cholera, meningococcus, pneumococcus, *Haemophilus influenzae* type B, poliovirus, influenza, and hepatitis A and B. Immunity produced by such inactivated vaccines may be short-lived because they do not have the ability to replicate in the recipient.

Finally, inactivated toxins (toxoid vaccines) are available that protect against tetanus and diphtheria—illnesses caused by bacterial toxins that invade the bloodstream. Newer cholera and pertussis vaccines are also based, in part, on inactivated toxins.

Manufacturing vaccines

Until very recently, vaccines were manufactured by relatively crude methods. For most of history, smallpox vaccine was made by inoculating cowpox virus into the skin of young cattle, then scraping off and bottling the pustular material. Presently, most viral vaccines are produced by inoculating living viruses into cultures of cells that are grown on the inside surface of glass bottles. The virus released into the nutrient fluid is collected, purified, and bottled as vaccine. Some killed viral vaccines are grown in fertile eggs. Most bacterial vaccines are produced by the so-called fermentation process, in which bacterial cultures are grown in large stainless steel vats; then the cultures are inactivated by the addition of chemicals (*e.g.,* formaldehyde).

In all industrialized countries and an increasing number of less developed countries, vaccines are carefully monitored at every stage of their manufac-

Large-scale manufacture of vaccines must maintain exacting standards. The facility shown here is designed to generate large quantities of vaccine material under ideal conditions; air is filtered to remove any potential contaminants, and all equipment is precisely calibrated and regularly inspected. These measures ensure that vaccine products are safe, effective, and of consistently high quality.

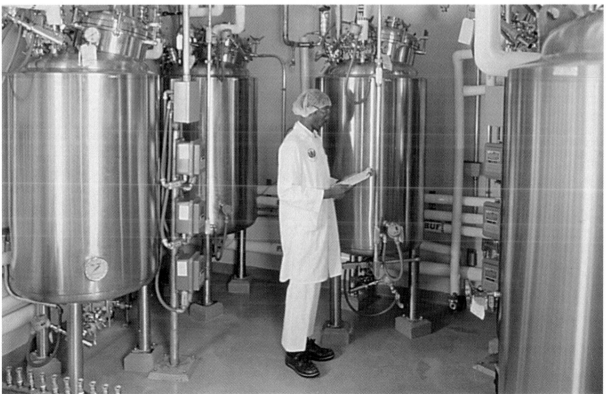

Lederle-Praxis Biologicals

ture—produced in facilities that must comply with so-called good manufacturing practices. Air is filtered to remove any potential contaminants, and all equipment used is carefully calibrated to maintain exacting standards and result in vaccines that are of high uniformity, purity, and safety.

In recent years vaccine research has taken a quantum leap forward, thanks to the biotechnology "revolution." The full genetic code for most pathogenic (disease-causing) microorganisms is now known, and genes can be purposefully selected and used to create peptide or protein antigens that can be manufactured accurately and in very large quantities. Moreover, the fruits of modern molecular biology can take advantage of viral mechanisms for the purpose of inducing immunity. It is now possible to insert selected genes into viruses such as an attenuated vaccinia virus; when inoculated into the skin, the vaccinia virus induces the infected cell to produce its own viral genetic products as well as the products (antigens) from the inserted genes. In this way a single "carrier" virus might, for example, be developed to induce immunity to rabies, measles, and perhaps the human immunodeficiency virus (HIV), the virus that causes AIDS. (Carrier vaccines are discussed more fully below.)

Child survival

By the 1960s and 1970s, long-term economic development, reliable water and sanitation, antibiotics, and vaccines against diphtheria/pertussis/tetanus (DPT), polio, measles, mumps, and rubella had eliminated or greatly reduced the incidence of many childhood diseases in the United States and other developed countries. In poor nations investments in economic development were also beginning to bring some infectious diseases under control, reducing childhood death rates. However, rapid population growth from continuing high fertility rates placed insupportable burdens on the poor, threatening to counteract the progress that had been made in improving child survival. High infant mortality results when babies are born to mothers who are "too young or too old," are born in rapid succession

Living standards are important determinants of child health and survival. Rates of child mortality are especially high in poor nations where people live without access to a safe water supply or adequate sanitation. In these conditions people are susceptible to waterborne and parasitic infections, such as childhood diarrhea (a leading killer of children in the less developed world), cholera, and malaria. In the 1960s and '70s, major investments in economic development, including improvements in sanitation and the provision of safe water, helped reduce infant death rates in many less developed countries. With improved living conditions, more children survived and were then at high risk of contracting common childhood infections for which medicine has no cures. Consequently, in 1974 the World Health Organization launched the Expanded Program on Immunization (EPI), with the interim goal of vaccinating 80% of the world's children against six preventable childhood killers—diphtheria, pertussis, tetanus, tuberculosis, measles, and poliomyelitis—by 1990.

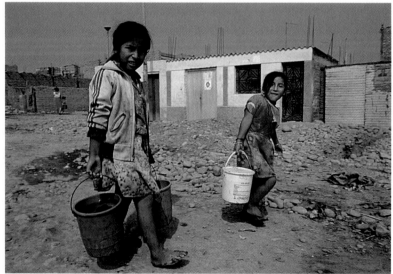

Alejandro Balaguer—Sygma

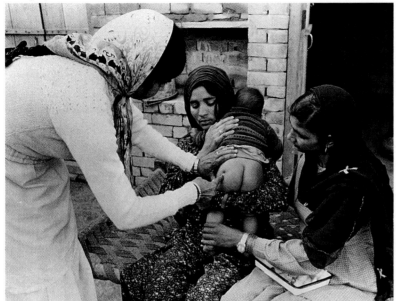

Immunizing babies: EPI* vaccination schedule	
vaccine	age
BCG and oral polio	birth
DPT and oral polio	6 weeks
DPT and oral polio	10 weeks
DPT and oral polio	14 weeks
measles	9 months
*Expanded Program on Immunization	

A child in India is immunized in a rural health center in 1980. One of the goals of the EPI was to reach children in remote parts of the world.

("too close"), or are born late in the birth order ("too late"). Clearly, reduced fertility rates are a key component of child survival.

Increasingly, it was recognized that high death rates in infants and children led parents to target their family size at levels that would compensate for expected losses. Thus, if infant and child mortality rates are in the vicinity of 50%, parents may choose to have six children if they wish to have three offspring survive to adulthood. Countries that had the highest infant mortality rates in the early 1960s subsequently had the lowest rates of decline in crude birth rates by the late 1980s, and vice versa.

Living standards and fertility rates are important determinants of child survival, but if children survive they are then subject to many infectious diseases for which there are no cures. However, many of these serious infections can be prevented. In 1974, when it was clear that the global campaign to eradicate smallpox was going to succeed (officially accomplished in 1977, when the last case of endemic smallpox was recorded in Somalia), WHO took a bold step. It decided to apply the lessons of the smallpox campaign more broadly, creating the Expanded Program on Immunization (EPI). The goal: to immunize the world's children against six major infectious diseases—diphtheria, pertussis, tetanus, tuberculosis, measles, and poliomyelitis. (The accepted target when this goal was set was full vaccination of 80% of children by 1990. To achieve full immunization, each child must receive five separate injections and four swallows of oral polio vaccine, all in the first nine months of life. As EPI director Ralph H. Henderson noted at the time, the six targeted diseases shared two outstanding features: they killed young children, and young children could be protected against them by vaccinations.

When the EPI began, fewer than 5% of the world's children were fully immunized. Ten years later, in 1984, this number had risen—but only to 25%. It was then clear that something substantial had to be done if

31

Expanded Program on Immunization: realizing the goal*

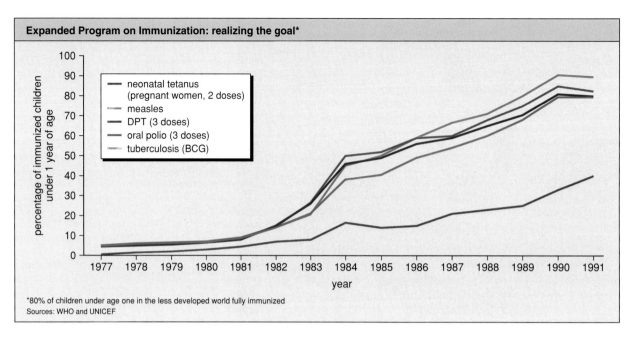

*80% of children under age one in the less developed world fully immunized

Sources: WHO and UNICEF

the 1990 goal was to be realized. In 1983 the United Nations Children's Fund (UNICEF) declared "a Children's Revolution," emphasizing four cost-effective means to reduce childhood mortality in the less developed world: growth monitoring, oral rehydration for diarrheal diseases, breast-feeding, and immunization (GOBI). The next year, at the urging of Jonas Salk, developer of the inactivated (injected) form of polio vaccine, and Robert McNamara, who served as president of the World Bank from 1968 to 1980, the Children's Revolution was launched. Immunizations were selected as the leading weapon, as it was recognized that the use of vaccines could be measured and the impact of vaccination programs evaluated. In March 1984 WHO, UNICEF, the United Nations Development Program (UNDP), the World Bank, and the Rockefeller Foundation created the Task Force for Child Survival at a conference held at the Rockefeller Foundation's Bellagio Conference Center at Lake Como, Italy. There the decision was made to accelerate the global immunization campaign. At that conference William Foege, a veteran of the smallpox campaign and former director of the Centers for Disease Control (CDC) in Atlanta, Georgia, was selected to lead the task force. Further resources for the stepped-up global immunization efforts were mobilized in the following years at conferences in Cartagena, Colombia; Talloires, France; Bangkok, Thailand; and Montreal, Quebec.

The campaign that followed fully justified the hopes of its sponsors. On Oct. 8, 1991, at United Nations headquarters in New York City, Hiroshi Nakajima, director-general of WHO, and James Grant, executive director of UNICEF, announced that the 1990 goals of fully immunizing 80% of the world's children had been achieved. Indeed, immunization was saving the lives of 3.5 million children in the less developed countries each year. Emboldened, WHO then announced plans to eliminate neonatal tetanus, eradicate poliomyelitis, and reduce measles deaths by 95%—all by the year 2000!

Vaccine use in developed countries: successes and failures

The discovery and successful use of polio vaccines in the mid-1950s ushered in what has been called "the vaccine era." In less than a month after it was released for general use in 1955, four million doses of Salk's inactivated polio vaccine were given in the U.S. alone. Over the next four years more than 450 million doses were given, and the incidence of paralytic polio was reduced from 18 to 2 per 100,000 population. In the 1960s and '70s, under the auspices of the CDC, not only polio but measles and rubella vaccines were given in mass campaigns and their use enforced by school-entry laws in every state. By 1975 poliomyelitis had been successfully eradicated from the U.S., and for a time measles also seemed destined to disappear (reaching a low of 1,497 reported cases nationwide in 1983). Similar successes were recorded in virtually all industrialized countries.

Unfortunately, the very success of immunization bred failure. To be fully immunized, children in the U.S. and most developed countries require some 17 different inoculations and six visits to a clinic or physician's office during the first 15 months of life. With the fading images of the March of Dimes poster children and iron lung machines, complacency developed about the threat of epidemics and the potential severity of readily preventable childhood diseases. The result: many parents simply "forget" to have children vaccinated; current immunization rates of U.S. children under age two are well below those in many less developed countries, including some of the poorest (*see* Sidebar, pages 34–36).

Yet nearly all American children are born in hospitals. If a comprehensive and long-lasting immunization series could be given at birth, parents' failure or reluctance to have their children vaccinated might be reduced, as would the cost and effort involved in the existing system for administering multiple vaccines and boosters.

Less developed countries: the immunization challenge

The EPI helped most of the world's less developed countries build vaccine-delivery infrastructures that work. As Donald A. Henderson, who had led the successful smallpox-eradication campaign, noted in 1989, "There are far larger numbers of trained health staff; radio, telephone, and even television are found in areas where none existed 20 years ago; and air and

(continued on page 37)

Resurgence of preventable childhood infectious diseases (U.S.)			
	lowest number of cases (year)	number of cases in 1991	rise in incidence (%)
measles	1,497 (1983)	9,488	533.8
mumps	2,982 (1985)	4,031	35.2
pertussis	1,248 (1981)	2,575	106.3
rubella	225 (1988)	1,372	509.8

Source: Centers for Disease Control and Prevention

Children Unprotected: A U.S. Emergency

by Samuel L. Katz, M.D.

By 1990, more than 80 per cent of the developing world's children were being brought in four or five times for vaccinations even before their first birthdays. As a result, Calcutta, Lagos, and Mexico City today have far higher levels of immunization of children at ages one and two than do New York City, Washington, D.C., or even the United States as a whole.

—James P. Grant, executive director, UNICEF,
Foreign Policy #91 (Summer 1993)

In communities from New York to Los Angeles, members of thousands of local organizations came together to make National Preschool Immunization Week [April 24–30, 1993] a success.... The heartache is, what can happen for seven days can happen every day—with help from a Congress that understands every day an immunization opportunity is missed, more children are put at risk of serious illness, even death. That is our definition of an emergency.

—Patricia Schroeder (Dem., Colo.) and Gary Goldberg,
letter to *Chicago Tribune,* May 15,1993

The prevention of infectious diseases by vaccines has been one of the great triumphs of modern preventive medicine. In the United States the reported cases of vaccine-preventable diseases (diphtheria, tetanus, whooping cough, paralytic polio, measles, mumps, and rubella) in 1992 were reduced by more than 97–99% from those numbers that occurred in years of peak incidence.

These remarkable records of achievement, however, have been eroded on a number of occasions, with major disease outbreaks occurring because access to vaccines and other elements of health care has been restricted for some deprived population groups. As recently as 1989–91 the country witnessed an alarming recrudescence of measles. The great majority of the 55,000 patients who acquired measles were unvaccinated; many of them suffered its complications and required hospitalization, and the three-year epidemic claimed 132 lives. These young victims are tragic examples of the nation's failure to provide effective preventive health measures that reach *every* infant and child.

The U.S., along with Japan and other wealthy, industrialized nations, has provided leadership in the development of new vaccines. Their availability, however, does not ensure their administration to infants and children at risk. Vaccines are of no use if they sit in refrigerators in clinics or the offices of physicians.

Samuel L. Katz, M.D., is Wilburt C. Davison Professor of Pediatrics, Duke University School of Medicine, Durham, North Carolina, and Chairman, Advisory Committee on Immunization Practices, U.S. Centers for Disease Control and Prevention.

Regulations in all 50 U.S. states require that children receive all the recommended vaccines by ages five and six years, so that 98% of school-entering youngsters have fulfilled these requirements. It is youngsters under two years of age, for whom nearly all the basic vaccines are recommended by the ages of 15 to 18 months, who have the poorest immunization records. In 1993 some 37–56% of the nation's two-year-olds—about four million children—were not immunized. Even in the 11 states where vaccines are provided free to all, only 55–65% of two-year-olds had received all the recommended immunizations.

These low rates are not a matter of cost alone; rather, the problem is a complex one that involves inadequate parental education, lack of access to clinics and/or physicians administering vaccines, immunization schedules that are not "user friendly," inadequate registries and the lack of a tracking system that provides immediate access to any child's immunization record so that families can be notified when a child has fallen behind, and a major decline of the U.S. public health infrastructure during the 1980–92 Reagan and Bush administrations.

Boxes of polio vaccine, kept refrigerated to prevent spoilage, are readied for shipment from an Indiana warehouse. Less than a month after its release for general use, millions of doses of "Salk" vaccine were given in the U.S.

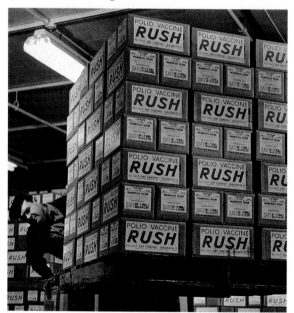

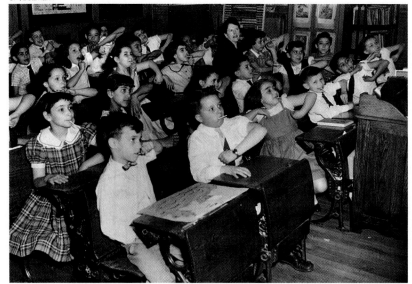

In a single week in May 1955 tens of thousands of New York City schoolchildren received polio shots—and lollipops—as the city's mass immunization program got under way. The stunning success of polio vaccine campaigns in the U.S., reducing polio incidence to near-zero levels in just a few short years, stands as one of the great triumphs of modern preventive medicine.

Because the failure to immunize young children and its consequences are now well recognized, a number of innovative remedial actions have been initiated in some parts of the country. These include mobile vans taking immunizations to children who live in underserved areas, the integration of immunization facilities with entitlement programs (such as the Supplemental Food Program for Women, Infants, and Children and Aid to Families with Dependent Children), and the establishment of convenient clinics—for example, in housing developments or in schools.

But many more measures are needed. To assist single parents or families in which both parents work, immunization clinics need to offer evening and weekend hours. To assist non-English-speaking families, culturally appropriate and imaginative educational programs need to be mounted to explain the importance of vaccination and attract parents to the vaccine programs for their children. The provision of a national registry would enable a health provider on any contact (such as an emergency-room visit) to determine a child's need for any or all vaccines and to provide them on the spot. Failure to administer recommended vaccines often occurs because providers are misinformed about when and whether children should receive immunizations. However, even infants who are breast-feeding and those with infections and fever *can* be safely vaccinated in most circumstances.

Many parents today consider childhood infections to be a thing of the past; they have not seen paralytic polio, measles, or whooping cough and their devastating effects on young infants and children. American society's very success in this regard has also been its enemy.

It is economically wasteful as well as morally unconscionable that many health insurance programs and employer health programs provide reimbursement for costly hospital care and complex technological procedures but fail to reimburse a few dollars for preventive measures such as childhood vaccines. Yet the cost-effectiveness of vaccines is always cited whenever medical interventions that are economically positive are highlighted. It is estimated that for every $1 spent on immunization, $10 to $14 are saved because future diseases have been prevented.

A heartening example of a new vaccine and its impact is the *Haemophilus influenzae* type B conjugate product that became available in the U.S. in 1989. The most common cause of meningitis among infants and children has been strikingly reduced as a result of wide use of this vaccine, initially for children under five years and more recently for infants beginning at age two months. In only three years the disease *H. influenzae* meningitis, which was common in pediatric wards and was responsible for the death or severe permanent neurological damage of tens of thousands of U.S. children, has almost disappeared. This dramatic reduction is due in large part to the competitive efforts of different pharmaceutical firms working aggressively to develop this product and make it widely available over the past five years.

Presently, efforts are being directed toward combining multiple vaccines into single injections, sparing infants and children the larger number of shots currently required. Most recently (March 31, 1993) a combined vaccine (Tetramune) that includes four different antigens (diphtheria, tetanus, pertussis, and conjugated *H. influenzae* B) was licensed, reducing the number of infant injections required from eight to four. Efforts are now under way to incorporate hepatitis B and inactivated polio, among other antigens, in similar combined products.

Early in his administration, Pres. Bill Clinton proposed a number of bold initiatives to prevent further events such as the measles outbreaks of 1989–91. These would provide: free vaccines for families that lack health insurance or otherwise are unable to afford them, a national registry, increased personnel for public health clinics, educational programs for families and for health professionals, and negotiated vaccine prices that aim to lower the overall cost but still provide sufficient funding for research and development that will lead to newer and better vaccines.

In the spring of 1993 the national Centers for Disease Control and Prevention (CDC) issued new "Standards for Pediatric Immunization Practices," emphasizing *access* (making vaccines readily available to all youngsters), *delivery* (efficient vaccine administration), *documentation,* and *education.* These new standards are meant to overcome existing barriers and ensure that all preschoolers get the protection they need.

Ever rising costs of vaccines are one factor accounting for the decline in U.S. immunization rates. More important, without the threat of epidemics, many parents have become lax about seeing that their youngsters are protected.

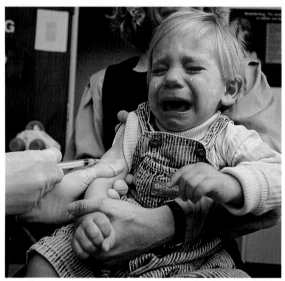

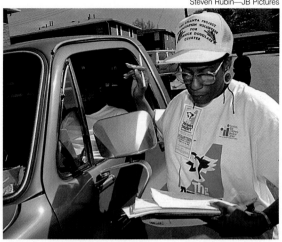

A program in Atlanta, Georgia, is doing something about the alarming decline in childhood immunization. Volunteers go door-to-door in neighborhoods to locate youngsters who need their shots and then to see that they get them.

Another encouraging effort was the first National Preschool Immunization Week, sponsored by the CDC and a host of other partners, April 24–30, 1993. Future immunization weeks that will be held annually are intended to stimulate activities at national, state, and local levels—the goal being to achieve permanent improvements in childhood immunization nationwide.

A prime example of the ever present threat posed by the failure to immunize children was the outbreak of paralytic polio (due to type 3 virus) that began in late 1992 among members of a Calvinist religious group in The Netherlands and subsequently spread throughout the country. Six months later the same virus strain was isolated from as many as 21 children in the Canadian province of Alberta, although no polio cases had occurred. Nonetheless, those youngsters who were not immunized remained highly vulnerable, and the virus could easily find its way into the U.S. A similar situation developed in 1979 when polio in The Netherlands spread to Ontario and then to several Amish groups in Pennsylvania, Missouri, and Iowa, who, for religious reasons, had not had their children immunized.

Immunization for vaccine-preventable diseases is an essential cornerstone of child health programs that should be made available to every infant and child in the United States and throughout the world. Removal of the threat of these infectious diseases offers assurance that all children will have the chance to achieve their full potential, which should be an essential right of *every* child.

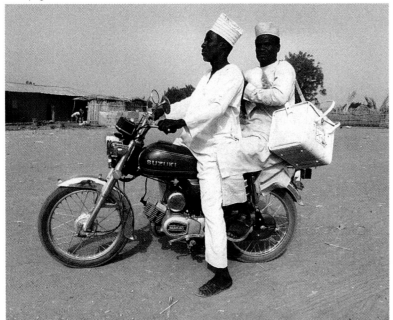

In Nigeria a UNICEF-supported mobile vaccination team carries immunizations, stored in special refrigerated containers that are shielded from light and heat, to rural outreach sites that have no health facilities. Most existing vaccines are easily destroyed by heat, and each has its own special storage requirements; moreover, owing to their limited shelf lives, vaccines often go to waste before they reach the children who need them. A vital step in the EPI was establishing a "cold chain"—a system that ensures that vaccines are delivered at the right place at the right time and that they do not lose their potency along the way.

(continued from page 33)

road transport leave few populated areas on the globe which are truly inaccessible." The EPI required less developed countries to exercise their health systems as never before. The task was formidable. In 1991 it was estimated that 238 million doses of BCG, 523 million doses of DPT, 305 million doses of measles, and 689 million doses of polio vaccines moved from central storehouses to "the periphery" (the mouths, arms, and buttocks of children). Accomplishing this required major strategic planning.

Perhaps the single most important step—the "lifeline of EPI"—was establishing a vital "cold chain," a system to ensure that vaccines arrive at the right place at the right time in sufficient quantity and that their potency is maintained along the way. To preserve vaccines at the appropriate temperature from manufacturer to the most remote clinic, special equipment had to be designed and manufactured, and the capacity to prevent breakdowns and repair equipment had to be strengthened up and down the line. Essential cold-chain equipment includes solar and kerosene-driven refrigerators. Because heat can easily destroy the potency of most vaccines, temperature-sensitive chemical monitors were invented. These monitors change color each time a vaccine shipment is exposed to excessive heat, and a special indicator then informs program managers at a glance whether vaccines have always been kept at the required temperature.

Other equipment was designed to make vaccination safe. "Auto-destruct," single-injection vaccinating devices prevent the reuse of needles or syringes—a practice that could result in the spread of blood-borne diseases such as AIDS or hepatitis B.

Despite its successes, the very magnitude of the EPI has brought to light several important deficiencies. The following hurdles still need to be surmounted before universal childhood immunization can be realized.

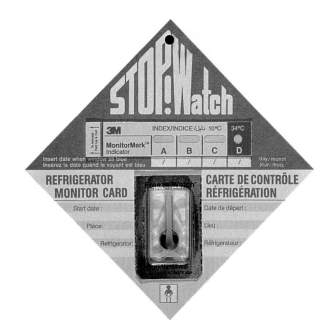

Reaching the missing 20%. The attainment of the EPI's 1990 immunization goals—80% of children in less developed countries immunized against six diseases—was a remarkable accomplishment. Nonetheless, 20% of the world's children still are not being reached. They are among the poorest and most inaccessible and consequently the most vulnerable to severe childhood infections. Without major new interventions, more than 100 million children in less developed countries will die from infectious diseases before the end of the century.

To achieve their optimal protective effect, all vaccines in the EPI program except BCG and measles require booster doses following the primary series. Many children who receive a first dose of vaccine fail to return for subsequent doses ("dropouts"). In addition, many potential opportunities

A voluntary physician immunizes rural villagers in Djibouti. Reaching "the missing 20%"—those who live in the most inaccessible parts of the world's poorest countries—is a major hurdle that still needs to be surmounted in order to prevent nearly 100 million children from dying of vaccine-preventable infectious diseases before the end of the century.

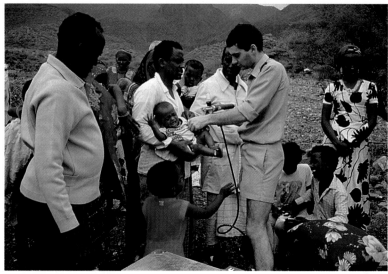

Sygma

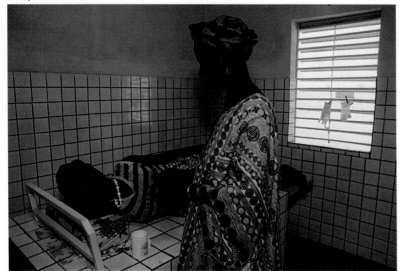

Jeremy Nicholl—JB Pictures

for immunization are missed. A particular problem is the failure to immunize eligible children who are taken to health facilities when they are ill since immunization services are often not available at clinics that provide primary health care services. This is often because it is difficult to have vaccines available at all times, owing to their limited shelf life (discussed below). A major step toward achieving universal immunization coverage would be to give needed immunizations to *all* children who are taken to clinics—for whatever reason—as these acute care visits may be their only encounter with the health system.

A child's access to vaccines is still further limited by the necessity of injection. If vaccines could be easily administered at home by any adult, many more children would be protected.

Shelf life and wastage. Three of the six EPI vaccines are made from living organisms: tuberculosis (BCG), measles, and oral poliovirus vaccines.

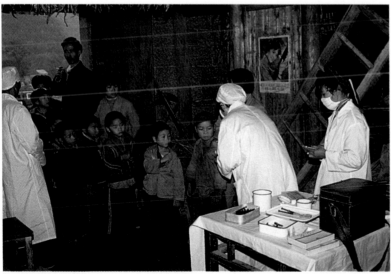

Sean Sprague—UNICEF

The others are complex proteins. Each has special storage and temperature requirements for optimum stability. BCG and DPT will remain potent for up to one year at refrigerator temperatures, but DPT loses potency if frozen. Measles and polio vaccines, on the other hand, require freezing temperatures ($-15°$ to $-25°$ C [$5°$ to $-13°$ F]) for long-term storage.

Most measles vaccine is freeze-dried and bottled; this product then has a shelf life of many years at refrigerator or freezer temperatures. To be administered, dried measles vaccine is reconstituted in sterile water; this suspension, however, must then be used within 24 hours. It is far cheaper to package measles vaccine in multidose rather than single-dose vials. Since clinics may not be open daily, reconstituted vaccines from multidose vials are often wasted. It is estimated that at least 25% of UNICEF-supplied measles vaccine is wasted.

Polio vaccine presents different problems. It must be stored frozen but cannot be freeze-dried and later reconstituted. Though it remains stable for weeks at refrigerator temperatures, it can stand at room temperature for only a matter of hours before losing its potency. Clearly, the present need to maintain both refrigerator and freezer temperatures in the cold chain is difficult and expensive; it can and does result in storage of vaccines at the wrong temperature, causing a loss of potency. Vaccines that lose potency will not be effective and must be discarded. If temperature barriers could be overcome, vaccine wastage could be minimized, vaccine delivery could be simplified, and more children would get the protection they need.

Neonatal tetanus. Another important immunization challenge is the prevention of neonatal tetanus, which causes some 740,000 newborn deaths each year. Neonatal tetanus results from bacterial contamination of the umbilical stump shortly after birth. It occurs when unsterile methods are used to cut the umbilical cord or germ-laden materials such as cow dung or mud are applied to the stump after cutting to stop the bleeding. Once infected with the bacterium that produces the tetanus toxin, the newborn loses muscular control and thus the ability to suck and obtain nourishment. Soon the infant's swallowing and breathing capacities deteriorate. About 85% of newborns infected with tetanus die in the first weeks of life.

With the persistence of unhygienic living conditions as well as ongoing reliance on traditional birth practices, the most practical strategy for preventing neonatal tetanus in many less developed countries is to immunize prospective mothers with a series of tetanus toxoid shots. The mother's immune system will make protective antibodies against this toxoid, and during gestation these antibodies will be transferred across the placenta into the growing fetus. While five doses of tetanus toxoid are optimal for inducing immunity, at least two doses are required for producing an immunologic response. Yet in 1990 barely 25% of women of childbearing age in less developed countries received even two doses of this vaccine. Utilizing every contact that women have with the health care system to provide tetanus toxoid vaccination would surely help to improve coverage. A far better way to ensure that newborns are protected from this often fatal disease would be to develop a tetanus toxoid vaccine that could be given to pregnant women prior to delivery in just one dose.

In Kavre, a rural district in the mountains of Nepal, where tetanus infection of newborns is prevalent, nurse-midwives advise prospective mothers about the need for several doses of tetanus toxoid immunization and the importance of giving birth in a clean place. In parts of the world where unhygienic living conditions persist, neonatal tetanus kills some 740,000 newborns a year. Infection results from bacterial contamination of the umbilical stump shortly after delivery. Once infected with the bacterium, infants develop severe muscle spasms that prevent normal breathing. The Nepalese nurse-midwives use dolls to demonstrate safe cord-cutting techniques, which will help prevent infection.

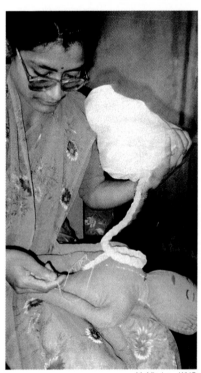

M. Minden—WHO

40

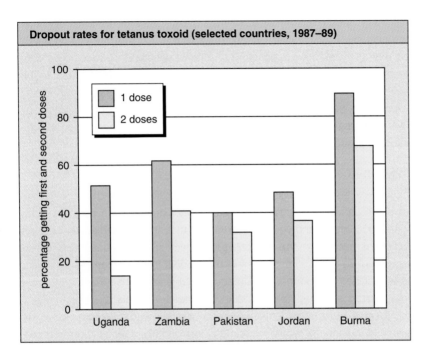

Dropout rates for tetanus toxoid (selected countries, 1987–89)

y-axis: percentage getting first and second doses

Legend: 1 dose, 2 doses

Countries: Uganda, Zambia, Pakistan, Jordan, Burma

Maternal antibody and measles. Although circulating antibodies transferred from the mother to the unborn child are an important defense against infectious diseases such as tetanus, in some cases such antibodies can interfere with an infant's immune response to a vaccine. This situation occurs with the administration of live-attenuated measles vaccine; if administered to a child while he or she still has maternal measles antibodies, the vaccine may not "take." Therefore, measles vaccination is generally delayed until nine months of age, when maternal antibodies will no longer interfere with the response. As a result, measles vaccination, the last in the EPI series, requires an additional visit to an immunization clinic.

In the case of measles, the earlier an infant loses maternal antibody and becomes susceptible to the disease, the more severe the infection. This seems to be particularly true in countries where many infectious diseases are endemic. The severity of infection may also reflect the child's nutritional status—those children with vitamin A deficiency being especially vulnerable. Indeed, measles continues to kill 1.4 million children annually— a majority of these deaths occurring in Africa, where, among other factors, maternally transferred antibody has a particularly short life.

National vaccine production. Although there is substantial variation among countries, 71% of tetanus toxoid, 61% of measles, and 60% of DPT vaccines that are administered to children in EPI programs are locally produced. It is important to note that vaccine coverage rates correspond to the availability of locally made vaccines; 92% of infants are immunized when a vaccine is produced locally, whereas only 70% are covered when the same vaccine is donated. Furthermore, there is less wastage of locally produced vaccines than imported and donated vaccines. Countries with local production, therefore, not only are more self-sufficient in terms of vaccine availability but also have improved coverage.

41

While this degree of independence is clearly desirable in terms of reaching children, it also raises concerns about the vaccine quality and safety as well as economies of scale. The issue of substandard-vaccine production was addressed at an international meeting of vaccination experts in November 1992. It was estimated that globally the quality of about 50% of vaccines is not known. However, significant efforts are being initiated by less developed countries and donor agencies to strengthen national regulatory and quality-assurance capabilities in vaccine-producing countries.

Why the Children's Vaccine Initiative?

Each year about 10 million children die from infectious diseases, many of which can be prevented with existing vaccines. By one estimate more than 8,000 infants and young children lose their lives—needlessly—to such infections each *day!* The EPI delivery system created a base from which significant new gains in protecting the world's children can be achieved; new vaccines—some that are already available and those that might come into existence—could readily be incorporated into this system. Many of the barriers to universal childhood immunization would be removed if the vaccines developed would remain stable for many days at room temperature and if a single dose (or reduced dose) multiantigen vaccine were created that could be given at or near birth, when contacts with the health system are optimal. Vaccine wastage, dropouts, and missed immunization opportunities would all be substantially reduced or eliminated by either or both of these tactics. Furthermore, if a single-shot tetanus toxoid vaccine were developed, the rate of immunizing women of childbearing age against tetanus would markedly improve.

Of course, none of this is likely to be accomplished if costs are prohibitive. Vaccine manufacturers have estimated that it can cost up to $200 million to bring a licensed vaccine to full-scale production in developed countries, and vaccine prices will undoubtedly be affected by these enormous investments. According to WHO figures, a full course of the existing vaccines in the EPI schedule costs about $1 per child, but the expense of getting the vaccines to a child is an additional $13 when transportation, refrigeration, communication, and staffing requirements are factored in. Vaccines that would require fewer contacts with the health system would, therefore, stretch available funds considerably. UNICEF studies have shown that there would be important cost savings if the number of contacts could be reduced from the current five to three. If an 80% coverage rate with three contacts could be maintained over a 20-year period, there would be about a 15% reduction in costs from those of delivering the present six vaccines, or a cumulated savings of $5.1 billion to $6.4 billion.

New vaccines using new technology are not necessarily more expensive. According to a recent report of the International Task Force on Hepatitis B Immunization, when hepatitis vaccines first became available in 1982 at over $40 per dose, they were considered to be too expensive to be of practical use, especially for the poorest countries. But competition from vaccine producers in newly industrialized countries and bulk purchases by governments brought the cost to less than $1 per dose.

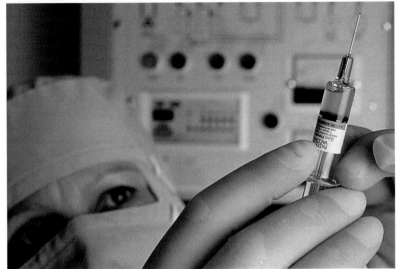

In 1988 Pasteur Vaccins of France launched its recombinant-DNA-based immunization against hepatitis B virus (HBV), a chronic infection that affects hundreds of millions of people worldwide. Thanks to the biotechnology revolution, vaccine development has taken a quantum leap forward in the past decade, resulting in products that can be manufactured inexpensively and in vast quantities. The first HBV vaccines in the early 1980s were made from purified blood of infected persons and cost about $40 a dose. Mass immunization against HBV is now practical in less developed nations, where it is especially needed, because competition among manufacturers and bulk purchases of vaccine by governments have brought the cost to under a dollar a dose.

What is needed most to produce a "children's vaccine" is an applied research program designed to move vaccines for children in less developed countries from the "[laboratory] bench to the bush" faster and more efficiently than is now possible. In June 1990, at a WHO-sponsored conference in Geneva ("Innovative Approaches for the Development of Third-World Vaccines"), the concept of a reduced-dose, multiantigen vaccine quickly won support. Less than three months later, on September 10, in New York City, international donors and scientists together issued the Declaration of New York, which officially called for the CVI. Then, in February 1991 at a meeting at Mount Kisco, New York, attended by representatives of some 15 international organizations, foundations, and assistance agencies, the CVI consultative group was formed. The CVI's immediate goals are to develop a single-dose tetanus toxoid vaccine, a heat-stable oral polio vaccine, an improved measles vaccine that will be effective when administered early in life, and combined vaccines composed of multiantigens that can be administered together. Many of the technical solutions to creating these new vaccines are already available or have already been envisioned.

Microencapsulation: reducing the need for booster doses

The process known as microencapsulation is now enabling scientists to develop new children's vaccines by containing antigens in a core reservoir that is surrounded by an outer polymer (plastic) shell (microcapsule) and released in a "pulse" when the shell, or wall, is breached. The specific polymers used are DL-lactide and glycolide (poly-[DL-lactide-co-glycolide]: DL-PLG). DL-PLG is in a class of biodegradable and biocompatible copolymers from which resorbable sutures and surgical clips as well as several controlled-release drugs are made. Thus, the polymers themselves have a well-established record of safety in humans. After introduction into the body, DL-PLG induces a minimal inflammatory response and biodegrades through a chemical process (hydrolysis) in which its ester linkages yield lactic and glycolic acids, normal body metabolic products.

43

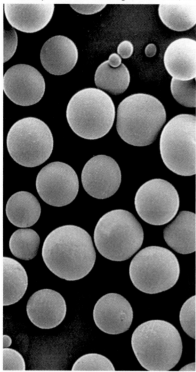

Many of the barriers to universal childhood immunization—the need for booster shots, vaccine wastage, and high dropout rates—would be removed if a single-dose, "one-shot," vaccine that would offer lifelong immunity were available and could be given to all newborns. The same is true for immunizing mothers against tetanus. The Children's Vaccine Initiative is currently supporting work toward such ideal products. Already there has been significant progress in the development of a tetanus toxoid vaccine that could be given to women in a single dose (instead of the two to five doses that are now needed). The technology that is making such a vaccine possible is known as microencapsulation— in which antigens are integrated into injectable, biodegradable, controlled-release microcapsules (above). After injection, these polymer (plastic) capsules release the entrapped antigen in such a way as to mimic repeated (booster) injections.

Following administration of such a vaccine, the antigens that are encapsulated in DL-PLG spheres of 10 micrometers or less in diameter are ingested by macrophages and serve to increase the immune response. When these antigens are encapsulated, they are not targets for preexisting antibodies such as those acquired by the fetus from the mother during gestation. Moreover, the process of coating dried antigen with DL-PLG results in a vaccine that has an extended shelf life and does not require stabilizers or a cold chain.

The rate at which DL-PLG biodegrades—and thus releases antigen—is a function of its chemical composition, specifically the ratio of lactide to glycolide. When microcapsules of differing chemical composition are mixed together, the antigen will then be released at different intervals. Delayed-release vaccines can be formulated to include both unencapsulated antigen that stimulates an immediate, or primary, antibody response and any number of encapsulated "pulsed" booster doses of the same antigen that are released over a period of up to two years. Furthermore, with this technology it is now possible to envision a formulation consisting of a mixture of microcapsules, each containing different antigens, that is administered at one time but is designed so that each antigen is released on a schedule that is optimal for induction of lifelong protective immunity.

An additional advantage of microencapsulation is that it makes possible the development of oral vaccines. DL-PLG effectively protects protein antigens from the harsh gastrointestinal environment. Microcapsules that protect their antigen core are taken up by intestinal macrophages, which then migrate to regional lymph nodes and stimulate the production of systemic antibody. This route of antigen delivery and presentation to the immune system also results in the stimulation of the mucosal immune system, leading to the production of antibodies in saliva, respiratory tract secretions, tears, and breast milk. Such secretory antibodies help to protect against enteric and respiratory tract infections. As previously noted, breast milk can be an important source of passively transferred antibody protection for suckling infants.

In early 1993 several different microencapsulation processes using various formulations of DL-PLG were being evaluated for a single-dose tetanus toxoid vaccine. These new products will first be tested in animals to determine which produces the best antibody response. Cost and ease of production are factors that will be considered in selection of a manufacturing process since it is desirable not only to keep the price of these vaccines low but to enable currently existing manufacturers in less developed countries to adopt the chosen process. Once an optimal formulation has been achieved, immunogenicity and safety tests will be performed, first in animals and then in human subjects, to ensure that these preparations do not result in untoward effects, such as allergic reactions.

Genetic engineering: the promise of vaccination early in life

Although a safe and effective live-attenuated vaccine for measles has been available for over 30 years, the use of this vaccine is limited since it is inactivated by the presence of maternal antimeasles antibodies in young infants. As a result, measles vaccination is given at around age nine months, when these antibodies have waned.

Now scientists may have a way around this problem. Genetic engineering techniques have made it possible to insert genes from a number of infectious agents, including measles, into unrelated live viruses or bacteria—for example, vaccinia, BCG, or salmonella. Thus, a live "carrier" vaccine serves as a vehicle to deliver antigens against multiple infections. Once safely incorporated into a permissive cell, the relevant gene induces the production of antigens that are expressed on cell surfaces, thereby stimulating antibody production. Because the antigens appear only after they have been produced by the recipient's cells, these engineered vaccines will not be inactivated by maternal antimeasles antibody.

Combined vaccines: prospects for a single-shot vaccine

In addition to creating microencapsulated vaccines that do not require boosters for achieving full protection, combining vaccines offers another way to reduce the number of contacts in immunization programs. Fortunately, the practice of combining vaccines is already well established. DPT, as a combined bacterial vaccine, has been in use since 1949, and oral polio vaccine includes three different immunogenic polioviruses. In many industrialized countries a combined live-attenuated viral vaccine for measles/mumps/rubella (MMR) is standard. Clinical experience has shown that there is no diminished immunologic response to individual antigens in such a combined vaccine, nor are adverse reactions increased. In industrialized countries recent advances in vaccine development have already produced DPT-based vaccines with additional antigens, such as hepatitis B and *H. influenzae* type B, and additional components will soon be included

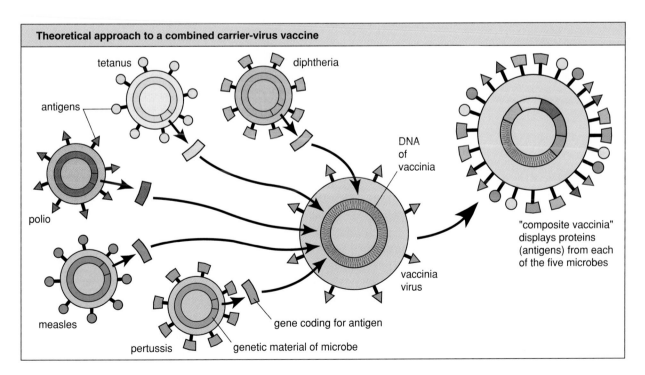

Theoretical approach to a combined carrier-virus vaccine

tetanus

diphtheria

antigens

DNA of vaccinia

polio

"composite vaccinia" displays proteins (antigens) from each of the five microbes

vaccinia virus

measles

gene coding for antigen

pertussis

genetic material of microbe

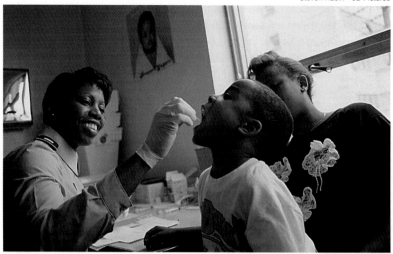

In Atlanta, Georgia, a National Guard reservist helps combat low immunization rates, giving children oral polio vaccine at a neighborhood clinic. It is ironic that the very success of childhood immunization in developed countries bred failure. In the U.S., current immunization rates, especially for children under age two, are well below those in many of the poorest less developed countries. Not only is preventing disease far more cost-effective than treating illness, but when children are protected by immunizations, the sometimes tragic effects of childhood infectious diseases are virtually eliminated.

as well. Over the next decade a major objective of the CVI is to improve DPT manufacturing in less developed countries.

Many—but not all—of the infectious diseases that cause the death of children can be prevented by existing vaccines. Vaccines still must be developed to protect children against the major causes of diarrhea and pneumonia, to offer better protection against tuberculosis, and to protect against malaria and AIDS, among others. Today, with advanced biotechnology methods, scientists can envision how inactivated antigens for many infections might be produced in a combined form. For example, a multicomponent single vaccine that would protect against diphtheria, pertussis, tetanus, pneumococcus, *H. influenzae* type B, influenza, hepatitis A and B, Japanese encephalitis, and meningococcus types A and C is a theoretical possibility.

Realizing the dream

Many strategies must be explored in order for the best combination vaccines to be created. To be fully effective in saving lives, especially those of children in less developed countries, the ultimate children's vaccine will have to be one that is affordable for global use.

Immunization remains one of the most powerful tools that medical science has for disease prevention. UNICEF Executive Director Grant has described the global efforts to develop and deliver new vaccines as "the greatest peacetime mobilization of forces in history." On April 7, 1987, Halfdan Mahler, then director-general of WHO, said, "Planet Earth can no longer accept that, in the age of modern technology, children should still die by the millions of diseases which can prevented by available vaccines." That same year the British physician and disability expert Sir John Wilson predicted that "the new generation of vaccines which are now being developed are likely to have a range in effectiveness which could change the whole future pattern of mortality and morbidity." He went on to hope that the day would come "when people will demand the right to immunization with the same passion with which they now demand the right to vote."

46

On July 1, 1993, when the Committee on the Children's Vaccine Initiative of the National Academy of Science's Institute of Medicine issued its report, *The Children's Vaccine Initiative: Achieving the Vision,* the committee chairman, Jay P. Sanford, commented:

Today, it is clear that . . . new and improved vaccines are within our grasp. . . . The United States, which has enormous capabilities and scientific expertise . . . does not have a track record in developing and selling childhood vaccines for developing country markets. . . . The reason is simple: private companies are reluctant to invest in costly and difficult research-and-development ventures when the likelihood of returns on investments varies from unpredictable to slim or none. . . . It is the committee's view that the greatest contribution that the United States can make toward the achievement of the Children's Vaccine Initiative is to harness the significant scientific and technical capabilities embodied in the U.S. public and private sectors toward the development and production of needed childhood vaccines.

A "children's vaccine" is beginning to take shape. The jury of scientific experts that will find the technical solutions in order to carry such a lifesaver into production is likely to be one selected by the CVI. When the dream is realized, every mother—whether in Bangladesh, East Los Angeles, or elsewhere on the globe—will be able to rest assured as she takes her newborn infant to breast that *her* child will have every chance to survive as well as to thrive.

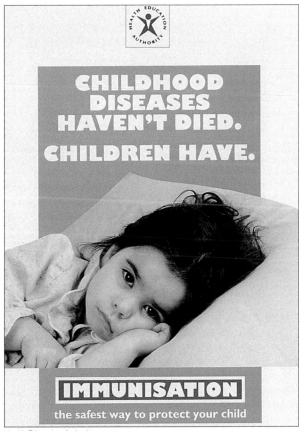

Health Education Authority

James Grant, executive director of UNICEF, has described the global effort to develop and deliver new and better vaccines as "the greatest peacetime mobilization of forces in history." Removal of the threat of childhood infectious diseases would ensure that children the world over had the opportunity to achieve their full potential—which should be every child's essential right.

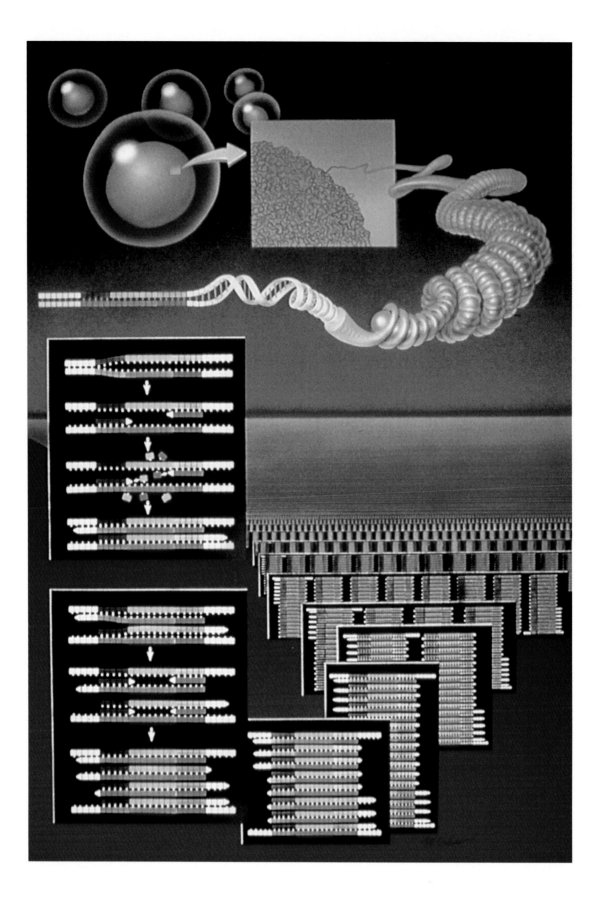

PATHOLOGY:
Saving Lives Behind the Scenes

by Frank Gonzalez-Crussi, M.D.

Let us suppose that you undergo surgery at a large medical center hospital for a lesion suspected of being a tumor. You are probably aware that the surgeon will be central to the outcome of your treatment. The qualities demanded of him or her are almost superhuman: keen perception, unfailing acumen, bold action, manual dexterity, decisive intervention, and readiness to cope with the unexpected—all in a flash and under conditions of great stress. But the surgeon, of course, is only the best publicized member of a complex team on which your well-being utterly depends. Without the participation of the anesthesiologist, the operation would simply not be possible; without the expertise of radiologists, the suspicious mass could not be accurately localized; and without the dexterous care provided by informed nursing services before, during, and after the operation, all the sophistication of the specialists might be in vain.

The best surgeons readily acknowledge that the operative act itself is but one factor in the patient's outcome and that ultimately the patient's fate rests in the thoroughness of preoperative investigation and the appropriateness of postoperative care. Nonetheless, it is the surgeon upon whom the brightest rays of the spotlight fall, while other members of the team stand in the peripheral glimmer. The dimmest light of all falls on a team member who generally lacks direct contact with the patient altogether: the pathologist.

Who are pathologists and what do they do?

Though unbeknownst to most patients, a pathologist probably *is* present in the operating room. The extent of the surgery itself may in fact be based on a pathologist's assessment. For the patient the happy news that a lesion is not a tumor will originate with the pathologist. On the other hand, if the less fortunate diagnosis of a tumor is confirmed, not only is its benign or malignant nature determined by the pathologist, but the need for or dispensability of additional treatment after the operation is likely to rest entirely upon his or her consultation.

Frank Gonzalez-Crussi, M.D., is Head of Laboratories, Children's Memorial Hospital, and Professor of Pathology, Northwestern University Medical School, Chicago. He is the author of several books, including Notes of an Anatomist *(1985),* On the Nature of Things Erotic *(1988),* The Five Senses *(1989), and* Day of the Dead *(1993).*

(Opposite) A symbolic representation of the polymerase chain reaction (PCR), a technique that makes it possible for the tiniest sample of DNA to be amplified many thousands of times in a remarkably short time. Thanks to PCR technology, pathologists now have a tool that enables them to do work that previously was impractical or, in some cases, may have been undreamed of.
(Illustration) Cetus Corporation—Peter Arnold, Inc.

The pathologists who are probably most familiar to the public are those who work in the service of the law, whose efforts are centered upon the postmortem examination, or autopsy. It is the forensic *pathologist (often in the role of coroner or medical examiner) who establishes whether a death was accidental, was due to natural causes, or occurred by violent means (homicide or suicide).*

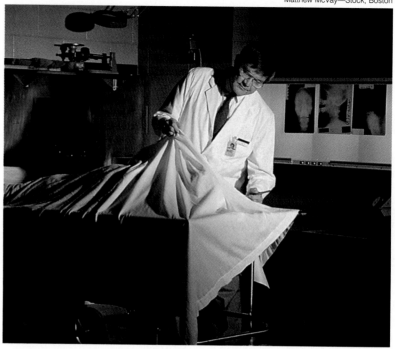

It is not really surprising that the nature of the pathologist's job may seem confusing to the layperson. The popular media not infrequently portray only those pathologists working in the service of the law, namely *forensic pathologists,* by whose toils innocence or culpability is assigned to persons suspected of wrongdoing. The work of forensic pathologists is largely centered upon the autopsy, or postmortem examination, and directed toward the ascertainment of the causes of death. The administration of justice in most cases cannot proceed until it has been decided whether an individual's death was due to suicide, homicide, accident, or natural causes.

While in the public's mind the pathologist's work is indissolubly linked to the performance of autopsies, some pathologists do not perform autopsies at all. The focus of their tasks is on the interpretation of cells or tissues removed from *living* patients. In the past, cell and tissue samples could be obtained only by surgery or at autopsy. Today, however, these may be procured by other means, such as needle aspiration (a biopsy that is done on deep tissues with a fine hollow needle and a syringe). Furthermore, surgical advances now allow exploration and sampling of almost any bodily tissue. Hence the need for pathologists who function as vital members of the "treatment team," supplying information of immediate surgical utility, and who are capable of conversing with surgeons in their own terms. It is the *surgical pathologist* who recognizes the multifarious appearances that diseased tissues may adopt; indeed, years of practice at this activity often allow these specialists to develop an uncanny facility, which it is not far-fetched to compare to the skill of a virtuoso concert performer.

The emergence of surgical pathologists is a relatively recent development. In fact, some surgical pathologists were originally surgeons.

Prompted by intellectual curiosity (and perhaps impatience at the stubbornly nonsurgical viewpoints of conservative pathologists), they decided to look for themselves at the ways in which tissues removed at surgery could be studied with the microscope. Some were so bedazzled by what they saw that they never returned to the operating room. Pathology was thus strengthened by excellent contributors who were originally "undocumented aliens" in the field.

Still other pathologists have nothing to do with microscopic interpretation of tissues, whether removed at autopsy, during surgery, or by needle aspiration biopsy. *Clinical pathologists* apply the powerful, largely automated, resources of biotechnology to the study of other specimens—most commonly bodily fluids such as blood, urine, and cerebrospinal fluid. These specialists generally work in hospital laboratories, and they rely on tools and techniques drawn from many scientific disciplines. Typically, the modern clinical pathology lab is large, bustling, and furnished with automated equipment to handle an enormous volume of work since certain tests are performed routinely in almost all hospitalized patients. Here, because no single clinical pathologist can hope to master the formidable amount of knowledge that is required today for achieving minimal competence in more than one biomedical domain, there are likely to be sections headed by professionals with expertise in fields as diverse as chemistry, microbiology, hematology, immunology, and virology. Some of these specialists may not have the traditional anatomy-oriented training of pathologists, and in some cases they may not be physicians.

Much to the layperson's puzzlement, some pathologists do not perform autopsies, do not interpret surgical biopsies, and do not diagnose diseases through the varied technologies available in the clinical pathology labora-

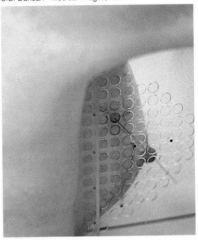

Nowadays the technique known as needle aspiration biopsy enables deep bodily tissues to be sampled without the performance of surgery. Thus, a tiny, nonpalpable breast lump detected by mammographic X-ray can be precisely pinpointed; then, with a fine hollow needle and syringe, a few cells are removed for the pathologist's expert analysis.

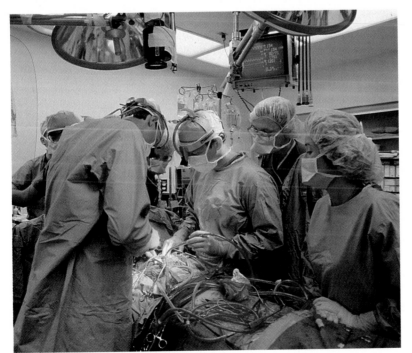

In the operating theater the brightest rays of the spotlight unquestionably fall on the surgeon, whose manual dexterity and bold actions are framed in drama. To a lesser extent, light shines on other members of the surgical team—those who directly assist in the operation itself—while the dimmest light falls on a team member who may have no direct contact with the patient. Yet it is this vital specialist—the surgical pathologist—who examines and interprets the tissues or cells that are removed during the surgery; in the case of a tumor, it is he or she who determines whether it is benign or malignant.

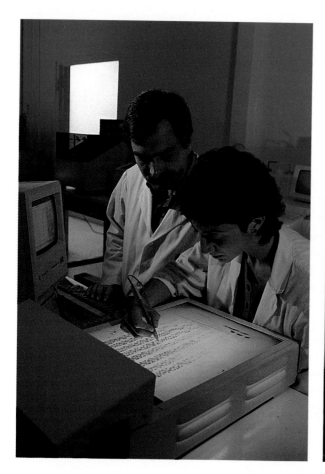

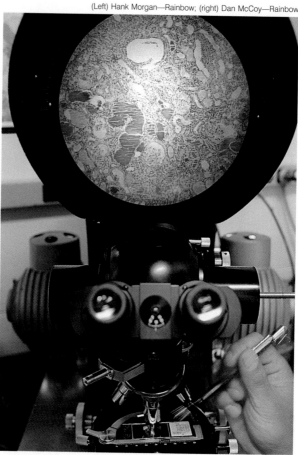

Some pathologists neither perform autopsies nor examine tissue specimens that are removed during postmortem examination. Clinical *pathologists use the powerful automated resources of biotechnology to examine bodily fluids (e.g., blood, urine, cerebrospinal fluid). (Above) Workers in a clinical pathology lab analyze protein fractions in serum, which have been separated by the technique of electrophoresis—often used to screen for diseases in which there is an excess or deficiency of specific immunoglobulins.*

Studying ill-understood abnormalities in order to clarify the nature of specific disease processes is the bailiwick of the experimental *pathologist. In some cases these research-oriented scientists confine themselves to studying animals. (Above right) A researcher uses the electron microscope to examine rat skin tissue.*

tory. In fact, the central concern of these pathologists is not to come up with the correct diagnosis for any individual patient but to understand the mechanisms of disease and the manner in which the organic abnormalities identified by their diagnosis-conscious colleagues come to be produced. These are *experimental pathologists*—that is to say, researchers. Their goal is to explain or clarify the concrete nature of diseases, shunning all explanations that merely substitute one unknown for another, as is often done in assigning abstruse technical terms to ill-understood abnormalities. Experimental pathologists are expected, of course, to avail themselves of the techniques of pathology, but they will draw evidence from any quarter so long as it is informative. As researchers, they are engaged in a creative occupation, and as in all creative activities, no cut-and-dried rules may be laid down to promote the success of their endeavors. Thus, some experimental pathologists work with cells and tissues obtained from patients and others entirely with experimental animals; some are pathologists by training, but others have come to pathology from widely disparate fields, even outside medicine.

A testimony to the vitality of pathology is its ability to attract excellent minds in such diverse subspecialties. Pathology as a discipline stands at the crossroads between clinical medicine and laboratory investigation, providing a link between basic science and clinical observations to ex-

52

plain disease processes. This uniquely advantageous position constitutes pathology's greatest strength.

Hard to define

Pathology is by no means easy to define. Pathologists themselves often complain that the proposed definitions are either too narrow or too broad. Among the former are definitions that reduce the scope of the discipline to "the study of the body's altered structure in disease." Among the latter are such vague definitions as "the study of disease," based sheerly on the etymology of the word (from the Greek *pathos,* "passion," meaning "disease or ailment," and *logos,* "work, discourse, or reason"). Despite such disagreement, in most parts of the world *pathology* has come to mean "the appearance of cells, tissues, and organs that are devastated by disease." In fact, the field itself is very commonly known as "pathological anatomy," or anatomic pathology.

It may be suspected that many if not most pathologists are directly concerned with morphology; *i.e.,* the study of structure in general and abnormalities of anatomic structure in particular. (The British, often prone to pithy and compendious utterance, use the term *morbid anatomy,* with the unfortunate side effect that its practitioners become "morbid anatomists"!) Indeed, very few areas of medicine can boast such a brilliant record of dis-

Experimental pathologists utilize the full array of techniques and equipment of pathology but also draw upon methods of other disciplines. The range of their researches is wide and their endeavors largely creative. (Below left) Some may be interested in investigating the human immunodeficiency virus, the virus that causes AIDS (top), and the means by which it compromises the body's immune defenses, while others may study the process of metastasis, whereby cancer cells spread to normal tissues (bottom). Still others may use tools of molecular biology such as two-dimensional protein analysis (below) to carry out research into genetic defects.

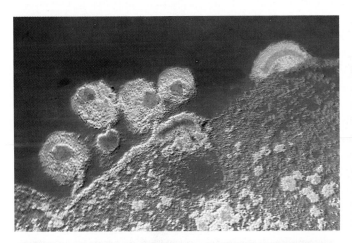

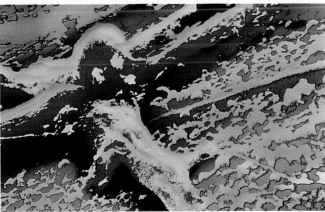

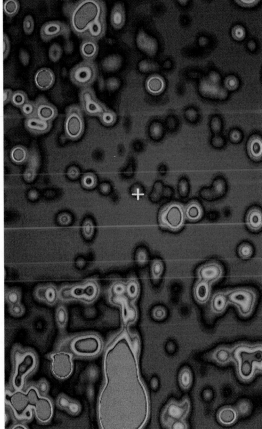

(Top left) Montagnier—SPL/Photo Researchers; (bottom left) Omikron/Photo Researchers; (right) Peter Menzel

coveries achieved by patient recording of the structural changes wrought in the body by disease—in other words, by description of pathological anatomy. However, simple observation, no matter how detailed, is not in itself science. The massive accumulation of facts about misshapen organs or abnormal tissues and cells could only produce volume after volume of irrelevant knowledge.

Revelations and guesses

For observations to acquire scientific relevance or coherence, they must be put at the service of a dominating idea—that is, they must be subserving to a hypothesis. Pathologists may be wont to claim that exciting hypotheses are "deduced" from their observations, but as philosophers point out, nothing "new" can ever be "extracted" from observations. Observations may trigger the birth of new ideas, but these were not *contained* in the observations; an idea cannot be extracted from an observation as juice is from an orange.

Critics of such morphology-prone traditionalism therefore tend to disparage the descriptive, observational approach as stagnant and unscientific; they would much rather test hypotheses by *active* experiments. It cannot be disputed that the most fruitful way to conduct scientific exploration is through a sound experimental design that is meant to provide an unambiguous answer to a clearly formulated question and that is carried out under rigorously controlled conditions. However, what critics of descriptive pathology sometimes forget is that, as the Nobel laureate Sir Peter Brian Medawar once wrote, "A 'mere observation' may be an experiment, and if activity is insisted upon as a criterion, it may be answered that even the merest observation cannot be made from a supine position." Just as astronomers discovered a new planet by the simple experiment of directing their telescopes to a certain *predicted* area of the sky, so pathologists have often gained new insights by directing their microscopes to certain *predicted* structures. *Predicted* here is a key word, implying that the observations could not have been entirely random but were guided by some idea; *i.e.,* a hypothesis. But how did the hypothesis originate in the first place?

Medawar was among those who grappled with the difficult question of the origin of hypotheses. If these are not derived or deduced from facts, how then do new hypotheses arise? Medawar thought that this "leap upstream of the flow of deductive inference" was akin to poetic inspiration, almost like a "revelation." The English philosopher Bertrand Russell, Medawar's contemporary, was less apt to use words redolent of mysticism; he saw the activity of formulating hypotheses as "making plausible guesses." Otherwise stated, devising hypotheses is a creative act and, like all creative acts, cannot be fully accounted for.

One way to approach all this is to look at the observation of structure in the style that is so dear to pathologists—as an activity uniquely suited to promoting that intuitive mental act by which hypotheses are born. The following example may go a long way toward clarifying what may otherwise seem abstruse and confusing.

54

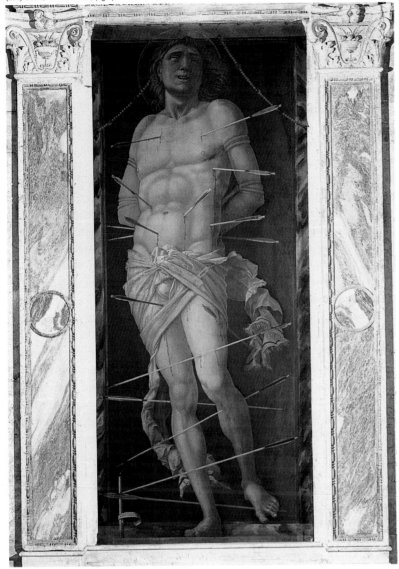

The work of pathologists is not simply to observe abnormalities and describe what they see; rather they must reach certain conclusions and make predictions. In other words, they make "plausible guesses" that go beyond what they actually observe. When a pathologist looks through a microscope at a cell and sees unfamiliar inert fibers jutting out, he or she cannot know for certain whether such protrusions are going into or coming out of the cell. The same might be said of Andrea Mantegna's portrayal of the martyrdom of Saint Sebastian; however, few people looking at the painting would reach the conclusion that the saint's body is ejecting arrows.

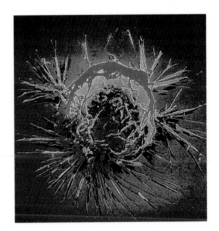

A pathologist observes a cell under the electron microscope. Slender fibers, not known to be a constitutive part of any cell type, are seen partly immersed in the cell's cytoplasm and partly sticking out into the extra-cellular environment. It is almost automatic to think that the cell is being pierced, or "impaled," by the fibers. Strictly speaking, though, no inference is warranted, since the image produced by the electron microscope is a static document; it captures an instant frozen in time and cannot say whether the fibers are being introduced into or ejected out of the cell. Yet the suggestiveness of images makes the former possibility, namely that the fibers are incoming and not outgoing, seem a very "plausible guess." When a pathologist showed just such a picture to his colleagues at a scientific meeting, he remarked that "when we see a painting of the martyrdom of Saint Sebastian, many ideas may occur to us, but not the idea that the body of the saint is miraculously secreting arrows."

Visual observation is like no other cognitive method; it stirs a certain turbulence in the mind and imparts to it a specific direction. Seeing is an elementary form of knowing; experiment may later prove that the direction suggested was wrong, which then forces a change of course.

Autopsy: birth of an anatomic bias

From a contemporary perspective, it seems natural to suppose that knowledge gleaned about parts of the body grew along with the idea that disease is the result of disordered bodily parts, but things were not so simple. The rationalist premise that disease originates from malfunctioning organs is a relatively modern acquisition. For a long time it was thought that supernatural or otherwise ethereal, unintelligible influences were the true causes of disease, so to search for them in dead bodies was as futile as it was contemptible. Curious persons, however, decided to see for themselves. The moment this decision was made, the autopsy was born. Indeed, the pristine sense of the word *autopsy* is precisely to look for oneself, to carry out a personal inspection. The historical development of this effort deserves at least a brief consideration.

In the Middle Ages biomedical science was reduced, in the expression of a distinguished historian, to "the understanding of texts." The latter were chiefly treatises inherited from the 2nd-century Greek physician Galen and from Aristotle (of the 4th century BC). Although anatomic dissection was done for the first time since antiquity in the late medieval period at the great universities at Salerno, and later at Bologna and Montpellier, this practice remained infrequent. Presumably, this was because dissection was not expected to throw light on the philosophical debates of the *medici*, the physicians of the time. It should be noted that recondite metaphysical

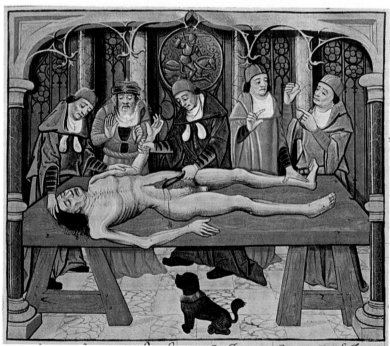

In the late medieval period at universities such as those at Salerno, Bologna, and Montpellier, dissections of human cadavers were carried out as a part of medical teaching, and anatomic studies began to be recognized as a worthy and dignified pursuit.

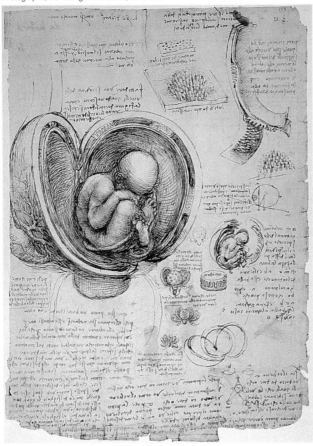

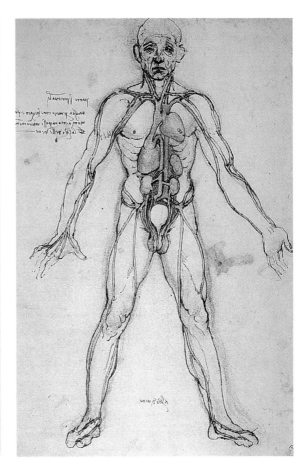

questions were the chief, if not the only, preoccupation of the medical profession in those times. This is not to deny that there were important achievements, not the least of which were the introduction of dissection as part of medical teachings and the legitimization of anatomic studies as a worthy and dignified pursuit. But no momentous theoretical innovation took place, and the origins of the science of pathology have to be looked for in later periods.

Most persons who have encountered great art are familiar with the beautiful anatomic drawings of Leonardo da Vinci. These remarkable works, executed over the course of some 30 years, starting in 1487, were based on his own dissections of cadavers. However, they had little if any influence on the study of gross anatomy, much less on pathology, because they were kept by the scientist-artist as private notebooks—and obscured by cryptic "mirror-image" notations. Nevertheless, the Renaissance had started, and artists (including Leonardo's rival Michelangelo) may have influenced the accretion of knowledge in subtle ways, simply by focusing attention so directly on the body.

Antonio Benivieni (1443–1502), a Florentine physician and contemporary of Leonardo and Michelangelo, was a refined erudite and, like most *medici,* a friend of poets and philosophers. Benivieni, however, distinguished himself by writing a treatise in which, apparently for the first time,

"Whoever succeeds in reading these notes of Leonardo will be amazed to find how well that divine spirit has reasoned of the arts, the muscles, the nerves and veins, with the greatest diligence in all things," wrote Giorgio Vasari in Lives of the Painters. *Indeed, the great Renaissance genius Leonardo da Vinci was not content to portray the human figure merely as he saw it. Rather he sought to understand the body's functioning as well as its form. On the basis of his own dissections carried out over a period of some 30 years, he produced drawings that are unrivaled in concept as well as execution. However, these masterful illustrations and the artist's cryptic notes were kept in private notebooks and were unpublished at the time and so had little influence on the study of anatomy or the development of pathology as a science.*

57

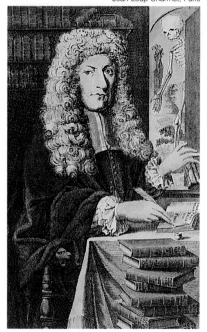

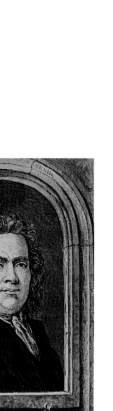

the symptoms of patients and the findings of the autopsy were collected. In *De abditis nonnullis ac mirandis morborum et sanatationum causis* ("The Hidden Causes of Diseases"), Benivieni documented in sketchy, concise narratives 110 cases in which he either performed the autopsy himself or stood by as an onlooker. Some of his descriptions were so sharp as to evoke specific diagnoses, clearly recognizable to the reader some five centuries later. For instance, he described a patient wasted away as a consequence of persistent vomiting: "it was found that the stomach had closed up and it was hardened down to the lowest part, with the result that nothing could pass to the organs beyond, and death inevitably followed." Little medical sophistication is needed to infer a diffuse, infiltrating cancer of the stomach (which today's oncologists recognize as *linitis plastica*— often called "leather-bottle stomach").

While no major discovery is to be found in Benivieni's work, the Florentine physician had pointed the way, and many who followed strove to emulate his methods. One of these was Théophile Bonet (Théophilus Bonetus), who lived from 1620 to 1689. This Genevan physician has been called "one of the great medical compilators of all time." During a period of convalescence in his late years, Bonetus wrote a hefty work in which he discussed over 3,000 autopsies. Usually known as *De sepulchretum,* the first two words of its forbiddingly long title, the work is considered a veritable treasure trove of anatomopathological experience, which historians of medicine have yet to fully explore. This opus contains lengthy and much fuller descriptions than those of Benivieni, of such pathological states as acute pyelonephritis, probable bronchopneumonia, and peritonitis.

By this time it was clear that observations at autopsy could have some meaning, even though the nature of the message was still obscure. At the beginning of the Enlightenment, the Dutch physician Hermann Boerhaave (1668–1738) of Leiden expressed the opinion that "everything pertaining to the case must be listed; not the least thing neglected which a critical Reader might rightly seek to understand the malady." Faithful to his professed principle, in describing a case Boerhaave was not content to note that a patient had eaten a copious meal. He went on to specify: "veal soup with fragrant herbs . . . ; a little white cabbage boiled with sheep; spinach; calf sweet bread lightly roasted; a little duck, thigh and breast; two larks; a bit of apple compote and bread; and dessert consisting of pears, grapes and sweetmeats"—a description that appears to say more of the gluttony of aristocrats at the time than of the mechanisms of disease. Shortly after this overabundant meal, the patient described by Boerhaave experienced great pain, as if "something near the upper part of his stomach was ruptured, torn, or dislocated." The Dutch physician deserves great credit; to this day, accounts of "idiopathic" rupture of the stomach sometimes mention him as the first observer ever to document this unhappy occurrence, which has no clear cause.

Boerhaave's clinicopathological experience was compiled in two monographs: the first published in 1724, entitled *Atrocis, nec descripti prius, morbi historia* ("Account of Dreadful Diseases Not Previously Described"), the second in 1728, *Atrocis, rarissimique morbi historia altera* ("Description

58

of Another Dreadful and Unusual Disease"). In both may be found sharp observations but also reflections of the limitations of the era.

Nor were the intellectuals of those times uniformly supportive of the gleanings of anatomic dissection. The Englishman Thomas Sydenham, an acknowledged genius among 17th-century physicians, condemned autopsies outright, sarcastically alluding to those medical men who had "pompously and speciously prosecuted the promoting of this art by searching into the bowels of dead and living creatures." Evidently, a respectable segment of the intelligentsia still believed that the true seat of disease was outside the body.

A "science" at last

First in unhinging the rigid and excessively speculative ways of looking at the body in disease was the genial professor at the University of Padua, Giovanni Battista Morgagni (1682–1771). By his detailed descriptions and his insistence on correlating clinical symptoms with pathological manifestations, Morgagni may be said to have inaugurated the era in which

Known as a "great medical compilator," the 17th-century Genevan anatomist Théophile Bonet (opposite top) offered lengthy descriptions of disease based on more than 3,000 human dissections. The charismatic 18th-century Dutch physician Hermann Boerhaave (opposite bottom) was the author of several works in which he accounted for seemingly every last detail of every "dreadful and unusual disease" he encountered. Boerhaave's copius observations were based on autopsy studies carried out in the anatomic theater at the University of Leiden (below).

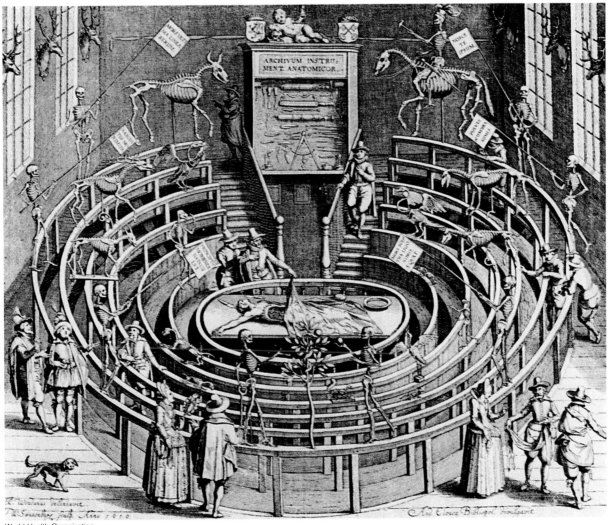

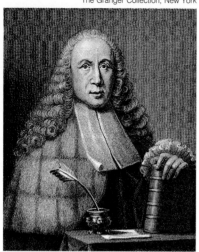

Giovanni Battista Morgagni, professor at the University of Padua in the early 18th century, was a true scientist, who correlated clinical symptoms with pathological evidence. Morgagni sought to understand not only the seat of disease but its causes. His erudite contributions earned him the well-deserved title "father of pathology."

pathology first became a scientific discipline. Unswerving in his opposition to Galenic dogma and untiring in his advocacy of keeping close to the observations, this Italian is widely regarded as the "father of pathology."

Morgagni summarized his experience with 700 cases in his most famous work, *De sedibus et causis morborum per anatomen indagatis* ("The Seats and Causes of Diseases Investigated by Anatomy"), and thenceforward there could be no doubt that the practice of autopsies could be informative not only about the *seat* of disease but also about its causes. Interestingly, the book has two separate indexes; one correlates the anatomic alterations with the symptoms, the other the symptoms with the anatomic findings. Thus, with Morgagni started the "modern" approach of regarding clinical symptoms as expressions of disordered organs.

As to his personal attributes, Morgagni is said to have been a gentlemanly, unassuming, delicate man. There is a widespread assumption that habitual exposure to the dissection of cadavers requires an unfeeling detachment, or callousness, in its practitioners. Such was not the case with Morgagni. (It is said that on two notable occasions he refused to perform an autopsy: once in Vallinsieri, who had been a colleague, and once in a bishop whom he had known as a friend.)

During much of the 18th century, the center of learning for anatomic pathology had been in Padua with Morgagni. In the first part of the 19th century, it moved to Paris. There Jean-Nicholas Corvisart (1755–1821), physician to Napoleon, and René-Théophile-Hyacinthe Laënnec (1781–1826), inventor of the stethoscope, among other things, distinguished themselves by adding to the observations of their predecessors. Marie-François-Xavier Bichat (1771–1802) deserves a place of honor in the history of anatomic pathology. With little more than simple chemical techniques, genius, and intuition—certainly not with the aid of the microscope, which he hardly ever used—he identified more than 20 different kinds of "tissues," the specialized structures that enter into the composition of organs and bodily parts. Bichat's extraordinary discoveries were to be largely confirmed by the studies of the Germanic school of pathology that flourished in the second half of the 19th century. Among the many deserving notice, only two major figures will be mentioned here.

Karl Rokitansky (1804–78) has been called by modern commentators "the most indefatigable autopsist of all time." He may have supervised 70,000 autopsies and personally performed 30,000: 2 a day on average, 7 days a week, for the 45 years that he toiled, unremittingly, on the first floor of Vienna's famed hospital, the Allgemeine Krankenhaus. Modern pathologist-historians have sometimes lamented the approach taken by this "intense, dark, melancholy man." His professed aim was to establish the study of pathology "on a purely anatomic basis." Accordingly, he and his collaborators examined meticulously every organ of the thousands of bodies they dissected but often without equally meticulous attention to the clinical manifestations present in life.

Rudolf Virchow (1821–1902), in contrast, may be said to have seen "the whole picture." He was a man of true genius, and the universality of his mind astonished not only his contemporaries but also his successors. His

60

accomplishment has been said to be no less than an attempt to establish "the scientific basis of medicine." Rokitansky's toils had yielded huge amounts of morphological data, but Virchow's vision went much farther. He warned against the exclusive dominance of pathological anatomy, believing that pathology, "in order to maintain its significance as the basis of practical medicine, will have to turn from the dead to the living and transform itself into pathological physiology." By this he meant that in addition to dissecting cadavers, the pathologist should be concerned with making "bedside" observations of patients and with conducting experiments in animals. Virchow was convinced that the pathologist must not be solely confined to the study of the end results of disease but should explore *mechanisms*—how the disease in question came to be—in other words, the conditions under which normal bodily functions go astray to produce this lesion or that.

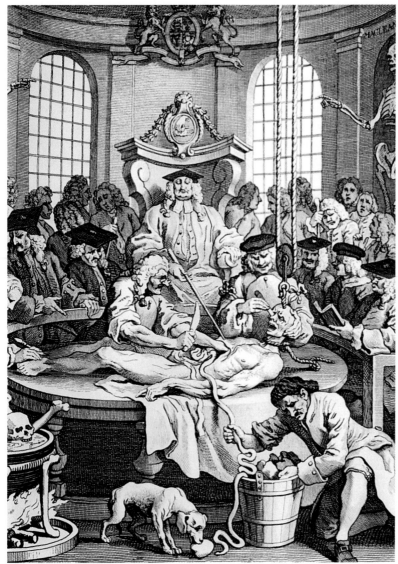

Ann Ronan Picture Library/Image Select

Even as the autopsy became established as a worthy scientific pursuit that could shed much light on the nature of human disease, there were many intellectuals and medical men who continued to doubt its value or had outright contempt for the practice—the English physician Thomas Sydenham (1624–89) among them. In fact, up until the 19th century, corpses were not widely available for autopsy studies, and some anatomists resorted to unlawful means to obtain them. (Left) William Hogarth conveys little esteem for London surgeons, whom he caricatured in the act of dissecting the body of an executed criminal (1751).

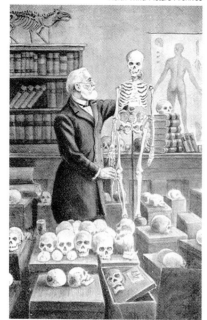

North Wind Picture Archives

Virchow's "cellular theory" was a milestone in the history of the biological sciences, not just in medicine. Virchow postulated that "there is a general principle for building all organisms, and . . . this principle is the formation of cells." He proceeded to demonstrate that all cells are fundamentally the same, that they are the smallest units capable of manifesting all the features of life, that complex organisms are formed of aggregates of cells and their products, and that cells exist individually and have a life of their own even though they participate in the formation of multicellular organisms. The absurd notion of spontaneous generation had been long abandoned, but prominent scientists continued to maintain that cells could build themselves out of noncellular material present in the organism. This fallacy was definitively put to rest by Virchow's demonstration that cells can arise only from cells. His ideas were expounded fully in his famous *Cellularpathologie,* published in 1858.

Sound as they were, even Virchow's fundamental postulates did not lack detractors. The ability of present-day biological research to probe into the smallest subcellular structures has prompted the notion that cells, after all, are but biochemical domains and that it is the constitution of the *molecular* and *subcellular* universe that should be the focus of study. Nevertheless, there are dangers in losing sight of the whole. As the distinguished contemporary Mexican pathologist Ruy Perez-Tamayo has commented: "A complete catalogue of all intracellular molecular transactions would read like a telephone directory: lots of people but little or no action. The missing element would be the cell as a unit, both as an individual and as a program. The point here is that molecular information conveys valuable knowledge . . . but that biology is more than molecules."

With earlier workers, from Morgagni to Rokitansky, pathology became an indispensable but still subordinate field of study, "the handmaiden of clinical practice." With Virchow it became the scientific study of disease—its processes, consequences, and mechanisms. For whatever else may be

Rudolf Virchow, depicted in his Berlin laboratory (above), was the embodiment of the German "Professorismus" and one of the most brilliant pathologists ever to live. Virchow's cellular theory, set forth in his highly regarded opus Cellularpathologie *(1858), was a milestone in the history of biological studies. His accomplishments spanned many fields, and he traveled widely during his lifetime. In 1900 (right) the professor stands, rapt in attention, at the head of a patient during a brain operation in Paris.*

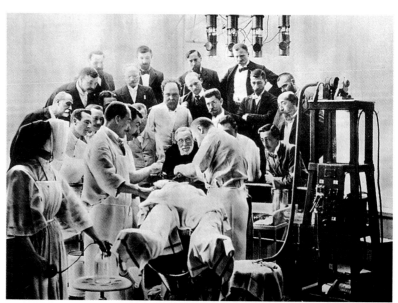

The Bettmann Archive

associated with disease, it was in the vital processes taking place within the cells themselves that researchers had to find the actual explanation for all morbid conditions.

Virchow was nearly 81 years old when he died in Berlin; indeed, his life had been so rich in accomplishment it might have earned him enduring fame even *without* his scientific discoveries. In 1848, when he was 27 years old, he was commissioned to investigate an outbreak of typhus in Upper Silesia. Public health in his country improved as a consequence of his report, but he used the latter to express his political ideas, which were highly critical of the government and by no means endeared him to authorities. Shortly thereafter he was elected to the National Assembly, and the impetuosity of his youth brought him into open conflict with the rigid authoritarianism of Prussian power. When asked by government officials about the influence of heredity in disease, Virchow is said to have answered, "I know a family, a very exalted one, in which the grandfather had softening of the brain, the son hardening of the brain, and the grandson no brains at all." It was well understood that Virchow was speaking of three kings of Prussia: Frederick William II, III, and IV.

Virchow continued to be a thorn in the side of the Prussian government in his mature years. Gray-haired, with thick, round, metal-rimmed spectacles, he was the very embodiment of the German "*Professorismus*" that Otto von Bismarck so vehemently detested. Perhaps it is not the least of his distinguished accomplishments that he so outraged Bismarck during the 1865 debates of the Prussian Chamber that the "iron chancellor" challenged him to a duel. Luckily for science, the professor was not about to pick up the gauntlet.

Further scientific burgeoning

From the above, one can see that pathologists of the 19th century appear to have belonged to one or the other of two diverging tendencies: one, perhaps best represented in the ideas of Virchow, who would have liked there to have been less emphasis on morphology and greater attention paid to dynamic studies, including chemistry, clinical observations, and experimentation; the other, the more stringently "anatomic" path, in which various types of disease were viewed as fundamentally morphological entities. Current disagreements on the very definition of *pathology* reflect the degree of emphasis that individual pathologists would like to see placed on each of these historical paradigms. For the most part, however, pathology as a medical science has achieved its many contributions by conforming to one model or the other according to need. But it is nonetheless true that pathology evolved largely as a specialty based on the study of altered structure in disease, as "morbid anatomy."

One obvious reason it took this course is that the earliest pathologists were anatomists, and their professional descendants were in a strict sense anatomists, too, since they continued to be in charge of the performance of autopsies. In the process of documenting systematically every pattern of structural deviation, pathologists found themselves more and more insulated from clinical medicine, much to the dismay of Virchowians.

For a while the anatomically minded approach yielded extraordinary results. Its cultivators must have thought they had struck gold, and it is difficult to persuade the miner to abandon the site at which he has just seen, or thinks he has seen, a rich ore. One example, among many possible ones, may serve to illustrate the early compelling power of the anatomy-based approach.

The parathyroids are tiny glands present in the neck whose minute dimensions and appearance render them almost indistinguishable from the surrounding fatty tissue. Upon first consideration it seems difficult to believe that organs so tiny that they are often overlooked or unrecognized should be in charge of controlling the state of calcification of the entire human skeleton. But this, in fact, is the case. Thousands of autopsies performed by pathologists of the Germanic tradition (and described with Teutonic compulsiveness) clearly established that every time that a patient had brittle bones with frequent fractures and blood-filled cysts in many areas of the skeleton, the parathyroids were abnormal. What for centuries had been confusing, chaotic manifestations of bone disease suddenly acquired unity and order. The malady that is now known as von Recklinghausen's disease was discovered in 1882 by Friedrich von Recklinghausen to be a disorder in which the parathyroids function abnormally as a result of a tumor or excessive cellular growth, wreaking devastation throughout the skeleton. Knowledge thus derived from autopsy studies allowed the performance of surgery on the parathyroid glands, in some cases resulting in cure of a cruel and otherwise fatal disease.

The above example is a testament to the power of anatomic studies in developing concepts of pathology and applying them to the treatment of diseases. Other developments enabled the science to grow and flourish in other directions. In the second half of the 19th century, the industrial production of aniline dyes was perfected in Germany, and techniques were developed that permitted cut tissues to be stained and prepared in a way that made them suitable for microscopic examination. Thus, a vast new universe lay open for morphologists; the microscopic intricacies of diseased tissues were amenable to detailed and systematic description for the first time, and generations of pathologists saw before them a new and exciting challenge.

Here it is pertinent to note that the microscope was hardly a new invention. As early as 1614 Galileo was able to see details of the anatomy of insects with a primitive optical instrument that preceded Antonie van Leeuwenhoek's invention in 1656. Nevertheless, 250 years passed before the microscope became a tool for scientific exploration of human tissues.

Why such a time lapse? Historians have offered a number of explanations for the late blooming of microscopy in human medicine. One is that the earliest versions of the microscope were difficult to produce and therefore very expensive. Buyers tended to be the idle rich, who were interested in the instrument more as an expensive "toy" or gadget than as a serious scientific tool. The contemporary pathologists Guido Majno and Isabelle Joris at the University of Massachusetts Medical School at Worcester give an additional reason: the perceived unreliability of the microscope. With

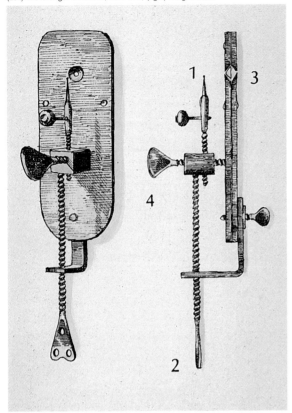

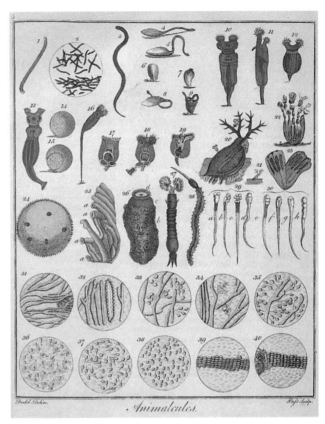

Animalcules.

rudimentary lenses, a lack of condensers, and imperfect systems of illumination, most microscopes that were built (up until about the first half of the 19th century) were apt to introduce optical artifacts that misled observers into seeing things that were not really present in the examined specimen.

Eventually, however, technical advances removed all these obstacles, and alluring new vistas were opened up, which pathologists could not resist. To this day much of their work continues to be based on microscopy techniques, which over the past century have become greatly refined in their accuracy, sensitivity, and specificity. Then, just as outcries were beginning to be heard about the folly of clinging to a morphological approach with methods that seemed close to being exhausted, along came *electron microscopy*. The extraordinary power of magnification of the new tool enabled the observer to study not merely tissues and cells but the subcellular components, the "organelles," of individual cells. Thus, pathologists could now perform "the autopsy of a cell." Accordingly, starting in the 1950s and over the subsequent two decades, a vast amount of information was collected on the ultrastructural abnormalities that cells exhibit in disease.

The fate of the autopsy

What happened in the meantime to the conventional autopsy—the dissection of cadavers—undertaken for the sake of unveiling "the seats and causes of disease" as first propounded by Morgagni? A look at its course in the United States is instructive.

The microscope is unquestionably one of the essential tools of pathology. Up until the early 19th century, however, the instruments were imperfect and sometimes introduced optical artifacts; thus, pathologists were often misled by what they observed. The devices (above left) were invented by the renowned Dutch microscopist Antonie van Leeuwenhoek (1632–1723). Although Leeuwenhoek's studies lacked organization, his astute observations (mostly of various low forms of animal life) enabled him to make discoveries that influenced other scientists for many generations. Among other things, he was the first to observe and describe spermatozoa (from insects, dogs, and humans). The meticulously rendered observations of animal life above (c. 1795, "after Leeuwenhoek") show "very little animalcules," including sperm, which the Dutchman had described over a century earlier.

65

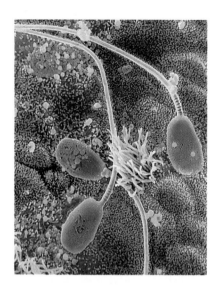

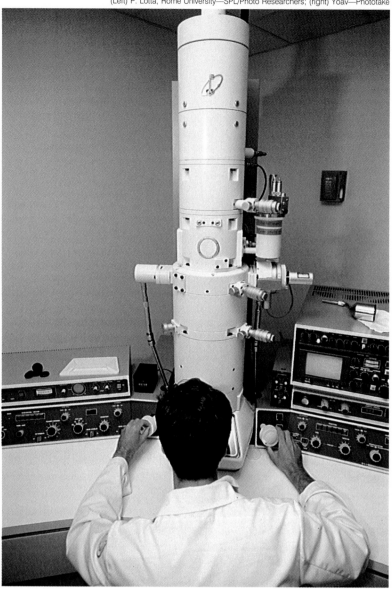

The invention of the electron microscope in the 1950s enabled pathologists to peer deeper into cells than they ever could before—to view the subcellular components (organelles) of individual cells. Whereas previous microscopes depended on light for illumination, the electron microscope uses electrons, producing images with stunning levels of magnitude and resolution. The scanning electron microscope (right) uses a beam of electrons to provide a three-dimensional image of the surface of a specimen, which has a depth of focus up to 500 times greater than is possible with a light microscope. The scanning electron micrograph (above) captures human sperm migrating up the uterus on their way to fertilize an egg.

In 1910 a comprehensive survey of the state of American medical education, known as the Flexner Report, was carried out. One of its conclusions was that physicians who learned their trade through apprenticeships with other practitioners, as was then often done, sorely lacked that firm medical understanding that can be acquired only by anatomic studies. A true revolution in medical teaching followed, and the practice of autopsies became common. In metropolitan Chicago only 10% of hospitalized patients who died in 1919 were autopsied; by 1930 the figure was 26%, and in 1960 it had reached 49%. At Mount Sinai Hospital in New York City, the autopsy rate rose from 20% in 1920 to 55% in 1955. Across the U.S. by the 1950s, the autopsy rate was approximately 50%, but in university-affiliated teaching hospitals, which serve as training grounds for physicians, the majority of patients who died—75%—were autopsied.

66

As early as 1950, however, a declining trend was noted in some places. The decline became pronounced and generalized, and by 1979 only 15% of patients dying in a hospital in the Chicago area were autopsied. In some hospitals in the United States, rates of 4% or less were not uncommon, and similar declines in autopsy rates were also being observed in other industrialized countries.

Why this decline? Probably the most comprehensive contemporary analysis has been done by Rolla B. Hill and Robert E. Anderson. In their book, *Autopsy: Medical Practice & Public Policy* (1988), they cite the following as some, but not all, of the reasons for the decline: financial costs, ignorance of autopsy's potential benefits and uses, physicians' and hospitals' fears of litigation based on autopsy findings, physicians' obstinate refusal to confront their own misdiagnoses or treatment failures, perceived legal and procedural obstacles in obtaining permission from the patient's next of kin to perform postmortem studies, the harried pace of today's medical practice, and a diminished emphasis on autopsy studies in medical school curricula.

It is important to stress, however, that the decrease in the number of autopsies performed does not necessarily reflect a disenchantment with its utility. The value of the autopsy in medical education and research continues to be regarded as inestimable by enlightened sectors both within and outside the medical profession. Indeed, hundreds and perhaps thousands of disease processes have been defined or clarified by postmortem studies. In fact, a recent survey easily listed close to a hundred diseases that have been either discovered or critically clarified only in the last half of the 20th century as a result of the autopsy. Among these are cardiomyopathies (chronic heart muscle disorders); numerous congenital malformations; the common hereditary disease cystic fibrosis; Zollinger-Ellison syndrome (a type of gastrointestinal ulcer associated with a hormone-producing tumor of the pancreas); angiosarcoma, a rare tumor of the liver, induced by the chemical vinyl chloride; toxic shock syndrome; collagen diseases such as relapsing polychondritis (a disease affecting cartilage throughout the body); Whipple's disease, a malady affecting the small intestine, named for the American pathologist and Nobel Prize winner George Hoyt Whipple (1878–1976); Legionnaires' disease; embolism of the amniotic fluid; and such perinatal conditions as congenital biliary atresia and congenital chromosomal disorders (*e.g.,* trisomy 18, fragile X syndrome).

In addition, diseases that are already familiar to doctors become better understood through autopsy studies. For example, certain risk factors for sudden infant death syndrome and many of the complications of AIDS have been so identified. Just as importantly, when new drugs, innovative prosthetic devices, or new surgical treatments are first tried, the long-term effects on patients can be thoroughly assessed *only* by means of complete autopsy studies.

Nor can it be said that the autopsies of patients treated by conventional means are uninformative. At least 10 different studies done within the last 15 years, each by an independent group of investigators, have concluded that in approximately 10–15% of patients who were diagnosed by the most

Second-year medical students remove the skin from the head of a cadaver in order to study the underlying blood vessels, nerves, muscles, and bones. The value of the autopsy in medical education and research has always been—and continues to be— inestimable. In the United States a true revolution in medical teaching occurred in the 1930s through the '50s, when the practice of autopsy became routine. In the latter half of the 20th century, however— for complex reasons—there has been a trend toward the abandonment of this vital learning experience.

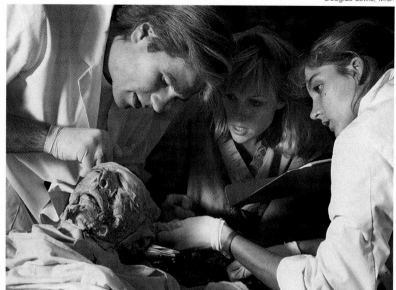

sophisticated modern diagnostic tools and techniques, the autopsy was still capable of disclosing major discrepancies that, had they been known during the patient's lifetime, might have modified the treatment. An additional 10–20% of the autopsies disclosed lesions that remained unknown before the patient's death but that would not have modified the treatment even if they had been more opportunely discovered.

Only a supine complacency, if not outright arrogance, can explain the attitude of physicians who deny the value of the autopsy on the premise that "everything we wanted to know about the case was already known." By the same token, reluctance or inability to employ advanced investigative techniques, and stubborn adherence to sterile, obsolete practices that render the autopsy uninformative, is a fault that falls to the lot of some pathologists.

Pathologists working in a hospital morgue perform a postmortem examination. Even when the most sophisticated diagnostic tools have established the nature of an illness, the autopsy is rarely uninformative. Not only can it disclose the precise cause of death, but in many cases it reveals information about a patient's illness that was not evident or available while he or she was alive.

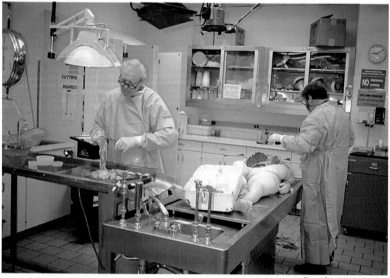

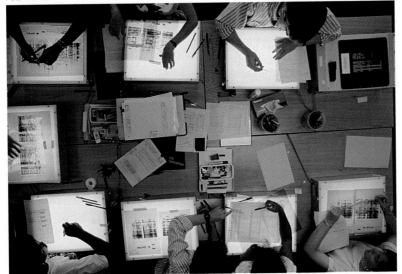

Peter Menzel

Technicians at the Cellmark Diagnostics laboratory, Oxford, England, determine paternity by matching DNA of children with that of alleged fathers. So-called DNA fingerprinting has revolutionized forensic investigation, making it possible to ascertain with great accuracy whether cells collected as evidence belong to one individual or another.

Exciting new vistas

Quite apart from individual human failings, the field of pathological anatomy, which is far from restricted to the autopsy, will remain a strong and viable specialty. Without a solid grounding in pathology's anatomy-oriented base, physicians cannot aspire to understand disease; their efforts are mere aimless gropings, a chasing of shadows. But it is also reasonable to predict that the face of pathology will change, without loss of its morphology-inclined personality. Perez-Tamayo has predicted "not a decrease in the different methods for study of disease, but rather an integrated accretion of those currently used in neighboring medical specialties, in related biologic disciplines, and even in remote or completely unrelated areas of science."

A curious example may be cited that bears out this prediction. It is the application of—of all sciences!—entomology to the service of pathology. Forensic pathologists have recently attracted notoriety by taking advantage of the biology of insects in their efforts to solve crimes. Maggots swarming in decomposing flesh are a loathsome sight, but their existence is governed by basic biological laws. The larvae of flies, beetles, and various creatures that feed on decomposing remains evolve according to predictable time schedules; their life cycles have been well studied and can be experimentally reproduced in the laboratory. Therefore, study of these life forms permits the forensic pathologist to determine with accuracy the time of death of persons killed and left to rot outdoors. Drugs or poisons may be recoverable from the body of worms or maggots long after the hope of retrieving them from the body of the deceased has been abandoned. Recently a suspected rapist was convicted when, in the face of his persistent denials, his presence at the scene of the crime was established by demonstration that insects known to breed solely in that area were trapped in his clothing and in the radiator of his car.

The incorporation of the powerful techniques of molecular biology into the scientific study of disease constitutes one of the most important advances in the recent practice of pathology. It is justified to predict that all

The vitality of the specialty of pathology is greater today than ever before. Although the autopsy will never diminish in importance, pathologists now have many powerful new tools that offer vast opportunities for discovery. Such discoveries will ultimately lead to cures for disease and the relief of human suffering.

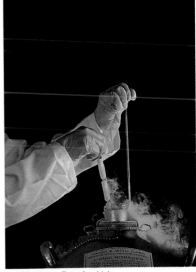

Matt Meadows—Peter Arnold, Inc.

69

branches of medicine will feel the impact of this development. The DNA molecule, as is well known, is the basic genetic material—the sequence of nucleotides in this compound reflecting the uniqueness of every individual human being. Hence, ascertainment of the chemical conformation of this essential molecule now allows the pathologist to determine—with a degree of accuracy heretofore undreamed of—whether cells from blood, sperm, or any other DNA-containing specimen belong to one individual or another. Consequently, so-called DNA fingerprinting has revolutionized forensic investigation by bringing scientific precision into a realm traditionally fraught with vagary, subjective opinion, and "reasonable doubt."

Not only cells but bacteria and viruses contain DNA (and RNA, whose single-stranded nucleotide sequences that relay genetic information encoded in the DNA to the rest of the cell are uniquely individual or species-specific). Accordingly, pathologists have at their disposal the means to diagnose viral or bacterial diseases when their causative agents (microorganisms) are not visible even with the most powerful microscopes or when they fail to grow in appropriate culture media—the latter being, until recently, the definitive way to diagnose bacterial or viral disease.

Nor is securing a large specimen required in order for the new molecular biological technologies to be of enormous value. The ingenious polymerase chain reaction, or PCR, uses an automated procedure to amplify a tiny amount of DNA at an exponential rate in a remarkably short time (often just a few hours). Starting with an infinitesimally small DNA sample—on the order of magnitude of mere molecules—that serves as a "template," researchers are able to end up with as much DNA as suits their particular needs. The power of PCR methodology is illustrated by its ability to track transmission of the human immunodeficiency virus (HIV), the virus that causes AIDS. PCR amplification, for example, recently enabled pathologists to determine that at least six patients had become infected with HIV during dental procedures performed by a dentist in Florida, who subsequently died of AIDS. With PCR, pathologists in all the subspecialty fields previously mentioned have a new tool; the technology is currently being applied to solve forensic problems, study genetic diseases, diagnose bacterial and viral illnesses, and scrutinize the genomic alterations of cancerous and noncancerous cells.

What will these recent and remarkable advances that are having such a profound impact on the specialty of pathology mean for the autopsy? Will the trend of the past several decades persist? Hill and Anderson have admonished: "Even if pathologists were to fuse the magic of cell and molecular biology with classic morphology, the autopsy would continue to languish unless students were extensively involved, clinicians became interested and modified their attitudes, and the public was convinced of the enormous benefits [to] society."

In conclusion, nothing can ever diminish the autopsy's value for understanding human disease and making possible medicine's vast array of stunning cures. May reason, prudence, and good counsel soon prevail and reverse the more ominous trends that now threaten the speedy relief of human suffering.

ANATOMY REVEALED

Two venerable collections and a future museum

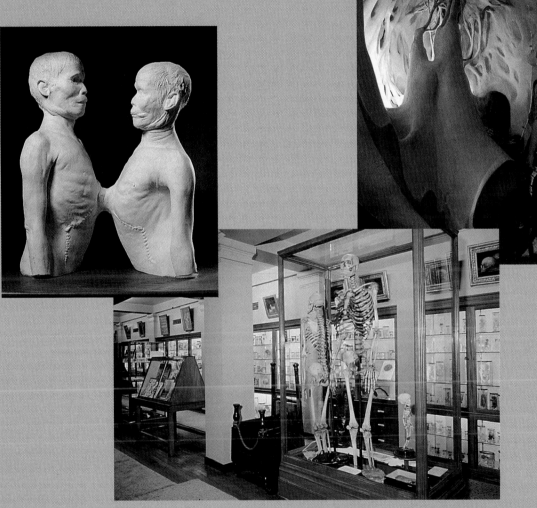

Photographs, (top left) plaster cast of the torsos of the celebrated Siamese twins, Chang and Eng, in the collection of the Mütter Museum, College of Physicians of Philadelphia; (top right) walk-through human heart in the Museum of Science and Industry, Chicago; (bottom) display case in the Hunterian Museum containing the skeleton of Charles Byrne, the "Irish giant," with kind permission of the trustees of the Hunterian Collection, Royal College of Surgeons of England, London

John Hunter's Extraordinary Legacy

by Elizabeth Allen, M.I.Biol.

The Hunterian Museum is among the greatest medical museums in the world. It is housed in the same porticoed building that is home to the Royal College of Surgeons of England, on a historic London square, Lincoln's Inn Fields. The Hunterian is named for its founder, the 18th-century Scottish surgeon John Hunter. Regarded as the father of scientific surgery, Hunter was also the founder of pathological anatomy in England and an early advocate of scientific investigation and experimentation.

The development of surgery, then no more than a crude craft, was severely hampered in the 18th century by the absence of anesthetics, lack of antiseptic technique, and, not least, absence of any organized system of teaching. Surgeons of the day did not study to become doctors of medicine, nor did they enjoy the esteem with which physicians were regarded. Surgical training was by apprenticeship, but the more fortunate students, particularly those in London, could attend privately run anatomy schools and "walk the wards" behind eminent surgeons. Hunter played a vital role in establishing an organized course of training and raising the professional and social status of the surgeon in Britain. One of his pupils claimed that he did more than anyone else to make surgeons "gentlemen." Hunter himself regarded surgery as a mutilation of the patient and an admission of medicine's failure to effect a cure. He advised his students that "surgeons tend to forget that they are not masters but only servants. They can assist the natural powers within all living flesh but cannot replace them."

Hunter's early career

Hunter was born in 1728 on a farm near Glasgow, Scotland. He appears to have had little inclination for formal schooling. He did, however, have an insatiable interest in the natural history of the surrounding fields and woods. A short period in his late teens during which he worked with his brother-in-law, a cabinet-maker, may have provided training in manual dexterity, a skill that he used to great effect later in life.

In 1748 he traveled to London to assist his older brother William, a prominent obstetrician and the proprietor of a private anatomy school. Hunter immediately showed considerable aptitude for dissection

Elizabeth Allen, M.I.Biol., is George Qvist Curator, Hunterian Museum, Royal College of Surgeons of England, London.

and was kept busy preparing teaching specimens for William's classes and supervising the pupils in the dissecting room. He also studied surgical technique, first under William Cheselden at Chelsea Hospital and then under Percivall Pott at St. Bartholomew's Hospital—both renowned surgeons of the day. In 1756 he was appointed house surgeon at St. George's Hospital, but his eagerness to continue his researches and anatomic studies apparently prompted him to resign after only five months.

In October 1760 Hunter was commissioned staff surgeon to the British army and was stationed on Belle Isle, off the coast of France. On the basis of his experience in the management of gunshot wounds gained during his military service and further work after his return to London, he wrote what is considered his greatest work, *A Treatise on the Blood, Inflammation, and Gun-Shot Wounds* (published posthumously in 1794). Later, having been posted to Portugal, Hunter, when not attending the sick and wounded, spent his time studying the natural history of the area. Among the many subjects he investigated were the acuity of hearing in fish, the regeneration of lizard tails, and the geologic structure of the Portuguese countryside. His interest in geology and paleontology led him to speculate on changing climatic conditions, changes in sea levels, and the possibility of dating geologic strata by their fossil contents. Most important, these researches led him to conclude—contrary to the prevailing belief of the day—that the Earth had to be many thousands of centuries old. Material brought back from his tenure in Portugal formed the nucleus of the collection of specimens to which he would devote much of the rest of his life.

Innovator and pioneer

When Hunter returned to London in 1763, his place in his brother's school had been filled, and he needed to supplement his army retirement pay. He started his own private surgical practice and also took in pupils. His study of teeth, gained through his association with the Spences, a family of prominent dentists, resulted in the publication of the first scientific work on dentistry in the English language; *The Natural History of the Human Teeth* (1771) covered the anatomy, development, diseases, and transplantation of teeth.

Hunter's interest in transplantation prompted him to attempt a series of experimental grafts, including the transplantation of a spur from a cock's leg to its comb. Subsequently, he attempted to transplant a human tooth into a cock's comb. Although one such procedure was successful, Hunter believed his inability to repeat it was "due to some natural cause"; he thus anticipated the problem of tissue rejection faced by modern transplant surgeons.

Hunter was in every sense an innovator. Most of those who instructed in human anatomy in this period taught structural anatomy. Hunter, however, believing that the "principles of life" were vital to the study of anatomy, taught *functional* anatomy—stressing the relationship between structure and function. Whereas most of his contemporaries employed specimens for demonstration during lectures, Hunter amassed a vast "museum," which he made available to his students for private study.

Unwritten book

Hunter's museum is often and appropriately referred to as his "unwritten book," as it contains evidence of a wide range of unpublished research. It differed from similar collections in existence in the 18th century in being not merely a series of exhibits but an illustration of Hunter's theories—in particular, his ideas about the continual adaptation of living things.

Hunter took each anatomic system and demonstrated the increasing complexity of the organs from the lowest life forms (plants and lower animals) to the highest (mammals, including humans). More important, he illustrated how the body could adapt to changes in the environment and changes due to trauma or disease. He believed that the future of surgery lay at least partly in assisting the body in compensating for disease or injury rather than in routinely excising or amputating diseased parts.

The collection, which numbered nearly 14,000 specimens at his death in 1793, was divided into three main sections. The first part demonstrated comparative anatomy and physiology, focusing on adaptations and mechanisms concerned with ensuring the day-to-day survival of the individual organism. This part of the collection included specimens from Hunter's animal experiments demonstrating bone growth and remodeling. One of the more arresting exhibits consists of tissue from the biceps muscles of a man whose left arm was shortened by a fracture that had healed improperly. Whereas many surgeons of the day would have advised amputation of the nonfunctional limb, Hunter advocated waiting to see what would happen and, over a period of time, the muscle of the affected arm compensated by shortening, and the man eventually regained the use of the arm.

Hunter's interest in circulation led him to seek permission from King George III to experiment on the royal deer in Richmond Park. He believed that cutting off the blood to the "velvet," the soft, highly vascular hot skin that covers and feeds the growing antler,

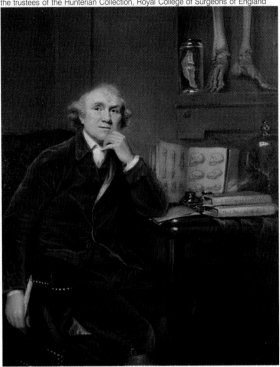

John Hunter (1728–93), considered the father of scientific surgery, was the first in Britain to study pathological anatomy. He assembled an impressive collection of anatomic specimens during his career as a teacher, clinician, and scholar.

would have a detrimental effect on the antler. He tied off the external carotid artery, which supplies blood through the deer's neck to the velvet, expecting to see the velvet wither and the antler fail to grow (or possibly even be shed); but when he returned a month later, he was surprised to find the velvet again hot to the touch and the antler still growing. By killing the animal and dissecting the blood vessels, he showed that a collateral, or secondary, circulation had formed, restoring the blood supply to the antler.

Also among the items in his comparative anatomy and physiology collection are numerous examples of electric and luminous organs in marine animals, including the electric ray, eel, catfish, and torpedo. Hunter was the first to publish an account of such organs; in 1773 he presented his "Anatomical Observations on the Torpedo" to a meeting of the Royal Society, remarking, "The magnitude and the number of nerves bestowed on these organs in proportion to their size must on reflection appear as extraordinary as the phenomenon they afford."

It was his interest in abnormal growth that led Hunter to include what is undoubtedly the best-known exhibit in his museum, the 2.4-meter (7-foot 10-inch) skeleton of Charles Byrne, the famous "Irish giant," who, during his short lifetime, advertised himself as being over 2.44 meters (8 feet) tall, claiming he was the tallest man in the world. Byrne, who died in his mid-twenties, in fact had not finished growing. When his skull was X-rayed in the 1920s (at the instigation of U.S. neurosurgeon Harvey Cushing), it was confirmed that the giant had had a pituitary tumor.

The second section of the museum contained Hunter's collection of pathological specimens, which he used to illustrate his theories on the nature of disease. Hunter is regarded today as the father of surgical pathology. Microscopy and tissue-staining techniques were undeveloped in the mid-18th century, and the study of diseased tissues, so-called morbid anatomy, was limited to visual examination. Little existed in the way of records correlating symptoms during life with the appearance of the organs after death. Hunter's pathology collection commenced with the demonstration of basic processes such as healing and tumor formation and then progressed to diseases specific to certain organs. He studied tumors, benign and malignant, in some depth and included in his collection probably the earliest recorded case of metastasis (cancer's spread). Also included was a section of a 4.1-kilogram (9-lb) benign tumor that Hunter had removed from a patient's neck. According to his notes, the operation took 25 minutes, during which the patient did not once cry out—a remarkable occurrence in the preanesthetic era! Hunter produced a very acceptable cosmetic result, and there was, apparently,

A watercolor depicts the Hunterian Museum as it appeared c. 1860 and suggests the broad range of Hunter's interests. The collection is more than an assemblage of objects; it illustrates his pioneering scientific theories.

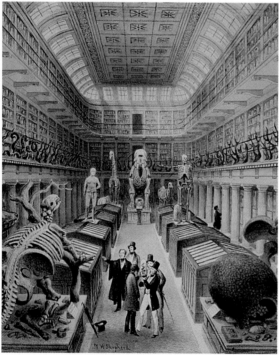

no recurrence of the tumor or damage to the facial nerves.

Of particular importance is the specimen that demonstrates Hunter's most outstanding contribution to operative technique, his development of the classic method for alleviating popliteal aneurysm (weakening and swelling of the artery just behind the knee joint). If the condition was untreated and the aneurysm was allowed to burst, the condition was invariably life threatening. Although surgeons had attempted to open the aneurysm, remove the blood clot, and resuture the artery wall, amputation was regarded as a less dangerous option! Having demonstrated the development of collateral circulation in deer and in further experiments on dogs, Hunter revolutionized the management of this kind of aneurysm by tying the healthy part of the artery (a process called ligation) high up in the thigh and allowing the secondary circulation to take over in the lower leg. His first three patients recovered from the operation but died of unrelated disease within a year or two; his fourth patient, a 36-year-old coachman, survived, with a healthy leg, for another 50 years, outliving his surgeon. After the patient's death the leg was dissected by another surgeon and mounted for inclusion in Hunter's collection. "Hunter's ligation" for popliteal aneurysm has saved thousands of lives and can still be used in cases where a lengthy graft procedure is not advisable.

Hunter included in his museum specimens of diseases he could not identify—many of which probably represent the earliest record of such diseases—in the belief that future generations of students would classify and learn from them. As many of these specimens show very advanced states of diseases that are now cured or controlled at an early stage, the collection serves as a valuable resource of material that is no longer available to the modern medical practitioner.

Hunter was also interested in cryonics (the practice of freezing dead animals in hopes of future restoration). Before unsuccessfully trying to freeze and revive a freshwater fish, Hunter had considered persuading a healthy man to be frozen for 100 years, thawed out for a short period, and then refrozen, this process to be repeated for the next thousand years or so—to observe how civilization developed! He did not attempt this experiment but consoled himself by freezing a rabbit's ear; although he noted the inflammation and increased vascularity of the ear on thawing, he did not fully understand the damage caused by ice crystals.

The third section of the museum illustrates adaptations in living things designed to ensure the continuation of the species. It includes fetuses of such exotic animals as the aardvark, sloth, and kangaroo. The series of human fetuses illustrates the different stages of gestational development; it also contains the fetuses of female quintuplets. Most of this section of the Hunterian collection remains much as it was

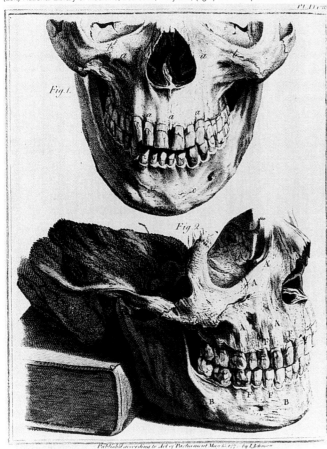

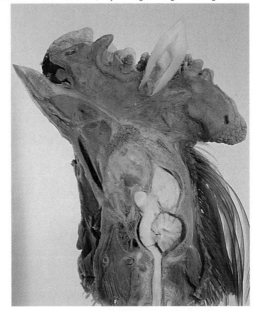

Hunter's The Natural History of the Human Teeth *(left) was the first scientific work on dentistry in the English language. To prove that teeth were living structures, he attempted to transplant a freshly extracted human tooth into a rooster's comb. His dissection of the bird's head (above) clearly shows the development of blood vessels, which confirmed the viability of the grafted tissue.*

in its collector's lifetime and is therefore considered one of the most valuable and interesting parts of the present museum.

Extraordinary legacy

It was Hunter's wish that the collection he had amassed over a period of more than 30 years be kept intact for future generations of students. In his will he left the entire collection to his executors, his nephew (and respected anatomist) Matthew Baillie and his brother-in-law Everard Home, to be offered for sale "in one lot" to the British government. After strenuous efforts on the part of the executors, £15,000 was granted by the government for this purpose some six years after his death. The question of placement of the collection led to much further deliberation; it was finally offered to the Company of Surgeons, which in the following year was reorganized and renamed the Royal College of Surgeons in London (becoming the Royal College of Surgeons of England in 1843). The collection remained at Hunter's house in Leicester Square until suitable accommodation could be designed and built at the College.

The new museum was opened in 1811, but the collection expanded so rapidly that the original building was demolished and rebuilt twice the size in 1837; further rooms were added in 1855 and 1891. This phenomenal expansion was necessary to house gifts from fellows of the College and other scientists, although the museum's growth must be credited in part to the efforts of its many eminent conservators.

By the outbreak of World War II, the museum held approximately 65,000 specimens in five large rooms. In May 1941 the building suffered extensive bomb damage, and nearly 75% of the collection was destroyed. The present museum, which opened in 1963, contains more than 3,600 surviving Hunterian specimens (including 2,104 demonstrating "normal" anatomy and 1,547 "morbid anatomy" preparations), which are, as far as possible, as they were originally arranged by Hunter.

Hunter's collection was, and still is, unique; it provides a valuable resource for anatomists and biologists and for research on many diseases that are now treated or cured at an early stage. The museum is not open to the public—admission is restricted to members of the medical, nursing, and veterinary professions and to bona fide biological scientists, all of whom must apply in writing for the privilege of viewing Hunter's extraordinary legacy to medical science.

Pathological Treasures of the Mütter Museum

by Gretchen Worden

On May 20, 1856, Thomas Dent Mütter wrote to the College of Physicians of Philadelphia that ill health was forcing him to resign his post as professor of surgery at Jefferson Medical College. Mütter also informed the College that he wished to offer it guardianship of the unique anatomic and pathological materials he had collected for his personal "museum."

Mütter had been appointed to the chair of surgery at Jefferson in 1841, just 10 years after receiving his M.D. degree from the University of Pennsylvania. Following his graduation he had spent a year in Paris, the medical Mecca of the period. At that time physiology—the study of organ and system function—was becoming a true science, based on recently acquired knowledge of chemistry and physics, and pathologists were beginning to correlate clinical findings with pathological anatomy. From his exposure to the finest medical minds in Europe, Mütter returned to the U.S. with an understanding of the latest French techniques in orthopedic and plastic surgery and a firm belief in a system of teaching medicine based on close observation of actual cases. The inspiration for his museum probably dated from that time. He subsequently amassed a large assortment of specimens for use in his classes. The time and effort his colleagues devoted to writing and publishing, Mütter spent in collecting, making the museum his legacy to the profession.

August—and enduring—institution

The organization to which Mütter offered his collection (and of which he was a member) was a private medical society founded in 1787 by 24 of the leading physicians of Philadelphia, among them Benjamin Rush, a signer of the Declaration of Independence. The College was established for the purpose of gathering the latest scientific and medical knowledge, promoting the use of this knowledge for the public welfare, and encouraging the highest standards of professional practice and conduct among its members. Toward these ends it had started a library in 1788 and a small "cabinet of pathological specimens" in 1849. The College's stated purpose and its stability and standing in the medical community explained Mütter's choice of repository; it has proved to be a fortunate one in

terms of guaranteeing both the museum's longevity and its accessibility to the public. Similar collections in medical schools and teaching hospitals of the 19th century—and intended only for the eyes of medical students—were largely dispersed or discarded in the 20th century as they lost relevance to modern medical education and competed with the higher priorities of classrooms, laboratories, and hospital beds.

The Mütter Museum's continuation was assured by an endowment of $30,000 that accompanied the collection, the income from which was to pay for the services of a curator and a lecturer and for the care and enlargement of the museum. In addition, the College, which until that time had met in rented quarters, was required to erect a fireproof building to house the collection. The institution signed the agreement with Mütter in 1858 and in 1863 moved into its first real home, a brick and granite structure (since demolished) near the heart of downtown Philadelphia. Mütter himself died in 1859 at age 48 before he could see his full plans realized.

Dispatched to the new building from Jefferson Medical College in 1863 were bones; air-dried, varnished anatomic specimens; plaster casts; specimens preserved in alcohol and other liquids; wax and papier-mâché models; and oil and watercolor paintings—more than 1,700 items in all—which joined the 92 specimens in the College's existing collection. Many of the items that today's visitors find most impressive and memorable were among those given by Mütter himself: the bladder stones removed from Chief Justice John Marshall by Philip Syng Physick (the "father of American surgery") in 1831; a wax model of a 15¼-centimeter (6-inch)-long horny protuberance (*cornu cutaneum*) that projected from the forehead of a Parisian widow; and the deformed skeleton of a woman whose rib cage had been compressed by the tight lacing of her corset. Around this nucleus the museum grew rapidly as desirable material was purchased abroad with funds from Mütter's endowment. Fellows of the College—individuals elected by their colleagues for their eminence in American medicine—also contributed specimens from their private and hospital practices.

Linked livers, educational ears

In 1874 the museum acquired several noteworthy additions. Members of the College had performed the autopsy of Chang and Eng, the world-famous Siamese

Gretchen Worden is Director, Mütter Museum, and Associate Director, Francis C. Wood Institute for the History of Medicine, College of Physicians of Philadelphia.

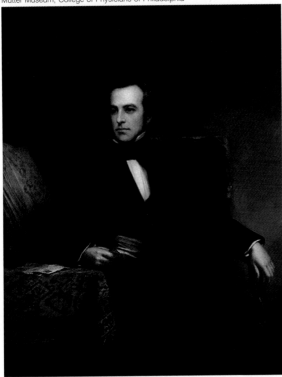

Before his death in 1859, surgeon Thomas Dent Mütter offered the College of Physicians of Philadelphia his unique collection of anatomic and pathological specimens. This generous bequest formed the nucleus of the present-day Mütter Museum.

twins, and the museum was allowed to retain their connected livers along with a plaster cast of their torsos showing the band of skin and cartilage that connected them. (The bodies themselves were returned for burial to North Carolina, where the pair had lived with their wives and numerous children.)

The same year saw the successful culmination of negotiations with anatomist Joseph Hyrtl of Vienna, resulting in the purchase of his collection of 139 skulls illustrating the anatomic variation among ethnic groups of central and eastern Europe. Also bought from Hyrtl were dried placentas illustrating obstetric anomalies, wax corrosions (specimens prepared by injection of wax into hollow organs and vessels, the surrounding tissue then being corroded away) demonstrating the circulatory system, and specimens of the ossicles and labyrinths of the ears of humans and other animals—the latter having taken Hyrtl 14 years to assemble. Two years later the College would acquire another superb otologic collection from Vienna, this being the series of normal and abnormal tympanic membranes and other parts of the ear meticulously prepared by the renowned Austrian otologist Adam Politzer. This prizewinning collection had been exhibited at the 1876 Centennial Exhibition in Philadelphia, where it enabled practitioners to see for the first time minute internal structures of the ear; the display of Politzer's specimens prompted vast changes in the practice of American otology.

The "Soap Lady" and other wonders

In December 1874 came the preserved corpse of a woman who is now known as the "Soap Lady." The adipose, or fatty, tissue of her body, of which there was a considerable amount, had decomposed after burial into a stable brownish- or grayish-white fatty wax known as adipocere, similar in chemical composition to soap. The body, discovered during the relocation of a cemetery in the older part of Philadelphia, was acquired by Joseph Leidy, a prominent anatomist, who donated it to the museum. Leidy presented a similarly preserved male body from the same site to the Wistar Museum of the University of Pennsylvania, which specimen has since been transferred to the Smithsonian Institution in Washington, D.C. Originally it was thought that both of these individuals had died of yellow fever in 1792 (which was actually a year before the great epidemic in Philadelphia), but the machine-made pins on her shroud, discovered during a recent X-ray study, showed that the Soap Lady's death must have occurred later than was originally believed—probably in the first half of the 19th century.

In 1877 Leidy was responsible for another of the museum's prized acquisitions, the skeleton of a 2.3-meter (7-foot 6-inch) giant from Kentucky, whose remains he had seen on exhibit at the Academy of Natural Sciences in Philadelphia. Leidy recommended that the College purchase this specimen from the purveyor of biological materials who owned it, and thus, for $50 and no questions asked, the museum acquired the largest human skeleton on public display in North America. The individual was a male in his early twenties; certain features of the skull—lengthening of the face and enlargement of the frontal sinuses—indicate that he suffered from acromegaly (chronic hyperactivity of the pituitary gland). Because of the severe curvature of his spine, his total height is less than it might have been.

More miscellania medica

The museum continued to follow the pattern set by Mütter's original collections until 1871, when the College passed a resolution to begin gathering obsolete medical instruments as well. These now constitute the major part of the museum's current acquisitions—items reflecting changes in the technology of medicine and memorabilia of past practitioners. Outstanding among these items are Rush's medicine chest; a wooden stethoscope said to have been made by the great French clinician René-Théophile-Hyacinthe Laënnec himself, who is credited with invention of the device; Florence Nightingale's sewing kit, used by the nursing pioneer while she served at Scutari, Turkey, during the Crimean War; a quartz piezoelectric electrometer (an instrument that measures ionizing radiation) devised by Pierre Curie and his brother in about 1898 and used by Pierre and his wife, Marie, in their earliest work with radium (personally presented by Marie Curie to the College in 1921); a 1949 Emerson iron lung, a poignant reminder of the prevaccination ravages of polio; and a full-scale model of the first successful heart-lung machine, devised and used in Philadelphia by surgeon John H. Gibbon, Jr., in 1953.

One of the museum's most popular exhibits is the collection of more than 2,000 objects removed from the throats and airways of patients by pioneer broncho-esophagologist Chevalier Jackson and his colleagues and presented by Jackson in 1924. The drawers full of toy jacks, dentures, safety pins, and pieces of food show the stunning variety of items that people accidentally swallow and that could be removed nonsurgically by the special instruments Jackson devised.

Many of the items in the Mütter's various collections reflect the interest and involvement of Philadelphia physicians in national and international affairs. In 1893 Philadelphia surgeon W.W. Keen assisted in an operation to remove a cancerous growth from the jaw of Pres. Grover Cleveland. Unlike today's well-publicized presidential medical procedures, this operation took place in secret on a private yacht steaming up Long Island Sound on the pretense of taking the president to his summer home. The country was in the middle of a financial crisis precipitated by the inflationary Sherman Silver Purchase Act of 1890, and any perceived weakness on the part of Cleveland would have jeopardized his efforts toward repeal of the act. The

full story of the operation was not publicly revealed until Keen published it in the *Saturday Evening Post* in 1917 (Cleveland had died in 1908), at which time he presented the museum with the tumor and the laryngeal mirror and cheek retractor used in the operation.

The U.S. Civil War brought specimens and photographs of battle injuries, contributed by the Army Medical Museum (now the National Museum of Health and Medicine) in Washington, D.C. In 1865 a messenger from the U.S. surgeon general conveyed to the museum a specimen connected with one of the nation's most tragic events, described in a museum label as a "piece of the thorax . . . of J. Wilkes Booth . . . assassin of President Lincoln." This tissue, removed at autopsy by army surgeon and Philadelphian Joseph Janvier Woodward, is currently the focus of much attention because of the continuing controversy about whether Booth was killed on April 26, 1865—as alleged by the government—or whether he escaped. In the opinions of some researchers, historical inconsistencies raise sufficient doubts about the identity of the body autopsied as Booth's to warrant a comparison of DNA from the Booth specimens in both the Mütter and the National Museum of Health and Medicine with DNA samples from Booth family descendants. Negotiations to conduct such a study were under way in 1993.

The steady increase in the museum's collections during the 19th century, as well as the growth of the College's library, led the Fellowship to have a new facility built for the College on 22nd Street between Chestnut and Market streets, to which the institution moved in 1910. The move allowed the museum to continue acquiring new material.

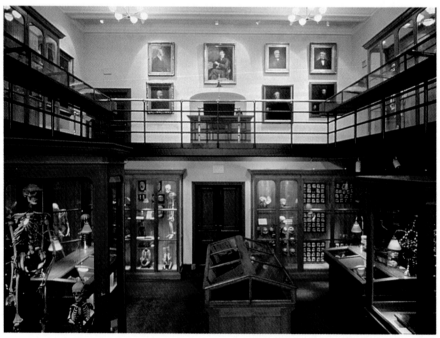

In 1910 the Mütter Museum moved to its present-day home on 22nd Street in the same building that houses the College of Physicians of Philadelphia. The collection had rapidly outgrown its previous home, thanks in part to the contribution of surgical and postmortem specimens from many distinguished fellows of the College.

Mütter Museum, College of Physicians of Philadelphia

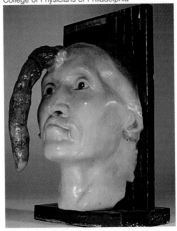

One of the items from Mütter's personal collection was this lifelike wax model of a French woman who had a curious hornlike growth (cornu cutaneum) protruding from her forehead.

Recent additions

In comparison with the numbers of instruments and items of medical equipment, the pathological specimens acquired in recent years are few but choice. Among them is the skeleton of a man who died in 1973 of fibrodysplasia ossificans progressiva, a very rare and incurable disorder in which bone forms in muscles and ligaments, eventually immobilizing the joints. The abnormal-fetal-development collection—which already contained representative examples of cyclopia (development of only one eye), neural tube defects and associated disorders (anencephaly, spina bifida, hydrocephaly), and conjoined twins—has been expanded by the addition of rare anomalies such as ADAMS (amniotic deficiency, adhesion, and mutilation syndrome), which produces abnormal development of the lower body; thanatophoric dwarfism, in which limbs and lungs are undersized; caudal regression, a condition often associated with maternal diabetes and characterized by incomplete growth of the body below the navel; and acrania, in which a portion of the skull over the brain is missing.

The museum's wax model collection was also augmented recently by the acquisition of approximately 100 historical models, bringing the present total to 276. Lifelike anatomic and pathological models in wax were created from the 17th through the late 19th century to take the place of hard-to-preserve, and often difficult-to-obtain, soft tissue specimens for the instruction of medical students. The additions came from a collection that had been purchased between 1850 and 1910 in England and Europe by professors from the University of Pennsylvania; it included examples from such outstanding artists as Joseph Towne of London, Fritz Kolbow of Dresden, Germany, and Alfons Kröner of Breslau, Germany (now Wrocław, Poland). Though primarily dermatologic—illustrating ulcers, eczemas, and the various stages of syphilis and smallpox lesions—the recently acquired models also depict conditions such as breast cancer and gouty toe.

A still-vital mission

In the early years of the museum, most of the visitors were medical students, fellows of the College, and visiting physicians. The various collections were never as heavily used for formal teaching as Mütter had envisioned, though they were occasionally used in lectures and lent out for exhibit at medical meetings. During the course of the 20th century, however, students in biology, nursing, pharmacology, and medical technology have been visiting in increasing numbers, making use of not only the museum's collections but also other resources of the College, such as the historical collections and public services divisions of the library and the Francis C. Wood Institute for the History of Medicine.

The collections also hold interest for modern researchers in a variety of fields. For example, a firm involved in the research and development of medical instruments recently examined the museum's collection of urologic catheters and dilators, in part, to see whether any forgotten aspects of the instruments might be incorporated into modern products, thereby avoiding the "reinvention of the wheel."

In 1976 the tumor that had been removed from President Cleveland was reexamined, this time by pathologists armed with modern knowledge of oral cancers. As a result of their study, the tumor was identified as a verrucous carcinoma, a generally non-metastatic type of cancer. Earlier pathologists had failed to agree on the exact nature of the lesion. This new finding enabled medical scientists finally to explain why Cleveland's cancer never recurred—a fact that had puzzled modern surgeons considering the relatively primitive state of surgical technique in 1893 and the usually metastatic nature of oral cancers. Another researcher has proposed testing the specimen to see if it contains any evidence of human papillomavirus (HPV), which is known to be associated with this type of cancer; Cleveland's tumor could provide the earliest known example of HPV in human tissue. The proposed DNA study of the tissue specimen from Lincoln's assassin could, in a similar fashion, add important information to the historical record. Herein lies the value of such museums of preserved human material: they may hold the answers to questions that today have not even been formulated but tomorrow may be very important.

The Mütter Museum was created at a time when such museums were part of every medical student's education. This museum has survived where most others did not because it became part of an institution with a broader mission, one that included the education of the general public. The Mütter Museum today remains a source of enlightenment to visitors of all backgrounds and ages, confirming that medicine and its fascinating history are a vital part of everyone's heritage.

Anatomy for Everyone

by Richard R. Andrews, M.D.

Most people would like to know more about how their body is built and why it functions as it does—*without* going to medical school or getting a Ph.D. in anatomy! Even those who do acquire such specialized knowledge would appreciate a tool that further facilitates learning and would be useful for the exchange of ideas with professional colleagues. Being able to walk through a grand-scale three-dimensional human body model could be "just what the doctor ordered."

Larger than life

This concept of a colossal model of the human body, in fact, is not new. According to the French archaeologist R.A. Schwaller de Lubicz, author of *Temple in Man: Sacred Architecture and the Perfect Man,* the 18th-dynasty Great Temple of Amon at Luxor at one time was laid out in the shape of a body, with a "heart room," a "stomach room," and a "head room." Over the years there has been no lack of interest in larger-than-life body models. Probably the two best-known examples from more recent times are in Chicago's Museum of Science and Industry and Philadelphia's Franklin Institute Science Museum; both institutions can boast decades-old walk-through hearts. Some physicians report having been so impressed with these models as children that they were motivated to enter the healing profession.

Other walk-through anatomy exhibits include a tooth at the Cleveland (Ohio) Health Education Museum and a pelvis in the department of anatomy at Harvard Medical School in Boston. In every instance these educational exhibits have been great attractions. Such popularity was undoubtedly the motivation for a whole-body amusement park at Walt Disney World's Epcot Center, Lake Buena Vista, Florida. In 1989 an entire pavilion, some 9,300 square meters (100,000 square feet) in size and devoted to dramatizing the intricacies of the human body and making the subjects of health and disease come alive, was opened. The exhibits in the Wonders of Life pavilion include "Body Wars"—a simulator-assisted trip through the human body and the chance to witness an "inner-space" conflict in which bacteria invade the bloodstream and are attacked by the immune system's powerful scavenger

Richard R. Andrews, M.D., is President, the International Museum of Anatomy, and Medical Director, Delmarva Rural Ministries, a service organization for migrant farmworkers, Nassawadox, Virginia.

and killer cells; "Cranium Command," which allows visitors to get inside the brain of a 12-year-old boy; and the not-to-be-missed "Sensory Funhouse," with its hands-, feet-, ears-, and eyes-on displays.

Even Hollywood has got in on the act. Probably the concept was best realized in the memorable 1966 movie *Fantastic Voyage,* in which Raquel Welch, who plays a medical technologist, is injected along with her scientist-colleagues into the bloodstream of a Czech scientist to help with an "inside job" of removing a blood clot from his brain. In the process the team makes its way through the valves of a powerfully beating heart only to confront a huge and threatening white blood cell; they discover trouble in the sacs of the lungs; and, for a time, they get caught in the mucus of the nose. In a similar "vein" was the more recent *Innerspace* (1987), with its gripping action taking place within a treacherous hydrochloric acid vat (more commonly known as the stomach). Other motion pictures have brought the body to life—each in its own unique way—Woody Allen's *Everything You Always Wanted to Know About Sex (But Were Afraid to Ask),* with its larger-than-life reproductive organs; *Honey, I Shrunk the Kids,* with its special-effects antics that make "innocent" children the size of insects; and its sequel, *Honey, I Blew Up the Kid,* in which an eccentric father inadvertently turns his baby into a 34-meter (112-foot) monster.

Museum of the future

In 1988 the concept for the not-yet-realized International Museum of Anatomy (IMA), eventually to be housed in Washington, D.C., and to contain the ultimate walk-through body model, was born. The intent is to build a Statue of Liberty-sized human body in a recumbent or semirecumbent position such that visitors will be able to stand inside virtually every major organ or structure of importance. This future museum will offer models that will be detailed and sophisticated enough to be of interest to even the most knowledgeable physician-visitor. Yet the five-year-old child will also be able to learn more than ever before was possible in a direct, experiential way. In such a learning environment even the person with a disability such as dyslexia, which makes "book learning" difficult, would be at considerably less of a disadvantage.

The gigantic model will teach normal anatomy (body *structure*), normal physiology (body *function*), and, of course, pathology (body *disease*). The exhibits within the body will serve many purposes. Schoolchildren, for example, will be able to learn about substance abuse in a no-nonsense way; a "field trip" through the brain will show exactly what damage a drug such as cocaine can do to the "pleasure center" of this complex organ and why, once the harm has been done, chronic users of the drug often find themselves unable to experience any pleasure at all. Meanwhile, in another part of the body, physicians would be able to stand inside a series of progressively healing body sores and address some of the therapeutic controversies concerning wound treatments.

In 1992 a smaller-scale, single-organ prototype for this eventual body-building project was begun—construction of a 3 × 3-meter (9.9 × 9.9-foot) fiberglass eyeball. By late 1993, when the eyeball opens its lid to the public, visitors will be able to walk through this first-of-its-kind organ, located in Northampton county, Virginia. The team that conceived and designed the eye included a practicing ophthalmologist, a family practice doctor, a nurse/carpenter, teachers, and artists. How better to become a "pupil" than to actually be inside a pupil and discover how this adjustable opening in the center of the iris (the eye's colored portion) regulates the passage of light? It is more than just a black dot after all! To get to the pupil, one will have stepped through the transparent structure at the front of the eye (the cornea). From the pupil one can proceed to the posterior chamber—passing through the biconvex lens into the jellylike vitreous and eventually arriving at the all-important retina—the eye's "essence"—which, one will learn, has direct extensions (the retinal nerves) to the brain. Viewers will "see" for themselves what causes nearsightedness, glaucoma, and cataracts. They will also discover where tears come from and where they go, besides down the cheeks. A hint: ever wonder why people have to blow their noses after crying?

It is likely that the enthusiasm of body tourists who visit the Northampton county eyeball will breathe life into the next-planned organ model in the same state. Support is growing for the construction of a 10 × 30-meter (33 × 99-foot) walk-through human lung to be strategically located in Richmond. Some Virginians are already looking forward to the day when their capital city is known as the "lung capital of the world" rather than the "tobacco capital." Perhaps by then some healthier agricultural product will have replaced the state's current leading cash crop. Such a model may well provide the most effective deterrent to smoking, or the best incentive for quitting, that medicine has to offer—better than Surgeons General's reports or the most stringent antismoking legislation and lessening the need for such cures as nicotine gum or patches. Young and old will be able to walk through and discover how a pink, healthy lung looks and works; then they will see—from the inside—how emphysema, bronchitis, and lung cancer develop in the charred, black lungs of a smoker. If "a picture is worth a thousand words," this model should be worth *ten thousand* words on the prevention front.

Other individual organs and body parts are envisioned. Meanwhile, full efforts are being devoted to achieving the necessary technological developments to bring the grand plan for the IMA into being. The District of Columbia-based body will take advantage of state-of-the-art computer technologies such as laser holography, virtual reality, and touch-sensitive video screens that provide menu-guided access to each anatomic part—in many languages and at various levels of sophistication. To learn about the pancreas, for example, one visitor might select "Ph.D./Swahili," another "second-grade/English." In this ultimate "classroom" neurosurgeon and schoolchild alike will be able to discover previously unimagined wonders of human anatomy.

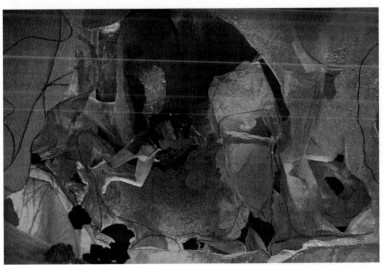

Actor Stephen Boyd navigates the windy sacs of the lungs as he and four coscientists, including Raquel Welch, set out to do an "inside job" of removing a blood clot from the brain of the eminent Czech scientist Dr. Benes, played by Jean Del Val. The concept of being able to get inside the human body—so "fantastically" realized on the screen of the motion picture Fantastic Voyage—*is the motivation behind an envisioned walk-through Statue of Liberty-sized human body model, to be housed in the future International Museum of Anatomy in Washington, D.C.*

The Curious Phenomenon of the Double

by Richard M. Restak, M.D.

How would you feel if you had to go through what I experience? Every other time when I return home I see my double. I open the door and see myself sitting in the armchair. I know it is an hallucination the moment I see it. But isn't it remarkable? If you hadn't a cool head wouldn't you be afraid?

Such was the confidence imparted to a friend by the 19th-century French writer Guy de Maupassant in a moment of candor. Maupassant was not the first writer to describe the phenomenon of autoscopy—the experience of seeing a "double," an exact duplicate of oneself. In one of the earliest written accounts of autoscopy, Aristotle told how a certain Antipherone had encountered a hallucinated vision of himself while on a walk. The German poet Goethe, while suffering from an acute depression, witnessed himself dressed in unfamiliar clothing and approaching on horseback. "I shook myself to get rid of this hallucination, and I no longer saw anything," he wrote of the phantom.

That this phenomenon of the double is universal is evident by its appearance not just in literature but in cultural myths and folklore from around the world. In ancient Egypt the *ka,* depicted hieroglyphically as uplifted arms, represented the personification of those physical and intellectual qualities constituting a person's individuality. The Egyptians believed that the *ka,* a kind of double, survived the death of the body and could reside in pictures or statues of the deceased. In parts of Europe for many centuries, it was a common folk belief that an encounter with one's double portended imminent death. The German *Doppelgänger* ("double-goer"), a ghostly counterpart or companion of a living person, has become an accepted idea in Western thought.

With the advent of modern medicine, doctors began observing the experience of the double in neuropsychiatric conditions marked by excessive fatigue, anxiety, fright, or other forms of emotional distress. Autoscopy and related phenomena are also well-documented features of several distinct

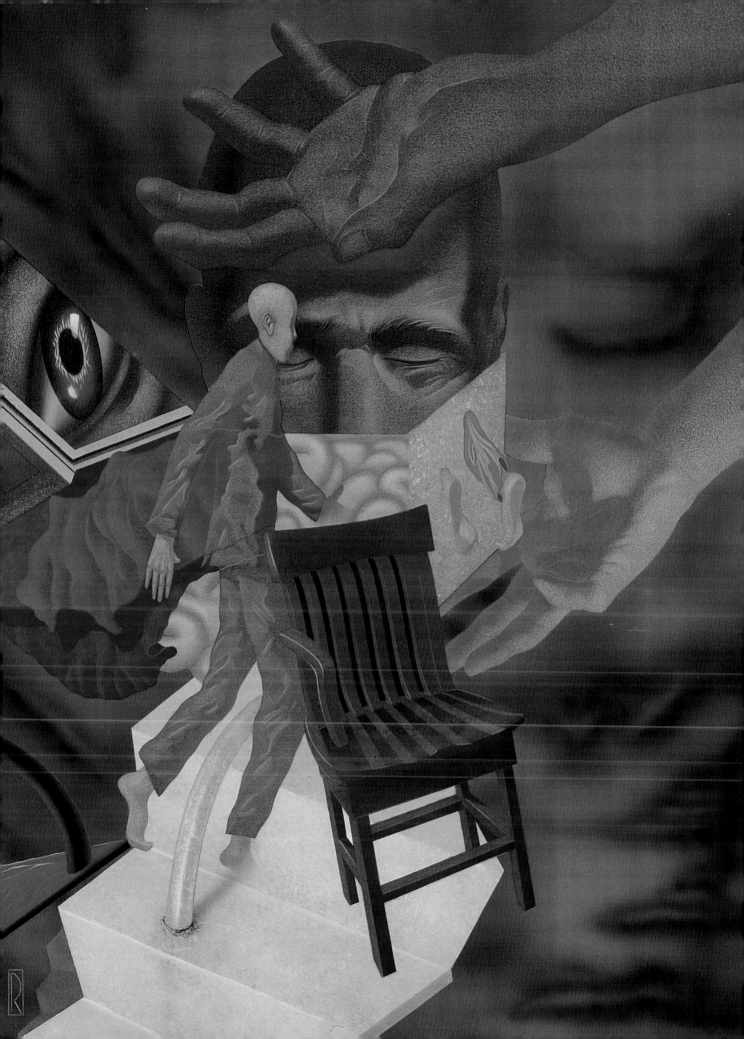

brain disorders, among them epilepsy, and psychiatric syndromes. While doubles are noteworthy simply because of their dramatic and disturbing nature—who would not be startled to gaze into the face of a stranger and see himself or herself staring back?—their existence has long fascinated both philosophers and scientists. The following examples from literature shed some light on this curious phenomenon.

Phantoms in fiction

The double was a particularly appropriate theme for the American poet and short story writer Edgar Allan Poe, in whose works—and, indeed, personality—strange dualities abounded. In the story entitled "William Wilson," the protagonist tells of a lifetime of pursuit and oppression by a mysterious man who shares his name. Finally, in a fury of rage and frustration, Wilson corners this unknown enemy at a masquerade ball and thrusts his sword into the man's body. Fearful of being discovered in the act of murder, he turns to lock the door of the chamber, and a bizarre scene ensues:

But what human language can adequately portray *that* astonishment, *that* horror which possessed me at the spectacle then presented to view? The brief moment in which I averted my eyes had been sufficient to produce, apparently, a material change in the arrangements . . . of the room. A large mirror,—so at first it seemed to me in my confusion—now stood where none had been perceptible before; and as I stepped up to it in extremity of terror, mine own image, but with features all pale and dabbled in blood, advanced to meet me with a feeble and tottering gait.

Thus it appeared, I say, but it was not. It was my antagonist—it was Wilson, who then stood before me in the agonies of his dissolution. His mask and cloak lay . . . upon the floor. Not a thread in all his raiment—not a line in all the marked and singular lineaments of his face which was not, even in the most absolute identity, *mine own!*

In Oscar Wilde's *The Picture of Dorian Gray,* a double is encountered in a painting rather than a mirror. Upon viewing his handsome likeness in a portrait, Gray, a vain, corrupt young aristocrat, wishes that the face in the picture might grow old while his own would remain eternally youthful. The wish comes true, but eventually Gray can no longer bear to look upon the aging, dissolute version of himself in the painting:

Once it had given him pleasure to watch it changing and growing old. Of late he had felt no such pleasure. It had kept him awake at night. When he had been away, he had been filled with terror lest other eyes should look upon it. It had brought melancholy across his passions. Its mere memory had marred many moments of joy. It had been like conscience to him.

Richard M. Restak, M.D., is Associate Clinical Professor of Neurology, Georgetown University School of Medicine, Washington, D.C. He is the author of numerous books, the most recent of which is The Brain Has a Mind of Its Own: Insights from a Practicing Neurologist *(1991).*

(Overleaf and pages 85 and 90) Illustrations by Ruben Ramos

Gray impulsively decides to destroy the portrait in the belief that this action will free him from the evil deeds he has committed. But stabbing the picture with a knife results not in absolution from his sins but in Gray's own death and terrible transformation. Thus, his servants, upon entering the room, witness an incredible sight:

Hanging upon the wall [was] a splendid portrait of their master as they had last seen him, in all the wonder of his exquisite youth and beauty. Lying on the floor was a dead man, in evening dress, with a knife in his heart. He was withered, wrinkled, and loathsome of visage. It was not until they had examined the rings that they recognized who it was.

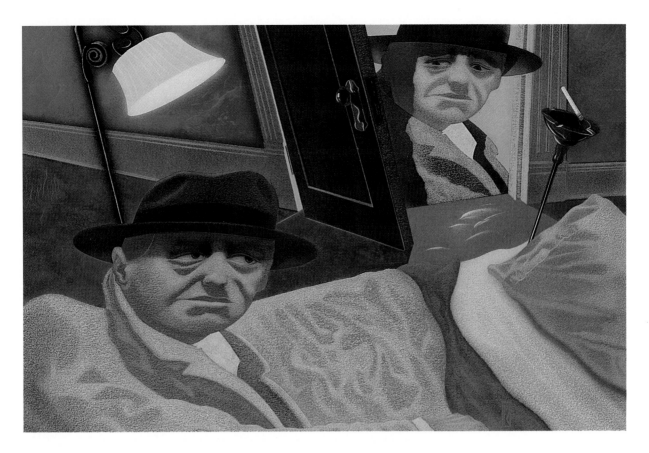

Perhaps the most brilliant depictions of the double in literature are encountered in the works of Dostoyevsky, especially in his novels *The Double* and *The Possessed*. In the former the character Golyadkin, a lowly clerk who leads a solitary existence punctuated by periods of manic excitement, tortured self-recriminations, and a belief that unspecified "enemies" are intent on destroying him, flees from a ball at which he has publicly humiliated himself. Making his way home through a dank, misty November night, he encounters a man "dressed and muffled exactly like Mr. Golyadkin from head to foot." Later, upon returning to his apartment, he finds sitting on his bed "none other than himself—Mr. Golyadkin. . . . Another Mr. Golyadkin, but exactly the same as him. . . . It was, in short, his double, as they call it, in all respects."

So real, so close—so elusive

In real life as in fiction, accounts of experiences with doubles share many common elements. Typically, the double is described as appearing quite suddenly; it may take the form of an entire body, the bust, or only the head. Often its occurrence is preceded by the feeling of an unseen "presence" in the surroundings, usually somewhere in back of the subject. Subsequently, the "presence" materializes into a clearly visualized figure, usually in three dimensions. It may appear gray or fully colored; solid or semitransparent; normal sized, enlarged, or shrunken. On occasion, the phantom seems so real and close that the beholder reaches out to touch it, only to see it fade away. If no attempt is made to engage it, the double may stare intently at the subject or, more frequently, mirror his or her facial expressions and movements—*e.g.,* if the subject lifts his left hand, the double lifts its right hand.

The most striking and characteristic feelings associated with the experience are fear and distress based on a powerful affinity with the image. Some have described a shared consciousness between themselves and their double, which often appears sad, tired, or even as if in agony. Doubles may materialize only rarely, perhaps once or twice in a lifetime, or they may exert an almost continuous presence. And although they may appear at any time of the day or night, the most common occasion is at twilight or at dawn.

Many theories about the origin of doubles have surfaced over the years. Included among them is a narcissistic overconcern with one's body, health, or internal state. The appearance of a double has also been attributed to disturbances in the integration of sensations from various parts of the body into a cohesive "body image." Still another theory is that the double occurs when, under extreme stress, one reverts to primitive thought patterns. While any or all of these factors may play a role in individual instances, none provides a completely satisfying explanation.

From all that is presently understood, it seems safe to say that the experience of the double in its extreme manifestations is a symptom of brain dysfunction, either temporary or permanent. Among the conditions that may precipitate the experience are schizophrenia, depression, migraine headache, extreme stress, lack of sleep, and head injury. The brain dysfunction may also result from illnesses elsewhere in the body that have a secondary impact on the brain (such as influenza), conditions affecting the middle ear, and alcoholic liver damage. In Maupassant's case, his unnerving hallucinations are now attributed to the effects of dementia paralytica (syphilis of the brain), which ultimately killed him. Poe's reputation as an alcoholic is well known, although any connection between his drinking binges and his literary creations—especially his penchant for portraying phantoms and wraiths—can only be speculated upon. In all likelihood Dostoyevsky's eerily compelling depictions of the double were a consequence of his temporal lobe epilepsy.

Epilepsy and the brain: seized by a sense of strangeness

Epilepsy is a brain disorder that has been widely misunderstood. The Greeks, who referred to it as the "falling sickness," blamed it on supernatural causes. Over the centuries epilepsy sufferers were feared, rejected, shunned, and physically attacked. Even during relatively enlightened periods, epilepsy was associated with various forms of mental illness, and as recently as the early years of the 20th century, epileptics were confined to institutions for the insane. One reason for epileptics' being treated as if they were mentally deranged is that certain forms of the disease are marked by sometimes bizarre disturbances of thought, emotion, and behavior. This is particularly true of epilepsy originating in the temporal lobe and its connections to the rest of the limbic system, which is responsible

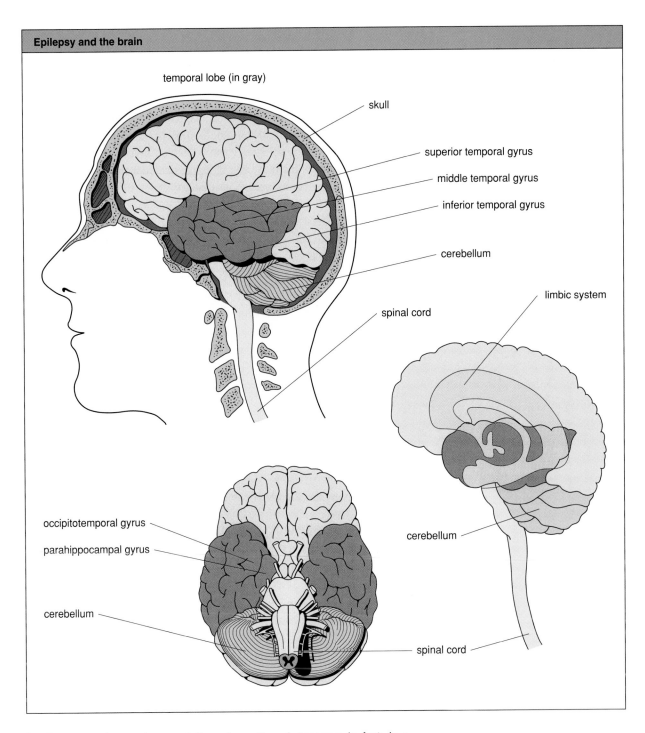

temporal lobe (in gray)

skull

superior temporal gyrus

middle temporal gyrus

inferior temporal gyrus

cerebellum

spinal cord

limbic system

cerebellum

occipitotemporal gyrus

parahippocampal gyrus

cerebellum

spinal cord

for the expression and appreciation of emotion. Autoscopy, in fact, is a manifestation of disturbances in this area of the brain.

Anatomically, the temporal lobe is not a separate segment but rather an arbitrarily defined region of the brain. It consists of five major folds, or gyri. The superior, middle, and inferior temporal gyri are located on the lateral surface of the brain and are easily seen. The occipitotemporal gyrus (linking the temporal lobe to the occipital lobe behind it) and the parahippocampal gyrus (joining the temporal lobe to parts of the older, more primitive limbic system) are on the underside of the brain. The functions that are most notably associated with the temporal lobe are hearing, language processing, and emotional experience and expression. It is this last function that goes so dramatically awry in temporal lobe epilepsy.

Temporal lobe seizures frequently begin with a vague and ill-defined sensation of fear, depression, or anger. This "aura" quickly gives way to the main aspect of the seizure, which is marked by major disturbances of thought, perception, memory, and other mental functions. One of the most common features of the seizure is déjà vu, the feeling that a new and unfamiliar person, place, or occurrence has been encountered before. At other times the epileptic experiences *jamais vu* ("never before seen"), the uncomfortable sense that one's familiar surroundings are novel, altered, or otherwise unfamiliar. Some patients in the midst of a temporal lobe seizure report that they are compelled to think certain thoughts; often these have philosophical or religious themes. For example, the patient may have intensely disturbing yet seemingly irresistible thoughts about the Final Judgment or the destruction of the world. Of all epilepsy sufferers, about 7% will at some time in their life experience autoscopy; the vast majority of these will have epileptic disturbance originating in the temporal lobe.

Studies of the human brain reveal that the temporal lobe is a center for vivid memories extending over an individual's entire lifetime. It is the area of the brain that provides people with feelings of certainty about their own identity and about the constancy of the outer world; it also affords the capacity for deeper, more profound human experiences such as those of the sacred and the awesome. Temporal lobe disorders typically induce a sense of strangeness about oneself or the world at large—feelings akin to the depersonalization experienced when a person encounters a double.

Impostors everywhere: delusions of misidentification

Whatever its origin, the experience of the double exists along a continuum extending from the normal everyday certainty of one's own uniqueness to, at the other extreme, the full-fledged experience of confronting someone who appears to be a duplicate of oneself or, in some cases, of another familiar person. At the farther end of the continuum—and definitely within the realm of neuropsychiatric illness—are the so-called delusions of misidentification. Each of these usually occurs as part of a more widespread psychotic delusion or hallucination.

The most common delusion of misidentification is the neurological disorder known as Capgras syndrome, which involves the belief that an important person in the patient's life, usually a spouse or close relative, is not who he or she claims to be but an exact replica, an impostor impersonating the original. The first case, described in a French medical journal in 1923 by psychiatrists Joseph Capgras and J. Reboul-Lachaux, was that of a woman who claimed that a large number of doubles had been substituted for her husband. Although such afflictions are not common, neither are they rare, and most neurologists and psychiatrists have encountered them in the course of their practice.

One of my patients, an elderly woman, complained that someone had taken away her son and replaced him with an imposter; another patient claimed that "something strange" had been done to her dog and that the dog now living with her was not her own but another, identical animal. Quite similarly, at the very end of Dostoyevsky's *The Double,* Golyadkin misidentifies his imagined persecutor, Dr. Rudenspitz: "This wasn't Dr. Rudenspitz! Who was it? Or was it him? It was! Not the earlier Dr. Rudenspitz, but another, a terrible Dr. Rudenspitz." In *The Possessed* the idiot Marya Tinofeyona becomes convinced that her husband, Stavrogin, has been replaced by an imposter, to whom she remarks, "You are very like him, very like him, perhaps you are a relation—only he is a bright fellow and a prince, and you are an owl and a shopman."

Another delusion of misidentification is the Fregoli syndrome, named after a 19th-century European actor who possessed remarkable abilities to alter his facial appearance onstage. In this delusional belief the patient's imagined persecutors have altered their faces so that they look like familiar persons. In my own practice I treated a young schizophrenic who declared that a co-worker had taken on the appearance of his (the patient's) brother in order to harm and rob him. Another of my patients—a man about the same age—believed in the existence of machines that could manufacture copies of minds of others, including his own. He claimed that copies of his mind had been placed in the bodies of different people and that he could identify these people because their mannerisms were similar to his own.

The syndrome of intermorphosis is a psychiatric condition in which the patient believes several persons are changing places with one another: Mary becoming Jane, Jane becoming Barbara, Barbara becoming Mary. In the original case described in 1932, the afflicted woman claimed that the people and things around her were undergoing frequent changes in both appearance and identity.

The case of Mrs. B. illustrates still another variation of a delusion of misidentification. Mrs. B. reported to her psychiatrist that another Mrs. B. had replaced her and was now the object of Mr. B.'s affections. In support of her claim, Mrs. B. mentioned a lessening of her husband's physical attraction toward her. She reasoned that since Mr. B. was no longer attracted to her, he must have someone else—but since Mr. B. was married to Mrs. B., the someone else must be another Mrs. B. She also expressed fears that she would cease to be herself if the "other" Mrs. B. was accepted by others as the true Mrs. B. This is an example of the delusion of subjective doubles. Most instances of subjective doubles involve claims like Mrs. B.'s that one's physical self has been replaced. In rare instances the afflicted person claims that his or her personality has replaced that of the person whose body he or she is using. In order for this belief to emerge, the individual must lose the capacity for recognition of his or her own body.

The right time, the right place

Doubles can also occur in more subtle forms, not associated with illness—psychiatric or otherwise. Indeed, given a state of clear, albeit heightened, awareness, it is possible for simple autoscopy to arise in a totally healthy

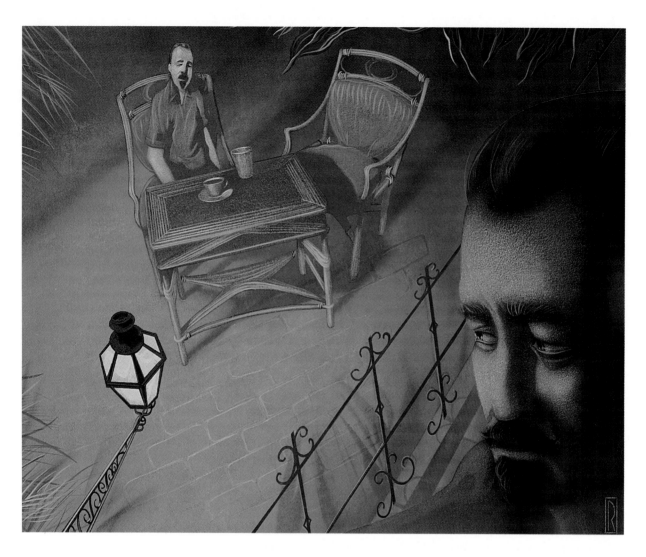

person. In order for this to take place, however, certain external and internal conditions must exist: a particularly conducive setting and time (often late evening or at dawn); a psychological predisposition marked by fatigue, isolation, stress, and some slippage from one's usual state of mind; and a brief but intense emotional identification, perhaps lasting only seconds. I personally have had two such experiences.

The stranger with my face. The first incident occurred some years ago during a trip to Caracas, Venezuela, when I happened to be excessively tired. Before retiring for the night, I ate a solitary meal in a restaurant. While waiting for my order to arrive, I looked up and observed a man sitting on the balcony of the restaurant. After a few moments the stranger looked down at me (no doubt in response to my staring up at him). He wore a van Dyke beard similar to my own and, also in common with me, was informally dressed. As we exchanged looks, I had for the briefest moment the distinct and uncomfortable sensation that the stranger was none other than myself. I looked away, anxious and confused. Within seconds the feeling passed, not to recur again.

90

That's my wife! Another "double" experience occurred when I was traveling—this time in Munich, Germany. I was taking a walk the evening before I was to deliver a lecture. I had arrived from Washington, D.C., earlier that morning after an all-night flight and, having remained awake throughout the day, had not slept for more than 24 hours. Suddenly, as I walked at dusk along a fashionable street, a woman stepped out of a department store into a waiting limousine. Though I could not have seen her for more than a few seconds, her looks, gait, and style of dress convinced me that my wife had come to Munich to surprise me. I speculated that she had rented the limo in order to do some shopping—an extravagance that would have been most uncharacteristic of my wife. Further, I was equally convinced that when I returned to my hotel room, she would be waiting there for me. So strong was my emotional identification with this stranger that I considered running up to the vehicle, tapping on the window, and surprising her. But as the limousine pulled away, the psychological linkage to the woman abruptly faded, leaving me with a searing feeling of loneliness and the realization that I had to spend the night alone in this alien city where I knew not a soul and could speak not a word of the language.

What distinguished the above two experiences from the common, everyday occurrence of simply noticing physical similarities between two people was the intensity of the identification. Both of these unsettling incidents conform in many respects to the conditions commonly associated with the appearance of doubles. In Munich the experience occurred at dusk; I was in a state of sleep deprivation; and I was both anxious (worried how my talk would be received the next morning) and lonely. What distinguished my experience from a fully evolved pathological phenomenon was the fact that I was not hallucinating; I had simply had an intense illusion that another woman was my wife. Moreover, the misidentification of the strange woman did not arouse the dismay or feeling of the "abnormal" that would have accompanied my seeing someone come out of the store who appeared to be myself. Likewise, in Caracas the man on the balcony *was* physically present, and thus my experience was illusory rather than hallucinatory. Nonetheless, because of the intensity of the feelings aroused, I remained acutely uncomfortable and would not have approached the man under any circumstances.

Variations on the double

Most people, in fact, can probably call to mind similar encounters with such "attenuated" forms of the double. For example, Mr. J., a middle-aged businessman, was walking to his office one morning and passed an elderly man who instantly reminded him of a dear friend he had not seen for some time. The stranger looked exactly as Mr. J. imagined his friend would look 20 years hence. This triggered in Mr. J. a series of melancholy reflections about his own aging. It was as if he had encountered a "double" that forced him to confront the prospect of growing old.

Dreams and dreamlike states. A contemporary authority on the double, psychoanalyst James Grotstein, a professor at the University of California at Los Angeles, believes that the continuum from normal states of "temporary hyperidentification" to autoscopy should include not only experiences like mine and Mr. J.'s but also encounters that take place in dreams and daytime fantasies. Grotstein, in fact, would include among autoscopic phenomena "the entire spectrum of self-consciousness from normal to abnormal." Of course, there are differences. Unlike the full-fledged experience of the double, daydreams do not arise suddenly or intrusively, against one's wishes, nor do they necessarily appear to be "real."

The correspondence of autoscopy with dreams that arise in sleep, or just before it, is somewhat closer, however, as is illustrated by the case of a man who, in the twilight state between waking and sleeping, perceived the person lying beside him to be a former girlfriend. He experienced her presence with an intensity and immediacy that he said he had not felt in many years. He then woke up to the temporarily disorienting discovery that the woman in bed with him was not his old flame but rather his wife.

Some dreams share with the autoscopic experience an emotional intensity that carries over into the waking state. For example, people commonly report meeting a long-deceased spouse or parent in dreams and, upon awakening, vividly reexperience the grief of their loss.

Then again, in Charles Dickens' *A Christmas Carol,* Ebenezer Scrooge's poignant encounters with his past and future selves share qualities of both dreams and daydreams. Conducted by the Ghost of Christmas Past to the school he attended as a child, Scrooge observes the following scene:

The door at the back of the house . . . opened before them, and disclosed a long, bare, melancholy room, made barer still by lines of plain deal forms and desks. At one of these a lonely boy was reading near a feeble fire; and Scrooge sat down upon a form, and wept to see his poor forgotten self as he had used to be.

Doubled in death. Autoscopy also regularly occurs during those profound, often ineffable mystical occurrences reported by people who have had so-called near-death experiences—that is, they have come close to clinical death or have actually "died" and been revived. The following case history is typical: A 31-year-old woman who suffered a severe head injury in an automobile accident recalled that after the crash she "left her body" and observed it from above, lying in a pool of blood in the car. The victim then watched herself get out of the car, walk around it, and start banging on the driver's window. She felt that her mind was completely separate from her body and did not share with it any emotion, intellect, or sense of physical connectedness. A man then told her body to get back into the car. The body obeyed and assumed its original position. A friend of the victim who witnessed this accident and remained at the scene until rescue workers arrived reported that the injured woman never left the car—and that she was found in exactly the position she had described her unconscious body to be in.

Felt but not seen. On other occasions the double may take the form of a haunting "presence." A woman who engaged in so-called automatic writing (wherein her hand would seem to write words without voluntary effort on her part) described to the renowned 19th-century Harvard psychologist William James the "presence" of a double in this way:

92

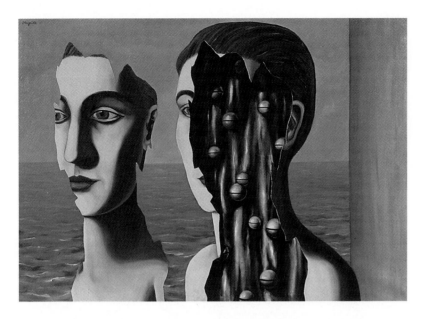

"Le Double Secret" ("The Double Secret")
by René Magritte, 1927

Oil on canvas, 45 x 64 inches, Musée National d'Art
Moderne, Paris; photograph, Giraudon/Art Resource

Whenever I practice automatic writing, what makes me feel that it is not due to a sub-conscious self is the feeling I always have of a foreign presence, external to my body. It is sometimes so definitely characterized that I could point to its exact position.

One of my patients began a journal of automatic writing while in the midst of a severe depression. She subsequently reported to me that she had "discovered" that her mother, dead for many years, was guiding her hand. Later, upon being shown a page from the journal, I pointedly asked her, "Did you write this?" She responded, "My hand did the writing, but my mother told it what to write."

Experiencing the "presence" of a double sometimes involves sharing some of the qualities of fear and dread described by those who claim to have met with ghosts or apparitions. Other, more benign examples of felt rather than directly apprehended presences include "guardian angels" and imaginary childhood companions.

"New" families: three cases

Variations on the experience of the double have been reported in the aftermath of injury to the brain. A striking example of this is the case of Martin, a 44-year-old man who suffered traumatic brain injury in a car accident. After the neurosurgeons removed a large blood clot from Martin's brain, along with severely damaged portions of the right frontal lobe, a computed tomography scan showed additional damage to the left frontal lobe. Following a difficult and prolonged postoperative recovery during which he was hospitalized for nearly a year, the patient was finally allowed to go home on a weekend pass. Upon his return to the hospital, Martin calmly announced to his doctor that a different but nearly identical family now lived in the same house as his previous family. Rather than being dismayed or upset by this exceedingly strange turn of events, he seemed totally unconcerned, as is illustrated by the following excerpt from his conversation with the doctor.

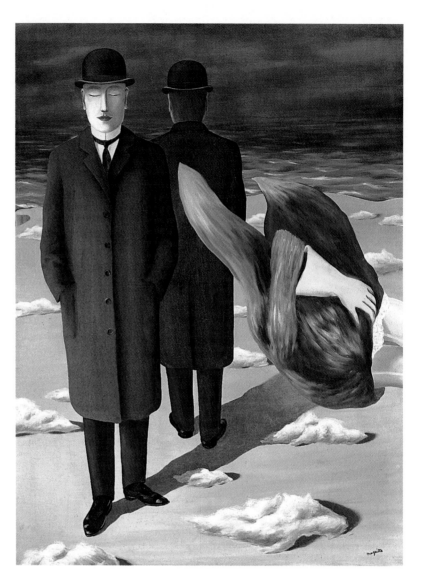

"Le Sens de la nuit" ("The Meaning of Night") by René Magritte, 1927

Oil on canvas, 54½ x 41½ inches, The Menil Collection, Houston; photograph, Janet Woodward

Doctor: So all of a sudden you came out of the hospital, and you went back in the same house with a whole different family.

Martin: Well, that's about the size of it, yes.

Doctor: How can you account for that?

Martin: I don't know. I tried to understand it myself, and it was virtually impossible to understand it.

While Martin was discussing this situation, which by his own admission he found "extremely hard to believe," his voice was, according to his doctor, "full of laughter, joyous acceptance, and bonhomie." Conspicuously missing from his reaction were those cognitive functions an intact frontal lobe enables: the ability to monitor, assess, evaluate, and adapt. Thus, Martin made no attempt to search for his "first" wife or evaluate how and why such a substitution had occurred. Interestingly, his "second" family was exactly like the first, with one telling exception: the children of the second family appeared to be about a year older than those in his true family.

94

Martin's experience after frontal lobe injury is reminiscent of an episode in one of Nobel Prize-winning author Isaac Bashevis Singer's tales of Chelm, the town of fools. In this fictional "case" the hero, Shlemiel, who lives in Chelm, decides one day to take a trip to Warsaw. Along the way he stops for a nap and, in order to be sure of taking the right direction upon awakening, turns his boots so that the toes point toward Warsaw. But while Shlemiel is asleep, the blacksmith, a prankster, comes along and turns the boots around. Upon awakening, Shlemiel sets off and is soon back in Chelm, where the streets and houses and people seem familiar to him. He concludes that he has arrived at a second Chelm exactly like the first. At his own house, where his wife and children greet him, he says, "Mrs. Shlemiel, I am not your husband. Children, I am not your father." His wife responds, "Have your lost your mind?" But he continues to assert, "I am Shlemiel of Chelm One, and this is Chelm Two."

Real-life sufferers from delusions of misidentification have been known to resort to behavior that is far from comical. Psychiatrist J. Arturo Silva has described one such case: Mr. A. became convinced that his father, sister, nephew, brother, and brother-in-law had died and that their bodies had been taken over by clones. Further, Mr. A. believed it was God's will that he, Mr. A., destroy the wicked people who had entered the bodies of his family. He shot and killed his father and seriously wounded the nephew. He intended to kill other "cloned" family members but could not locate them. While searching for these other relatives, he encountered a young man on the street whom he identified as an accomplice of the evil impersonators. Mr. A. shot and wounded the young stranger as punishment for assisting in the murder and impersonation of his relatives, events he was convinced had actually taken place. At trial Mr. A. was found not guilty by reason of insanity.

What to conclude?

Fortunately, the experience of the double rarely results in violence or murder. And most such experiences are not associated with neurological or psychiatric disorders.

Can anyone encounter a double? "Experts" believe that those most likely to experience autoscopy are people who exhibit enhanced powers of visual imagery coupled with an intense involvement with their health, their appearance, or the workings of their inner mind. Writers seem to be especially prone—even more so than visual artists, an indication that talents for visualization alone are not sufficient. But not just any writer: the tendency is most marked in those with a distinctly inward, introspective, even morbid orientation.

From the scientific point of view, autoscopy is fascinating because it offers the possibility that researchers may one day pinpoint a neurological basis for personal identity. At the same time, it serves as a useful reminder of the continuity that exists between normal mental functioning and madness. From a nonscientific point of view, it challenges deeply held notions of the uniqueness of the individual and raises intriguing questions about the nature of the familiar.

Health on the Reservation

by
Everett R. Rhoades, M.D.,
George Brenneman, M.D.,
and Mathuram Santosham, M.D., M.P.H.

William Wood, an Englishman visiting Massachusetts in 1633, observed, "The Indians be of lusty and healthful bodies, not experimentally knowing the catalogue of those health-wasting diseases which are incident to other countries, as Fevers, Pleurisies, . . . Consumptions, Subfumigations, . . . Pox, . . . Measles or the like, but spinne out the thread of their days to a faire length, numbering three score, four score, some a hundred years, before the universal summoner cites them to the craving Grave." Echoing this same theme, an English sea captain wrote in 1698 that the Indians in the area of what is now New York state "generally live to the age of 80, or 90 or 100 years without hardly a headache." From these and other early accounts by European settlers in North America, a tradition has grown up portraying the native inhabitants of the continent as a robustly healthy people.

The archaeological and historical evidence, however, tells a different story about the lives—and deaths—of these first Americans. Knowledge about the health of American Indian peoples prior to the arrival of Columbus is sketchy, but it is apparent that they suffered from maladies not unlike those that have plagued humankind for centuries. The occurrence of arthritis, anemia, malnutrition, dental problems, birth defects such as spina bifida, and certain infectious diseases is amply demonstrated in Indian art, healing traditions, and skeletal remains.

Infectious scourges: a European import

Whatever the health status of indigenous Americans in pre-Columbian times, there can be no doubt about the fact that devastating epidemics of infectious diseases followed rapidly upon contact with Europeans. Illnesses such as measles, cholera, pertussis (whooping cough), diphtheria, and others reduced many once-populous tribes to mere remnants of their former numbers. In addition, epidemic diseases played an important role in the subjugation of Indian peoples. One history of smallpox among the American Indians states that this dread disease was "more feared by the Indian than bullets."

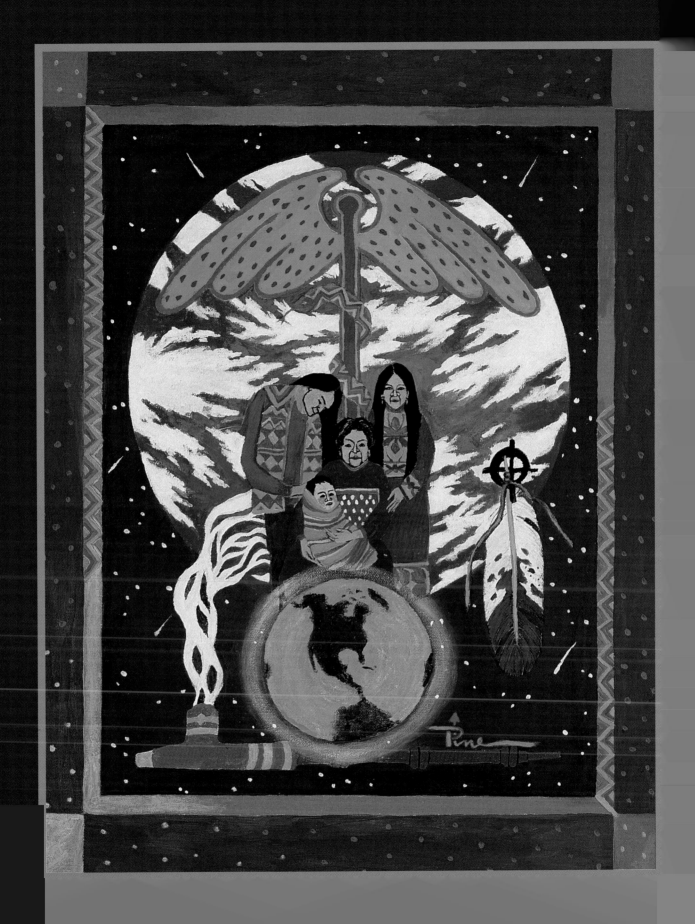

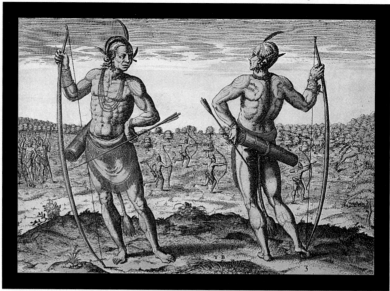

An engraving, c. 1590, depicts the indigenous inhabitants of Virginia as the vigorously healthy specimens typically described by European travelers of the day. Such idealized accounts of the native population created the long-held myth that disease was virtually unknown in the Americas prior to the arrival of whites. The archaeological evidence, however, reveals that the Indians were subject to many of the same ailments that have afflicted humans throughout history.

Everett R. Rhoades, M.D., *is Adjunct Professor, Department of International Health, Center for American Indian and Alaska Native Health, Johns Hopkins University School of Hygiene and Public Health, Baltimore, Maryland, and Acting Associate Dean for Community Affairs and Professor of Medicine, University of Oklahoma College of Medicine, Oklahoma City. He was formerly Assistant Surgeon General, U.S. Public Health Service, and Director, Indian Health Service, Rockville, Maryland.*

George Brenneman, M.D., *former Maternal and Child Health Coordinator, Indian Health Service, is Associate Director, Center for American Indian and Alaska Native Health.*

Mathuram Santosham, M.D., M.P.H., *is Director, Center for American Indian and Alaska Native Health.*

(Overleaf) Illustration by Eugene Pine (Chippewa and Winnebago)

Smallpox was one of the earliest and most extensively described diseases to affect the Indian population. It touched nearly all tribes and took an enormous toll. The Spaniard Toribio de Benevente wrote in 1540 that "when the smallpox began to infect the Indians, there was so much sickness and pestilence among them in all the land that in most provinces more than half the people died."

Exactly when smallpox first appeared in Indian populations has not been clearly established; one authority, Henry F. Dobyns, reports that it was carried to the New World on Spanish ships about 1516 and that the first known transmission to native Americans occurred on the island of Hispaniola. There is some disagreement as to whether the disease was imported from Spain or from Africa. Smallpox was known to be prevalent in Africa in the 16th century, and some historians speculate that it was introduced into the West Indies via the Spanish slave trade. A Spanish explorer, Panfilo de Narváez, who left Cuba in 1520 to replace Hernán Cortés as ruler of Mexico, reportedly took with him a black slave who was infected with smallpox. This incident—documented in several histories—is the basis for the often-quoted observation that "a handful of Spaniards and one Negro with smallpox conquered Mexico."

Dobyns lists 41 separate outbreaks of smallpox in the American Indian population, beginning in 1520 and extending into the early years of the 20th century. One of the most devastating of these epidemics spread across the Great Plains in the late 1830s. Its awful impact was described by James Mooney in his *Calendar History of the Kiowa Indians:*

The great smallpox epidemic . . . swept the whole plains north and south, destroying probably a third, if not more, of the native inhabitants, some whole tribes being nearly exterminated. . . . In this instance the disease first broke out among the passengers of a steamer in the Missouri river above Fort Leavenworth, and although every effort was made to warn the Indians by sending runners in advance, the sickness was communicated to them. It appeared first among the Mandan about the middle of

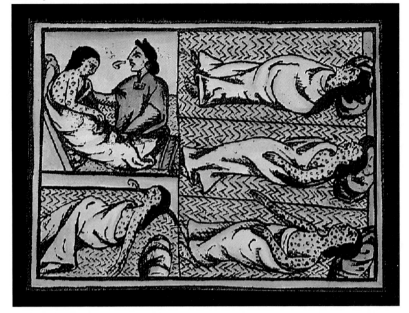

Drawings from an Aztec codex, or illustrated history, document the progression of smallpox in one patient, from the ministrations of the medicine man to utter prostration and, finally, death. Of the many infectious diseases Indians were exposed to through contact with Europeans, this scourge was perhaps the most devastating, with epidemics occurring from the 1500s into the early 20th century.

July, 1837, and practically destroyed that tribe, reducing them in a few weeks from about sixteen hundred to thirty-one souls. Their neighboring and allied tribes, the Arikara and Minitari, were reduced immediately after from about four thousand to about half that number. . . . From the Mandan it spread to the north and west among the Crows, Asiniboin [sic], and Blackfeet. Among the last named it is estimated to have destroyed from six to eight thousand. . . . In 1838 it reached the Pawnee, being communicated by some Dakota prisoners captured by them in the spring of that year. . . . It seems probable that at least two thousand Pawnee perished . . . about double the whole population of the tribe today.

The fatality rate in this epidemic was astounding. Among the Mandan, one of the hardest-hit tribes, approximately 98% of those who were infected died.

The vulnerability of the Indians to smallpox and other infectious diseases was a result of lack of previous exposure—and therefore absence of immunity—but was compounded by ignorance about the transmission and prevention of contagious illness. An example of the unwitting role played by the Indians themselves in spreading the disease is described by the historian Herman J. Viola:

In 1781, Blackfeet scouts chanced upon a Shoshone village on the south bank of the Bow River and, as it was strangely silent, watched for some time. No people were visible, although horses grazed among the tipis. At first, the scouts suspected a trap, but curiosity finally overcame caution: venturing into camp, they discovered that all the people in the tipis were dead. Overjoyed at their luck, the scouts looted the camp and returned home heavily laden. Unfortunately for the Blackfeet, the Shoshones had died of smallpox, and the easily acquired prizes were contaminated. As many as two-thirds of the Blackfeet tribe died within weeks.

Dobyns' demography of the North American Indians also lists 17 separate epidemics of highly lethal measles that ravaged the Indian population. A measles epidemic in 1531–33 involving tribes far to the north of the

The ravages of smallpox are clearly visible in this photograph of Running Face, a Mandan Indian and survivor of the catastrophic epidemic that killed most of his people in the late 1830s.

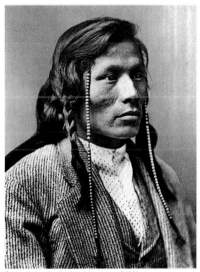

colony of New Spain resulted in millions of deaths. Influenza or influenza-like diseases, occurring alone or in conjunction with related illnesses, produced 10 epidemics between 1559 and 1918, with an estimated fatality rate greater than 90%. Other known epidemic diseases that exacted a high toll on Indians included bubonic plague, diphtheria, typhus, cholera, and scarlet fever.

The most important contagious epidemic disease of Indians in the 20th century has been tuberculosis (TB). Fortunately, TB in the Indian population has yielded to established public health practices, and although the incidence continues to be disproportionately high among Indians, the disease is largely controlled in this group. Trachoma, an infectious eye disease that often results in blindness, also plagued American Indians well into the 20th century.

Casualties of war

Hostilities with European settlers resulted in further Indian deaths and disruption of the Indian way of life. The settlement of Virginia, for example, was marked by inevitable clashes between the settlers and Indians arising from misunderstandings and encroachments of settlers onto Indian lands. In New England, trade and territorial disputes had devastating consequences for the local Indian groups. After the murder of a Boston trader in 1636, a punitive expedition was sent against the Pequot Indians by members of the Massachusetts Bay Colony; the main Pequot village and its inhabitants were destroyed. In the 1670s a particularly bloody conflict between New England Indians and English settlers, known as King Philip's War, took the lives of about 3,000 Indians. Entire villages were massacred and tribes decimated. The extent of casualties on both sides and destruction of property led one historian to characterize this as "the most costly war in American history."

By the end of the 17th century, warfare between Indians and European settlers had resulted in the coastal tribes along most of the Atlantic seaboard being dispersed, destroyed, or subjected to European control. Similar dramas occurred in the following century involving the Creeks, Choctaws, Chickasaws, Cherokees, Iroquois, and others. The physical and social disruption of these wars affected both the Indians and the colonists. However, the balance ultimately favored the colonists, whose losses were replaced by new immigrants.

The actual number of Indians killed in these and other conflicts is not known, and there is no way to measure the effects of war-related injury, physical and mental trauma, and social dissolution. In a 1973 article entitled "How Many Indians Were Killed? White Man Versus Red Man: The Facts and the Legend," historian Don Russell contended that from about 1800 on, no more than 3,000 Indians lost their lives in skirmishes with federal troops. "Even if all the wildest claims be taken at face value," Russell concluded, "the total would not exceed 6,000." Considering overall mortality from warfare and disease combined, however, it is surprising that any Indians at all survived. In fact, by the end of the 19th century, a number of tribes had been extinguished.

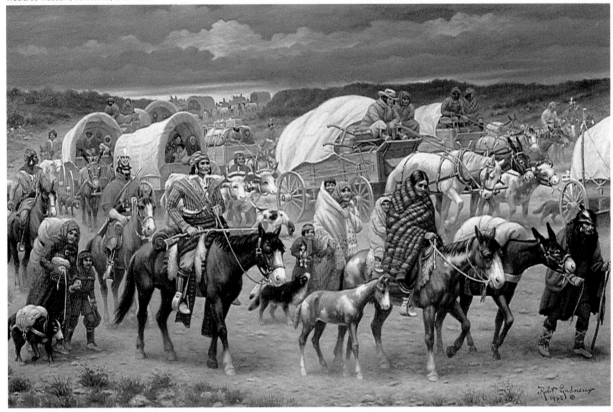

Forced removal: trails of tears

At the beginning of the 19th century with the expanding settlement of the eastern U.S., the survival of the tribes east of the Mississippi River, especially those in the southeastern states, depended upon the provision of a safe haven where they might remain free from encroachment and unmolested. Under the Indian Removal Act of 1830, the U.S. president was authorized to negotiate with the tribes, granting them unsettled western prairie lands in exchange for their desirable eastern territories.

Tragically, for some tribes resettlement proved at least as destructive as the wars that they had suffered in the preceding century. Under the policy of removal, many thousands of Indians from several tribes were forcibly moved to various temporary locations and finally to the newly created Indian Territory (roughly, the present-day state of Oklahoma). These removals took place in severe weather and under arduous travel conditions, often with only the barest of necessities. The French statesman, writer, and renowned traveler Alexis de Tocqueville described the crossing of the Mississippi in the winter of 1831 by a band of Choctaws on their way to take up new lands in the Indian Territory:

The Indians had their families with them, and they brought in their train the wounded and the sick, with children newly born and old men upon the verge of death. They possessed neither tents nor wagons, but only their arms and some possessions. . . . There was . . . no cry, no sob . . . all were silent. . . . Their calamities were of ancient date, and they knew them to be irremedial.

"The Trail of Tears" depicts the anguished exodus of the Cherokees from their ancestral home in the southeastern United States to the Indian Territory. Thousands of Indians died of exposure, exhaustion, starvation, and disease during the forced migrations that removed them from lands being settled and developed by whites.

101

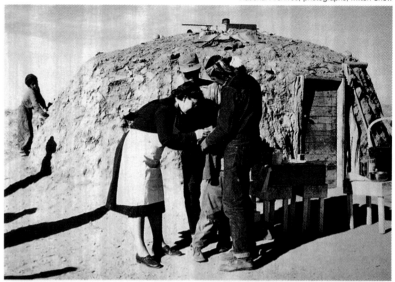

A public health nurse immunizes a child outside the family hogan on the Navajo reservation in the early 1950s (top). Government provision of health services to American Indians began in the early 1800s with occasional care provided by military physicians. By the mid-20th century a comprehensive health care system had been established by the federal government for the tribes. One of the first to promote Indian self-responsibility for health was Annie Wauneka (bottom), shown explaining an exhibit on tuberculosis— the major infectious disease of American Indians in the 20th century—at a Navajo fair.

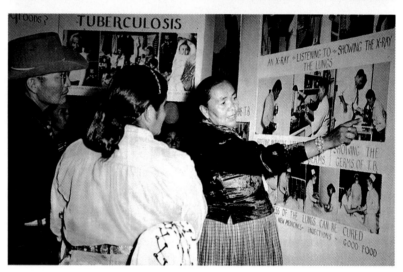

The eviction of the Cherokees from North Carolina and Georgia and their forced march westward was so marked by tragedy that the episode came to be known as the Trail of Tears. Although the casualties suffered during the removal of the southeastern tribes are those most widely described, many other tribes across the country endured similar trials. Some were moved more than once. As many as 25% of the Indians died in the process.

Indian health: a federal responsibility

The remainder of the 19th century was marked by continued warfare on the plains and in the west and completion of the resettlement of the Indian population on reservations. Reservation life, which brought abrupt and dramatic changes in the Indians' daily habits and activities, carried its own set of health risks—for example, enhanced conditions for the spread of tuberculosis. One crucial outcome of the events of the 19th century was the establishment of federal initiatives to provide health care for the tribes.

In the early 1800s occasional care was provided to Indian people by military physicians, who offered such services as they might have available. Among the first organized health care efforts was a campaign to vaccinate Indians living near military forts against smallpox. The first appropriation by the U.S. Congress for Indian health services—a sum of $12,000—was set aside in 1832 to provide for smallpox immunizations. Four years later the federal government began a program of providing health services and physicians to the Ottawa and Chippewa tribes.

In 1849 the Bureau of Indian Affairs (BIA), which had been administered by the War Department, was transferred to the Department of the Interior. In subsequent decades, in return for the cession of vast tracts of Indian land and other concessions, the federal government gradually assumed an increasing obligation to provide health care to the tribes. The first federal hospital built specifically to care for American Indian people was constructed in the 1880s in Oklahoma. Professional medical supervision of health activities for Indians began in 1908, when the post of chief medical supervisor was established within the BIA. The bureau began providing dental services in 1913 with the assignment of five itinerant dentists to visit reservations and Indian boarding schools.

The ceding of Indian lands to the United States by treaty formed the basis for the concept that the provision of health care to Indians by the federal government was not "free" but rather constituted a prepaid health plan. The various treaties, legislative acts, and court decisions have resulted in a government-to-government relationship between certain Indian tribes and the U.S. government. It is this unique relationship, in which the tribes function as sovereign entities, that continues to distinguish American Indians from other minority groups with whom they share certain socio-economic characteristics.

In 1920 U.S. Secretary of the Interior John B. Payne convinced the Congress that a senior officer from the Public Health Service (PHS) should be detailed to the BIA to advise on health matters. The following year, faced with growing concern about the alarmingly poor state of health of the Indian population, Congress passed the Snyder Act, which for the first time formulated a broad Indian health policy and authorized regular appropriation of funds for Indian health. Under this act the secretary of the interior was directed to "expend such monies as the Congress may from time to time appropriate . . . for the relief of distress and the conservation of health . . . of Indians throughout the United States." Interestingly, the language of this directive, with its specific reference to health "conservation," predated the broader American emphasis on health promotion and disease prevention by some 50 years. The act resulted in the creation within the BIA of a Health Division, which was a forerunner of the Indian Health Service (IHS).

Indian Health Service: mission and mandate

A milestone was reached in 1954 with the passage of a law that transferred the responsibility for Indian health care from the BIA to the PHS, which was itself a division of the Department of Health, Education, and Welfare (now the Department of Health and Human Services). The IHS came into being the following year. Granted agency status in 1988, it is now one of eight agencies of the Public Health Service.

The IHS currently serves just over one million Indians (about half of the total American Indian and Alaska Native population), residing in counties within or near reservations in 33 states. From its headquarters in Rockville, Maryland, the IHS oversees the workings of 12 administrative areas (*see* map) that operate a total of 50 hospitals and 552 health centers and stations. IHS facilities provide both curative and preventive services to the approximately 500 sovereign Indian nations in the U.S. The agency's budget for fiscal year 1993 was $1,855,000,000.

Given the size of its staff—some 15,000 employees—its unique mission, the diversity of the sovereign peoples it serves, and its emphasis on comprehensive community-based care, the IHS may be the most complex of all U.S. health agencies. Its staff represents a full range of health professionals, including more than 900 physicians and 2,000 nurses, along with laboratory technicians, pharmacists, dentists, and all of the ancillary personnel required for the operation of a health care delivery system. In addition, the IHS employs proportionally more sanitarians, engineers,

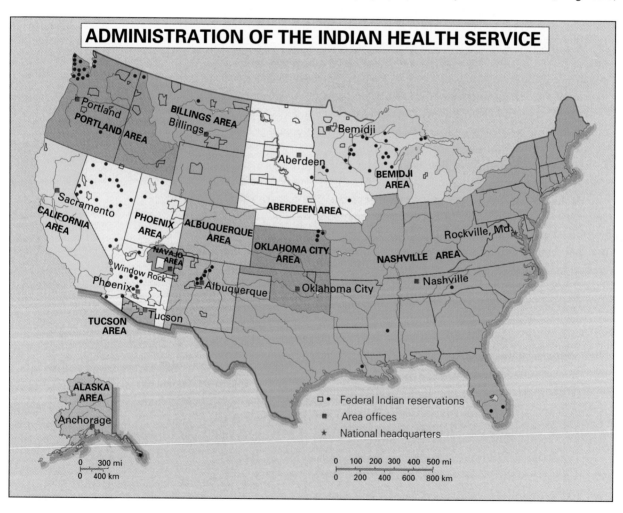

ADMINISTRATION OF THE INDIAN HEALTH SERVICE

Portland
PORTLAND AREA
BILLINGS AREA
Billings
Bemidji
Aberdeen
BEMIDJI AREA
ABERDEEN AREA
Sacramento
CALIFORNIA AREA
PHOENIX AREA
ALBUQUERQUE AREA
OKLAHOMA CITY AREA
Rockville, Md.
NASHVILLE AREA
NAVAJO AREA
Window Rock
Phoenix
Albuquerque
Oklahoma City
Nashville
TUCSON AREA
Tucson

ALASKA AREA
Anchorage

☐ • Federal Indian reservations
■ Area offices
★ National headquarters

0   300 mi
0   400 km

0   100 200 300 400 500 mi
0   200   400   600   800 km

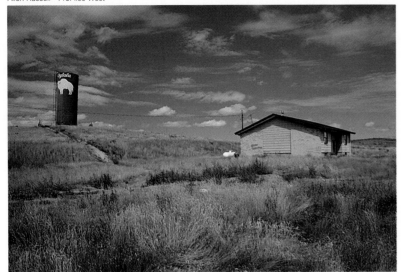

Most of the residents of the remote Pine Ridge Reservation in South Dakota, home of the Oglala Sioux, are unemployed, and two-thirds live below the poverty level, making Pine Ridge the poorest place in the United States. The population served by the Indian Health Service consists primarily of people living on or near reservations, most of which are rural areas much like this one.

injury-control experts, and health educators than any health care system in the private sector.

The mission of the IHS arises from a single goal, affirmed by Congress in the Indian Health Care Improvement Act of 1976 (reauthorized in 1992): to raise the health status of Indians to the highest possible level. Pursuit of this goal has resulted in a unique health care delivery system that maintains the delicate balance between integration and decentralization. IHS headquarters coordinates and integrates the multitude of services, sets priorities, allocates resources, and designs programs. Programs are managed locally, however, and considerable operational decision making is reserved for the local units that actually provide medical services to tribal members. This unique model, with its strong emphasis on continuity and consistency of health care delivery, is frequently studied by countries seeking to develop systems that provide efficient comprehensive care to large populations.

IHS services are available at no personal cost to members of federally recognized tribes. Because services have generally been directed to those who live on or near reservations, the population served is predominantly rural. When Indian people move to urban areas, they often lose access to federal health services (discussed further below). At present the IHS supports 34 urban programs, providing selected outreach, medical, and dental services. Nonetheless, Indian city dwellers, who now outnumber rural Indians, do not have the same kind of health care available to them as do those who live on reservations.

The number and kinds of services made available by the IHS have grown enormously since its inception. For example, in 1990 the IHS recorded nearly 5 million ambulatory patient visits, an 800% increase since 1955; dental procedures rose from 180,000 in 1955 to 2,369,000 in 1990, an increase of more than 1,200%. The IHS also spends approximately $300 million annually contracting with other health care providers, private and public, for additional ambulatory and hospital services.

In addition to its myriad regular services, the IHS has developed several initiatives to respond to special health problems such as infant mortality, fetal alcohol syndrome (FAS), otitis media (a middle ear infection that often leads to deafness and is especially prevalent in the Indian population), and—most recently—AIDS. The Indian history of unusual susceptibility to infectious diseases makes the threat of infection with human immunodeficiency virus (HIV), the virus that causes AIDS, all the more urgent to Indian communities and their health care providers. By 1988 the IHS had developed a comprehensive program of HIV testing and clinical treatment; it was also sponsoring vigorous AIDS information and education efforts. Some highly creative and culturally sensitive educational materials—posters, pamphlets, videos—have been produced to appeal to the values and beliefs of the Indian community. Other special initiatives of the IHS have targeted the needs of the Indian elderly, a growing segment of the population.

A demographically distinctive population

The Asian peoples who migrated across the Bering Strait an estimated 10,000 to 15,000 years ago became the ancestors of today's American Indians. As might be expected, the gene pool of the descendants of these aboriginal people differs somewhat from that of the rest of the U.S. population. Some of the distinctive genetic characteristics of the Indian population include differences in expression of the Rh blood factor; absence of the digestive enzyme lactase; a rapid physiological response (skin flush) to alcohol ingestion; dry ear wax; incisors (front teeth) that have a concave inner surface; and certain anatomic characteristics of the eustachian tube (the passage that connects the middle ear and throat), a difference that probably accounts for much of the high prevalence of middle ear infections in American Indians. With the exception of the Rh factor difference—which protects against a serious form of anemia in newborns—and possibly eustachian tube structure, these traits are not known to be linked with predisposition to or protection from any specific disorder. Nonetheless, as more

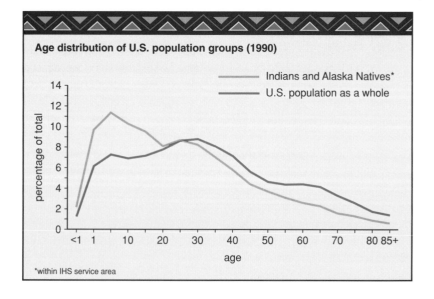

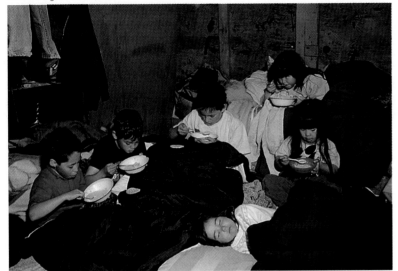

The children of an Alaska Native family share a meal in their cramped home. Compared with the U.S. population as a whole, Indian people are disproportionately young and have high rates of poverty and unemployment.

is learned about the role of genetic factors in causing disease, knowledge about genetic differences between Indians and other population groups may contribute to increased understanding of specific disease processes. Certainly, this is likely to be true for conditions such as diabetes, in which genetic factors play a prominent part.

More significant in terms of health than these genetic features are the distinctive demographic characteristics of American Indians. Compared with the general U.S. population, the Indian population has a much greater proportion of young people and a smaller proportion of elderly. In 1990 the median age of Indians served by the IHS was about 23 years (compared with the median age of 33 for the general U.S. population), and one in three Indians was younger than 15 years (compared with approximately one in five for the general population). At the same time, only about 6% of Indians were 65 years of age or older—compared with twice that percentage for the general population. These demographic characteristics are the result of a higher birthrate and an earlier age at death among American Indian people.

Also affecting the health status of Indians is their generally lower standard of living—a result of higher rates of poverty and unemployment and lower levels of education. According to estimates from the 1990 U.S. census, one in three Indians does not complete high school, compared with one in five of the general population. Fewer than one in 10 Indians obtains a bachelor's degree, compared with one in 5 in the rest of the population. Fifteen percent of Indian males and 13% of females are unemployed, compared with an average of 6.3% for both sexes in the general population. The median Indian household income is $20,000 ($10,000 less than that of the U.S. population as a whole). Finally, 30% of Indian people live below the poverty level, compared with 13% of the general population. On some reservations in remote and economically depressed areas, an even greater proportion of the residents have incomes below the poverty threshold. In fact, the Oglala Sioux reservation in Pine Ridge, South Dakota, has the highest rate of poverty in the U.S., with at least 60% of its residents living below poverty level.

Today a majority of American Indian people reside in urban areas, where opportunities for education and employment are greater than on reservations. At the same time, however, their access to government-sponsored health care, as previously noted, is diminished. Although the IHS is able to provide modest support for a number of urban programs, limited resources and an absence of individual entitlement to services (*i.e.,* it is Indian *tribes,* rather than individuals, that are entitled to government-provided services) mean that thousands of urban Indians are without adequate medical care. Since the mid-1970s a number of public and private urban health projects have with great industry and ingenuity found ways to help Indian city dwellers obtain access to basic medical services. However, the future of health care for urban Indians is likely to lie with improved accessibility of health care to all American citizens rather than with expansion of services by the IHS.

Indian versus general-population health: some comparisons

In spite of a number of improvements in health and living conditions and the virtual elimination of many epidemic diseases, the health of American Indians remains poorer than that of the U.S population as a whole. Conditions to which Indians are especially susceptible include diabetes, alcoholism, suicide, and injuries; Indians are also at greater risk for tuberculosis, pneumococcal disease, and other infections. Heart disease, cancer, stroke, and chronic obstructive pulmonary disease—leading causes of death among non-Indian people in the U.S.—tend to occur less frequently among the Indian population, although this lower rate may in part be the result of mistakes in racial classification on documents such as death certificates. The high incidence of several common and serious conditions among Indians—for example, cirrhosis of the liver and diabetes—is attributed to a combination of socioeconomic conditions, high-risk behaviors, and as-yet-undefined genetic factors.

One disease that deserves special mention because of its increased risk among Indian infants is infection with *Haemophilus influenzae* type B. Infection with this bacterium results in an incidence of complications—pneumonia, meningitis, and bloodstream infection—that is severalfold higher in American Indians and Alaska Natives than among the rest of the population. However, as a result of the recent introduction of new vaccines for this childhood infection, the incidence of serious complications has fallen dramatically.

Shorter lives. Although the life expectancy of Indians has increased dramatically—by more than 10 years, in fact, since 1970—to 72 years, it is still lower than that of the U.S. population as a whole (75 years). Not only do Indians have a higher overall death rate (574 deaths per 100,000 population) than Caucasians (509 per 100,000), they also die younger. For example, only one-fifth of all Indian deaths occur in those aged 65 years or older, whereas two-thirds of all deaths occur in this age group in the general population. Moreover, the ratio of age-adjusted death rates for

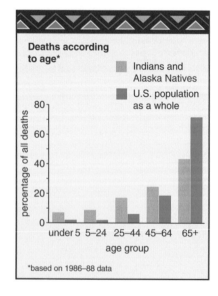

Deaths according to age*

- Indians and Alaska Natives
- U.S. population as a whole

percentage of all deaths

age group

*based on 1986–88 data

108

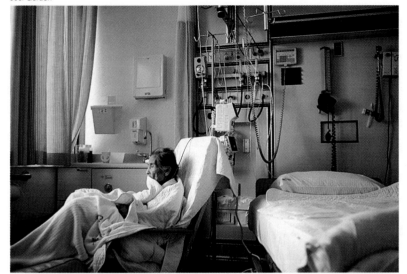

Joel Gordon

An elderly patient receives treatment in a hospital operated by the Indian Health Service (IHS). As a result of improved nutrition and medical care, the life expectancy of American Indians has increased in recent decades—although it remains below that of the U.S. population overall. With more Indians living longer, the IHS has expanded its services to meet the needs of the aging population.

young Indians is nearly three times greater than for young people in the general U.S. population, an excess that continues until about 55 years of age, when Indians begin to experience death rates that are actually lower than those of the rest of the population.

Differences in death rates. An examination of the differences in death rates and causes of death for specific age-groups reveals some interesting patterns. For example, among Indians the neonatal mortality rate (deaths among newborns from birth to 27 days) is equal to or lower than that for the general population. In contrast, the postneonatal mortality rate (deaths in the period from 28 days to 11 months) for Indians is 42% higher than that of the general population. The leading causes of postneonatal deaths among both Indians and non-Indians are sudden infant death syndrome (SIDS), birth defects, and injuries. SIDS, also known as "crib death," is

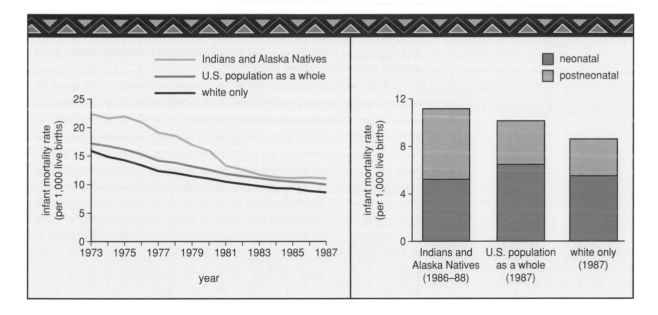

A health worker on the Navajo Reservation in Arizona checks one of her young patients for signs of middle ear infection. Such infections, which can lead to deafness if untreated, are more prevalent in American Indians than in the rest of the population.

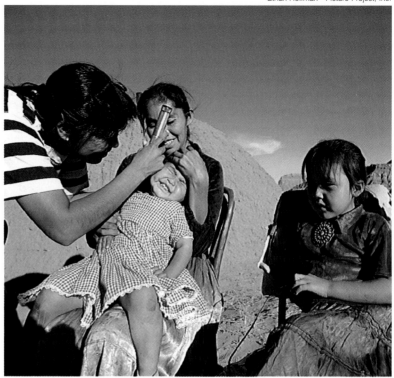

a condition of unknown cause in which an apparently healthy infant is discovered dead in its crib. On average, SIDS incidence is 40% higher among Indians than in the general population. Curiously, however, the rate of SIDS varies enormously among different groups of Indians in different locales. The rate among Indians in the Southwest is about one per 1,000 live births—less than the general U.S. rate—while among Indians in the Northwest and Alaska, three to five SIDS deaths occur for every 1,000 live births. A number of investigators are trying to discover the reasons for these differences.

Whereas the causes of death among Indian children and young adults aged one to 24 are much the same as those in the same age groups in the general population, about twice as many Indians aged 15 to 24 die from injuries as do their counterparts in the general population. It is generally recognized that alcohol plays a dominant role in deaths due to injury in all populations. In Indian communities, however, the influence of alcohol on the rate of injury is compounded by other factors. For example, because alcoholic beverages may not be sold on many reservations, obtaining them means traveling to a distant location. Consequently, many alcohol-related injuries involve pedestrians and vehicles traveling on rural highways.

The leading causes of death among Indians aged 25 to 44 are injuries and chronic liver disease and cirrhosis—compared with injuries and cancer in the general population. While injuries contribute significantly to deaths of both Indians and non-Indians in this age group, the death rate from injuries among Indians—108 per 100,000 population—is three times that of the general population. At the same time, the cancer mortality rate among

110

Indians of this age group is 30% less than that of the general population.

In the 45–64 age-group, heart disease and cancer are the leading causes of death among Indians and non-Indians alike. Compared with the general population, however, Indians experience 10% fewer deaths due to heart disease and 40% fewer cancer deaths. Among Indians aged 65 and over, the causes of death are similar to those of the general elderly population, but the rates differ; Indians are less likely than non-Indians to die from cardiovascular diseases and cancer but twice as likely to die from diabetes and injuries.

Important insights. The purpose of these many statistical comparisons is twofold. First, by examining the differences between Indian disease and death rates and those of the rest of the population, epidemiologists (scientists who study the incidence and prevalence of disease) hope to be able to find ways to improve Indian health. Second, research into the differences in patterns of disease among Indians and non-Indians may eventually result in a better understanding of underlying disease processes and better care for all Americans. The impressively low neonatal death rate in the Indian population, for example, is evidence of the effectiveness of the comprehensive prenatal care provided by the IHS, a public health measure that, if extended to other economically disadvantaged groups, might result in a lowering of the country's overall infant mortality rate, which is higher than that of nearly all other industrial nations.

The reasons for the lower death rate among Indian adults from heart disease and cancer, while not well understood, are nonetheless intriguing to scientists. The apparently lower Indian vulnerability to coronary heart disease may be a consequence of differences in the metabolism of lipoproteins such as cholesterol in Indians, although further research is necessary before conclusions can be drawn. Studying the differences in distribution of certain cancers in the Indian and non-Indian populations may help clarify many of the still poorly understood causes of this disease. Investigations

(Below left) On the streets of Gallup, New Mexico, an intoxicated Indian receives assistance from a member of a special patrol that offers protective custody for those who have had too much to drink. A trauma team (below) works to stabilize an injury victim in the emergency department of an IHS hospital on the Crow Indian Reservation in Montana. Along with cirrhosis and other liver diseases, injuries—often involving the use of alcohol—are a leading cause of death among American Indians aged 25 to 44.

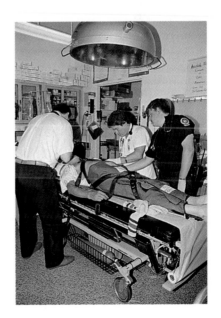

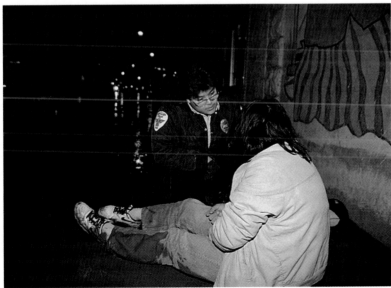

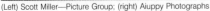

(Left) Scott Miller—Picture Group; (right) Aiuppy Photographs

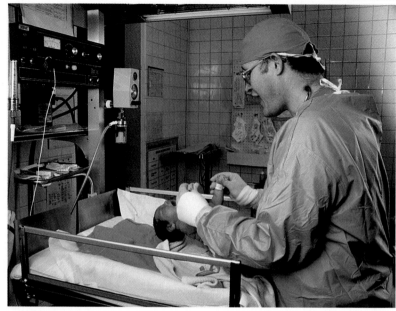

of diabetes among Indian groups such as the Pima and Maricopa—in whom the disorder is extremely prevalent—have greatly increased medical scientists' understanding of the relation of diabetes to diet, obesity, and insulin metabolism.

A revelation arising from these health statistics is that while a number of health problems affect Indians and non-Indians alike, many of these conditions are associated with higher death rates when they occur in Indians. Examples are alcoholism, in which the Indian death rate is six times higher than that of the general population; diabetes (two and a half times higher); and injuries (three times higher).

Impressive health improvements

In the 35 years since the IHS began collecting data, many indicators of Indian health have shown dramatic improvement. By 1989, for example, the Indian infant mortality rate had fallen by more than 85% and maternal mortality by 91%. Deaths associated with pneumonia and influenza had decreased by 71% and gastrointestinal diseases by 86%. Life expectancy of Indians born in 1987 was 72 years, an increase of 20% since 1950.

While control of infectious diseases is probably the major factor accounting for these gains, at least four other specific developments appear to have contributed. First, with a better-organized system of health care, access to antibiotics was increased, thus reducing deaths from bacterial infections such as meningitis, pneumonia, and especially tuberculosis. In the early 1960s the IHS found it necessary to devote entire hospitals solely to the care of Indians with tuberculosis; by the mid 1970s, however, the availability of effective drug treatment had effected a decline in the incidence of active TB to a level that no longer warranted reserving special IHS hospital beds solely for TB patients.

Second, community health workers succeeded in setting up effective

Under the dental program of the IHS, emphasis on preventive and corrective care has helped bring about significant improvement in the oral health of American Indian people.

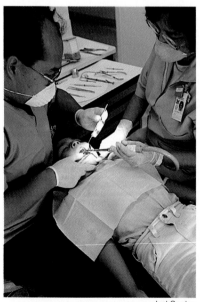

Joel Gordon

112

immunization programs that reached nearly every Indian family. Today immunization levels among Indian infants and young children served by the IHS are approximately 90%, a much better record than in the general population and certainly among the highest levels reported in any group of youngsters in the U.S.

A third factor contributing to improved Indian health was the establishment of an effective regional hospital system that provides high-quality health care and is generally accessible even to remote and isolated Indian communities. Currently, more than 95% of Indian births occur in a hospital; hospitals offer high-technology perinatal services for premature and low-birth-weight babies; and kidney dialysis is available on most reservations or is accessible within hours.

Finally, a law enacted in 1959, the Indian Sanitation Facilities Act, provided the authority and funding for the development of safe water and waste disposal in Indian communities. As a result, since 1960 more than 176,000 Indian homes have been provided with water and sanitation facilities. Sanitation remains a problem in some communities, however, notably in Alaska.

The success of the IHS probably owes as much to Indian acceptance of modern health care—which often was foreign to traditional Indian ways—as to the effectiveness of the care itself. Visionary Indian leaders have been instrumental in securing acceptance for up-to-date curative and preventive medicine among their people and helping to integrate essential features of Western medicine and traditional Indian practices. This willingness to adopt new methods was particularly important when it came to such strange—to Indian thinking—treatment modalities as the complex drug regimens and lengthy sanitarium stays required for the control of TB. In addition to receiving support from community leaders, IHS health care professionals were also encouraged to work toward integrating traditional Indian healing methods into their own programs. Western medicine is now coming to

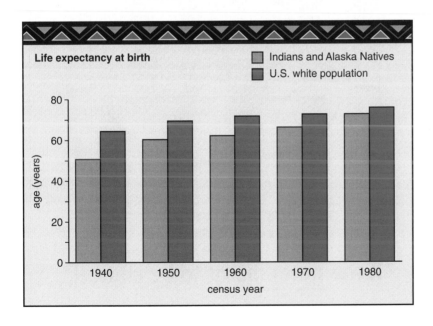

acknowledge the value of the Indian way, with its focus on the whole person rather than on an organ or a disease.

Unhealthy behaviors

Despite this remarkable record of success in health improvement, the efforts of the IHS have not yet resulted in parity between American Indians and the rest of the population. There is still a long way to go. Moreover, as the incidence of infectious and other kinds of disease has declined, an array of more complex conditions—heart disease and cancer, homicide, suicide, child and spouse abuse—has emerged. These pose particular dangers to the health of Indian people and special challenges to their health care providers.

Of course, similar changes have been experienced by the U.S. population as a whole, but some of these emerging problems have special significance for Indians. Whereas the major killers of all Americans today have more to do with lifestyle than with contagious diseases, this situation is especially true among Indians. Their major causes of premature death—including postneonatal infant mortality, injuries, cirrhosis, and diabetes—

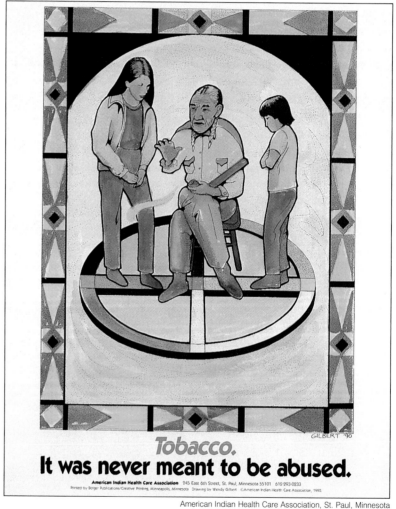

American Indian Health Care Association, St. Paul, Minnesota

are clearly linked to social and behavioral risk factors. High rates of infant death in the first year of life, for example, are associated with maternal risk factors such as cigarette smoking, alcohol abuse, and poor nutrition during pregnancy, as well as adolescent pregnancy.

It is interesting to note that there are striking differences in smoking behavior and disease incidence in different Indian groups. Smoking is uncommon among adults of southwestern tribes such as the Navajo and Apache—a recent study indicated that only about 13% of Navajos smoke—and these tribes also have a very low incidence of lung cancer, heart disease, and chronic lung disease. On the other hand, in the northern plains states, where as many as 50 to 70% of Indian adults smoke, heart and lung diseases are much more prevalent. Smoking—and lung cancer—rates are nine times greater among Oklahoma Indians than among their southwestern counterparts.

The substitution of high-fat, high-sugar, and low-fiber foods for the traditional Indian diet—in which corn and beans were staples—along with adoption of a more sedentary lifestyle, has increased the incidence of obesity and related conditions such as diabetes. Where injuries and cirrhosis are concerned, the most important contributing behavior is alcoholism. Indeed, it is widely believed that alcoholism contributes significantly to most of the 10 leading causes of Indian deaths (see Table).

Despite considerable study, the strong association between Indian people and alcoholism still is not completely understood. Although American Indians share with Asians a characteristic physiological response to alcohol ingestion—rapid flushing of the skin—genetic explanations for the devastating effects of alcohol in Indians have not been conclusively demonstrated. Weekend and binge drinking are thought to be more prominent among Indians than among the rest of the U.S. population, and FAS is emerging as a major cause of mental retardation in American Indians. (See Sidebar, pp. 120–123.) Some believe that the reported higher rates of alcohol-related deaths among Indians reflect the fact that Indian deaths are more likely to be registered as "alcohol related" than is the case for non-Indian deaths. Whether or not this is true, Indian people themselves designate alcoholism as the major health problem facing them today. A variety of initiatives—health-promotion activities, campaigns to educate pregnant women about the risks of drinking, substance-abuse treatment programs—provide encouraging evidence of a growing resolve among many tribes to end the alcoholism "epidemic" in the Indian community.

New activism

Emphasis on the dismal living conditions of many American Indians and their associated illnesses serves to perpetuate a distorted picture of Indian health. It causes discouragement among health professionals who care for Indians, and it instills in Indian communities a sense of low self-esteem—the latter further contributing to self-destructive behaviors.

A truer picture of contemporary Indian life shows that today, as for centuries past, the extended family and the community remain the center of life for most Indian people, and even those living outside the tribal community

Ten leading killers of Indians and Alaska Natives

1. heart disease
2. injuries
3. cancer
4. cerebrovascular disease (stroke)
5. chronic liver disease and cirrhosis
6. diabetes
7. pneumonia and influenza
8. suicide
9. homicide
10. chronic obstructive pulmonary disease

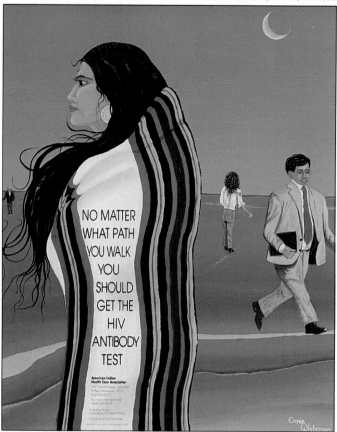

draw on and add to this source of strength. American Indian philosophy embraces the concept of wholeness: the health of an individual depends on the spiritual, social, cultural, and emotional context of the family, the community, and the natural environment. Renewed recognition of this view is helping Indian leaders deal with the complex social and behavioral factors that are adversely affecting the health of their people. As a result, Indian communities are becoming increasingly involved in their own health programs and services. Moreover, many communities are adopting tribal policies that address health risks such as drinking and smoking. The following are some specific examples of this growing sense of responsibility of Indian people for their own health.

• Since 1975, under the provisions of the Indian Self-Determination and Education Assistance Act, 8 of 50 hospitals, 331 of 452 outpatient facilities, and many additional health programs have been transferred from IHS administration to tribal management.

• Nearly every IHS health area and service unit now has an advisory health board that includes representatives from the tribes served. These boards review and comment on program implementation and approve or disapprove all health-related research proposed in their communities. The IHS is providing training and technical assistance to tribes and communities in order to increase their ability to manage their own health care programs. One example of this cooperative approach is found on the

116

Whiteriver Apache reservation in Arizona, where active collaboration between the tribe and researchers from Johns Hopkins University, Baltimore, Maryland, has led to the development of an *H. influenzae* vaccine that provides immunity in Indians.

• Nearly every tribe served by the IHS manages a community outreach program that employs community health representatives. These are local Indians, chosen by the tribe, who receive training in basic health services and who make regular home visits to recently discharged hospital patients, monitor blood pressures, organize community cleanup campaigns and programs of rabies vaccination for pets, and provide various other services. In addition, they encourage people to visit the clinic and often provide transportation. Their efforts are coordinated with those of public health nurses. In remote regions of Alaska the community health program trains selected village residents to function as community health aides. These individuals provide all first-line primary health care and handle local emergency care, consulting as necessary—by telephone or radio—with physicians at field hospitals or clinics.

• Many tribal health boards have declared their board meetings smoke free, setting an example for their membership, and many Indian communities control access to alcohol. More and more, celebrations and other social functions sponsored by Indian organizations and all social functions associated with IHS-sponsored meetings are alcohol free.

• The IHS both respects and encourages traditional Indian healing practices. One member of the national headquarters staff, A. Paul Ortega, a Mescalero healer and teacher, instructs other IHS employees about the values and principles of traditional healing. In most communities IHS doctors and nurses work in concert with traditional healers for tribal members desiring both approaches. Even in many of its hospitals, the IHS sets aside special areas for traditional healing practices. At the Gallup (New Mexico) Indian Medical Center, for example, a ceremonial hogan was constructed on the hospital grounds.

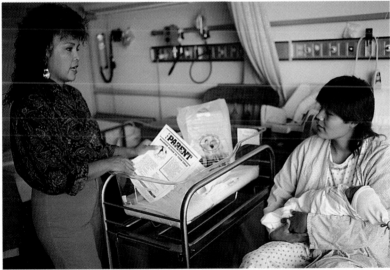

Joel Gordon

At the IHS hospital in Chinle, Arizona, on the Navajo Reservation, a community outreach worker encourages a young mother to attend a parenting class sponsored by the local school district. Outreach workers are an integral part of many tribe-run programs that provide a variety of health and health-related services for American Indian people.

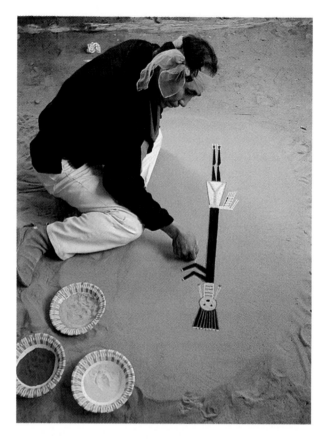

Devoted leaders—past and present

Over the years, in the effort to promote Indian involvement in health, leadership has been provided by a number of outstanding individuals, at least a few of whom deserve mention.

● In the 1950s Annie Wauneka, a community leader and chairperson of the Navajo Tribal Health Committee, was instrumental in bringing TB under control on the reservation. Among other things, Wauneka provided support and encouragement for those who were reluctant to follow the prolonged TB treatment regimen.

● Susie Yellowtail, a nurse and member of the Crow tribe, worked locally and nationally for decades to secure improved health care for Indian people.

● Arta Karlow, an Oglala Sioux, pioneered in the eradication of TB among her people and later took the lead in other health-promotion efforts.

A new generation of leaders is now taking up the cause of improving the health of Indian people—individuals like Cecilia Fire Thunder, a contemporary Oglala Sioux, who has become a national advocate for Indian self-responsibility in maintaining wellness and, on her own Pine Ridge Reservation, has initiated programs emphasizing both individual and community responsibility for health. Fire Thunder's efforts led to the requirement among the Oglala Sioux that individuals who are candidates for tribal office have a history of sobriety.

Many examples can be cited of individuals whose innovative actions have changed their fellow tribe members' attitudes toward health. Among

118

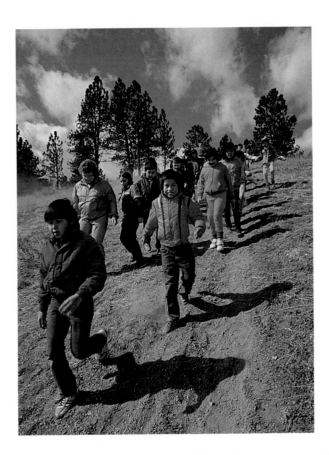

Youngsters on the Northern Cheyenne Reservation in Lame Deer, Montana, participate in "Walkway to Good Health," a fitness program sponsored by the IHS. By adopting an active lifestyle at a young age, these children may be able to avoid such health risks as obesity, heart disease, and diabetes and are more likely than any previous generation to live long and healthy lives.

Aiuppy Photographs

the Cheyenne River Sioux, tribal chairman Wayne Ducheneaux insisted on finding more constructive methods than incarceration in the reservation jail for dealing with intoxicated individuals. His tribe achieved a milestone in December 1987 when the council passed a resolution declaring the tribe's intention to become alcohol free by the year 2000. Another example of community mobilization is the program of fitness instituted at Zuni Pueblo in New Mexico. Though at first there was little interest in physical activity programs, Bruce Leonard, an IHS health educator, managed to garner enthusiasm for an aerobics class at the local gymnasium. Currently the Zuni tribe is in the forefront of community attention to fitness. Leonard's efforts are a testimony to the value of persistence even when initial interest seems slight or nonexistent.

It is this grass-roots leadership and emerging community involvement that appear to be producing a new paradigm for the long-standing partnership of the various tribes and the federal government. The IHS is responding to this changing situation with some changes of its own. Today the agency functions increasingly as a facilitator, supporting and encouraging local health promotion and health care delivery.

The progress since 1955 has been remarkable. The IHS's dedication to the "relief of distress and the conservation of health" and the programs that developed as a natural outgrowth of this commitment have been resoundingly successful. Many current trends bode well for the continuation of this laudable record of success.

The Tragedy of
Fetal Alcohol Syndrome:
A Father's Reflections

by Michael Dorris

Unlike so many good people—social workers, health care professionals, elected officials—who have chosen out of the kindness of their hearts and the dictates of their social consciences to become knowledgeable about fetal alcohol syndrome (FAS), to work with its victims, to demand its prevention, I was dragged to the subject blindfolded, kicking and screaming. I am the worst kind of expert—a grudging, reluctant witness, an embittered amateur, above all else, a failure. I am the adoptive parent of one child with FAS and two others who suffer from fetal alcohol effect (FAE). Like me, my adopted children are of American Indian descent and therefore come from a group that is, owing to various socioeconomic factors, at especially high risk for this condition.

My family's experience provides a living, breathing encyclopedia of what does *not* work in curing or reversing the damage to a child prenatally exposed to too much alcohol. We have tried special education and psychological counseling but to no avail. Anticonvulsant drugs were helpful but were not the answer. Brain surgery did not work. Anger did not work. Patience did not work. Perhaps most frustrating of all, love did not work.

* * *

Fetal alcohol syndrome is a group of birth defects, physical and mental, that can afflict the offspring of women who drink alcohol during pregnancy. The condition was first identified in France in 1968, and a few years later it was described by U.S. researchers, who introduced the term *fetal alcohol syndrome*. Except in its most extreme form, however, FAS is still difficult for many physicians to diagnose. Statistics suggest that the full-blown syndrome occurs in about one in every 750 U.S. births.

FAE, a partial and variable constellation of FAS symptoms, is approximately five times as prevalent. More subtle in its manifestations, FAE is no less debilitating over the course of a lifetime. While its victims

Michael Dorris, author of The Broken Cord—*named best nonfiction book of 1989 by the National Book Critics Circle— is a past recipient of the Indian Achievement Award and a member of the National Advisory Council to Save the Children. He is also the author of several works of fiction and is Adjunct Professor at Dartmouth College, Hanover, New Hampshire, where in 1972 he established the Native American Studies Program.*

may appear to be "normal" physically, they are almost always sorely burdened by learning and behavioral problems.

FAS babies are often born prematurely, have a low birth weight, and are slow to mature. Physically, they exhibit a typical pattern of facial abnormalities that includes small eye openings, short, upturned noses, and thin upper lips. In fact, this pattern is so characteristic that whatever their racial origin, victims of FAS have a tendency to broadly resemble one another. If exposed to excessive amounts of alcohol during the first or second trimester of development, victims may suffer deformities in the major organ systems, especially heart defects. At all ages their heads and brains are smaller than those of their non-alcohol-exposed counterparts, and it is not uncommon for them to experience recurrent dental, visual, and auditory problems. Many have curvature of the spine, suffer from seizures, and manifest poor motor coordination.

Third-trimester exposure often—but not always— results in brain malformation. Persons whose neurological development has been affected by alcohol may score low on IQ tests both as children and as adults (although some may test at normal levels); even more significantly, such individuals struggle with tasks requiring cognitive ability. They are hyperactive and easily distracted, have short attention spans and poor socialization skills, and seem at a particular disadvantage in the area of abstract reasoning, such as in the acquisition of math skills. It is also difficult for them to comprehend and apply many simple, basic rules of conduct. Moreover, as a study published in March 1993 in the British medical journal *The Lancet* revealed, although many of the physical abnormalities of FAS disappear or diminish over time, intellectual and psychological impairment persists.

Widespread—and worsening—problem

While it is presently impossible to ascertain the precise number of those who suffer to some degree from FAS or FAE, most experts conservatively estimate that between 50,000 and 70,000 Americans are born annually with permanent, lifelong damage sustained as a result of prenatal exposure to alcohol. Worldwide, FAS strikes one to two babies in every 1,000 live births and is the leading known preventable cause of mental retardation.

FAS is an especially insidious social problem be-

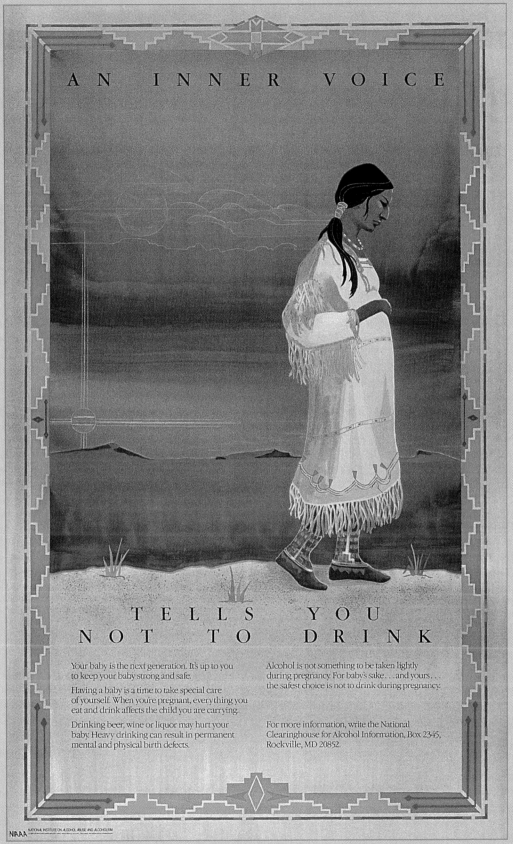

cause once girls with FAS (and FAE) reach maturity, they are likely to repeat the pattern of alcohol abuse during pregnancy. Because of their inherent inability to grasp the long-term consequences of their actions, these girls (and women) are less likely than others to use birth control, seek early prenatal care, or comprehend and follow advice about avoiding dangerous activities and substances during their pregnancies. Moreover, in the U.S. at least, some studies have shown that compared with other women of reproductive age, those with FAS and FAE begin childbearing younger and continue longer, conceiving and giving birth to appreciably more than the average number of offspring. Whether she is affected by FAS or not, any woman who has already borne one FAS baby has almost an 8-in-10 chance of doing so again if she continues drinking—and subsequent offspring are likely to be even more severely impaired than the first.

Intoxication and the embryo

The biochemistry of FAS is not terribly complicated for even a layperson to grasp. Ethyl alcohol, or ethanol, passes freely across the placenta. Therefore, whatever a pregnant woman drinks, the baby she is carrying drinks, too. It is that simple. Moreover, the fetus cannot eliminate alcohol nearly as quickly as the adult body can; when a woman drinks, the concentration of alcohol *in utero* is higher than in the rest of her system, and it persists twice as long. By the time the woman feels pleasantly relaxed or euphoric, the fetus may be comatose.

The degree of damage to the fetus depends on how much alcohol the mother consumes and when during the course of the pregnancy she consumes it, as well as on her age, metabolism, general health and nutritional status, and the use of other harmful substances (tobacco, licit and illicit drugs, etc.). Oddly enough, the medical establishment was slow to recognize the danger of alcohol to the fetus. The 1974 edition of a standard medical school text, *Pharmacological Basis of Therapeutics,* maintained that "alcohol gains free access to fetal circulation, but it does not seem to harm the fetus." And as recently as the early 1980s, many doctors were still prescribing daily "therapeutic" glasses of beer or wine to calm their pregnant patients.

Small, occasional doses of ethanol are unlikely to cause measurable harm to the fetuses of most healthy women. But because there is no known "safe" threshold, the American Medical Association, the American Academy of Pediatrics, and the surgeon general of the United States now recommend that women abstain completely from the time of conception through the cessation of breast-feeding. If a pregnant woman has continued to drink before learning of the potential hazards, she is advised to stop or drastically cut back as quickly as possible to ensure the best chance of

having a healthy, unimpaired child. All evidence suggests that regardless of any previous history of alcohol dependency, a woman will *not* bear a child with FAS or FAE if she refrains from drinking during the course of her pregnancy.

An "Indian problem"?

To what extent does this preventable scourge affect American Indian people? The answer, like so much about FAS, is ambiguous. On the one hand, prenatal exposure to ethanol impairs the individual fetus in exactly the same ways whether its mother is a member of a country club in Greenwich, Connecticut, or an inner-city woman on welfare. Nonetheless, the Indian population is disproportionately affected. A couple of years ago, when the state of South Dakota had no resident specialist in birth defects, it reported a total of two FAS births. During the same period, however, Jeaneen Grey Eagle, director of Project Recovery, an alcoholism-treatment program on a reservation in Pine Ridge, South Dakota, estimated that between one-third and one-half of the infants born in certain communities of her reservation were at high risk owing to heavy maternal drinking. Unfortunately, underdiagnosis does not equal small numbers. In a national study of birth defects conducted in the early 1980s, the prevalence of FAS among Indian children was found to be 30 times greater than among whites. Some tribes, especially those in the northern Plains area and in Alaska, report that more than one-third of all newborns are likely to eventually show indications of either FAS or FAE.

While FAS has been described in every socioeconomic class and ethnic group and in both urban and rural settings, it is obviously most pervasive and drastic in communities where chronic alcohol abuse is prevalent. Not surprisingly, FAS also emerges as a serious problem wherever cultural norms that discourage women from drinking have eroded. In the U.S. many Indian and Alaska Native communities qualify under both of these criteria. The Indian Health Service currently identifies alcoholism as the number one public health peril for the population it serves, and many tribes acknowledge it as their most pressing health problem.

The interpretation of these disturbing data must not be confused with the misleading folk belief that American Indian peoples are less resistant than other groups to either the effects or the allures of "firewater." Prior to contact with Europeans, there was virtually no use of fermented beverages among indigenous cultures north of the Rio Grande, and the irresponsible attitude toward alcohol stereotypically attributed to American Indians in fact echoes the drinking behavior of the European trappers who introduced alcohol to their native trading partners in the 17th, 18th, and 19th centuries. These men, rough and out of place in polite precincts of their own societies, drank in order to become intoxicated—and they encouraged similar behavior in those whose resources of furs they desired to purchase at the lowest possible cost.

In subsequent generations grinding poverty, economic exploitation, feelings of powerlessness, lack of employment, and the prohibition of traditional religious practices have created in some Indian communities an environment ideally susceptible to substance abuse and addiction. And, whereas in many tribes inebriation among women was traditionally frowned upon, in recent decades alcohol abuse by women—and especially by young women of childbearing age—has become more common.

While the experts may not completely agree on why alcoholism is such a serious problem for Indian people, they are unanimous on one point: the excessive consumption of beer, wine, or liquor on the part of a small but significant minority of American Indians has been disastrous for all concerned. Meanwhile, little progress has been made toward breaking the cycle of poverty and despair. Historically, public health programs on reservations have been among the first things cut when the federal budget gets tight; clinics are shut down, counselors laid off, preventive educational campaigns scrapped. For many tribal communities there is simply no access to family-planning services or chemical-dependency-treatment centers—two resources that could potentially have an impact on the incidence of FAS.

One family's struggle

But what of my own family? How have we coped with FAS? Not only was my son Adam, whose story I told in The Broken Cord, a victim of FAS, his adopted stepbrother and stepsister are, to a lesser and greater extent, affected by FAE. (Sadly, Adam was struck by a car in 1992 and later died of his injuries.)

In raising children unintentionally afflicted by their birth mother's use of alcohol, my wife and I and our extended families have had no choice but to become a kind of full-time social service agency. We have come to be specialists in referrals and know firsthand the admissions policies of rehabilitative institutions; the penalties meted out under the juvenile justice system; and the nightmares of dealing with uninformed, often smug, bureaucrats given, by default, responsibility for individuals who do not understand what is in their own best interests. We progressed from attending increasingly acrimonious meetings with teachers in the early grades to learning the intricacies of IQ scoring. We have become infinitely familiar with institutions such as Covenant House, Boys Town, Salvation Army shelters, and even prisons. We have paid out well over $150,000, not counting what our insurance has covered, for tuition to special schools, substance-abuse counseling, experimental medical procedures, Out-

ward Bound for Troubled Youth, and private camps for the learning disabled. We tried virtually every avenue that was suggested to us by well-meaning professionals who were in a position to know what might benefit our children. Yet nothing—nothing—consistently worked for more than a few weeks at a time.

Our two remaining adopted children are now adults or nearly so. Yet they cannot seem to function independently, hold jobs, consistently tell the truth, manage money, plan a future. Each has at one time or another been arrested or otherwise detained for shoplifting, inappropriate sexual conduct, and violent behavior. Despite all our efforts to protect them, they have periodically come under the influence of people who, for instance, worship Satan or take advantage of them physically, mentally, or financially. They maintain few enduring friendships, set few realistic goals, call upon no inner voice to help them distinguish right from wrong, safe from dangerous.

In the years since The Broken Cord was published, we have heard from parents rich and poor, religious and agnostic, of all ethnic groups and every economic stratum. The correspondence we have received has magnified exponentially our own family experience but has not contradicted it. The letter we have waited for but that has yet to arrive is the one that begins, "I've read your book and you're dead wrong" or "My child was diagnosed as having FAS, but we fixed it by doing the following things, and now, X years later, he (she) is perfectly fine."

Everyone's children, everyone's problem

My adopted sons and daughter are but three of the hundreds of thousands unnecessarily born blighted by FAS or FAE. Whether adopted or institutionalized, these children are ultimately society's victims and, therefore, its responsibility. But how to cope? How can a nation—especially in a tightening economy—pay the medical bills, build the prisons, construct the homeless shelters? How can it train special education teachers to function indefinitely with no hope of success? How can it persuade ordinary citizens to forgive behaviors that are irritating at best, threatening or dangerous at worst? How can it teach compassion for people who are likely to exhibit neither pity nor gratitude, who take everything society has to offer and have almost nothing constructive to give back? How can it redefine "not guilty by reason of insanity" to apply to seemingly heartless acts committed by people who are fundamentally incapable of comprehending the law?

This is a complicated and multifaceted problem but one for which a solution must be found—quickly. FAS is not a tragedy whose impact is restricted to its victims. It is not just a women's issue, not just the dilemma of a few Indian tribes. It knows no boundaries of ethnicity or income. These are everybody's children.

Pilgrims' Perils:
Breakdown in Jerusalem

by Eliezer Witztum, M.D., Moshe Kalian, M.D., and Daniel Brom, Ph.D.

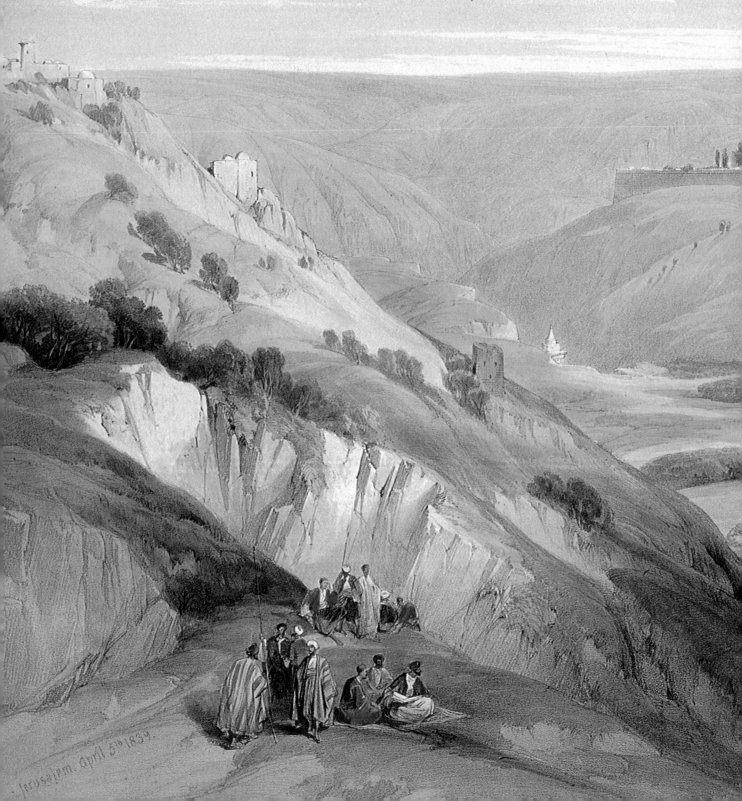

Jerusalem April 5th 1839.

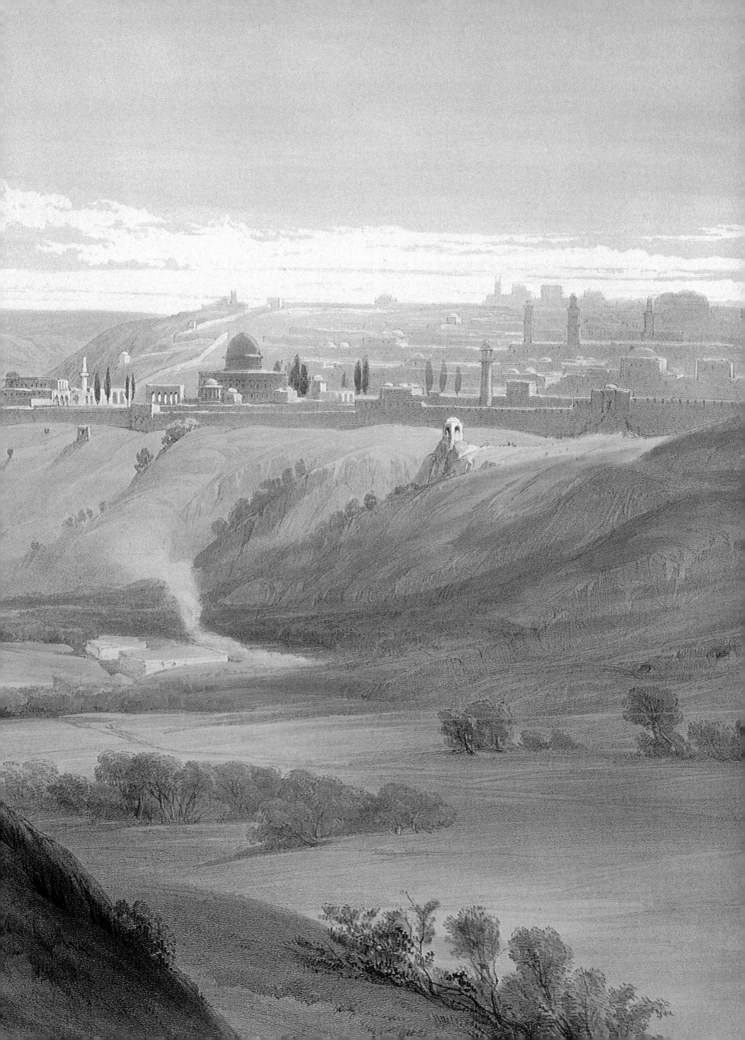

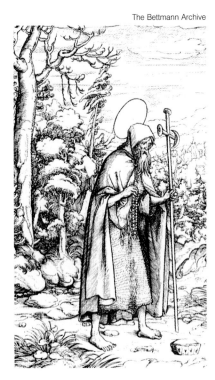

A barefoot Christian ascetic of an earlier century embarks on the long and arduous journey to the Holy Land. The hardships and hazards of such travel can scarcely be imagined by those who make the trip today in safety and comfort. Still, these ancient pilgrims had much in common with modern-day visitors to Jerusalem; some were motivated by piety, some by a spirit of adventure, and not a few by madness.

Eliezer Witztum, M.D., a psychiatrist, is based at the Community Mental Health Center Ezrath Nashim, Jerusalem. Moshe Kalian, M.D., is a psychiatrist at Kfar Shaul Psychiatric Hospital, Jerusalem. Daniel Brom, Ph.D., a psychologist, practices at the Latner Institute, Herzog Hospital, Jerusalem. All three have been involved in the treatment and study of emotionally disturbed tourists in their city.

(Overleaf) "Jerusalem from the Road Leading to Bethany" by David Roberts; collection, the Victoria and Albert Museum

And I saw the holy city, new Jerusalem, coming down out of heaven from God, prepared as a bride adorned for her husband.

—Revelation 21:2

My heart is in the East, and I am in the depths of the West.
My food has no taste. How can it be sweet?
How can I fulfil my pledges and my vows,
When Zion is in the power of Edom,
and I in the fetters of Arabia?
It will be nothing to me to leave all the goodness of Spain.
So rich will it be to see the dust of the ruined sanctuary.

—Judah ha-Levi (*c.* 1075–1141)

The noted historian of religion Mircea Eliade observed that every religious "cosmos" possesses a center, a site that is preeminently the zone of the sacred. The city of Jerusalem in the present-day country of Israel is sacred to three of the world's great religions, Judaism, Christianity, and Islam, and consequently has long been the destination of religious pilgrims. Jews have been drawn to the city ever since the building of the Temple, during the reign of King Solomon (in the 10th century BC); pilgrimage to the Holy Land became an accepted Christian institution in the 4th century AD; and although it is not mentioned by name in the Qur'an, Jerusalem is also sacred to Islam. The Dome of the Rock, a shrine on the Temple Mount, is said to mark the spot from which Muhammad ascended into heaven. Despite their very different beliefs, religious pilgrims of each of these faiths have gone to Jerusalem for much the same reasons—to immerse themselves in the geographic setting of their faith, to tread in the footsteps of the holy and revered, to experience spiritual regeneration—and for over a thousand years a steady stream of pilgrims has made its way to this holy city.

When reading of the religious pilgrims of earlier centuries, one cannot help but wonder what prompted them to venture forth at a time when to leave home meant to risk one's very life. Were they all extremely pious individuals? Or were some of them merely adventurers? And might not at least some of them have been mad?

The present-day equivalent of the pilgrimage is tourism, an activity that attracts hundreds of thousands of visitors to Jerusalem each year. If the pilgrimage is primarily a quest for contact with the sacred, tourism is prompted by much more complicated and heterogeneous motives. Travel is associated with curiosity, adventure, amusement, education, relaxation, status, and much more. In fact, virtually all of the motives that drive people in their daily life are part of the impetus to travel. The difference is that as tourists, people drastically alter their everyday routines. These changes sometimes have a dramatic impact on their mental or emotional state. The tendency of travel to destabilize is especially marked in certain highly susceptible individuals and in certain kinds of settings.

Travelers in distress

Psychiatric disturbances in travelers have been well if not widely documented in the medical literature. Typical cases are those of so-called airport wanderers—people who miss their flight connections, become disoriented, and are found wandering about airline terminals in a state of confusion. Mental breakdowns have also been observed in travelers to specific destinations, among them Florence and, not surprisingly, Jerusalem.

Since the mid-1970s psychiatrists Graziella Magherini and Augustus Zanobini and their colleagues at the hospital of Santa Maria Nuova in Florence have kept records on a number of cases of psychological distress in persons apparently overcome by emotions evoked by that city's historical and artistic treasures. The Italian researchers have given the name "Stendhal syndrome" to the constellation of symptoms they have identified—after the powerful emotional response the French novelist Stendhal (Marie-Henri Beyle) described upon his first visit to Florence in 1817. The subject of this report is a similar phenomenon observed among visitors to Jerusalem. The name "Jerusalem syndrome" was coined and the clinical phenomenon first observed by psychiatrist Yair Bar-El, director of Kfar Shaul Psychiatric Hospital in Jerusalem, where most of the data on the syndrome have been compiled.

"Chosen by God": a case history

Jeff, an unmarried American in his thirties, was taken to Kfar Shaul Psychiatric Hospital in Jerusalem by the police after an episode of violent behavior in the Church of the Holy Sepulchre. According to the arresting officers, Jeff had smashed icons and attempted to destroy liturgical objects in the church and then got into an altercation with priests who tried to stop him. Upon being handed over to the police, Jeff, who only a moment before had been shouting and struggling, became suddenly mute and motionless; according to the police report, the American had a "strange look" in his eyes.

To the hospital staff, Jeff appeared to be a nice looking, well-built young man with longish dark hair and a beard. He was clean and well groomed, although dressed somewhat unusually in garb reminiscent of biblical times.

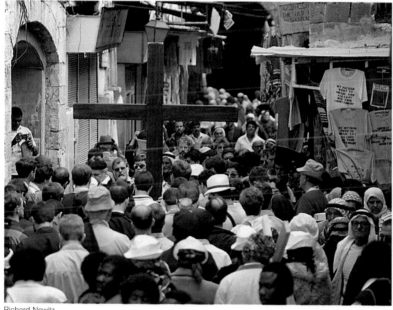

Richard Nowitz

A throng of 20th-century pilgrims makes its way along the Via Dolorosa during a Holy Week procession. According to tradition, this road marks the path Jesus followed as he carried the cross en route to Calvary, the scene of his crucifixion. For most Christians this is a deeply emotional journey, and many are distressed by the air of commercialism lent by vendors hawking T-shirts and other secular souvenirs.

Perhaps the most incongruous element of his physical appearance was the presence on his arms of numerous old, somewhat blurry tattoos. He seemed to be quite willing to cooperate with the doctors and answered their questions without hesitation.

Jeff characterized himself as a peace-loving, nonviolent person who was only fulfilling his "mission." Moreover, he described his actions at the church as simply carrying out "the will of God." He claimed it was not he but the priests who had been aggressive. In calling "earthly powers" (*i.e.,* the police) to assist them, the priests had exposed themselves as "false holy vessels," just as Jeff had expected they would. He explained his refusal to speak after the fight in the church as an attempt to distance himself from these "fraudulent unholy creatures." He was unsure why God had not allowed him to carry out his "mission" but speculated that perhaps "the time was not yet right."

Jeff had a somewhat unusual life story. As the middle son of an upper-middle-class urban Protestant family, he had led an unremarkable life up until the time he entered college. He then decided abruptly to "change course." He crossed the Atlantic and at the age of 18 started to live by himself in Europe, working as a musician and changing jobs often. He played rock and later "heavy-metal" music, formed his own band, lived a wild and irresponsible life, tried various types of drugs, and traveled extensively. Even on his best days, however, he was never happy, always feeling a kind of "inner emptiness" he could never fill.

After several years of this hedonistic lifestyle—of which his tattoos were an apparently shameful reminder—he again felt an urge to change direction; this time he immersed himself in religions and philosophies of the East. Yet his existential despair persisted, and Jeff felt that he was still searching for something. Then, upon turning to the Bible, he sensed "at once" that this was what he had been looking for. He decided to go to the Holy Land to strengthen his belief. He gave away all of his possessions, burned his record albums, and went to Jerusalem to "live a simple and humble life and study the ways of God."

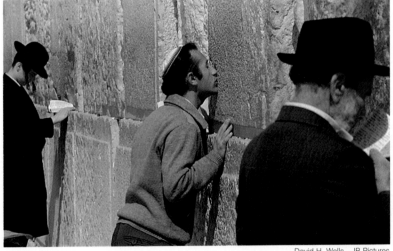

Pious Jews pray at the Western Wall in Jerusalem's Old City, one of the most sacred sites of Judaism. The wall is all that remains of the ancient Temple, destroyed by the Romans in AD 70. For centuries Jews have come from around the world to make their lamentations at this relic of the ancient spiritual center, earning it the designation "Wailing Wall."

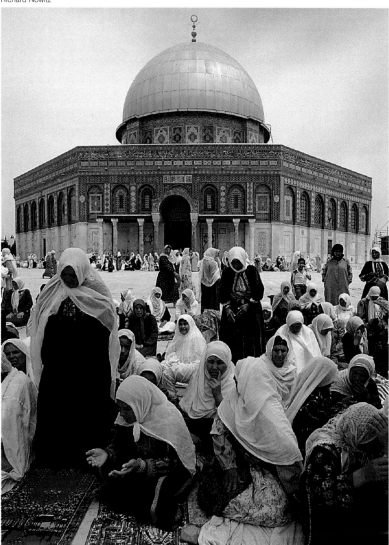

Women gather before the Dome of the Rock, a shrine on the Temple Mount in the Muslim Quarter of the Old City, said to mark the spot from which Muhammad ascended into heaven and long a sacred site for all believers in Islam.

He invented a religion of his own, based on spiritual elements of both Judaism and Christianity; not long afterward, he experienced a "purifying" personal revelation: God is living and loving. He decided to lead a celibate life until God sent him the right woman to marry. With mounting feelings of being a "chosen messenger," he spent his days touring the historical sites of Jerusalem. He visited churches, ate simple but healthy food, fasted once a week, and read both the Old and the New Testaments.

A short time after his arrival, he had visited the Church of the Holy Sepulchre for the first time and had found it disconcerting that such a simple, humble, and pure place should be under the patronage of so many different religious denominations. He felt there was something "dark" about this but could not define what it was.

About 10 days before the violent episode, he met a woman who was almost a "twin soul" and shared many of his ideas. They became very close, and although the relationship remained platonic, he started thinking

129

about her as a potential marital partner. Jeff said that during the week prior to his hospitalization, he had had trouble falling asleep. He felt that God was "testing" him.

The day after he was admitted, Jeff became very excited and tried to smash the ward television set after viewing a somewhat sexually provocative program. A mild dose of haloperidol (an antipsychotic drug) was administered, combined with structured, supportive psychotherapy. The therapist felt that Jeff's capacity for insight was limited. He refused the hospital's request for permission to contact his family. He was, however, able to admit having a long-standing identity crisis, which had resulted in the breach with his family and had also produced in him a strong desire to attain a unique status—"being chosen by God" to purify the Church of the Holy Sepulchre. During the course of his two-week hospitalization, Jeff did not give up his belief in his unique religion, but he showed improvement in reality testing (his ability to understand and foresee the consequences of his actions).

Vulnerable visitors

Since 1979 all tourists in Jerusalem requiring psychiatric hospitalization, as noted above, have been admitted to a single institution, Kfar Shaul Psychiatric Hospital. As in Jeff's case, most of these visitors drew the attention of authorities because of statements or behaviors of a religious nature in public. It seemed evident that they had been either attracted to or influenced by the religious significance of the city.

An average of about 50 travelers are referred for care at Kfar Shaul annually. In recent years comprehensive statistical data have been kept

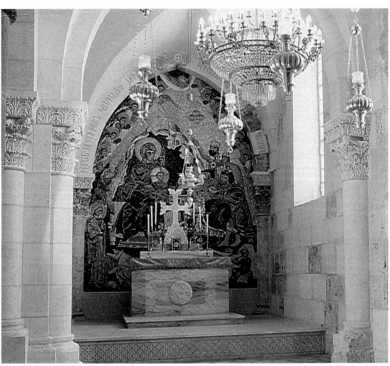

The Church of the Holy Sepulchre supposedly marks the site of the crucifixion and entombment of Jesus and is, therefore, one of the holiest places in all Christendom. Destroyed and rebuilt a number of times over the centuries, the building is architecturally undistinguished and is often disappointing to tourists. Also disconcerting to many visitors is the fact that various different Christian groups— including the Greek and Armenian Orthodox, Roman Catholic, and Coptic churches—control different parts of the present-day structure and regularly hold services in it.

Table 1: Religious participation				
religious faith	strictly observant	observant	nonobservant	total
Jewish	10	22	13	45
Catholic	5	8	5	18
Protestant	2	3	9	14
other	0	1	1	2
unknown				10
total	17	34	28	89

on these patients. The data on which this report is based were collected during 1986 and 1987. When the demographic characteristics of visitors treated during this period were compared with those of tourists hospitalized for psychiatric treatment between 1979 and 1984, no significant disparities were found with respect to age, sex, marital status, religion, country of origin, method of referral, or the number of previous visits to Israel. Therefore, it seems reasonable to assume that the data presented here represent a fair sample of visitors psychiatrically hospitalized in Jerusalem.

The patients hospitalized in 1986–87 included 32 women and 57 men; their mean age was 32.4 years. A majority—74%—were single, 15% divorced, and only 11% married. Fifty-two percent had received 13 or more years of education; 36% had between 8 and 12 years; and 7% had less than 5 years. Most tourists came from western Europe (44%) and North America (40%); the remainder were from eastern Europe, South America, South Africa, and elsewhere.

A wide range of tourist motivations were represented in this sample. Recreational tourism, in which the trip and the contact with another culture are a form of entertainment, was the mode for 30% of the group. Another 26% had reasons of a mystical-religious nature. About 15% were visiting relatives, and 7% had come to do volunteer work. Eleven percent of the travelers were seeking an alternative lifestyle. In terms of religious affiliation, half of the tourists were Jewish; among the Christians, Catholics slightly outnumbered Protestants. Seventy percent described themselves as either strictly or moderately observant of their faith (see Table 1). No Muslim travelers were treated at Kfar Shaul during the period in which this survey was conducted.

Psychiatric profile

Examination of the behavior of these patients immediately prior to their admission to Kfar Shaul shows that deviant behavior, including excessive preaching and vagrancy, was found in 33%. Aggressive acts, such as physically attacking others or threatening them with a weapon, led to the admission of 11%; another 11% were walking about naked when apprehended and taken to the hospital. Thirteen percent were admitted after attempting suicide, and 33% did not exhibit any specific aberrant behavior.

Table 2: Diagnosis	
schizophrenia	49
acute psychosis	14
affective psychosis (mood disorders)	11
personality disorder	7
dementia	2
other	6
total	89

Psychotic episodes, a category that includes the sudden onset of serious mental impairment as well as exacerbation of a chronic disorder, were by far the most important reason for hospitalization (see Table 2). There was no relationship between diagnosis and the religious background, sex, or age of the patients, except that patients suffering from dementia were much older than the others.

In general, then, tourists needing psychiatric hospitalization tend to be men and women of European or North American origin, young adults, with an above-average education. Half of them have a profession, but only a quarter are actually employed. Psychotic phenomena (e.g., delusions, hallucinations) are the predominant symptoms in about 80%; the rest suffer from personality disorders or other psychological disturbances.

All patients were asked if they had had a mystical experience preceding their admission, and 36 (40% of the sample) answered in the affirmative (see Table 3). Most, like Jeff, also believed themselves to be a mystical-religious figure. Twenty-four patients (27%) thought they were the Messiah; four believed they were God; three identified with Satan; and another seven patients thought they were biblical figures such as Abraham, the prophet Elijah, King David, or John the Baptist. Not unexpectedly, Jews tended to identify with Old Testament figures. Mystical experiences were more frequent among individuals from a Roman Catholic background than in Jewish or Protestant patients.

Comprehending the syndrome

Fortunately, for the majority of those hospitalized at Kfar Shaul, the stay was short and the outlook for a complete recovery good. In most cases the traveler's holiday was only temporarily interrupted.

In their attempt to understand the phenomenon of "Jerusalem syndrome," the psychiatrists at Kfar Shaul have observed a correlation between patients' psychotic symptoms and their cultural and religious backgrounds. Thus, the doctors note that during the psychiatric crisis, the individual's behavior is generally consistent with the norms dictated by his or her particular religious model. Of the 30% who identified with a messianic figure, for example, not one patient had committed the offense of public nudity.

Table 3: Religious delusions and mystical experiences		
delusional identification with:	number who had delusion	number who had mystical experiences
Messiah	22	20
God	4	3
Satan	3	2
other, mostly biblical figures	7	6
no identification	34	5
unknown	19	—

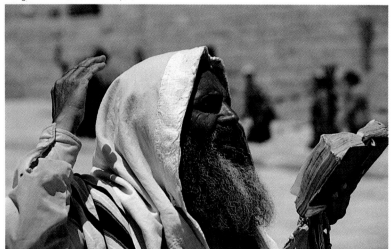

Public displays of religious fervor are not an uncommon sight in the streets of Jerusalem, a city that has the power to stir profound emotions. Whether the religious significance of the city has the capacity to upset the mental balance of individuals otherwise firmly grounded in reality is a question that mental health professionals are still seeking to answer.

Likewise, whereas Jewish patients commonly identified with prophets and other Old Testament historical figures, none imagined themselves to be God; this is consistent with the Jewish tradition, in which the deity generally is not concretely represented in human form.

Does Jerusalem's religious atmosphere actually *induce* psychiatric disturbance in the vulnerable visitor? These authors have not arrived at a definite answer. They point out that over a quarter of the patients in their sample were attracted to the city for clearly mystical-religious motives, and 40% had had mystical-religious experiences while in Jerusalem prior to admission to the hospital. Moreover, about a fifth of the sample had no history of psychiatric hospitalization before coming to Jerusalem, a fact that would seem to implicate the city's unique ambience as a precipitating factor in their psychological disturbance.

If Jerusalem does not actually cause the mental crisis, can it at least be said that the city exerts a special attraction for people with a history of psychiatric problems? In Jeff's case his history clearly suggested delusional beliefs as his motive for becoming religious; his decision to visit Israel was founded in his psychotic thinking. Ultimately, the religious significance of the Church of the Holy Sepulchre and Jeff's grandiose delusions of being a divinely chosen messenger combined to trigger the event that resulted in his hospitalization. The data presented above show that 40% of the disturbed visitors believed, like Jeff, that they were important religious figures and that they had a "mission." Jerusalem appealed to their grandiose ideas, and they came either with clear eschatological motivation or with vague notions of purpose that took shape once they arrived. Further insight into the part played by the city itself is provided by local hoteliers, who, when asked if they think that Jerusalem "draws" the mentally deranged, typically respond with a wry smile.

Early Arrival

Why Babies Are Born Too Soon and Too Small

by Barbara Luke, Sc.D., M.P.H., R.D., and Louis G. Keith, M.D.

One can see them in neonatal intensive care units all over the country: tiny babies hitched up to a bewildering array of tubes and monitors. Some are too frail even to wail. Most will live long enough to leave the hospital; the majority of the very tiniest will have neurological damage; and many will incur staggering medical bills.

The price some of their parents pay in emotional anguish, and that some of the babies may pay in physical pain, is of course beyond reckoning. Although a neonatal intensive care unit can be a place of joy, the smallest of these babies usually face a grim future—or no future at all.

—*New York Times* editorial, Oct. 21, 1991

Because of its frequency, prematurity—*i.e.,* birth at less than 37 completed weeks' gestation—is a major public health problem and an important factor in infant deaths and childhood disability. In the United States in 1990, the year for which the most recent figures are available, of the total 4,158,212 live births, 436,590, or 10.5%, were premature. During the past 20 years, both the total number of births and the number of premature births have increased, although not to the same extent. Between 1970 and 1990, total births in the U.S. increased by 52%, compared with a 114% increase in premature births. There are severalfold differences in prematurity rates by race. Among whites total births rose by 46% and premature births by 102%; among blacks total births rose by 64% and premature births by 131%. Among whites 88 per 1,000 live births in 1990 were premature, compared with 186 per 1,000 among blacks.

Prematurity in 1990 also accounted for 10.5% of infant mortality, up from 8.4% in 1980. More than half of all premature infants are also low-birth-weight babies. This combination of being both preterm and undergrown at birth places newborns at particularly high risk of dying; those who survive are likely to suffer severe growth and developmental problems, and many will have lifelong disabilities.

Historical perspective

In the early part of this century, a "premature infant" was defined in terms of both gestational age and birth weight. An infant was considered to be premature if born at less than 37 weeks' gestation or weighing less than 2,500 grams (one gram = 0.035 ounce). Because this definition combines

Barbara Luke, Sc.D., M.P.H., R.D.,
is Assistant Professor and Director,
Section of Reproductive and Perinatal
Epidemiology, Department of Obstetrics
and Gynecology, Rush Medical College,
Rush-Presbyterian-St. Luke's Medical
Center, Chicago.
Louis G. Keith, M.D., *is Professor of*
Obstetrics and Gynecology, Northwestern
University Medical School, and President,
the Center for the Study of Multiple
Birth, Chicago.

(Opposite page) Photograph, Ansell Horn—Phototake

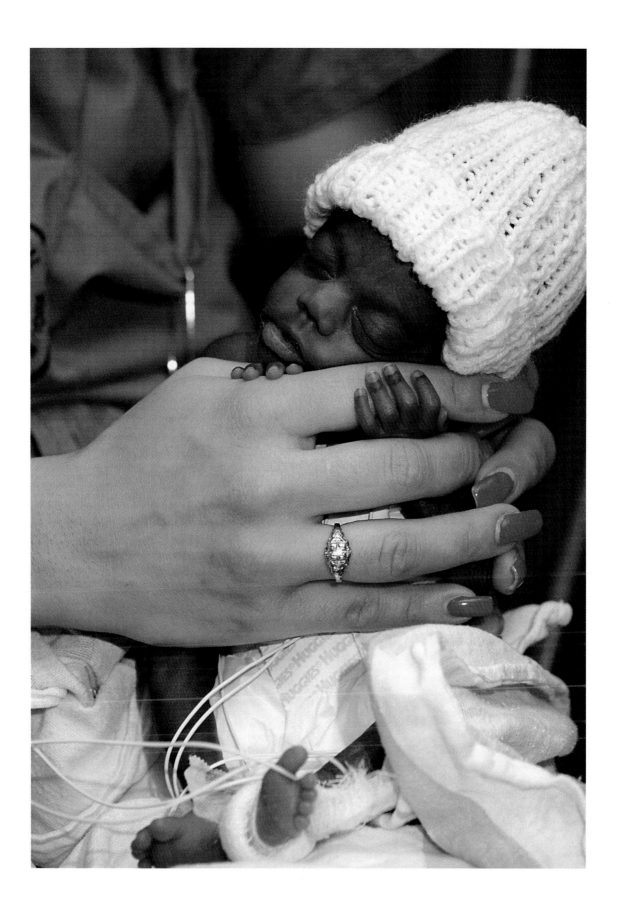

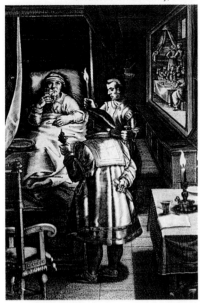

A syphilis sufferer confined to her bed sips broth and is attended at home at a time when little else could be done to spare the patient from the ravages of her disease. In the past, chronic infectious disease in childbearing women was the most common cause of prematurity.

the factors of immaturity and potential undernutrition, it was difficult to separate the causes from the outcomes.

In the United States the obstetrician Julius Hess was a pioneer in the care of premature infants. He wrote the first textbook on the subject and in the early 1900s founded the first U.S. center for the care of premature infants at Chicago's Michael Reese Hospital. At that time the most frequent cause of premature birth was chronic disease in the mother, most notably syphilis, which accounted for some 50 to 80% of all cases. Other maternal infections that contributed to prematurity included tuberculosis, smallpox, diphtheria, measles, typhoid fever, scarlet fever, and influenza.

In the 1890s Pierre Budin, a French pediatrician, first outlined the special needs of the premature infant. The most immediate need was to maintain body temperature. Because of the premature infant's inability to maintain its own body temperature, incubators were developed. The first such device was designed by Étienne Tarnier in 1889 for use at the Paris Maternity Hospital. Hess in the U.S. improved on this around 1915, designing the first practical incubator; his device, which enclosed the newborn in a water jacket, was widely used for the next 25 years. Other American pediatricians preferred an "incubator room" over individual incubators. In 1916, at Bellevue Hospital in New York City, the pediatrician Linnaeus LeFetra kept the premature infants' ward moist with a large pan of water simmering on an electric stove. The temperature was maintained between 24° and 27° C (70° and 80° F), while relative humidity in the room was 60 to 70%. Infants were wrapped in cotton, and hot-water bottles were placed at the bottom and sides of their cribs until they could maintain a stable body temperature without them.

Feeding posed another special problem. Human milk was considered by most pediatricians to be the best food, but even breast milk had to be diluted and fed by bottle to infants weighing less than 1,500 grams. If breast milk was unavailable, buttermilk or skim milk with added carbohydrates was used for the first three weeks, at which time some boiled whole milk was added. Not at all pediatricians considered breast milk ideal

Incubators were developed at the end of the 19th century in the hope of keeping infants born before 37 weeks' gestation alive outside the womb. The first such devices, designed by the French obstetrician Étienne Tarnier and used at the Paris Maternity Hospital, maintained the body temperature of these vulnerable infants, whose own bodies could not yet do so.

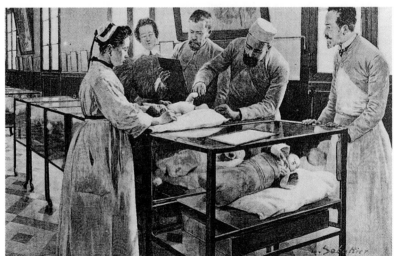

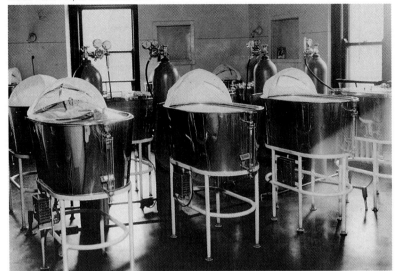

Incubator beds devised by Chicago obstetrician Julius Hess around 1915 were a significant improvement over earlier versions, providing a temperature-, humidity-, and oxygen-controlled environment for the preterm infant. Still, however, the survival rate for these high-risk babies was extremely low.

food for premature infants, however. The American pediatrician Thomas Rotch advocated a modified milk formula prepared in special laboratories. Its advantages were that the infant could be fed without being removed from the incubator, it was sterile, its constituents were balanced, and the proportions of protein, fat, and carbohydrate could be varied.

The survival rate for premature infants during the first half of the 20th century was very poor. In 1916 LeFetra reported that only 15% of premature infants born at Bellevue survived. In one 1921 study 30% of all low-birth-weight infants died within the first month of life. Other studies showed that mortality increased as birth weight decreased: 11% of infants born weighing between 2,000 and 2,500 grams died; 69% weighing 1,000 to 1,500 grams died; and 94% of those born prematurely at weights under 1,000 grams died. Gestational age also played an important part in contributing to infant deaths: 425 of every 1,000 premature infants died (42.5%), compared with only 233 per 1,000 (23.3%) full-term infants.

Prematurity today: many relevant factors

There is no single cause of prematurity. Social and economic factors are important; demographic factors play a role; both maternal employment and lack of it are influential; nutrition and exposure to toxic substances affect pregnancy outcome; and medical factors and complications that arise during the pregnancy influence the time of birth. The nature of the specific conditions within each of these broad categories is exceedingly diverse, and their relative effects are not always equal. More important, not all factors within each category are amenable to change.

Among demographic and psychosocial factors low socioeconomic status, race (black), marital status (single), low maternal age (variously described as under age 15, 16, or 18 years at the time of pregnancy), having less than 12 years' education, and short stature (height of less than 152 centimeters [60 inches]) cannot or are unlikely to be changed during pregnancy. In contrast, low prepregnant weight, stress (both physical and

137

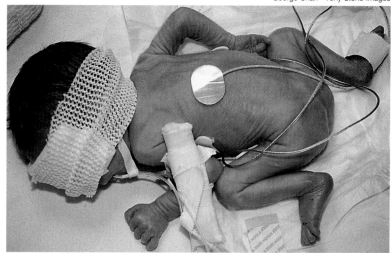

The survival odds for premature and low-birth-weight babies are dramatically higher today than they were just a few decades ago. Nonetheless, these infants remain at high risk for severe growth and development problems, and many will have lifelong disabilities.

emotional), physical carriage (posture), and prolonged or strenuous work often can be changed—either before or during pregnancy.

Whereas the increase in the number of live births in the 1970s and 1980s primarily reflects an increase in the proportion of the female population of reproductive age (15–44 years), the increase in the rate of prematurity—nearly twice that of the total number of births—reflects, among other things, the effects of adverse social factors, including increases in unemployment, poverty, numbers of childbearing women lacking health insurance, and unwanted pregnancies. It is instructive to examine these interrelated factors.

In 1991, 8.4 million persons in the U.S. were unemployed—1,550,000 more than in 1990 and 4,330,000 more than in 1970. The unemployment rate was 6.7% (6% for whites; 12.4% for blacks). The rate of unemployment affects the number of uninsured individuals and their ability to obtain routine medical and prenatal care. The cost of living also increased during these same years. The consumer price index, a measure of the cost of living, rose from 38.8 in 1970 to 136.2 in 1991. One of the major results of the simultaneous increases in the rate of unemployment and the cost of living is that more individuals presently live in poverty. In 1990, for example, 33.6 million persons, or 14% of the U.S. population, were living below the poverty level, compared with 25.4 million persons, or 13% of the population, in 1970. Nearly one-half of female-headed households had incomes below the poverty threshold. (In 1990 poverty level income for a three-person household was $10,419.) As with unemployment, poverty status profoundly affects the ability to obtain routine medical and prenatal care.

In 1993 about 37 million persons in the U.S., for one reason or another, had no health insurance. This factor directly affects the number of women who lack access to prenatal care or receive too little care too late in their pregnancies for the attention to be of medical benefit. In 1980, 5.1% of women who gave birth had late or no prenatal care; a decade later this figure was 6.4%. These figures translate to about 185,000 births a decade ago, compared with about 260,000 births in recent years—an increase of about 75,000 births in which prenatal care was deficient or absent.

The rate of unintended pregnancies has risen markedly in recent years. Unintended pregnancies often are associated with delays in getting prenatal care or not getting it at all and behaviors during pregnancy that increase the risk of adverse outcomes. In other words, women who do not want their babies are not likely to do what they can to ensure that the outcome of the pregnancy will be favorable. In a survey in Oklahoma conducted between 1988 and 1991, more than 44% of respondents reported that their pregnancies were unintended; of these, 31% were mistimed and 13% unwanted. Among women under age 20, more than two-thirds had pregnancies that were unintended, compared with one-half of women aged 20–24 and one-third of those aged 25 and older.

The rate of induced abortions provides a partial index of the number of unwanted pregnancies. In 1988, for example, there were 1,591,000 induced abortions in the United States, or 401 induced abortions per 1,000 live births. Four out of 10 women having an induced abortion in 1988 had at least one prior induced abortion. The number of abortions has risen each year since this procedure was legalized in 1973. The highest abortion rate is among women aged 19 or younger; 45% of all pregnancies in this age group are aborted. While abortion reduces the number of unwanted pregnancies that result in premature birth, multiple induced abortions are associated with an increased risk of prematurity in subsequent pregnancies that may or may not be intended.

All of the circumstances just described affect the health status of women. They all have a direct bearing on the rate of adverse pregnancy outcomes, including prematurity. Other circumstances that contribute to prematurity, described below, deserve special mention.

Obstetric considerations

Several obstetric factors related to a woman's pregnancy history are associated with prematurity. Opinion as to their relative importance, however, varies widely among obstetricians. Moreover, none of these can be changed. Such factors can include previous death of an infant, having had

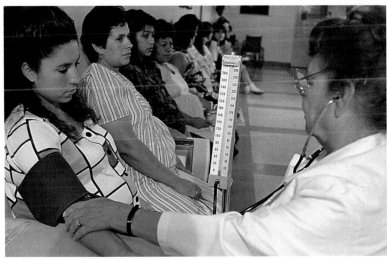

Alon Reininger—Contact Press Images

Soon-to-be mothers wait to have checkups in the crowded obstetrics clinic of a public hospital in Los Angeles. Demographic and social factors have a great deal to do with pregnancy outcome. Women of low socioeconomic status and those in minority groups often lack access to adequate prenatal care, or they get it only very late in their pregnancies—circumstances that contribute to their having babies who are born too early and are unhealthy from the start.

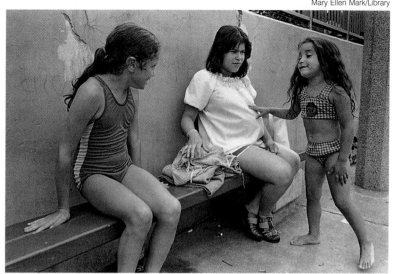

Recent studies have documented unprecedented numbers of unmarried teenaged women having babies. Low maternal age is one of the demographic factors contributing to prematurity. Moreover, a large majority of teen pregnancies are either unintended or unwanted. Young women who did not intend to become pregnant in the first place and who do not then abort are the group most likely to engage in behaviors that place their fetuses at high risk of being born too soon, at low birth weight, or both.

a spontaneous or an induced abortion, previous preterm delivery, short interval between pregnancies, abnormal (incompetent) cervix, and abnormality of the genital structures.

The obstetric factors in the current pregnancy that influence the risk of prematurity are even more diverse. They include: infection; preterm labor; early rupture of the fetal membranes; late or no prenatal care; twin or multiple gestation; and complications that arise at various times during gestation such as high blood pressure (preeclampsia), excessive vomiting (hyperemesis), increased uterine fluids (hydramnios), Rh incompatibility, and bleeding (placenta previa or abruptio placenta). The conditions that have been most extensively investigated are cervical incompetence and genital tract infections.

In the past, women who had repetitive acute, painless second-trimester pregnancy losses (occurring anytime from the 13th to the 24th week of gestation) without associated bleeding or uterine contractions were described as having cervical incompetence, characterized by the loss of structural or functional integrity of the cervix. More recently it has been suggested that this condition may result from a variety of factors—most importantly, acquired infection—which then lead to premature birth.

Evidence is rapidly accumulating that microbial colonization and inflammation of the lower genital tract are significantly associated with prematurity—especially very early prematurity, birth between the 24th and the 32nd weeks. Infection by anaerobic bacteria that normally reside in the vagina without causing symptoms and ubiquitous organisms such as group B streptococci may contribute. Several sexually transmitted organisms—*e.g., Neisseria gonorrhea, Chlamydia trachomatis, Trichomonas vaginalis*, and possibly the human immunodeficiency virus (the virus that causes AIDS)—have also been implicated. All can cause a local inflammation in the space between the fetal membranes and the uterine wall, which initiates a cascade of biochemical changes that alone or in combination with cervical dilatation and uterine contractions lead to preterm labor and premature

140

Babies born too soon: stages of development

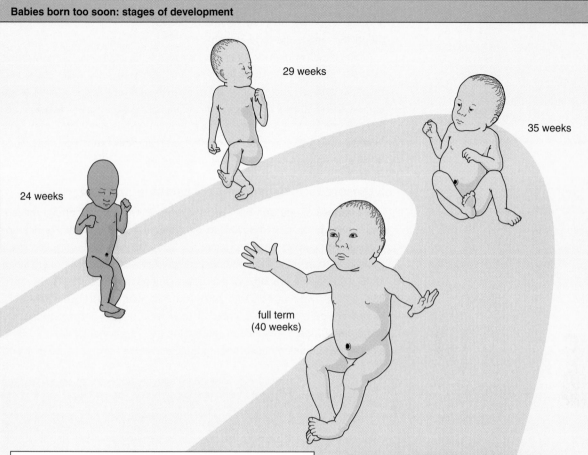

29 weeks

35 weeks

24 weeks

full term
(40 weeks)

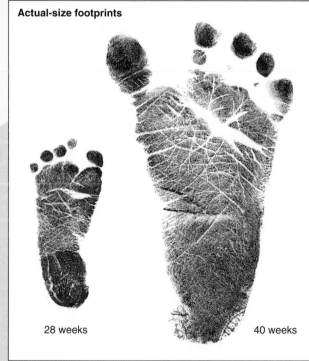

Actual-size footprints

28 weeks

40 weeks

Drawings illustrate the developmental stages of three premature babies and a full-term baby. A 24-week infant kept alive by neonatal intensive care technology weighs just over 500 grams (1¼ pounds), measures 33 centimeters (13 inches), and has skin that appears dark reddish, or dusky, because pigmentation has not yet begun. Eyes are still shut; lungs are only minimally developed; and the body is unable to regulate its own temperature or ward off infection. Chances for long-term survival are only 5–20%. At 29 weeks a 1,100-gram (2½-pound) preemie's lungs have developed to a stage that its chances of survival are 90–95%. Eyes are partly open and able to focus, and the infant may show some alertness and ability to suck. A 35-week infant has smooth pigmented skin with an underlying layer of fat; eyes are able to focus and recognize objects; and muscle tone and breathing, sucking, and swallowing capabilities have developed. A robust full-term baby, at 3,100 grams (7 pounds) and 50 centimeters (20 inches), is well nourished, protected from infection by antibodies from the mother, and ready to go home.

Footprints, courtesy of Michael Reese Hospital and Medical Center

birth. Specific maternal organs may also become infected during pregnancy and subsequently increase the rate of prematurity: kidneys (nephritis), liver (hepatitis), and lungs (pneumonia).

Although all women are theoretically at risk for such infections, women of lower socioeconomic status who are less well educated, black and Hispanic women, and sexually active women without a stable marital union appear to be at much higher risk, largely because sexually acquired infections are more prevalent in these women. In addition, they may lack medical insurance, access to health care, or both, and they may seek medical attention very late in their pregnancies.

Exposure to toxic substances: common and dangerous

Use or abuse of one or more toxic substances, including alcohol, tobacco, and a variety of illicit drugs such as marijuana and cocaine, is not uncommon in women during pregnancy. In the United States, government statistics document a 40% reduction in the overall number of smokers since 1965. The decline among women, however, has been less (32%). In 1991, 23% of U.S. women smoked. Moreover, smoking-prevalence rates were higher in younger females entering their reproductive years. During the same period, there was little decline in the use of alcohol by women. Both alcohol and smoking cause poor intrauterine growth and have been linked

The abuse of one or more toxic substances during pregnancy is clearly associated with adverse infant outcomes. In the United States several hundred thousand babies are born each year to mothers who drink alcohol, smoke cigarettes, and use illicit drugs. Moreover, studies have documented that the number of infants exposed in utero to such toxic substances has more than tripled in just the past decade. Alcohol and tobacco use increase the risk of babies' being born at low birth weights or having birth defects. Use of the drug cocaine during pregnancy is linked, directly or indirectly, to the onset of premature labor.

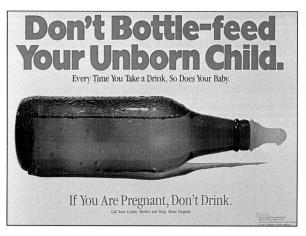

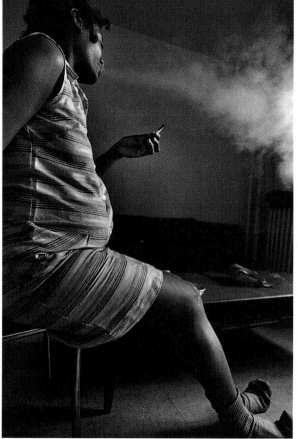

(Left) National Library of Medicine, Bethesda, Maryland; (right) Eugene Richards—Magnum

to birth defects and low-birth-weight infants but have not been specifically linked to prematurity.

Among commonly abused drugs, cocaine is most clearly associated with prematurity. The cause of this connection is not entirely clear. Cocaine may provoke intense spasms of uterine arteries; it may also induce uterine contractions that lead to premature separation of the placenta from the uterine wall. Regardless, the onset of premature labor frequently follows directly upon cocaine ingestion and does not appear to be dose related. It remains unclear, however, whether cocaine's effect on prematurity is potentiated by other factors—concomitant adverse conditions such as poor nutrition or having a sexually transmitted disease.

Another substance that may have a bearing on a woman's pregnancy, if she had been exposed to it *in utero,* is diethylstilbestrol (DES), a synthetic estrogen given to some three million to six million pregnant women in the U.S. during the 1940s and '50s to prevent spontaneous abortion and premature delivery. In fact, the reproductive performance of "DES daughters" is probably worse than that of their mothers. DES exposure is a specific iatrogenic (*i.e.,* inadvertently induced by treatment) cause of cervical incompetence and prematurity. Among the daughters first- and second-trimester spontaneous abortions are common, and the rate of preterm delivery—prior to 35 weeks—is high. This outcome is attributed to abnormalities of the cervical and uterine anatomy in DES daughters. The drug is no longer prescribed in pregnancy.

Work and prematurity

The association between hard physical work and adverse pregnancy outcomes has been known for many generations. However, it has been only during the past hundred years that this association has been studied scientifically. One of the first researchers to document a relationship between physical work and adverse pregnancy outcome was the French obstetrician Adolph Pinard, who studied women working in the laundries of Paris in the 1890s. These women worked under arduous conditions, standing for long hours, for little pay. Pinard made an astute observation: "The birth weight of an infant born to a woman who has been resting for two or three months during her pregnancy is 300 grams higher than that of a child born to a woman who has been working until her delivery." This connection between rest, particularly in the final weeks of gestation, and better pregnancy outcome for both the mother and the child was also seen on the other side of the Atlantic. In the early 1900s the U.S. National Child Welfare Association initiated a vigorous public health campaign advising pregnant women to rest in order to prevent complications of pregnancy such as miscarriage, stillbirth, and prematurity.

During recent decades women's participation in the U.S. labor force has increased dramatically. The proportion of women in the workforce increased by 60% between 1960 and 1990. Nearly 7 out of 10 women of childbearing age—both married and single—now work outside the home. A recent study by the Bureau of the Census compared employment among women during their first pregnancy during the years 1961–65 with the employment rate of women during first pregnancies in 1981–85. More women in the latter group were employed (65% versus 44%); fewer women quit their jobs (28% versus 63%); and more worked closer to the time of giving birth. More than 30% of employed women in 1981–85 worked to within one month before childbirth, compared with 10% in 1961–65.

In addition, there have been changes in the age distribution of U.S. women having children and in the spacing and overall numbers of births. First, owing to a rapid rise in the birthrate in the 1950s and 1960s, followed by a decline in the 1970s, the largest proportion of childbearing-age women presently are aged 35 or older (more than 28%, compared with 18% aged 20–34 and 16% aged 19 and younger). Second, more women are choosing to delay childbearing in favor of professional and educational pursuits. For example, the proportion of first births to women aged 30 and older increased from 4% in 1970 to nearly 18% in 1989. Such delays are associated with increases in educational attainment and greater numbers of young women who have career aspirations. These changing circumstances suggest that women have developed a greater commitment to working, and in turn this has resulted in increasing proportions who work while pregnant and who work longer into their pregnancies.

The increased prevalence of working through late gestation has heightened the social and scientific interest in the potential effect of work on reproductive outcome. Although physical activity in general—even participation in vigorous exercise such as jogging—does not appear to be detrimental to pregnancy outcome, certain types of strenuous work have been associated with preterm delivery and giving birth to low-birth-weight infants.

A group of contemporary French investigators, led by Nicole Mamelle of the National Institute of Health and Medical Research in Lyon, quantified this relationship; they devised a scoring method clearly demonstrating that increasing levels of work result in a parallel increase in the rate of prematurity. The addition of adverse medical factors to this score further

The association between hard physical labor and preterm delivery was established about a century ago. Women whose work is highly strenuous and who are on their feet for long hours, especially in the last trimester of pregnancy, are those at highest risk of going into labor early and giving birth before they are due.

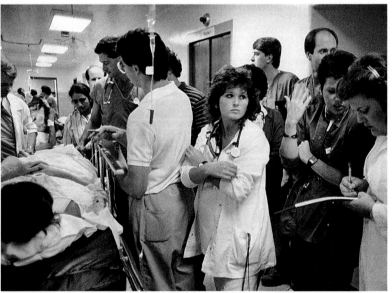

Andy Levin

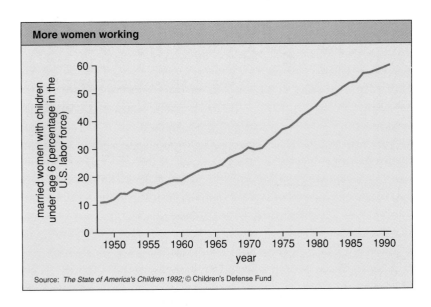

More women working

married women with children under age 6 (percentage in the U.S. labor force)

Source: *The State of America's Children 1992;* © Children's Defense Fund

magnified the prematurity risk. North American investigators demonstrated that the risk of prematurity is highest (7.7%) among women whose jobs require prolonged standing; this is compared with a risk of 4.2% in women with sedentary jobs; the lowest risk (2.8%) is among women with semi-active work involving intermittent walking on the job. In a recent study of a large group of nurses who worked during their pregnancies, the risk of prematurity was increased among those who worked more than 8 hours a day or 40 hours a week, stood more than 4 hours at a time on the job, or had a prior history of preterm birth.

In Europe governments have long recognized the favorable effects of work leave on pregnancy outcome. Most industrialized countries in the world and many less developed countries provide an entitlement for pregnant women that allows specified periods away from work both before and after birth, provides cash benefits during the leave period, and guarantees protection of job rights. In the United States the association between work and preterm birth and the therapeutic effects of work leave on pregnancy outcome have not been completely accepted, and prior to 1993 the U.S. had no work-leave policy. On Feb. 5, 1993, Pres. Bill Clinton signed the Family Leave Act (which had been vetoed three times by Pres. George Bush during the prior administration). Although the act allows a woman to take 12 weeks' leave during pregnancy, it does not provide for continuation of salary, nor does it afford protection of job rights.

Maternity-leave programs around the world share a number of common components, but the amount of leave before and after delivery varies, as does the proportion of continued salary. Work leave before delivery ranges from 11 weeks in the United Kingdom to 4 weeks in Hungary and Denmark. Work leave after childbirth varies from as long as nearly three years in Finland to six weeks in Canada and Israel.

In the United States a frequent argument against paid maternity leave is that women may not return to the workforce after giving birth. However, there is evidence that the opposite is true. Although the U.S. does not

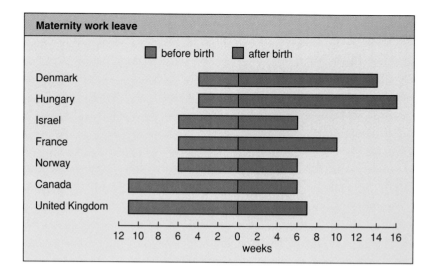

Maternity work leave

as yet have a maternity-leave policy comparable to those of most other industrialized nations, many private companies have formulated their own policies that enable pregnant women to take work leave and still retain benefits. The philosophy behind these policies is that such preventive investment in individual and family health pays off and therefore makes good "business sense." Though passage of the Family Leave Act is a step in the right direction, the country still has a long way to go in formulating a truly enlightened maternity policy that applies to all women.

Nutrition in pregnancy

Observations during World War II of the effects of famine conditions on reproductive performance were among the first studies to provide information about the role of nutritional factors in the etiology of prematurity. Although most of the reports focused on birth weight, these "natural experiments" provide valuable information on the effects of undernutrition on fertility and on the length of gestation. One reproductive effect, which had also been observed in Germany in World War I, was "war amenorrhea," loss of menses secondary to an inadequate food supply and harsh environmental conditions, which reduced the total number of pregnancies.

The effects of famine conditions on reproductive outcome were studied in detail both in Leningrad (now St. Petersburg) and The Netherlands. The siege of Leningrad lasted from August 1941 to August 1943, with famine conditions at their worst between September 1941 and February 1942. The city was bombed; there was no heating or public transportation; and the winter of 1941–42 was particularly severe. Not only was food scarce (bread rations between September 1941 and February 1942 ranged from 125 to 500 grams per person per day), but often what was available was not nutritionally adequate. Bread, for example, was often made from combinations of wheat flour and sawdust or other nonnutritional fillers.

Data from the Leningrad State Pediatric Institute indicated that the birthrate fell and the rates of prematurity, stillbirth, and neonatal death rose in 1942. During the first half of 1942, the stillbirth rate doubled and prematurity rose to 41.2%. Average birth weight dropped by 550 grams, and neonatal mortality rose to 9% for term and 31% for preterm infants.

In The Netherlands famine conditions existed from October 1944 until May 1945. Because of the excellent prenatal records and vital statistics maintained by the Dutch government before, during, and after the famine, these data have been studied extensively by many researchers. Although the dietary and environmental conditions were similar to those during the famine in Leningrad, the Russian women had been exposed to a much longer period of suboptimal nutrition and extreme physical hardship prior to the famine. Dutch women, on the other hand, were well nourished and were not subject to extreme physical stress before the German blockade. Nonetheless, as in Leningrad, amenorrhea was reported to be as high as 50% among urban Dutch women in famine-affected areas, and the birthrate fell to about one-third of normal.

The American epidemiologists Zena Stein and Mervyn Susser conducted the most detailed studies of the effect of the Dutch famine on women and their newborns. They evaluated the prenatal and newborn records from teaching hospitals in famine-hit areas (Amsterdam, Leiden, and Rotterdam) and from parts of the country that were unaffected by famine but where food rations were reduced (Groningen in the north and Heerlen in the south). The data indicated that the average length of gestation was reduced by only about four days in famine-affected women. Babies born to mothers who were exposed to famine in the third trimester had the lowest birth weights as well as the lowest birth lengths and head circumferences. Of all the indexes, maternal body weight was most affected, followed by infant birth weight. Length of gestation was the least affected.

Research in recent years has shown associations between prematurity and numerous nutrition-related factors: low maternal weight prior to conception (pregravid weight), low weight for height, and low gestational weight gain. The most consistent finding in clinical studies is the association between low pregravid weight and prematurity. While short maternal stature has been associated with prematurity, its effect is mediated through pregravid weight; i.e., as low weight for height. Data from the First British Perinatal Mortality Survey, which assessed the prematurity rate in 17,000 births in 1958, showed that the prevalence of premature births was nearly twice as great for women who were under 152 centimeters, compared with those 173 centimeters (68.7 inches) or taller, and nearly three times greater among women with pregravid weights of 50 kilograms (one kilogram = 2.2 pounds) or less, compared with those weighing 63 kilograms or more.

The second most important nutritional factor associated with prematurity is low gestational weight gain—inadequate total gain or rate of gain during the pregnancy. Low gestational weight gain and low pregravid weight appear to act indirectly on other nutrition-related factors associated with prematurity. A rate of weight gain of less than 0.23 kilogram per week after 20 weeks' gestation, weight gain of less than 4.3 kilograms after 24 weeks' gestation, or weight gain of less than 5 kilograms by 32 weeks have all been associated with an increased risk of prematurity. Fortunately, low gestational weight gain is a risk factor that may be susceptible to intervention.

Photograph, Lennart Nilsson from *A Child Is Born,* Dell Publishing Company

A fetus, photographed in utero *at 18 weeks' gestation, is at a crucial stage in development, when it depends on an adequate supply of oxygen and nutrients from the mother. Both low maternal weight at the time of conception (pregravid weight) and a low rate of weight gain during pregnancy may increase the risk of premature delivery. Women who do not have enough body fat when they become pregnant may lack the nutrient reserves that provide essential fetal nourishment, via the placenta, throughout gestation. Studies of pregnant women carried out during the famines of World War II demonstrated that nutritional deprivation and a low rate of weight gain, especially beyond 20 weeks' gestation, resulted in a depletion of maternal fat, which had direct consequences for the developing fetus: a lack of adequate nourishment owing to insufficient growth of the placenta.*

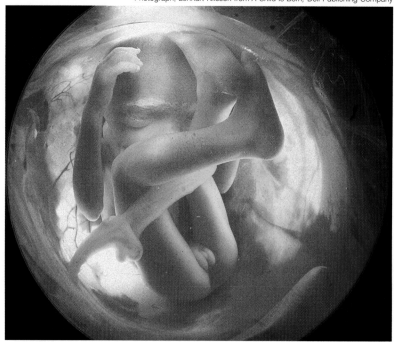

Maternal pregravid weight, alone or in combination with gestational weight gain, may exert its effect on pregnancy outcome through the presence (or absence) of maternal nutrient reserves, particularly maternal body fat. As a buffer against environmental fluctuations in dietary intake, maternal body fat may also play an important role in the hormonal and biochemical aspects of gestation. Increasing pregravid weight (an indirect measure of increasing body fat) is also associated with better intrauterine growth; this is reflected in higher infant birth weights, longer birth lengths, and larger head circumferences. As the earlier studies of well-nourished women whose pregnancies coincided with the Dutch famine of 1944–45 had demonstrated, this interrelationship is critical. Maternal body weight apparently absorbed the first impacts of the famine, preceding a decline in placental weight and newborn measures. Only after maternal weight reached a lower threshold, evidenced in a depletion of maternal body fat, did nutritional deprivation significantly affect the placental growth and subsequent development of the fetus. With the provision of food following the liberation, the nutritional needs of Dutch mothers were attended to; maternal body weight and placental subsufficiency were then quick to recover, and birth weights subsequently increased.

Studies have also demonstrated that fasting affects preterm birthrates and that such an effect may have a hormonal basis. This phenomenon has been demonstrated in the rhesus monkey: an imposed fast results in an initial decrease in maternal whole blood glucose, followed by an increase in maternal prostaglandin concentration; these hormonal fluctuations then result in an increase in the frequency of uterine contractions, leading to premature delivery. In women a doubling of the preterm birthrate following a 24-hour total food and water fast has been reported.

148

Other studies have examined the association between specific individual nutrients and prematurity. Vitamin A deficiency, alone and in combination with protein-calorie malnutrition, is prevalent in less developed countries. A case-control study comparing pregnancy outcome by income and social class in India showed a significant association between prematurity and women of lower income and low social class, where vitamin A intakes were low. A study from Cardiff, Wales, reported low folic acid levels in 83% of women who aborted, 61% who had malformed newborns, 49% whose infants were small for gestational age, and 18% who delivered preterm but in only 13% of women who had normal-term births. A double-blind randomized trial of prenatal magnesium supplementation found that fewer preterm births and longer median lengths of gestation occurred in magnesium-supplemented women than in women who were given a placebo. The magnesium supplementation was also associated with lower rates of postpartum maternal complications and with healthier newborns.

In a recent study of prenatal calcium supplementation, half the subjects received two grams of calcium carbonate and the other half received a placebo. The calcium-supplemented group had an average prematurity rate of 7.4%, compared with 21.1% in the placebo group, and mean length of gestation was 39.2 weeks in the former and 37.9 weeks in the latter. Among calcium-supplemented women 9.6% had low-birth-weight babies, compared with 21.1% in the nonsupplemented group, and the mean infant birth weights in the two groups were 3,129 grams and 2,939 grams, respectively.

Iron is probably the most important nutrient for women during pregnancy, and most require supplemental iron. Several large studies have evaluated maternal iron status and prematurity. Data from more than 50,000 pregnancies from the U.S. Collaborative Perinatal Project (1959–65) and nearly 55,000 pregnancies from the Welsh Cardiff Births Survey (1970–82) showed that both abnormally high and abnormally low levels of hemoglobin (the iron-containing pigment in red blood cells) and hematocrit measures (the ratio of red blood cells in whole blood) increase the probabilities of fetal death, prematurity, and low birth weight.

Length of gestation has also been studied in regard to differences in the fatty acid component of the diet. Dietary long chain (polyunsaturated) omega-3 fatty acids, found primarily in fish oils, inhibit the formation of prostaglandins from arachidonic acid. Recent studies have hypothesized that a high maternal intake of fish and other marine foods rich in these fatty acids increases birth weight and duration of pregnancy through such prostaglandin inhibition. One study evaluated pregnancy outcome and the ratio of omega-3 fatty acids to arachidonic acid in maternal red blood cells in Faroese and Danish women. Faroese women, who consumed a diet 20% higher in omega-3 fatty acids than that of the Danish women, experienced an increase in pregnancy duration of 5.7 days as well as higher mean birth weight. In an earlier controlled trial conducted in London, pregnant women were given a dietary supplement containing vitamins, minerals, and halibut liver oil. Women who took the fish-oil-containing supplements had longer pregnancies than controls who received no supplements.

149

Heme-rich dietary sources of iron	
food and serving size	iron content (mg)
oysters (raw, 1 cup)	7.8
spinach (fresh, cooked, 1 cup)	6.4
duck (roasted, 1/2 duck)	6.0
lima beans (cooked, 1 cup)	5.9
beef liver (fried, 3 oz)	5.3
liver sausage (braunschweiger, 2 slices)	5.3
refried beans (canned, 1 cup)	5.1
sirloin steak (lean, broiled, 5 oz)	4.8
lentils (cooked, 1 cup)	4.2
clams (canned, 3 oz)	3.5
beets (canned, 1 cup)	3.1
apricots (dried, 1/2 cup)	3.0
mushrooms (cooked, 1 cup)	2.7
potato (baked, with skin)	2.7
sardines (canned, 3 oz)	2.6
lamb chop (lean, broiled, 5 oz)	2.6
almonds (slivered, 1/2 cup)	2.5
peas (frozen, 1 cup)	2.5
fried chicken (5 oz)	1.8
pumpkin (canned, 1/2 cup)	1.7
shrimp (canned, 3 oz)	1.4

Source: *Nutritive Value of Foods*, Home and Garden Bulletin 72, U.S. Department of Agriculture, 1991

Possibilities for prevention

Just as there is not one single cause for prematurity, there is no one therapy or method of prevention. Factors associated with prematurity that are not amenable to change include the patient's age, race, education level, and height at the onset of pregnancy. Factors that are potentially modifiable and can be targeted for interventional therapy include changes in work, reduced stress, improved nutrition, weight gain, and avoidance or treatment of sexually transmitted diseases. Still other factors, such as exposure to alcohol, tobacco, or other toxic substances, can be totally eliminated.

Improved access to early prenatal care is clearly one of most important interventional tactics. In terms of cost, according to 1989 statistics, the average expense of medical treatment for infants born at term to mothers who received adequate prenatal care was $400, whereas the average expense of medical treatment for each infant born prematurely to mothers who had no prenatal care was $9,800. Pregnancies are that are unwanted or never intended may result from the lack of contraceptive use, especially among sexually active teenagers. How many unintended pregnancies result in prematurity, as opposed to induced or spontaneous abortion or full-term live birth, is difficult to know. Nonetheless, there is ample evidence to suggest that women whose pregnancies are unwanted or unintended are less likely to seek early or adequate prenatal care, and this type of health-care-avoidance behavior clearly influences the rate of prematurity. It is possible to prevent these pregnancies with the provision of sex education and wide access to family-planning services. Several attempts to reduce prematurity incidence by altering modifiable risks, where possible, are worth highlighting.

A French program that works. One very interesting French program, conducted on a nationwide basis, was aimed at lowering the preterm-delivery rate. This program was evaluated over the period 1971–82 in the city of Haguenau (in the northeastern region) and was based on the outcome of nearly 17,000 singleton births. The preterm-delivery rate (delivery at less than 37 weeks' gestation) was reduced by 30% (from 5.8 to 4%), and the early-preterm-delivery rate (delivery at less than 32 weeks' gestation) by 40% (from 2.8 to 1.6%). This reduction was achieved by application of several fundamental principles.

Prevention of preterm delivery was based on the realization that certain physical efforts and activities of daily life induce uterine contractions that in turn increase the risk of prematurity. This concept had been introduced in the 1970s by Émile Papiernik of Paris. The basic preventive intervention consisted of advising women to reduce their physical efforts, especially those women in whom a higher risk had been identified during the course of the present pregnancy (even if these women had not previously delivered prematurely and even if they did not have medical complications in their obstetric histories). Great importance was given to the recognition of the uterine contractions by the woman herself. Once she was able to recognize her contractions, she could be instructed to avoid the particular circumstances that caused them. Other specific interventions included a change in the number and objectives of the prenatal consultations, rest "prescriptions," cessation of work after 32 weeks in normal cases and earlier if the mother developed pregnancy-related complications, preventive hospitalization in high-risk cases, home visits by midwives, and provision of household help by a family member.

The costs of this French program included additional prenatal visits, hospitalizations, and disability or work leave. The savings included reductions

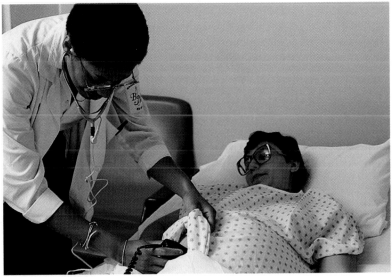

Ann Chwatsky—Phototake

Numerous studies have documented the importance of prenatal care in ensuring the birth of a healthy, full-term infant. The American College of Obstetricians and Gynecologists recommends that a pregnant woman have 13 to 15 physician visits—making the first visit early in the first trimester and then progressing to weekly checkups toward the end of the final trimester. Women with high-risk pregnancies need to see their obstetricians even more frequently.

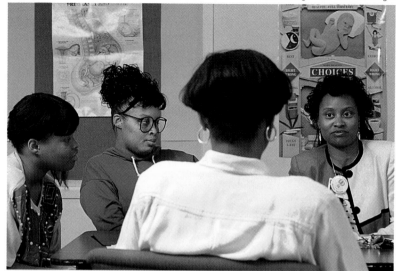

Low-income women enrolled in a health maintenance organization are paid $10 per visit to attend prenatal education classes run by a nurse-instructor. Maternal education—in addition to regular medical attention—is now well recognized as a crucial aspect of prenatal care. Women who take responsibility for their own well-being both before and during pregnancy are less likely to engage in risky behaviors that may endanger their fetuses and are more likely to recognize when something in the pregnancy is amiss.

in neonatal mortality, in neonatal intensive care unit stays, and in long-term handicaps in children. At the time the results of the French study were reported, an editorial in the *Los Angeles Times* speculated that if such a program were instituted in the U.S., for each $1 spent on prenatal care, it would be possible to save $3.50 on neonatal intensive care unit costs and another $6 on costs for long-term care of low-birth-weight babies and care for physical or mental disabilities that result from prematurity. Probably today the savings would be even higher. Unfortunately, the principle behind prevention as a cost-effective measure is not appreciated by third-party payers and government, at least at the present time.

More educated mothers-to-be. In the U.S. the educational components of many prenatal care programs have changed in two important ways in recent years. First, in many such programs the primary responsibility for patient education has shifted from physicians to nurses, and many physicians and clinics have hired nurse specialists or nurse midwives to serve in this role. Second, and perhaps more important, women themselves have begun to take greater responsibility for their own well-being during their pregnancies. These more enlightened women, who receive comprehensive prenatal care throughout their pregnancies, are aware that some of the discomforts of pregnancy—well known to but not understood by their mothers and grandmothers—may actually be signs of impending preterm labor, which could, if left unchecked, lead to a premature delivery of an immature infant. They are alerted that certain signs and symptoms such as back pain, cramps, mild contractions, and pelvic "heaviness" should be reported immediately to their medical care team. Moreover, mothers-to-be are now well informed about specific signs and symptoms that may indicate a problem at various stages of the gestational period. Often written materials accompany oral instructions, which helps ensure attentiveness to a wide variety of situations that may indicate that something is amiss.

The provision of this type of information is seen as a critical component of patient education, which significantly influences pregnancy outcomes.

Although maternal education had always been part of prenatal programs, in the past the patient often was expected to be a passive recipient of knowledge; thus, women were likely to watch for and report only the most dire developments—e.g., bleeding, leaking of amniotic fluid, or the onset of "hard" labor. The shift from passive to active patient participation means that there is a greater likelihood that an unfavorable outcome can be averted.

Better clinical care. One recent and remarkable change in prenatal care is the performance of vaginal examinations during the second half of pregnancy. The unquestioned value of vaginal examination at this stage is that subtle changes in length, consistency, and dilatation of the uterine cervix, which often precede preterm labor, can be detected. This knowledge is of great value for the clinician because it allows assessment of cervical changes in conjunction with other risk factors in the patient's pregnancy history and in the course of the current pregnancy. Any number of interventions can then be prescribed on a timely basis if warranted.

Routine vaginal examination had been used for more than a half century in European clinics but was not adopted in the United States because it was widely believed that these exams would lead to infection. Now many U.S. obstetricians appreciate that the benefits of assessment of cervical status far outweigh any real or theoretical risk.

Home uterine monitoring. Obstetricians have long realized that the uterus contracts throughout pregnancy despite the woman's general inability to perceive most contractions prior to the onset of labor. Some years ago it was determined that a crescendo of uterine activity occurred in the 24–48 hours before the cervix began to open, and thus the earliest clinical signs of labor could be recognized. U.S. investigators seized upon this information to devise technology that enables such contractions to be monitored on an ambulatory basis (preferably at home) and transmitted over the telephone to the pregnant woman's health care team (at a hospital, clinic, or satellite facility). Nurses who are trained to evaluate the frequency, intensity, and duration of these contractions can then inform the

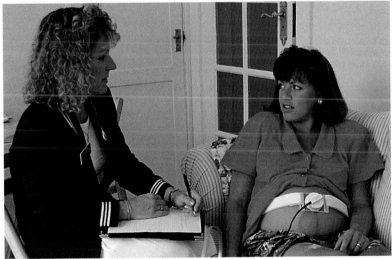

Karen Wollins

A registered perinatal nurse visits a woman at home to check her home-monitoring equipment. Because contractions occur throughout pregnancy, even though the woman herself may not be aware of them, technology was developed so that mothers-to-be who are at high risk for early labor can be continuously monitored at home. If at any time there is a crescendo of uterine activity, signaling that the cervix is about to dilate, a trained nurse or other specialist who receives the information over the phone can notify the woman's obstetrician. If necessary, she can then be admitted to the hospital, where medications that halt the contractions are expeditiously administered.

patient over the phone whether she should seek medical attention. The woman's obstetrician will determine whether she should be admitted to the hospital, where potent medications capable of stopping contractions can be administered if necessary.

Not all clinicians, however, agree about the value of home uterine monitoring. Those who are skeptical contend that the regular phone contact with a nurse or other health care provider is as valuable as the use of the monitoring equipment, if not more so. Insurance companies have also entered these debates, questioning the costs of home monitoring. As a consequence, a number of studies have been done. In 1990 three reports were published, all of which found home uterine monitoring to be a cost-effective measure when used for carefully selected, high-risk patients.

What price prematurity?

About 250,000 infants, the majority of whom are low birth weight, premature, or both, are treated annually in neonatal intensive care units in the United States. As noted earlier, in 1990, 10.5% of all U.S. births were premature, and about half of these infants were also low birth weight. Because the incidence of such adverse outcomes has not decreased, society is obliged to deal with the costs. In the most conservative terms, the annual cost to the nation of caring for these infants is no less than $12 billion.

Neonatal intensive care for very low birth weight (under 1,500 grams) ranks among the most costly of all hospital services; the lower the birth weight, the higher the costs. In 1988 a study conducted by the U.S. Office of Technology Assessment found the cost of caring for a single infant weighing less than 2,500 grams ranged from $12,000 to $39,000; the cost for an infant under 1,500 grams ranged from $31,000 to $71,000. Infants who survived with birth weights under 750 grams averaged the longest hospital stays (about 98 days) and incurred the highest costs—$62,000 to $150,000. By comparison, the average cost of hospital delivery for a normal-birth-weight, full-term baby in 1988 was $1,200.

Low-birth-weight infants have higher rates of respiratory, gastrointestinal,

In 1990, 10.5% of all infants born in the U.S. were premature—about half of them being low birth weight as well. The cost of keeping these babies alive in today's neonatal intensive care units can run as high as hundreds of thousands of dollars for a single infant. The annual cost to the nation for their care is no less than $12 billion. Clearly, prevention is a bargain.

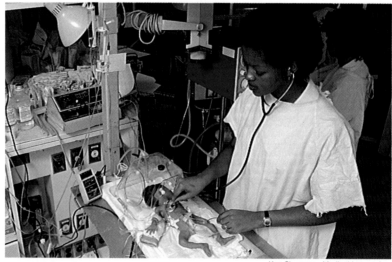

Ken Sherman—Medical Images Inc.

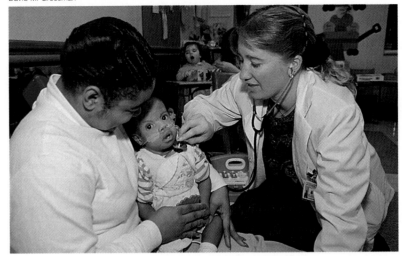

David M. Grossman

Though today's wonders of technology may enable the tiniest and frailest "preemies" to survive, they may face a future of lifelong health problems.

and infectious diseases than do infants born at normal weights. Low birth weight and prematurity result not only in initial hospitalization costs but in more frequent subsequent hospitalizations and the need for intensive health care due to chronic illness and disabilities. One study of rates of rehospitalization by birth weight in eight regions of the U.S. found that 19% of low-birth-weight infants who survived the first year were rehospitalized, compared with 8.4% of normal-birth-weight infants. Moreover, the average length of stay for rehospitalization for a low-birth-weight baby was three times that of a baby born at normal weight. Many of these children also incur long-term costs associated with institutional or foster care and special education.

Neonatal intensive care, along with improved obstetric practices, has been responsible for substantial reductions in birth-weight-specific neonatal mortality over the past 25 years. Mortality for infants with birth weights under 1,000 grams has fallen from 90% to about 50% and from more than 50% to only 10% for infants weighing 1,000 to 1,500 grams. Advances in medical technology have had a substantial impact on the treatment of infection, intracranial hemorrhage, and respiratory distress syndrome, which together occur in approximately 380,000 premature infants born in the U.S. each year. In the early 1990s the Food and Drug Administration approved two kinds of pulmonary surfactant, a lifesaving drug that has greatly increased premature infants' chances of survival. This means, however, that there are now larger absolute numbers of both normal and seriously handicapped survivors.

Unfortunately, the technology cannot determine at birth which infants are doomed to severely handicapped lives; an extremely premature infant's chances for survival and normal development are largely determined by where and under what circumstances the baby is born. Unquestionably, the best therapy for prematurity is prevention. As the *New York Times* editorial cited at the outset concluded, "Medical technology has met the challenge of keeping tiny babies alive. The greater challenge is to reduce the need for those marvelous machines."

HUNGER
IN THE MIDST OF WAR

by Michael J. Toole, M.D., D.T.M.&H., and
Daniel S. Miller, M.D., M.P.H.

They are walking carrion and die in daily lots of 50 in some places, 300 in others. Seldom are there mourners. Their deaths are either a relief for equally famished relatives or a matter of total indifference.
—Kenneth Freed, reporting from Kismaayo, Somalia,
Los Angeles Times, Dec. 22, 1992

It was food more than her exhaustion and fear that seemed to grip Mrs. Mutapcic as she lay in the snow. "My babies are hungry," she said.
—John F. Burns, reporting from Sarajevo, Bosnia,
New York Times, Jan. 15, 1993

On Dec. 9, 1992, American troops landed on a beach in Mogadishu, Somalia's capital, and quickly secured the airport. Authorized by a United Nations Security Council resolution, U.S. and other national military forces attempted to restore order to an anarchic nation to allow the distribution of food and medical supplies to a hungry and intimidated population. By permitting this military intervention, the international community took an unprecedented step toward guaranteeing the basic survival and human rights of people in countries where governance has totally broken down or where governments have intentionally blocked humanitarian relief efforts.

At the same time, the specter of hunger induced by war and civil conflict had emerged in Europe. In early 1993 in Bosnia and Herzegovina, heroic efforts were launched to deliver food to besieged communities in Sarajevo and the remaining Muslim enclaves in eastern Bosnia. More than 200 metric tons of food were flown into the dangerous Sarajevo airport every day, and road convoys, heavily guarded by UN troops, made their way through Serb-controlled Bosnia to deliver food and medical supplies to remote valleys where thousands of Muslims were trapped.

New world disorder

The military-supported relief operations in Somalia and the former Yugoslavia did not represent the first times that the UN had launched such

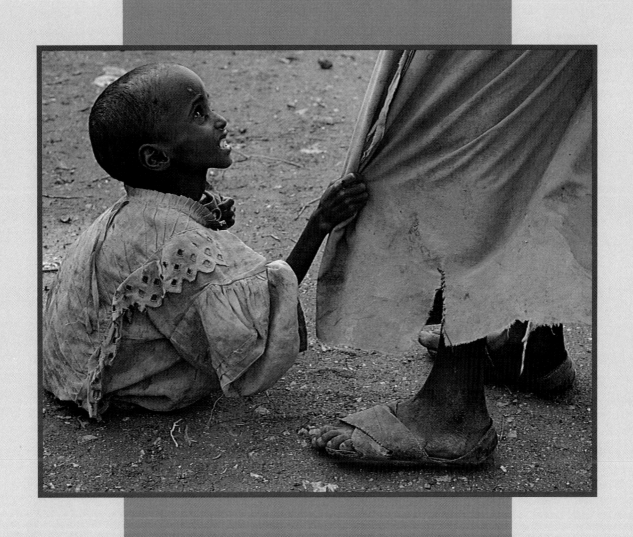

Michael J. Toole, M.D., D.T.M. & H.,
is a medical epidemiologist with the
International Health Program Office,
Centers for Disease Control and Prevention
(CDC), Atlanta, Georgia.
Daniel S. Miller, M.D., M.P.H., is a
medical epidemiologist, Division of Cancer
Prevention and Control, CDC.
This article was prepared in their private
capacity. No official CDC support or
endorsement is intended.

(Overleaf) Photograph, Andrew
Holbrooke—Black Star

interventions. A similar approach had been taken following the Persian Gulf war in early 1991, when half a million Kurdish refugees were trapped in the mountains of northern Iraq without adequate means of survival. The military forces that mounted the relief operation in Kurdistan in northern Iraq were provided by the same nations that had fought the war against Iraq. No such geopolitical self-interest, however, was apparent in the case of Somalia, and the scale of the operation—covering much of southern Somalia—was without precedent.

France was the first country to call for forceful intervention by the UN to ensure the delivery of humanitarian assistance. The French minister for health and humanitarian action, Bernard Kouchner, had for some time claimed that the global community has *le droit d'ingérence* ("the duty to intervene") in situations like those in Kurdistan and Somalia. Approximately 10 countries provided soldiers and military hardware to help with the Kurdish relief operation in 1991; by early 1993, 22 countries had pledged to do the same in Somalia. And soldiers from 10 countries guarded the relief convoys in Bosnia and Herzegovina, while both the U.S. and Germany airlifted food into the beleaguered country.

Clearly, a new era is dawning in which the international community may be more determined than ever before to safeguard the survival of civilians caught up in internecine warfare. It is not clear, however, if this principle of humanitarian intervention will be applied routinely and consistently wherever the need arises. Today there are already a dozen countries where such intervention could be justified by the desperate plight of geographically isolated or ethnically targeted communities. In southern Sudan, Mozambique, Liberia, Angola, Zaire, former Yugoslavia, Tajikistan, Armenia, Azerbaijan, Myanmar, Sri Lanka, and Bougainville (Papua New Guinea), many millions of people are deprived of much-needed humanitarian assistance because the international community cannot gain secure access.

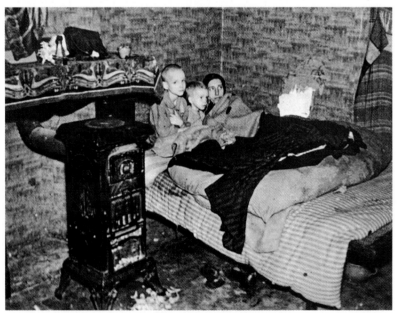

During the winter of 1944–45, members of a Dutch family try to keep warm by huddling in bed. A German blockade of The Netherlands during the last months of World War II caused that country to suffer one of the 20th century's most severe famines.

Rijksinstituut voor Oorlogsdocumentatie, Amsterdam, The Netherlands

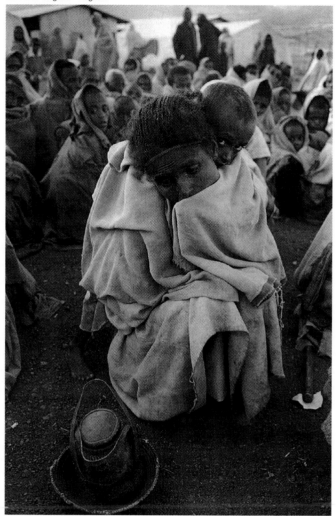

A starving mother and child wait for food to be distributed in a camp in Ethiopia. As often happens, the 1984–85 famine in that country was made worse by political rivalries—the Ethiopian government preventing delivery of food shipments to rebel areas.

Famine: not a "natural" disaster

Famine has been defined as a condition of populations in which a substantial increase in deaths is associated with inadequate food consumption. The key word in this definition is *consumption* since—contrary to popular belief—famines are not always due to problems of food availability. While natural catastrophes often act as a trigger, the underlying conditions within a population, which allow famine to develop, are generally human generated.

Lack of food for consumption arises as a result of any or all of the following circumstances: failure to produce food because of adverse climatic or other environmental conditions, such as drought, flooding, or locust plagues; failure to distribute food; and collapse of the marketing system, which, because of political, economic, or environmental crises, affects all or part of the population. While progressive deterioration of the ecological environment in the form of deforestation, overgrazing, and subsequent desertification and soil erosion has played a part in the evolution of some recent African famines, political upheaval and armed conflict have been

159

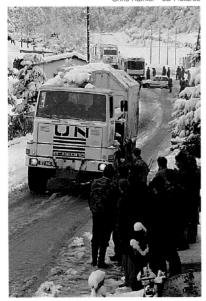

Famine may be the result of political crisis as well as crop failure. A United Nations convoy (above) attempts to deliver food in eastern Bosnia and Herzegovina, but the relief effort is thwarted by savage and ongoing fighting. A Bosnian prisoner of war (opposite page, top) in a Serb-controlled camp shows the ravages of hunger. In Armenia, embroiled in fighting with Azerbaijan over the enclave of Nagorno-Karabakh, a woman (opposite, bottom left) searches through garbage for food. In contrast, citizens of Malawi (opposite, bottom right) happily receive relief provided with the cooperation of the government.

common factors. The disastrous famines in Biafra, a region of Nigeria that had declared its independence (1969), Uganda (1981), Ethiopia (1984), Mozambique (1984), and The Sudan (1988) were all precipitated by civil war. The public generally associates famine with Africa and Asia; however, two of the worst famines of this century occurred in Europe. Severe famines in Leningrad in 1941 and The Netherlands in 1945 were the result of wartime blockades.

Most disturbingly, intentional starvation has apparently been used increasingly as a deliberate weapon of war by some governments and political organizations. While earlier historical examples of the use of food as a weapon include the Allied blockade of Germany in 1916–18, the practice has become more common in the past decade. In 1984–85 Ethiopian government forces prevented international food shipments from reaching civilians living in the rebel-controlled provinces of Tigray and Eritrea. Four years later both Sudanese government and rebel forces attacked and destroyed food convoys intended for starving civilian populations in southern Sudan. An estimated 250,000 southern Sudanese died in 1988 while efforts by international relief organizations such as the International Committee of the Red Cross (ICRC) were thwarted by rival military groups. Armed forces on all sides of the conflict in former Yugoslavia blatantly attacked or obstructed food deliveries intended for hungry civilians; night after night in early 1993, evening television news projected images of rows of trucks loaded with food standing idle at Serb checkpoints in snowbound eastern Bosnia.

World hunger, 1992–93

At the beginning of 1992 major food shortages were predicted in three regions of the world: the republics of the former Soviet Union, southern Africa, and eastern Africa. In the former Soviet Union predictions of famine were based on the rapid collapse of the economy, spiraling inflation, and political chaos. In southern Africa the worst drought in many decades caused major crop losses, even in countries that normally export large quantities of food, such as South Africa and Zimbabwe. In the countries of the Horn of Africa (Somalia, Ethiopia, Djibouti) and in The Sudan and Kenya, a severe drought and continuing political turmoil led the UN to forecast widespread food shortages. However, by the end of the year in all three regions, famine had actually occurred only in those countries where wars raged.

In the former Soviet Union very few deaths were attributed to food scarcity during 1992; only in Armenia and Azerbaijan, two republics that were fighting over the disputed enclave of Nagorno-Karabakh, had food shortages led to hunger. Farther south, in the republics of former Yugoslavia, starvation was intentionally used as a weapon in the campaign of regional "ethnic cleansing." Photos of emaciated prisoners of war in Bosnia and Croatia startled the world with their evocative reminders of World War II concentration camps. In January 1993 the World Health Organization (WHO) estimated that adults in Bosnia and Herzegovina had lost an average of 12 kilograms (26 pounds) of body weight since the turmoil began.

Almost one-third of children under five years of age were identified as moderately or severely malnourished. In the Muslim enclave of Zepa in eastern Bosnia, approximately 1,200 deaths occurred among the 33,000 residents between April 1992 and March 1993; 675 of the deaths were reported as "hunger related," and more than 400 resulted from war-related injuries. These deaths in Zepa represent an annual death rate four times higher than the death rate in that besieged enclave in the year before the fighting broke out.

In southern Africa famine was averted in Zimbabwe, South Africa, Zambia, Malawi, Botswana, Swaziland, and Lesotho by timely relief assistance provided by governments and international aid organizations. In Mozambique, however, aid efforts were hampered by continuing warfare; hundreds of thousands of hungry Mozambicans besieged relief centers, particularly in the provinces of Sofala, Manica, Gaza, and Inhambane. An estimated two million Mozambicans were displaced from their homes by the combination of war, drought, and economic collapse. The Mozambican Ministry of Health estimated that a basic survival diet for one person would cost 26,500 meticais (about $9) per month during 1992; thus, a family of five would require a monthly income of 132,500 meticais. The average family wage in the capital, Maputo, however, was calculated at 68,300 meticais, enough to purchase only one-half the family's minimal food requirements. More than 150,000 Mozambicans fled to the refugee camps of neighboring Zimbabwe and Malawi. The severe deprivation suffered by these refugees prior to leaving their country is illustrated by death rates in Zimbabwean refugee camps. During July and August 1992 the daily death rate among Mozambican refugees who had been in the Zimbabwean camp of Chambuta for less than one month was 8 per 10,000 population per day. This was 4 times the death rate of refugees who had been in the camp between one and three months and 16 times the death rate normally reported for nondisplaced populations in Mozambique.

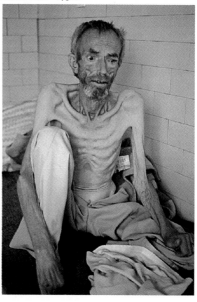

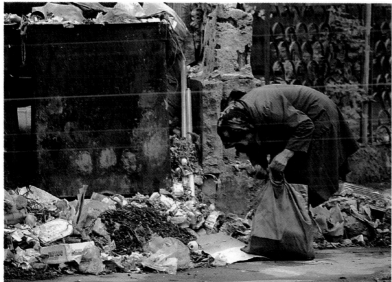

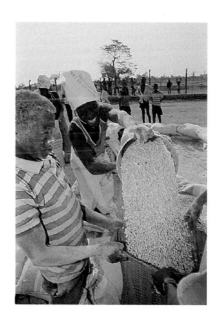

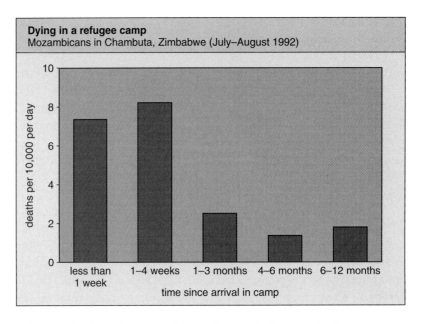

Dying in a refugee camp
Mozambicans in Chambuta, Zimbabwe (July–August 1992)

deaths per 10,000 per day (y-axis)

time since arrival in camp (x-axis): less than 1 week, 1–4 weeks, 1–3 months, 4–6 months, 6–12 months

In The Sudan, Kenya, and Somalia, predictions of famine were accurate—the deadly combination of drought and war affecting millions of people. Nevertheless, severe hunger was prevented in Ethiopia and Kenya by effective humanitarian relief distributed by the government, a consortium of UN relief organizations, the ICRC, and many private voluntary organizations. The escalation of armed conflict in Somalia and southern Sudan led to an increase in refugee flows that affected every country in the region. During 1992 an estimated eight million people in The Sudan, Ethiopia, and Somalia had either fled into neighboring countries (international refugees) or been displaced within their own country (internal refugees). It is this dangerous progression of events—war, hunger, and mass population displacement—that defines the current global hunger and humanitarian crises.

International refugees

In 1990 the plight of the world's refugees was critical. At that time there were approximately 14 million refugees who had fled their countries because they had a well-founded fear of persecution based on their religion, ethnicity, nationality, or political beliefs. Refugees are protected under several international legal conventions, and they are entitled to assistance from the Office of the United Nations High Commissioner for Refugees (UNHCR). Since the beginning of the decade, the cold war has ended and dramatic changes have taken place on the world map. Some civil wars that began prior to 1990 have stopped, in part because the main adversaries in the cold war (the Soviet Union and the United States) ceased to support the military forces that were engaged in those wars. Civil wars in Ethiopia, Mozambique, Nicaragua, and Cambodia have either ended completely or diminished in intensity. However, in other countries such as Angola, Afghanistan, and The Sudan, armed conflicts have been rekindled. In addition, new and ferocious conflicts have begun—most notably in former Yugoslavia, Somalia, Liberia, Tajikistan, and Azerbaijan. As a result of these new conflicts, the number of refugees dependent upon international assistance had increased dramatically to approximately 18 million by the end of 1992 (*see* Table 1).

While death rates among newly arriving refugees were high in some populations (*e.g.,* Somalis in Kenya and Bhutanese in Nepal), the situations usually improved relatively quickly as the international community mobilized its assistance. Within six months after refugees arrived in camps, death rates tended to return to near-normal levels. Such has not been

Table 1: International refugees, 1991–93			
place of origin	place of asylum	year of arrival	estimated population
Iraq*	Iran	1991	1,000,000
Iraq	Turkey	1991	450,000
Ethiopia	The Sudan	1991	51,000
Guinea	Sierra Leone	1991	170,000
Serbia, Bosnia and Herzegovina	Croatia	1991–92	288,000
Croatia, Bosnia and Herzegovina	Serbia	1991–92	463,000
Croatia	Bosnia and Herzegovina	1991–92	70,000
Croatia, Bosnia and Herzegovina	Montenegro	1991–92	64,000
Croatia, Bosnia and Herzegovina	Slovenia	1991–92	50,000
Croatia, Bosnia and Herzegovina	Macedonia (former Yugoslavia)	1991–92	32,000
Somalia	Kenya	1991–92	320,000
Somalia	Yemen	1992	50,000
Ethiopia	Kenya	1992	80,000
The Sudan	Kenya	1992	20,000
The Sudan	Ethiopia	1992	20,000
Mali	Algeria	1992	40,000
Myanmar	Bangladesh	1992	250,000
Bhutan	Nepal	1992	70,000
Mozambique	Malawi	1992	150,000
Mozambique	Zimbabwe	1992	60,000
Togo	Ghana	1993	80,000
Togo	Benin	1993	130,000
Tajikistan	Afghanistan	1993	60,000

*Kurdish refugees: most had returned to Iraq by the end of 1991

Source: United Nations High Commissioner for Refugees

Table 2: Refugees in their own countries (May 1993)	
country	estimated displaced population
The Sudan	5,000,000
South Africa	4,100,000
Mozambique	3,500,000
Somalia	2,000,000
former Yugoslavia	1,100,000
Philippines	1,000,000
Angola	900,000
former Soviet Union	750,000
Ethiopia	600,000
Liberia	600,000
Sri Lanka	600,000
Afghanistan	530,000
Myanmar	500,000
Peru	500,000
Iraq	400,000
Lebanon	400,000
Rwanda	350,000
Colombia	300,000
India	280,000
Cyprus	265,000
Cambodia	200,000
Sierra Leone	200,000
Uganda	200,000
El Salvador	155,000
Guatemala	150,000
Chad	100,000
Zaire	100,000
Turkey	30,000
Source: Refugee Policy Group, U.S. Committee for Refugees	

the experience of populations that have been trapped within their own countries by civil war, and the plight of internal refugees remains critical.

Internal refugees

During late 1991 and throughout 1992, up to two million Somalis fled their homes and sought shelter in makeshift displaced persons camps within the country. The same phenomenon occurred in The Sudan during the late 1980s; almost two million Sudanese fled the civil war in the south of their country and sought refuge in the slums that emerged on the edge of Khartoum, the nation's capital in the north. Despite the hostility of The Sudan's northern inhabitants, these internally displaced Sudanese were able to receive assistance from various international relief agencies based in the capital. Most of these same agencies were unable—or unwilling—to work in the southern war zones. In Mozambique an estimated two million to three million inhabitants were displaced by the combination of war and drought that created famine conditions in much of the country in 1992. Many camped along the main roads, or "corridors," that link Mozambican ports with landlocked Zimbabwe and Malawi, in the hope of benefiting from food distribution. In Liberia, Angola, Zaire, and Ethiopia, many hundreds of thousands of civilians were displaced—and continue to be—by long-standing civil conflicts.

The pattern in each of these countries is similar; a rebellion by an ethnic or regional minority is followed by an extensive period of "low-intensity" warfare. The normal income-earning and food-producing activities of the people are severely disrupted, and periodic drought sometimes exacerbates the problem. By the end of 1992 an estimated 25 million people worldwide were refugees within their own country (see Table 2).

Internal refugees are not unique to Africa. In Europe the situation has been complicated by the recent creation of new nation-states. In former Yugoslavia one million displaced civilians who would have been classed as internal refugees in Yugoslavia suddenly became international refugees in the newly separated states of Croatia, Slovenia, Serbia and Montenegro, Bosnia and Herzegovina, and Macedonia. The UNHCR estimates that a total of two million people are either international or internal refugees in one or another of the republics that used to constitute Yugoslavia. Hundreds of thousands of internal refugees have fled armed conflicts in several republics of the former Soviet Union; e.g., Armenia, Azerbaijan, Georgia, and Tajikistan. In Asia millions have been displaced by civil wars in Afghanistan, Sri Lanka, Myanmar, the Philippines, and Cambodia. Only in Latin America has the situation for the internally displaced improved since the end of the 1980s. Under the conditions of UN-supervised peace agreements between the various factions involved in civil wars in Guatemala, El Salvador, and Nicaragua, almost one million internal refugees in Central America have returned home.

Demise of public health

The public health consequences of war, hunger, and population displacement result from a fairly consistent chain of events. While the actual armed

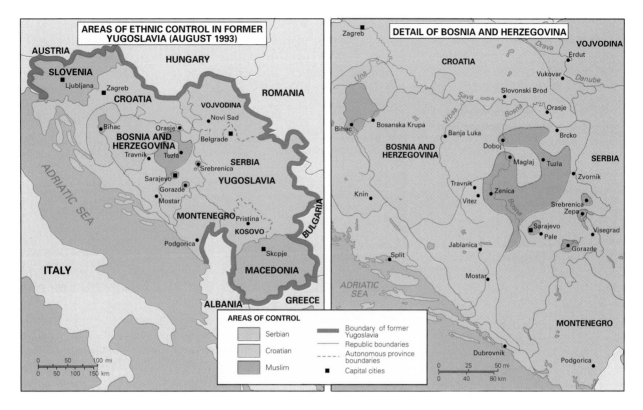

AREAS OF ETHNIC CONTROL IN FORMER YUGOSLAVIA (AUGUST 1993)

AUSTRIA
SLOVENIA
Ljubljana
Zagreb
CROATIA
HUNGARY
ROMANIA
VOJVODINA
Bihac
Orasje
Novi Sad
BOSNIA AND HERZEGOVINA
Belgrade
Travnik
Tuzla
Srebrenica
SERBIA
Sarajevo
YUGOSLAVIA
Gorazde
Mostar
MONTENEGRO
Pristina
KOSOVO
Podgorica
Skopje
ITALY
MACEDONIA
ADRIATIC SEA
ALBANIA
GREECE
BULGARIA

AREAS OF CONTROL

Serbian
Croatian
Muslim

Boundary of former Yugoslavia
Republic boundaries
Autonomous province boundaries
Capital cities

0   50   100 mi
0   50   100   150 km

DETAIL OF BOSNIA AND HERZEGOVINA

Zagreb
CROATIA
VOJVODINA
Drava
Erdut
Vukovar
Danube
Slovonski Brod
Una
Sava
Orasje
Bihac
Bosanska Krupa
Banja Luka
Brcko
Vrbas
Bosna
Doboj
BOSNIA AND HERZEGOVINA
Maglaj
Tuzla
SERBIA
Zvornik
Knin
Travnik
Zenica
Vitez
Bosna
Srebrenica
Zepa
Sarajevo
Pale
Visegrad
Jablanica
Gorazde
Split
ADRIATIC SEA
Mostar
MONTENEGRO
Dubrovnik
Podgorica

0   25   50 mi
0   40   80 km

conflict may directly cause many thousands of deaths from injuries, most civilian deaths are indirectly related to the violence. An estimated 14,000 Somali civilians died of injuries during the civil war in Mogadishu. By early 1993 more than 10,000 residents of Sarajevo had been killed as a result of Serb shellings from nearby mountains. Fear of violence often prompts communities living in proximity to the war zones to flee their homes. In many cases this violence is intentionally directed at civilians; for example, Muslim civilians in Bosnian enclaves were the targets of shelling, and the

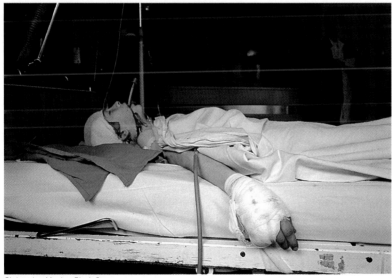

Christopher Morris—Black Star

A child injured in the fighting in Sarajevo receives treatment in a hospital. Tens of thousands of citizens of the Bosnian capital have been killed or wounded, largely during shellings of the city carried out by Serbs from the surrounding mountains; often the violence is intentionally directed at civilians.

Continuing warfare in Bosnia and Herzegovina prevents the planting and harvesting of crops and disrupts other basic activities, leading to widespread hardships for ordinary citizens. A man in a home for the aged (right) suffers from shortages of food and heat, and a woman desperately seeking drinking water in Sarajevo (below right) tries to shield herself from snipers.

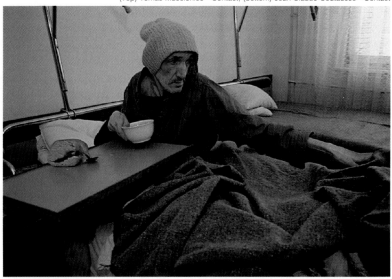

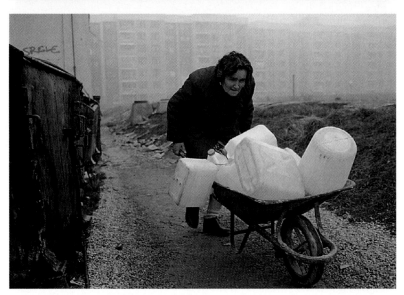

systematic rape of women in Bosnia and Herzegovina and Croatia has been well documented. Because of the uncertainty created by ongoing war, local farmers often do not plant crops as they normally would. Furthermore, the supply of seeds and fertilizer may be disrupted, irrigation systems may be damaged by the fighting, and crops may be intentionally destroyed or looted by armed soldiers. The resulting food shortages cause prolonged hunger and may eventually drive families from their homes in search of relief.

Displaced populations tend to migrate toward cities or large towns, where they set up temporary homes in makeshift camps where the supply of clean water is almost always inadequate and sanitation facilities absent. In these crowded and unsanitary conditions, epidemics of infectious diseases—such as measles, diarrhea, and meningitis—are common. The combination of malnutrition and infectious disease is a deadly one. Data

166

Table 3: Displacement and death*			
study site	date	deaths per 1,000 per month (displaced population)	deaths per 1,000 per month (nondisplaced population)
Mozambique (Gaza)	1983	8.1	1.4
Ethiopia (Korem and Harbu)	1984	60–140	2.0
The Sudan (El Meiram)	1988	90.0	1.7
Liberia (Monrovia)	1990	7.1	1.1
Somalia (Marka)	1991–92	13.8	2.0
Somalia (Baydhabo)	1992	51.0	2.0
The Sudan (Ame)	1992–93	17.0	1.7
The Sudan (Ayod)	1992–93	20.0	1.7
Bosnia (Zepa)	1992–93	3.0	0.7
*compiled from multiple sources			

collected in displaced persons camps in The Sudan, Mozambique, Liberia, and Ethiopia prior to the crisis in Somalia indicated that death rates were between 7 and 70 times higher than the death rates among nondisplaced populations in those countries (see Table 3). Surveys of such populations have repeatedly demonstrated that those most at risk are children under the age of five and the elderly.

The main causes of death tend to be similar in each population; measles, diarrhea, malnutrition, and pneumonia usually cause more than 80% of all deaths. Malaria may be responsible for many deaths in countries where it is endemic, and epidemics of meningitis, cholera, typhoid fever, and hepatitis occur often in the unsanitary camps that house displaced communities.

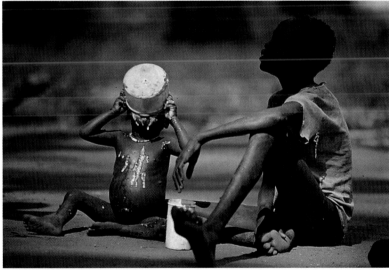

Derek Hudson—Sygma

Sudanese children eat food provided for them in a camp for displaced persons. Fighting in The Sudan and other African countries in the 1990s has created large numbers of persons displaced from their homes, many of them suffering from malnutrition and consequently highly susceptible to infectious diseases.

While protein-energy malnutrition is common among young children in these situations, displaced persons who rely on foreign donations of food (usually grains and vegetable oil) are also at risk for micronutrient-deficiency diseases that are relatively rare under normal conditions. These diseases, such as scurvy (caused by a lack of dietary vitamin C) and pellagra (caused by a deficiency of niacin) have been reported recently in many African refugee camps and in former Yugoslavia.

Women of childbearing age are particularly vulnerable to nutritional deficiencies. Studies of the distribution of scurvy in Ethiopian refugee camps and pellagra in Malawian camps, for example, have shown a much higher prevalence of these diseases in women than in men. It is also common for women in refugee camps to suffer from iron deficiency anemia, which places them at high risk for potentially fatal complications, such as severe hemorrhaging during childbirth.

Focus on Somalia

Failure to act now will result in a horror worse than the Ethiopian famine and more devastating than the tragedy of Biafra, and there will be more images to haunt the conscience of the international community.
—R. Coninx, medical coordinator for Africa, International Committee of the Red Cross, writing in *The Lancet,* Sept. 12, 1992

Just when you think it can hardly get worse in Somalia, it gets worse.
—Editorial, *New York Times,* Nov. 4, 1992

The most dramatic example of widespread hunger during the year 1992 occurred in the eastern African nation of Somalia. How did this human tragedy come about? How successful were the international community's unprecedented humanitarian and food-aid relief efforts that were mounted in order to alleviate the crisis? What ultimate toll have war and consequent severe famine taken on the Somali people?

Evolution of the disaster. Somalia has an ethnically homogeneous population that shares a common language but is characterized by distinct tribes, or clans, with long histories of rivalries and hostilities dating back centuries. Somalia endured both British and Italian colonial rule until the 1960s, when it had a brief experiment with independent democracy that ended in a military coup. For the next 24 years Somalia was governed by a military dictator, Muhammad Siad Barre, whose regime was marked by political oppression that inflamed and exploited interclan rivalries. During that time, in addition to extensive exploitation and corruption, there was intense military buildup for warfare with neighboring Ethiopia over disputed ownership of the Ogaden plains.

While Somalia's wealthy lived in seaside villas and many were related to Siad through tribal and family connections, the remainder of the country suffered widespread poverty and deprivation. Over the years one-party rule and the lack of outlets for public dissent resulted in growing armed internal opposition, especially in northern Somalia. In January 1991 various clans and factions banded together to oust Siad. The civil war took an estimated 14,000 combatant and civilian lives in Mogadishu alone. Ten months after Siad's departure, a second civil war erupted among the crumbling alliances of numerous rival clans and subclans. The country was plunged into chaos and fragmented into "ministates"—an Islamic fundamentalist region in the northeast; an independent Somaliland in the northwest; central Somalia, including the capital, Mogadishu, where two factions pitting a wealthy businessman, Ali Mahdi Muhammad, against a former general, Muhammad Farah Aydid, fought for control; and southwestern Somalia, where Siad's son-in-law attempted to regain control.

Infrastructure decimated, chaos reigns. In the process of the turmoil, the country's economy and social and political institutions—and its entire infrastructure—were destroyed. By 1992 electricity, running water, and sanitation facilities were absent in most areas. Transportation systems and schools were damaged beyond repair; fuel and spare parts were scarce. Agriculture and trade were disrupted as tens of thousands of farmers fled the countryside to avoid the warfare. Irrigation systems and water wells were blown up. Many hospitals and clinics were looted or completely leveled. Medical personnel were killed or exiled. There were no police, no

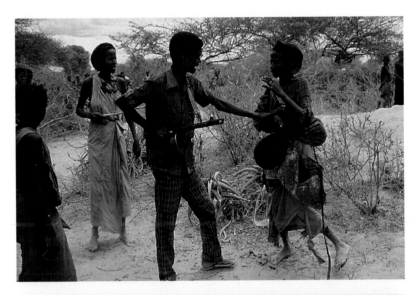

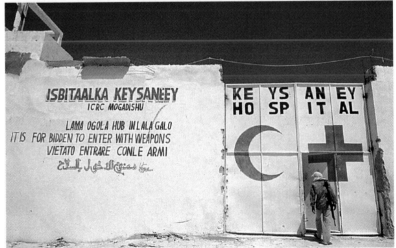

(Top) Andrew Holbrooke—Black Star; (bottom) Jose Nicolas—Sipa

In 1992 looting was a way of life and survival in much of Somalia, making relief efforts extraordinarily difficult if not impossible. An armed bandit (above left) holds up a woman for the food she has; the extent of the breakdown of order is apparent at an International Red Cross hospital in Mogadishu (left), where a sign forbids entry with weapons.

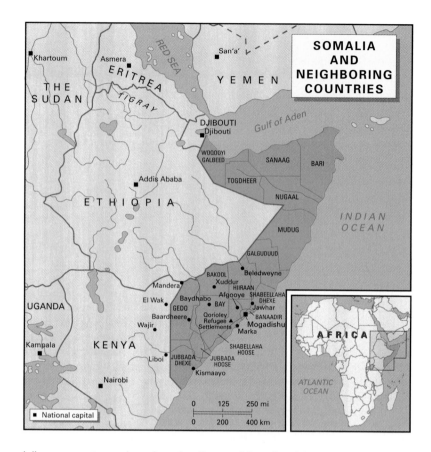

jails, no courts, and no law. Looting and banditry became a way of life and survival. Men and boys as young as nine years of age armed with AK-47 and Browning semiautomatic rifles cruised the streets of Mogadishu and the countryside in pickup trucks modified to carry machine guns and antiaircraft and antitank weapons. The arms were a legacy of the cold war of the previous two decades, when the Soviet and U.S. governments provided massive military aid to countries in the region.

Drought leads to famine. Superimposed on the warfare and chaos was a severe and prolonged drought, which began in late 1990 when the short rainy reason (*Der*) was lighter than normal; then the normally long rainy season (*Gu*) failed to arrive altogether in early 1991. Crops that were planted by the few remaining farmers were devastated. The combination of drought and social disintegration resulted in catastrophic famine. Consequently, there were massive population migrations of as many as 900,000 people out of war-torn rural and urban areas to refugee camps in Kenya, Ethiopia, Djibouti, and Yemen. Many of the refugees traveled on foot over hundreds of kilometers to cross the borders of Somalia in search of safety and food, and many reportedly died of hunger during their march. Others died in attempts to cross the Gulf of Aden or to escape to Kenya in small, desperately overpacked boats.

International aid stymied. During 1991 and the early part of 1992, the supply of international food relief within the borders of Somalia was at best erratic. By late 1990, during the height of the war to depose Siad,

170

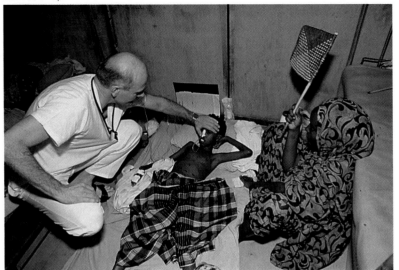

A French doctor with the group Médecins sans Frontières treats a child in a camp outside Mogadishu. Though numerous nongovernmental international relief organizations have attempted to give assistance in Somalia, their efforts are often prevented or disrupted by the country's continuing state of political instability.

scores of international embassy staff, relief workers from nongovernmental organizations, and all UN personnel had been evacuated from the country. The efforts of the few remaining relief organizations—the ICRC, SOS International, and Save the Children Fund (U.K.)—were severely restricted by the unremitting killing and destruction. It was not until mid-1991, as relative calm was restored, that relief organizations began to filter back into Somalia.

In June 1991 a report on the food-supply situation and crop prospects in sub-Saharan Africa prepared by the UN's Food and Agriculture Organization indicated that food stocks in urban areas of Somalia had been depleted.

Table 4: Nutritional status of Somali children: periodic surveys			
survey date	organization	region or town	prevalence of malnutrition (%)*
June 1991	International Committee of the Red Cross	Gedo Bay Mogadishu Marka	50 68 81 99
February 1992	Save the Children Fund/U.K.	area from Mogadishu to Afgooye	32
April 1992	Médecins sans Frontières (France) and Epicentre	Marka and Qorioley	43 (residents) 47 (displaced in town) 75 (displaced in camps)
January 1993	Center for Public Health Surveillance (Somalia)	Baardheere Jawhar	38 14
February 1993	Center for Public Health Surveillance (Somalia)	north Mogadishu	10
*children aged five and under			

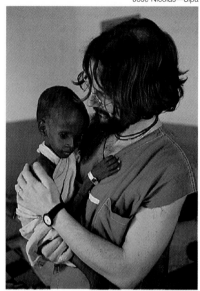

A relief worker holds an infant suffering from malnutrition. Mortality rates among children in Somali relief camps have been among the highest ever recorded anywhere.

Rural districts faced severe food shortages, with below-average aggregate food production and commercial imports at one-third of the previous year's level owing to a severe decrease in the country's purchasing power. At that time the ICRC made expeditions through south-central Somalia and observed widespread malnutrition (*see* Table 4, page 171) in western areas bordering Kenya (Gedo), the central region that was considered the agricultural breadbasket (Bay), Mogadishu, and the southern coastal town of Marka. During the latter half of 1991, the ICRC began general food-ration distributions, and Save the Children Fund (U.K.) opened supplemental feeding centers for malnourished children. The ICRC, Médecins sans Frontières (Doctors Without Borders, France), and the International Medical Corps (IMC) established surgical-training programs for Somali doctors and nurses in Mogadishu in an attempt to rebuild the medical infrastructure. Meanwhile, however, all national embassies except that of Egypt remained closed owing to the lack of an internationally recognized government in Somalia.

Then in November 1991 all aid efforts were again disrupted when the country exploded into another frenzy of warfare between two factions of the United Somali Congress. The small surgical units that had been trained by voluntary aid organizations became mobile army surgical hospital (MASH) units treating 150–200 cases of major trauma per day without the benefit of general anesthesia, adequate surgical supplies, or essential drugs. Many of the victims of warfare were women and children. The slaughter did not stop until March 1992, when a fragile and frequently violated truce was negotiated by the UN during Ramadan, the Islamic holy month.

Refugees' plight. During 1992 death rates among Somali refugees in the larger refugee camps of Liboi and Ifo that were officially sanctioned by the government of Kenya ranged between 1.5 and 2.4 per 1,000 population per month. (The normal average monthly death rate in Somalia is approximately 1.5.) Mortality tended to be much higher, however, among new arrivals from Somalia and among refugees in the "transit areas" or

A mother and her child head for a camp near Baydhabo. It has been estimated that as many as three million Somalis have been displaced from their homes, most of them settling in makeshift camps outside cities.

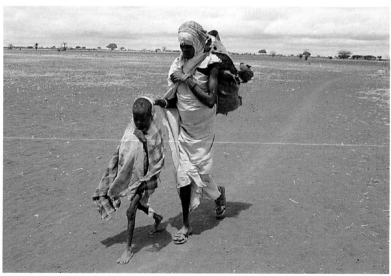

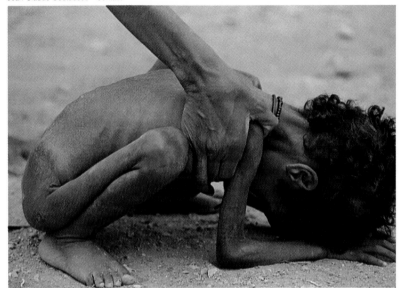

A Somali mother reaches to lift her starving child. Children under the age of five are the most ravaged by the combination of war and famine.

"receiving centers" that Kenya did not recognize as official refugee camps, such as El Wak (7.2 per 1,000 per month) and Mandera (11.4 per 1,000 per month). Lack of recognition meant that UNHCR had limited access to the camps and, therefore, refugees received fewer support services and less food and medical relief than those in the official camps. In addition, refugee-relief efforts by the government of Kenya, UNHCR, and nongovernmental organizations (*e.g.,* CARE, Catholic Relief Services, Médecins sans Frontières) were constrained by the need to assist indigenous populations of Kenya, who were also affected by the same severe drought.

Internally displaced. While almost one million Somalis had fled to refugee camps in neighboring countries, probably twice that number were displaced within Somalia. Having fled their homes because of violence or lack of food, these internally displaced families usually congregated in makeshift camps on the edges of large towns. Following the Ramadan "truce," close to one million displaced Somalis fled to Mogadishu, despite the dangers of living in a city where many of the inhabitants were heavily armed. Somalis displaced from rural areas and farms were drawn by the magnet of international food aid in the capital. They occupied almost every empty space in the city—areas in which the supply of clean water was inadequate and sanitation facilities were virtually nonexistent.

Starvation and death. Whereas ICRC surveys of displaced populations in mid-1991 had demonstrated malnutrition rates as high as 80%, surveys conducted in mid-February 1992 by Save the Children Fund (U.K.) found lower rates—approximately 30%. However, in April French relief workers completed a large random, population-based survey in Marka and Qorioley, south of Mogadishu, that covered 73,000 residents, 23,000 persons displaced in towns, and 7,000 displaced persons in camps. The results indicated widespread famine, with the highest risk of malnutrition or death being among displaced families (Table 4). In addition, the survey estimated that approximately 7% of the total population had died during the previous

173

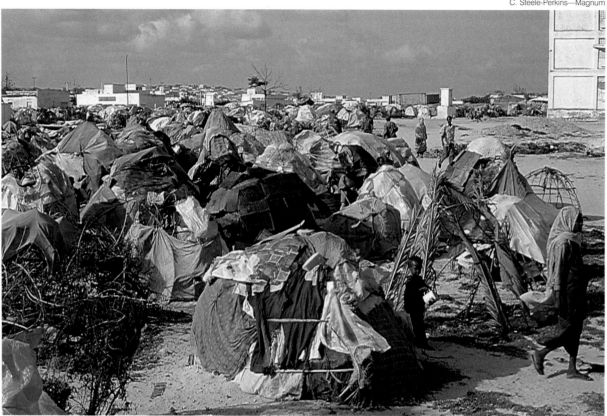

A camp in Mogadishu is home to an estimated one million displaced Somalis. Inadequate supplies of food and clean water and a lack of sanitation facilities make such places breeding grounds for disease.

year. The displaced in camps experienced the highest death rates, with children under five years being the most vulnerable (24% had died). The apparent improvement in nutritional status implied by Save the Children Fund surveys, therefore, might be explained by large numbers of deaths among the most vulnerable, leaving only the better nourished and healthier survivors to be measured in subsequent field surveys without there having been any real change in food availability or living conditions. Another explanation might be that the most affected members of the population had migrated out of the surveyed areas.

In late 1991 and early 1992, during the peak of the civil war, Médecins sans Frontières (France) surveys revealed that the leading causes of death were malnutrition and war casualties. In late 1992, however, infectious diseases such as measles and diarrhea were common, accounting for nearly 79% of deaths in the crowded and unsanitary displaced persons camps in Baydhabo.

Despite intensive relief efforts in some towns of south-central Somalia during 1992, field surveys in November revealed continued high death rates. For example, 39% of displaced persons in Baydhabo camps died between April and November 1992; in the same camps 70% of children under five years of age died—among the highest mortality rates ever documented anywhere in the world! In these camps it was not possible to obtain an adequate sample to measure the nutritional status of children because too few had survived.

174

By early 1993 various surveys of nutritional status and mortality suggested that malnutrition prevalence and mortality rates were finally decreasing, although baseline information from the surveyed areas was not available for comparison (Table 4). Data collected by the Italian relief agency Comitato Internazionale per lo Sviluppo dei Popoli (International Committee for the Development of Peoples; CISP), which operated maternal and child health clinics in northern Mogadishu, indicated that other major causes of illness among famine-affected populations in Somalia included respiratory infections (*e.g.,* pneumonia), malaria, intestinal parasites, skin infections, hepatitis, and tuberculosis. Vitamin A deficiency, which can cause scarring of the eyes and blindness, was also prevalent.

Relief efforts amid anarchy. In June 1992 the first television pictures of walking skeletons and fly-covered bodies, revealing the magnitude of the suffering and death in Somalia, were beamed into the living rooms of the developed world. Globally, the public was shocked. The resulting international response was massive. UN organizations such as UNICEF, the United Nations Development Program, the World Food Program, and a special envoy from the UN secretary-general returned to the country to attempt to coordinate aid efforts and to negotiate a lasting peace amid the anarchy. Numerous private relief agencies restarted operations or increased their personnel and scope of operations. However, all the aid organizations continued to work under extremely difficult circumstances, hampered by

Desperation forces homeless Somalis to attempt to survive in an overcrowded camp in Baydhabo.

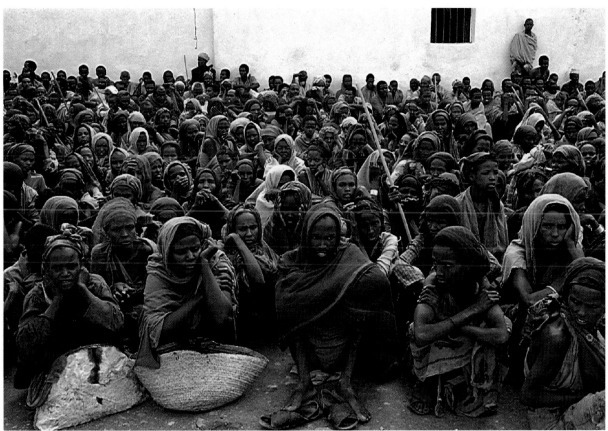

Andrew Holbrooke—Black Star

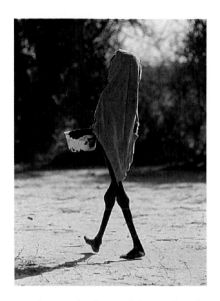

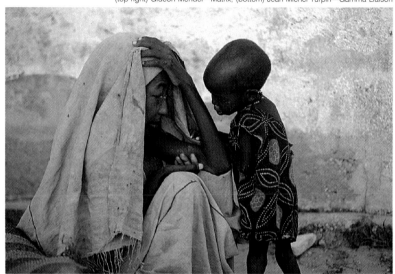

It was only after conditions in Somalia caught the attention of the media and reports of unprecedented numbers of starving, dying people reached television audiences that governments of other nations began to respond aggressively to the country's plight. People the world over were deeply affected by images of walking skeletons, starving mothers and children, and dead and abandoned bodies—all the innocent victims of civil unrest.

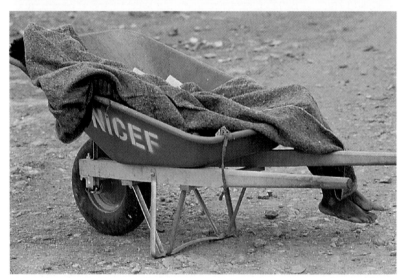

frequent random shootings, carjackings, armed robberies, and lootings, as well as intermittent skirmishes resulting from ever changing clan, family, and geopolitical alliances. The personal safety of the relief staff was always threatened because the warring factions neither acknowledged nor honored internationally sanctioned neutrality of humanitarian aid workers. Attempts to move food from the ports in Mogadishu or Kismaayo or across the border from Kenya into the interior were extremely dangerous undertakings and were often doomed to failure. It was estimated that 50–60% of all aid arriving in Somalia was looted from ports, warehouses, and transport vehicles before reaching its intended destination.

Military intervention. In August 1992, at the direction of U.S. Pres. George Bush, the United States military launched a massive airlift program to fly food and medical supplies directly to the communities in need. American C-130 Hercules aircraft flew hourly sorties from Mombasa, Kenya, into refugee camps in northern Kenya (Mandera and Wajir) and into towns in

176

south-central Somalia (Baydhabo, Beledweyne, and Xuddur), which had only unpaved or poorly paved landing strips. Air force planes from Canada, Germany, Italy, and Belgium joined the effort to supply Kismaayo and the now separate cities of north and south Mogadishu. The airlift, however, was limited to operating during daylight hours, was hampered by muddy landing strips during the rains, and was subject to intermittent armed attacks. Nonetheless, some of the food did eventually reach Somalis in need. On December 4 Bush authorized the mobilization of more than 30,000 U.S. troops to Somalia to ensure the safe delivery of relief supplies. Within days, relative calm was imposed on Mogadishu and, during the next two to three months, on most of southern Somalia. The U.S. troops were joined in the effort by soldiers from at least 20 other countries, including Italy, France, Belgium, Australia, Canada, Nigeria, and Egypt.

Food relief. Normally, famine-relief rations in one- to two-week supplies of dry commodities (rice, beans, etc.) would be distributed to families to be prepared in their own homes or shelters. However, in Somalia nearly half the rations were provided as daily meals of cooked rice and beans mixed with vegetable oil ("wet feedings") because recipients of dry rations were often attacked, robbed, and even killed. Moreover, the presence of large stockpiles of dry food would increase the likelihood of relief organizations' being attacked and looted. The ICRC became the major distributor of general food supplies in Somalia through a vast network of more than 750 kitchens serving cooked meals to approximately 750,000 to one million people a day.

Supplementary feeding centers were established by many relief organizations, including UNICEF, Médecins sans Frontières, Save the Children Fund, CISP, Action Internationale Contre la Faim (International Action Against Hunger; AICF), Irish Concern, and CARE, to provide additional caloric support to young children identified as being moderately malnourished. These centers provided daily or twice-daily meals consisting of

Attempts beginning in mid-1992 to airlift supplies into Somalia were hampered by armed attacks, but in December some 30,000 U.S. troops, joined by soldiers from other countries, were sent to restore order so that relief deliveries could be made. A U.S. soldier (below left) patrolling Mogadishu, where calm was quickly established, shakes the hand of a Somali boy. Sacks of food from France (below) are unloaded at the city's port for delivery by soldiers.

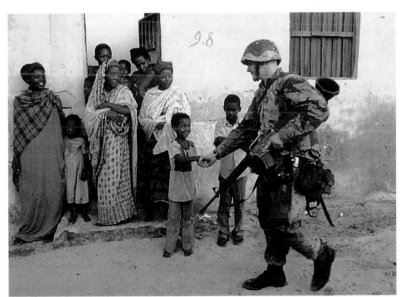

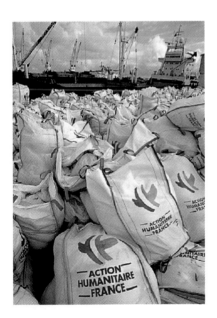

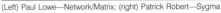

(Left) Paul Lowe—Network/Matrix; (right) Patrick Robert—Sygma

Once basic order had been restored in Somalia, sustained relief efforts could be undertaken. A baby (right) is given fluid to relieve dehydration. Residents of a camp near Baydhabo (far right) receive a meal at a local feeding center. A dying child is fed by a relief worker from Irish Concern (center), and a youngster is inoculated against measles (bottom) by a volunteer from the International Rescue Committee.

(Top left) C. Steele-Perkins—Magnum; (top right) Andrew Holbrooke—Black Star; (center) Betty Press—Picture Group; (bottom) Steve Lehman—Saba

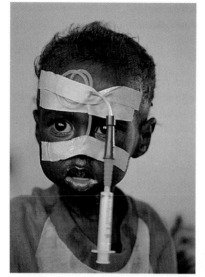
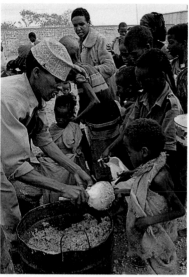
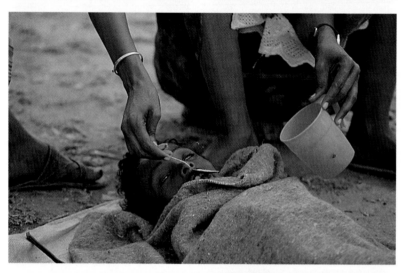
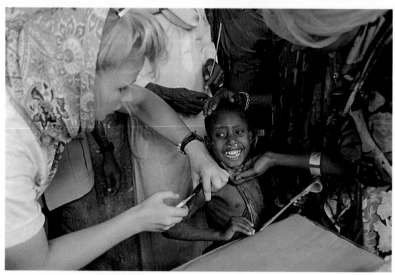

cooked porridge prepared from ground rice, ground beans, vegetable oil, and sugar. Unfortunately, because most families were unable to provide regular meals in the home, these "supplements" usually represented the only food that the affected children received each day. Many malnourished children in feeding centers did not begin to gain weight, despite intensive feeding, until concurrent infectious diseases were adequately treated. Therefore, most relief agencies routinely provided on-site medical support in the feeding centers, focusing on treating diarrhea with oral rehydration solution, giving antibiotics for respiratory infections, immunizing to protect against measles, and providing vitamin A supplementation.

A few therapeutic feeding centers were set up by AICF, Save the Children Fund, and Irish Concern to treat the most severely malnourished children, who are at the highest risk of dying. Unfortunately, it was too late for many such children to be saved; voluntary medical workers could provide only palliative care. CISP observed that nutritional rehabilitation of only moderately malnourished children required an average of three and one-half months. Moreover, in most feeding centers nearly 70% of children "defaulted"—*i.e.,* the children who were registered in the center attended for relatively short periods of time or only intermittently. The fate of these children is not known.

Restoring livable conditions. In addition to feeding centers and medical programs, some relief organizations focused their activities on helping to restore some degree of normalcy to life in Somalia. For example, Médecins sans Frontières workers from The Netherlands undertook demining of roads; British OXFAM workers began the rehabilitation of wells, pumps, and irrigation systems; and CARE distributed seeds and tools to encourage repatriation and the return of farmers to their land to reestablish an agricultural base. Reestablishment of a health care infrastructure was difficult and to a large extent impossible owing to the absence of a single, unified government. The northwest of the country declared its independence and established its own government and its own Health Ministry. In Mogadishu, although there were two separate Ministries of Health, an attempt was made to standardize public health programs and information collection through the establishment of a national Center for Public Health and Nutrition Surveillance, which was supported by UNICEF, WHO, and the U.S. Centers for Disease Control and Prevention.

Somalia's lessons

There are Somalias-in-waiting throughout Africa and the rest of the Third World.
—*The New Yorker,* Sept. 28, 1992

Relief officials say about 40,000 Sudanese who had taken refuge in the towns have fled into the bush and nearby swamps, where most are trying to survive on water lilies.
—Donatella Lorch, reporting from The Sudan,
New York Times, April 18, 1993

By March 1993 some semblance of order had been restored in most parts of Somalia; however, certain towns such as Kismaayo in the south of the country remained insecure. As the U.S. military began to hand over control to a multinational UN peacekeeping force, the quality of life for most Somalis had obviously improved greatly. Paradoxically, life had become more dangerous for foreign relief workers because the successful suppression of most looting had created intense resentment among the minority of the population that had profited from the earlier state of anarchy. Several foreign aid workers were the targets of vengeful snipers during the first few months of 1993. The drought was relieved by heavy rains in December 1992, and many farmers returned home to cultivate their fields. Nonetheless, Somalia remained a shattered nation; it will take many years to rebuild the country's infrastructure and to redevelop an effective national administration. This can happen only if and when a permanent peace is secured and a unified government created.

The lessons of Somalia need to be incorporated into the international community's collective consciousness. The world recognized the plight of the Somali people far too late to implement effective humanitarian aid measures to mitigate it. Ultimately, drastic action was necessary. In the future the early warning signs of impending famine need to trigger an automatic response from the world—one that comprises preventive interventions aimed at urgently ensuring both peace and the population's access to relief.

In early 1993, as U.S. troops began to depart from Somalia, reports of a massive humanitarian emergency were emerging from war-torn southern Sudan. Surveys of displaced Sudanese populations indicated that malnutrition rates were even higher than those recorded in Somalia during 1992. In March 1993 the acute malnutrition rates among children under five in Ame and Ayod were found to be 81 and 75%, respectively. In non-famine-affected populations in sub-Saharan Africa, acute malnutrition rates are normally less than 8%. The extent of the hunger in southern Sudan could be attributed only to the ongoing state of civil war. Yet despite this desperate situation, the world had not yet reacted to relieve the plight of the Sudanese.

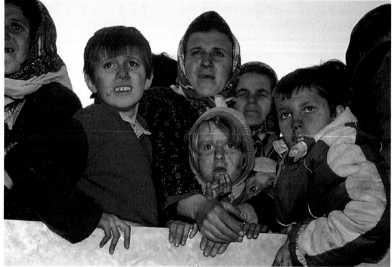

Courageous Bosnian civilians cling to the hope of safety and survival as a United Nations convoy carries them to Tuzla from their home in war-ravaged Srebrenica.

Chris Rainier—JB Pictures

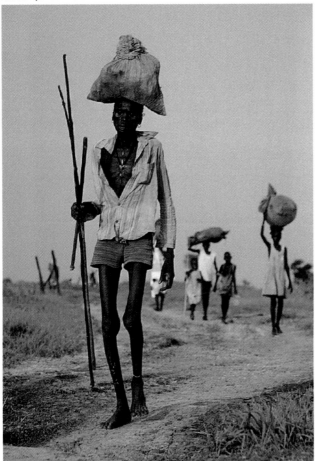

Uprooted from their homes, Sudanese trek toward a refugee camp. As civil war in this African nation continued in 1993, there were indications that starvation could reach levels even greater than those that occurred in 1992 in neighboring Somalia.

While the international community had mounted an extraordinary relief operation in former Yugoslavia, in March 1993 many food convoys were subjected to extended delays by Serb military forces, and the quantity of food that was being delivered was less than adequate for meeting even basic nutritional needs. Although the nutritional state of displaced Bosnians had not yet deteriorated to the level of Somalia and The Sudan, there were abundant warning signs that the situation could get much worse. Many hunger-related deaths were reported in the Muslim enclaves of eastern Bosnia.

Meanwhile, in Armenia, blockaded by its neighbors and overrun by refugees from adjacent Azerbaijan, elderly pensioners were close to starvation. Other countries that face crises potentially as serious as that of Somalia include Angola, Zaire, Mozambique, Liberia, Afghanistan, and Tajikistan. In all of these countries war is a major public health risk factor that will lead inevitably to hunger, displacement, crowded refugee camps, epidemics, and high death rates unless urgent action is taken. But humanitarian aid agencies cannot bear the entire burden of providing relief; without adequate security there can be no access to the affected populations and, therefore, no relief. What is clear is that in many parts of the world, hunger cannot be conquered without an enforced peace.

181

Hunger in America

by J. Larry Brown, Ph.D.

Hunger—defined as the chronic underconsumption of adequate nutrients for growth and proper maintenance of health—is a persistent problem in the U.S. It is also a growing problem. Recent figures suggest that 30 million Americans suffer from hunger. This number represents a 50% increase over that reported in 1985, when the Physician Task Force on Hunger in America alerted the nation that hunger had become a significant public health problem. Hunger in any wealthy nation is disturbing, but it is particularly so in the U.S., where the scope of the problem was dramatically reduced during the 1970s only to recur with a vengeance in the following decade.

Hunger is a serious matter to anyone who does not get enough to eat, but certain population groups are particularly susceptible to its ravages. Pregnant women, infants, and children, on the one hand, and elderly people, on the other, are likely to suffer the most grievous harm when food is inadequate. At any age, however, malnutrition can cause weakness and lethargy. It impairs the functioning of the immune system, making the victim more vulnerable to infectious disease. Absence or deficiency of specific nutrients causes a range of conditions—from anemia to rickets to blindness—affecting all the body's organ systems. In its most severe form, malnutrition leads directly or indirectly to death.

Unlike undernourished people in less developed countries, most hungry Americans receive enough calories to prevent overt emaciation. For this reason, hunger in America manifests itself quite differently from that in the Third World. Protein-calorie malnutrition, or marasmus, which is evident in the pictures of starving Somalian children, and kwashiorkor, characterized by extreme protein deficiency even when calories are adequate, occur rarely in the U.S. Instead, hunger in the U.S. tends to take the form the World Health Organization terms "silent undernutrition." It is reflected in the young child whose weight is several kilograms below the low end of the normal range on a growth chart. A layperson may easily miss this condition or simply see the youngster as a "skinny" child, but the trained professional will recognize that the child's size reflects growth failure. This form of hunger, though typically not as severe as hunger in less developed countries, is nonetheless significant from a health perspective.

J. Larry Brown, Ph.D., is Director, Center on Hunger, Poverty and Nutrition Policy, and Professor, Nutrition and Health Policy, Tufts University School of Nutrition, Medford, Massachusetts. He served formerly as Chairman of the Physician Task Force on Hunger in America.

Rural North Carolina, 1966; photograph, Bruce Roberts—Photo Researchers

182

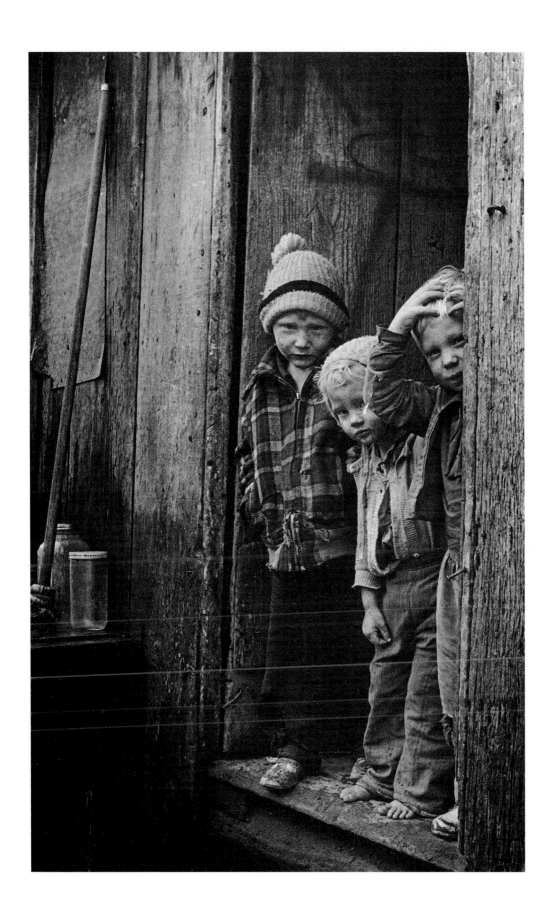

Hunger in recent times: a brief history

In 1967 a team of physicians was sent by the Field Foundation, a national nonprofit organization, to visit areas of endemic poverty in the U.S. These doctors, who visited Boston, Chicago, the hills of Appalachia, and Indian reservations of the West, reported observing children with the thin bodies and bloated bellies of kwashiorkor, along with cases of less severe malnutrition. In a report to Congress, the physicians described what they had seen:

If you go look you will find America is a shocking place. No other Western country permits such a large proportion of its people to endure the lives we press on our poor. To make four-fifths of a nation more affluent than any other people in history, we have degraded one-fifth mercilessly. . . . We do not want to quibble over words, but "malnutrition" is not quite what we found. They are suffering from hunger and disease and directly or indirectly they are dying from them—which is exactly what "starvation" means.

The '70s: a nation mobilized. The physicians' report on hunger in America received wide coverage in the news media and had a profound effect on the public conscience, compelling a national response. Political leaders including Presidents Lyndon B. Johnson and Richard M. Nixon, with strong bipartisan support from Congress, developed and expanded programs aimed at the elimination of hunger in America. One result was that the food-stamp program was expanded to serve more than 20 million people. Programs were also instituted to reach and feed the isolated elderly. The national school-lunch program was expanded and a school-breakfast program initiated so that poor children would have the nutritional base for academic success. To ensure the nutritional well-being of American children during the critical period of early growth, the so-called WIC program (Special Supplemental Food Program for Women, Infants, and Children), providing supplemental food for pregnant and lactating women, infants,

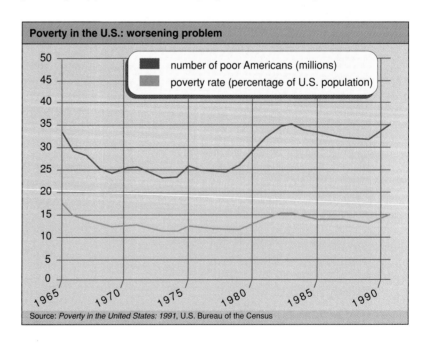

Poverty in the U.S.: worsening problem

- number of poor Americans (millions)
- poverty rate (percentage of U.S. population)

Source: *Poverty in the United States: 1991*, U.S. Bureau of the Census

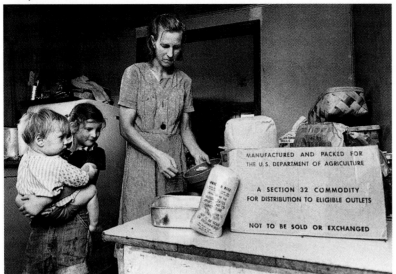

A mother in Appalachia prepares a meal using government surplus commodities. Hunger in this, the nation's poorest, section, encompassing parts of 11 states from southern New York to Georgia and Alabama, was a major target of the antipoverty programs of the 1960s during the administration of Pres. Lyndon B. Johnson.

and children, was developed. Collectively, these governmental responses virtually eliminated the condition of hunger during the 1970s—proving that hunger in the U.S. is indeed a "solvable" problem.

The '80s: ground lost. In 1981 Congress, at the behest of the administration of Pres. Ronald Reagan, began reducing these clearly successful programs as economic recession began to grip the nation. As early as 1982, signs of hunger were once again widespread. Increasing numbers of people going to churches and social-service agencies for aid admitted that they did not have enough food. Physicians in many parts of the country began to hear from patients who were hungry and to observe patients who manifested clinical conditions associated with hunger—among them anemia, tuberculosis, growth failure in children, and osteoporosis in adults.

More than 20 national studies were conducted between October 1982 and March 1986, the earliest being a report by the bipartisan U.S. Conference of Mayors that described hunger in America as "a most serious emergency." Other groups that surveyed and reported on the situation included the National Council of Churches, the U.S. Department of Agriculture (USDA), the Salvation Army, and the General Accounting Office. One of the most authoritative of these studies was that conducted by the Physician Task Force on Hunger in America, a national panel of experts assembled by the Harvard University School of Public Health. The group was composed of deans of schools of public health and medical schools, representatives of university nutrition departments, clinicians, and prominent leaders such as a former U.S. surgeon general and a former president of the American Academy of Pediatrics.

In its 1985 report entitled *Hunger in America: The Growing Epidemic,* this task force attributed the reappearance of domestic hunger to government policies and budget cutbacks. Following on the heels of other national studies, the task force report did much to reframe the debate over hunger in America. The group's estimate that some 20 million Americans were hungry provided—for the first time—a true sense of the scope of the

185

The number of children receiving federally subsidized meals in the school-lunch program was reduced by three million in the 1981–82 academic year, forcing many youngsters to go without enough to eat. Although some funding for school meals was restored between 1985 and 1988, hunger continued to be a growing U.S. problem.

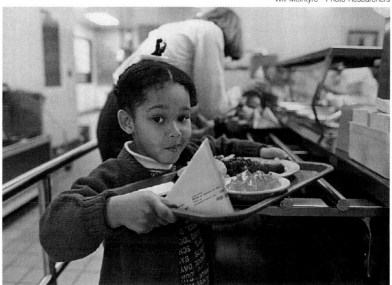

problem, enabling the public and Congress to grasp its significance. The report spelled out not only the devastating effects of hunger on the health of Americans but also its underlying causes.

Gradually, the evidence concerning hunger and its associated health effects began to make itself known. Leaders in Congress exhibited greater concern about the connection between public policies and the resurgence of hunger. Between 1985 and 1988 over $5 billion (to be spent over three-to-five-year periods) were added back to the food-stamp and school-meals programs. But these changes, while signaling a revived effort to respond to hunger, fell far short of the need. The lack of sufficient food programs, along with a faltering economy, resulted in the unabated growth of hunger during the remainder of the 1980s.

The '90s: a problem acknowledged. In April 1992 Vincent Breglio, Republican pollster for the *Wall Street Journal* and NBC News, conducted a nationwide opinion poll in which registered voters were asked to gauge the urgency of a variety of issues affecting the country. Ninety-three percent of those surveyed said that hunger was a serious national problem. The poll provided an indication of just how extensive hunger had become since the Physician Task Force released its 1985 estimate of 20 million hungry Americans. In testimony before the House Select Committee on Hunger, Breglio reported that 13% of survey respondents said someone close to them had experienced hunger during the past year. According to Breglio, that translated roughly into about 30 million people.

Following Breglio's testimony, Rep. Tony Hall (Dem., Ohio), chairman of the House Select Committee on Hunger, requested that the Medford, Massachusetts-based Tufts University Center on Hunger, Poverty and Nutrition Policy review existing data in order to more accurately estimate the number of hungry Americans. Two independent epidemiological models resulted in estimates that closely coincided with Breglio's. Notably, one of the models employed was the one first developed at the Harvard School of Public Health in 1985. Independent of the Breglio analysis, the updated

186

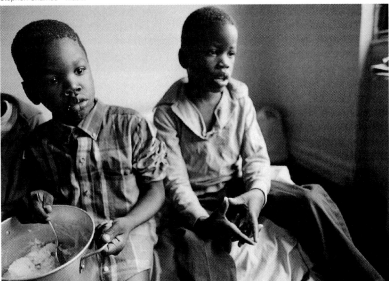

Harvard model reached the same conclusion—nearly 30 million Americans were hungry in 1992.

Undernutrition: cradle-to-grave effects

The health effects of chronic undernutrition—and the social impact of those health effects—make hunger a critical public health problem. Food is used by the body as energy to fuel all activities; it provides the building blocks for growth and development and enables the body to synthesize substances used to promote health and prevent or combat disease. Undernutrition, whether in terms of quantity of food or quality, may compromise any of these functions. The human organism is particularly vulnerable to hunger in periods of rapid growth, such as infancy and adolescence, and in old age.

Early life. The period of greatest risk from hunger is before birth; the

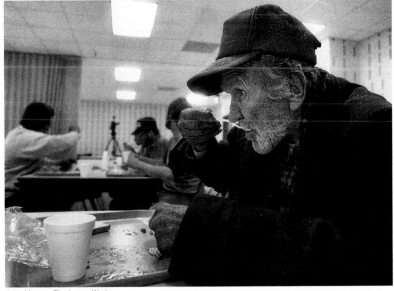

The impact of malnutrition on health is greatest in the young and the elderly. (Above) Youngsters living in a one-room apartment in a Brooklyn, New York, welfare hotel watch television as they eat a meager meal. Children who do not get enough to eat during the years of rapid growth are likely to suffer developmental deficits. (Left) Nutrient needs increase in later life. The inadequate diet of this Austin, Texas, senior could heighten his vulnerability to infection.

pregnant women needs extra nutrients to meet the needs of the developing fetus. When nutrition is inadequate during pregnancy, both the mother and the fetus are placed at risk. The greater risk, however, is borne by the fetus. Among the more serious consequences of poor nutrition during gestation are prematurity, defined as birth at less than 37 weeks' gestation, and low birth weight, weight of less than 2,500 grams (5.5 pounds). The infant born too early or too small is poorly equipped to adapt to extrauterine life. These babies are likely to suffer such complications as respiratory distress syndrome, weak immune response, and long-term growth and developmental problems. In fact, low birth weight is the third leading cause of infant deaths in the U.S., after congenital defects and sudden infant death syndrome; among black infants it is *the* leading cause of death.

Childhood. The rapid-growth years of early childhood constitute a second period during which poor nutrition may pose a grave threat to health. Because the human brain grows most rapidly from the first trimester of pregnancy through early childhood, the central nervous system is a critical locus of vulnerability in young children. After the preschool years, brain growth slows sharply until maturity (*i.e.*, adolescence). Nutritional deprivation that occurs before maturity—and especially deprivation occurring in early childhood—is associated with long-term developmental deficits.

Research suggests that even before growth problems become evident, a child's body may adapt to inadequate food consumption metabolically, by curtailing energy use. Since energy reserves are necessary for all the activities associated with normal development—play, learning, social interaction—the underfed child can suffer serious developmental delay.

The various risks associated with poor childhood nutrition have a synergistic effect. Thus, the low-birth-weight baby who receives inadequate nutrition may then be more vulnerable to infections, which in turn affect the infant's appetite and feeding behavior so as to reduce dietary intake. The result may be sharply delayed growth and development, often requiring medical intervention and frequent early hospitalizations.

Later life. After the childhood years, hunger's typical impact is to reduce the individual's ability to function effectively. Like children, however, adults of all ages who are poorly nourished are more vulnerable to infections and more likely to develop various deficiency diseases.

In old age the risks of malnutrition are once again heightened. During these years the impact of food on the maintenance of health and the prevention of disease is particularly crucial. The majority of elderly individuals suffer from at least one chronic condition, such as hypertension or diabetes, that requires a special diet. The potential for deficiency diseases increases the elderly person's requirement for certain nutrients—for example, calcium to prevent osteoporosis. And because some conditions of old age may impair digestion or the absorption of nutrients, it is all the more critical that older people eat nutrient-dense foods.

Sobering conclusions. The data on the association of malnutrition, illness, and mortality are not always easy to assess. In some cases scientists are hampered by a lack of baseline data, a factor that makes it difficult to evaluate trends over time. In other instances, they lack statistics on the

An inner-city youngster is weighed at Boston City Hospital's Failure to Thrive Clinic, which was established in 1984 when staff pediatricians began seeing children who were malnourished because their government-funded food provisions had been cut. Most American children receive enough calories to prevent the overt manifestations of malnutrition typically seen in less developed countries. Nonetheless, many suffer from "silent undernutrition," reflected in below-normal growth and developmental delay.

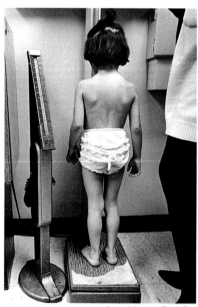

Lynn Johnson—Black Star

188

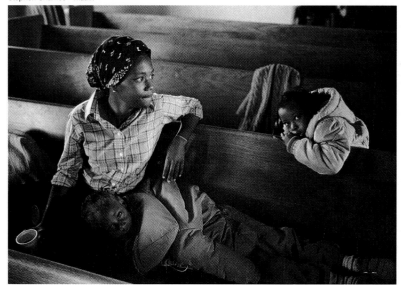

Homeless and hungry, a woman and her children prepare to spend the night on the hard wooden pews of a church in Venice, California. Poverty is the root cause of hunger in America.

prevalence of malnutrition in various socioeconomic groups. Nonetheless, several general conclusions may be drawn about poverty, hunger, and their impact on Americans:

● Compared with babies of middle-income and wealthy mothers, infants of poor mothers are more likely to die before birth as a result of maternal undernutrition.

● When they survive, these infants are at greater risk of low birth weight and its associated health impairments.

● Poor children are less likely than their better-off peers to be adequately nourished and are more likely to suffer growth deficits and cognitive deficiencies associated with undernutrition.

● Poor children are at higher risk of nutrition-related illness, including those illnesses associated with the more extreme forms of malnutrition seen in less developed countries.

● Poor adults are at greater risk of nutrition-related diseases and are more likely to die prematurely of such diseases than their better-off counterparts.

In short, experts who have studied the matter find that hunger is directly linked to poor health. Both are closely associated with poverty.

Hunger, poverty, and public policy

The clear relationship between poverty and nutritional status suggests that to understand the phenomenon of increasing hunger in the U.S., it is necessary to understand how certain economic variables affect the lives of low-income families. One such variable is the status of the nation's "safety net," the array of programs that assist people at or below the official poverty level. A second factor is the federal government's domestic nutrition policy. A third is the increasing "economic jeopardy" to which families, because of recession and unemployment, are being exposed.

The American safety net is weak compared with those of other industrialized nations. The U.S., for example, is one of only two such nations that have no program of national health insurance (the other being South

A 20-year-old woman with a newborn and a toddler waits her turn at a public medical clinic. The value of benefits paid by the Aid to Families with Dependent Children (AFDC) program—the primary source of support for impoverished single mothers—has fallen sharply in recent years. In 1991, 31 states froze AFDC benefits, and 9 reduced them. Most AFDC families qualify for food stamps, but these benefits do not enable them to meet the recommended dietary allowances for all basic nutrients.

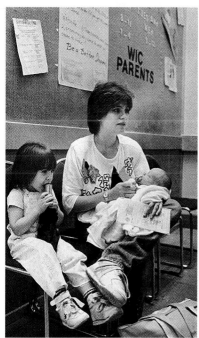

189

Africa). In many states poor families are denied public assistance if the father remains in the home, no matter how destitute the family may be. The federal program of Aid to Families with Dependent Children (AFDC), designed to protect children and families during difficult economic times, comes into play in the majority of states only if the family first breaks apart. Additionally, AFDC benefits for families and children have fallen sharply in recent years. When the figure is adjusted for inflation, benefits for a family of three with no other income were 23% lower in the typical state in 1991 than they had been in 1980. The inadequacy of the unemployment insurance program is another example of the failed safety net. The proportion of unemployed persons receiving unemployment insurance benefits set a record low for five of the six years from 1984 to 1989.

The food-stamp program, constrained by its restricted reach and limited benefits, is yet another instance of the inadequacy of the safety net. While not all impoverished people are eligible for food stamps (because of limits on the value of assets recipients may own), the ratio of poor Americans to monthly food-stamp recipients serves as a barometer of food-stamp availability among the poor. During the past decade or so, this ratio has varied widely—from a low of 59:100 (59 recipients for every 100 people in poverty) to a high of 73:100, a reflection of political and administrative factors that act to prevent a sizable proportion of needy and eligible families from receiving the protection of this key nutrition program. Moreover, food-stamp benefits are not high enough to allow recipients to meet the

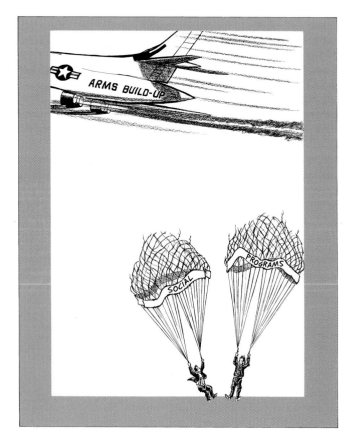

"When he promised us a safety net, I didn't know we were gonna use it like this!"

recommended dietary allowances for all basic nutrients. The USDA bases benefits on the so-called Thrifty Food Plan—a model budget for the best use of food stamps. Eighty-eight percent of individuals whose food expenditures equal the Thrifty Food Plan fail to receive the recommended dietary allowances.

In 1991 the number of Americans living in poverty grew to 35.7 million. (In 1991 a family of three was defined as "poor" if its total annual income was less than $10,860. The poverty threshold for a family of four was $13,924.) With a poverty rate of 14.2%, one in every seven Americans lived in poverty—the highest level in more than 20 years. The 1991 poverty rate represented an increase over previous years and was higher than the rate in any year of the 1970s or 1980s except for 1982–84, when unemployment was at especially high levels.

The steady increase in poverty is attributable in large part to a change in the distribution of income. Throughout the 1980s people at lower income levels were unfavorably affected by changes in distribution. Tax policies shifted income from the lowest and middle quintiles of the population into the highest quintile. In other words, the richest 20% of the population got richer, while the middle class and the poor got poorer. Another factor contributing to the rise in poverty levels is the decline in wages. More than at any time in recent history, substantial numbers of full-time workers earn wages too low for them to work their way out of poverty. For example, in 1990, 18% of full-time workers did not earn enough to lift a family of four out of poverty, an increase of about 6% since 1979.

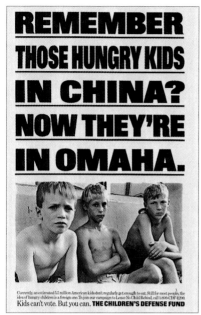

Legacy of neglect

Even as Congress took some steps to address hunger in the late 1980s, the Reagan and Bush administrations largely denied the extent of the problem and, in the case of the Reagan administration, its very existence. At the same time that economic vulnerability reached near records during the early part of the 1980s, the Reagan administration proposed further reductions in basic food and nutrition programs, beyond the $12 billion in cuts enacted in 1981 for the food-stamp and school-breakfast programs.

Moreover, the Reagan administration purported that the evidence of hunger was only "anecdotal." A rhetorical campaign to rally public opinion to such a notion continued even in the face of data from the federal government's own studies that hunger in America was a serious problem and, according to a 1983 USDA report, growing at "a frenetic pace." During the Bush administration Congress slowed the rapid growth of hunger by expanding food-assistance programs such as WIC and food stamps. But these increases were far too modest to begin to reduce the number of people actually going hungry.

The strong inclination of top governmental officials to ignore the problem—and even to divert public concern about it—stemmed from an ideology that held that the federal bureaucracy was already too large and a belief that "a rising tide lifts all boats." This latter concept became the justification of tax policies that throughout the remainder of the 1980s favored those with an income in the top 20%. As a result, income disparities in the

191

nation reached a record high, poverty remained unusually high for years of economic growth, and the extent of hunger failed to diminish.

"America can do better"

The publication on April 6, 1992, of the Medford Declaration to End Hunger in the U.S. signaled a renewed national commitment to address the problem of hunger in America. The declaration was cosponsored by a bipartisan coalition of national antihunger organizations, which set out to describe the economic costs and moral unacceptability of domestic hunger and outline how the problem could be ended. Key support came from Jean Mayer, then president of Tufts University and perhaps the nation's leading nutritionist. Prior to his death in early 1993, Mayer had been instrumental in framing policies to improve the health status of the U.S. population, including pioneering work to develop public programs to protect the poor from hunger and malnutrition. In the short term the Medford declaration recommends fully utilizing existing public programs to end hunger. As a second step the declaration recognizes the need to address the root causes of hunger by eliminating poverty and increasing self-sufficiency for all Americans.

To date, the declaration has been signed by the leaders of more than 3,000 U.S. organizations representing a broad array of political constituencies: Fortune 500 chief executive officers; union leaders; university presidents; local, state, and national officials; religious leaders; physicians; heads of national service organizations such as the American Association of Retired Persons, the Boy Scouts of America, and the National Urban League; and even Hollywood actors.

This unparalleled initiative to end hunger, coinciding with a new administration in the nation's capital, points to the possibilities for positive change. In one of his first statements on hunger, Pres. Bill Clinton declared that "hunger in America remains a terrible crisis." Clinton vowed, "America can do better, and . . . we must." As part of his platform to invest in people, the new president proposed to "fully fund programs that help disadvantaged families and children," and one of those he cited specifically was WIC. The president's proposed economic-investment package, presented to Congress in his first state of the union message, included strong support for initiatives to protect the minds and bodies of children from the ravages of hunger. This included not only expansion of WIC but reforms in the food-stamp program so it can reach more needy families, strengthening of the Head Start program, and initiatives to lessen poverty and promote the economic viability of families at greatest risk.

The larger question—the truly challenging one—remains how to eliminate the leading cause of hunger, poverty. The U.S. pays an enormous price for poverty, and hunger is only one part. Disease, despair, and shortened life-spans also figure into this grim accounting. From a public health perspective, available scientific evidence suggests that it is the height of folly for a nation to permit such a significant risk factor for illness and premature mortality to persist. From a moral perspective, the prevalence of poverty in the world's wealthiest country amounts to a situation that should not fail to rouse the collective social conscience.

192

From the 1993

ENCYCLOPÆDIA BRITANNICA

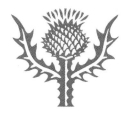

Medical Update from the 1993 Encyclopædia Britannica

The purpose of this section of the *Annual* is to offer readers newly revised and updated material from the latest edition of the *Encyclopædia Britannica.* This year the *Annual*'s editors have selected the timely subject "Anatomy of the Human Nervous System," a portion of the *Britannica* article NERVES AND NERVOUS SYSTEM. This seemed an apt choice because the 1990s have been officially recognized as "the Decade of the Brain." More has been learned about the brain and nervous system in the past dozen or so years than in all of previous history, and neuroscientists now predict "spectacular advances" in the diagnosis and treatment of many human nervous system disorders by the end of the century. Very basic to such anticipated advances is an understanding of the anatomy of the highly complex nervous system, which, the *Annual*'s editors believe, the following selection provides.

ANATOMY OF THE HUMAN NERVOUS SYSTEM

Development

Almost all neurons are generated during prenatal life, and they are not replaced by new neurons during postnatal life. Morphologically, the nervous system first appears about 18 days after conception, with the genesis of the neural plate. Functionally, it appears with the first sign of reflex activity during the second prenatal month, when stimulation by touch of the upper lip has been shown to evoke an avoidance-withdrawal response of the head. Many reflexes of the head, trunk, and extremities can be elicited in the third month.

During its development the nervous system undergoes remarkable changes to attain its complex organization. In order to produce the estimated one trillion neurons present in the mature brain, an average of 2.5 million neurons must be generated per minute during the entire prenatal life. This includes the formation of neuronal circuits comprising 100 trillion synapses, as each potential neuron is ultimately connected with either a selected set of other neurons or specific targets such as sensory endings. Moreover, synaptic connections with other neurons are made at precise locations on the cell membranes of the target neurons. The totality of these events is not thought to be the exclusive product of the genetic code, for there are simply not enough genes to account for such complexity. Rather, the differentiation and subsequent development of embryonic cells into mature neurons and glial cells are achieved by two sets of influences: (1) specific subsets of genes, and (2) environmental stimuli from within and outside the organism. Genetic influences are critical to the development of the nervous system in ordered and temporally timed sequences. Cell differentiation, for example, depends on a series of signals that regulate transcription; this is the process in which DNA molecules give rise to RNA molecules, which in turn express the genetic messages that control cellular activity. Environmental influences derived from the embryo itself include cellular signals that consist of diffusible molecular factors (see below *Neuronal development*). External environmental factors include nutrition, sensory experience, social interaction, and even learning. All of these latter are essential for the proper differentiation of individual neurons and for fine-tuning the details of synaptic connections. Thus, the nervous system requires continuous stimulation over an entire lifetime in order to sustain optimal functional activity.

NEURONAL DEVELOPMENT

The embryonic disk

In the second week of prenatal life, the rapidly growing blastocyst (the bundle of cells into which a fertilized ovum divides) flattens into what is called the embryonic disk. This soon acquires three layers: the ectoderm (outer layer), endoderm (inner layer), and mesoderm (middle layer). Within the mesoderm grows the notochord, an axial rod that serves as a temporary backbone. Both the mesoderm and notochord release a chemical molecular factor that instructs and induces adjacent undifferentiated ectoderm cells to form the neural plate. This includes a population of neural precursor cells, known as neuroepithelial cells, which develop into the neural tube (see below *Morphologic development*). Neuroepithelial cells then commence to divide, diversify, and give rise to immature neurons and neuroglia, which in turn migrate from the neural tube to their final location. Each neuron forms dendrites and an axon; axons elongate and form branches, the terminals of which form synaptic connections with a select set of target neurons or muscle fibres.

The remarkable events of this early development involve an orderly migration of billions of neurons, the growth of their axons (many of which extend widely throughout the brain), and the formation of thousands of synapses between individual axons and their target neurons. This migration and growth are dependent, at least in part, on chemical and physical guidance cues. The growing tips of axons (called growth cones) apparently recognize and respond to various molecular cues, which guide axons and some branches to their appropriate targets but eliminate other branches that try to synapse with inappropriate targets. Once a synaptic connection has been established, a target cell releases a so-called trophic factor (some of which have been identified) that is essential for the survival of the neuron synapsing with it. One example is nerve growth factor (NGF), a diffusable protein essential for the survival of sensory and sympathetic neurons. Physical guidance cues are seen in the migration of immature neurons along a preexistent scaffold of glial fibres through a process called contact guidance.

In some regions of the nervous system, initial synaptic contacts are precise and stable, indicative of an initial specificity of neuronal recognition. In other regions the initial contacts are not precise and stable and are followed later by an ordered reorganization, including the elimination of many synapses. The instability of some synaptic connections persists until a so-called critical period, prior to which environmental influences have a significant role in fine-tuning many connections. Following the critical period, synaptic connections become stable and are unlikely to be altered by environmental influences. This suggests that certain skills and sensory activities can be influenced during development (including postnatal life), and for some intellectual skills this adaptability presumably persists into adulthood and old age.

MORPHOLOGIC DEVELOPMENT

By 18 days after fertilization, the ectoderm of the embryonic disk thickens along what will become the dorsal midline of the body, forming the neural plate and, slightly later, the primordial eye, ear, and nose. The neural plate

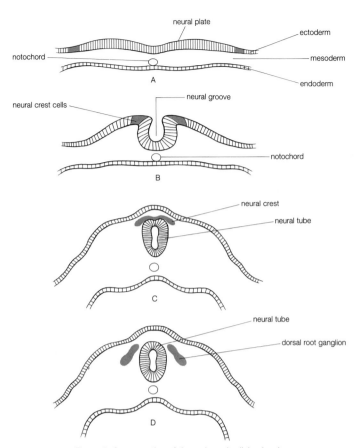

Figure 1: *Cross section of the embryonic disk, showing formation of the neural tube.*
(A) Thickening of the neural plate. (B) Infolding of the neural groove. (C) Closure of the neural groove to form the neural tube. (D) Development of the neural crests into dorsal root ganglia.

From M.B. Carpenter and J. Sutin, *Human Neuroanatomy*, 8th ed. (1983); Williams & Wilkins, Baltimore

The neural tube

elongates, and its lateral edges rise and unite in the midline to form the neural tube, which will develop into the central nervous system. The neural tube detaches from the skin ectoderm and sinks beneath the surface (see Figure 1). At this stage, groupings of ectodermal cells, called neural crests, develop as a column on each side of the neural tube. The cephalic (head) portion of the tube differentiates into the prosencephalon (forebrain), mesencephalon (midbrain), and rhombencephalon (hindbrain), and the caudal portion becomes the spinal cord. The neural crests develop into most elements (*e.g.,* ganglia and nerves) of the peripheral nervous system. This stage is reached at the end of the first embryonic month.

The cells of the central nervous system originate from the ventricular zone of the neural tube—that is, the layer of neuroepithelial cells lining the central cavity of the tube. These cells differentiate and proliferate into neuroblasts, which are the progenitors of neurons, and glioblasts, from which neuroglia develop. With a few exceptions, the neuroblasts, glioblasts, and their derived cells do not divide and multiply once they have migrated from the ventricular zone into the gray and white matter of the nervous system. With some exceptions, all neurons are generated before birth, although all are not fully differentiated. This effectively implies that an individual is born with a full complement of nerve cells. (One exception is that the neurons of the olfactory nerve are generated and replaced continuously throughout life.)

By mid-fetal life the slender primordial brain of the neural-tube stage differentiates into a globular-shaped brain. Although fully mature size and shape are not attained until puberty, the main outlines of the brain are recognizable by the end of the third fetal month. This early development is the product of several factors: the formation of three flexures (cephalic, pontine, and cervical; see Figure 2); the differential enlargement of various regions, especially

the cerebrum and cerebellum; the massive growth of the cerebral hemispheres over the sides of the midbrain and of the cerebellum at the hindbrain; and the formation of convolutions (sulci and gyri) in the cerebral cortex and of folia in the cerebellar cortex. The central and calcarine sulci are discernible by the fifth fetal month, and all major gyri and sulci are normally present by the seventh month. Many minor sulci and gyri appear after birth. By two years after birth, the size of the brain and the proportion of its parts are basically those of the adult.

The postnatal growth of the human brain is rapid and massive, especially during the first two years. The typical brain of a full-term infant weighs 350 grams (12 ounces) at birth, 1,000 grams at the end of the first year, about 1,300 grams at puberty, and about 1,500 grams at adulthood. This increase is attributable mainly to the growth of preexisting neurons, new glial cells, and the myelination of axons. The trebling of weight during the first year (a growth rate unique to humans) may be an adaptation that is essential to the survival of human beings as a species with a large brain. Birth occurs at a developmental stage when the infant is not so helpless as to be unable to survive yet is small enough to be delivered out of the maternal pelvis. If the brain were much larger (enough, say, to support intelligent behaviour), normal delivery would not be possible.

Postnatal growth

Between the ages of 20 and 75, it is estimated that an average of 50,000 neurons atrophy or die each day. In a healthy person, this loss is roughly equal to 10 percent of the original neuronal complement. Indeed, by the age of 75, the weight of the brain is reduced from its maximum at maturity by about one-tenth, the flow of blood through the brain by almost one-fifth, and the number of functional taste buds by about two-thirds. A loss of neurons does not necessarily imply a comparable loss of function, however; some loss may be compensated for by the formation from viable neurons of new branches of nerve fibres and by the formation of new synapses.

The central nervous system

The central nervous system consists of the brain and spinal cord, both derived from the embryonic neural tube. Both parts are invested by protective membranes called the

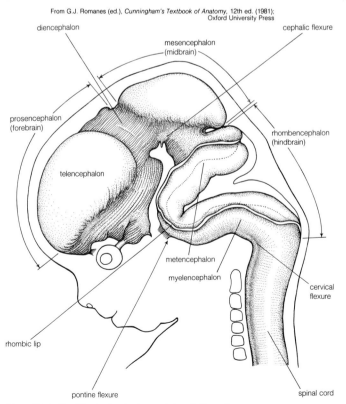

From G.J. Romanes (ed.), *Cunningham's Textbook of Anatomy*, 12th ed. (1981); Oxford University Press

Figure 2: Profile of the brain of a human fetus at 10 weeks.

meninges, and both float in a crystal-clear cerebrospinal fluid. The brain is encased in a bony vault, the neurocranium, while the cylindrical and elongated spinal cord lies in the vertebral canal, which is formed by successive vertebrae connected by dense ligaments.

THE BRAIN

The brain is a relatively small organ, weighing about 1,500 grams and constituting about 2 percent of total body weight. Three major divisions of the brain are recognized: (1) the massive, paired cerebral hemispheres (cerebrum), derived from the telencephalon; (2) the brain stem, from which all true cranial nerves emerge, consisting of the thalamus and hypothalamus, the midbrain, the pons, and the medulla oblongata (also known as the diencephalon, the mesencephalon, the metencephalon, and the myelencephalon); and (3) the cerebellum ("little brain"), derived from the pons, or metencephalon. The terms telencephalon, diencephalon, mesencephalon, metencephalon, and myelencephalon denote five distinct embryonic subdivisions derived from separate vesicles in the rostral neural tube (see Figure 2).

The cerebral hemispheres

Telencephalon. The paired cerebral hemispheres are mirror-image duplicates composed of a gray cellular mantle called the cerebral cortex, an underlying mass of white matter composed of myelinated nerve fibres, and collections of subcortical neuronal masses known as the basal ganglia. Each hemisphere receives impulses conveying the senses of touch and vision largely from the contralateral half (that is, the opposite side) of the body, while auditory input comes from both sides. Pathways conveying the senses of smell and taste to the cerebral cortex are ipsilateral (that is, they do not cross to the opposite hemisphere). In turn, each cerebral hemisphere supplies motor function to the opposite side of the body, the side from which it receives sensory input.

In spite of this arrangement, the cerebral hemispheres are not functionally equal. In each individual, one hemisphere is dominant, the dominant hemisphere being concerned with language, mathematical and analytical functions, and handedness. The nondominant hemisphere is concerned with simple spatial concepts, recognition of faces, some aspects of music, and emotion.

The hemispheres are partially separated from each other by the longitudinal fissure (see Figure 16), but in central regions this fissure extends only as deep as a broad interhemispheric commissure called the corpus callosum. It is through the corpus callosum that corresponding regions of the cerebral hemispheres are connected by various nerve projections.

Lobes of the cerebral cortex. The cortical mantle is highly convoluted; the crest of a single convolution is known as a gyrus, while the fissure between two gyri is known as a sulcus. Sulci and gyri form a more or less constant pattern, on the basis of which each cerebral hemisphere is divided into six so-called lobes: (1) frontal, (2) parietal, (3) temporal, (4) occipital, (5) central (or insular), and (6) limbic. Two important sulci located on the lateral aspect (that is, the side surface) of each hemisphere help to distinguish these lobes. The central sulcus separates the frontal and parietal lobes, and the deeper lateral sulcus forms the boundary between the temporal lobe and the frontal and parietal lobes (see Figure 3).

The frontal lobe, largest of all the lobes of the brain, lies rostral to the central sulcus (that is, toward the nose from the sulcus). The precentral gyrus, located rostral to the central sulcus, constitutes the primary motor region of the brain; when parts of this gyrus are given electrical stimulation in conscious patients (operated upon under local anesthesia), they produce localized movements on the opposite side of the body that are interpreted by the patients as voluntary. Injury to parts of this gyrus results in paralysis on the contralateral half of the body.

Parts of the inferior frontal lobe (close to the lateral sulcus) constitute Broca's area, a region concerned with neural mechanisms that convert thoughts into speech.

Sensory cortex

The parietal lobe, posterior to the central sulcus, is divided into three parts: (1) a postcentral gyrus, (2) a superior parietal lobule, and (3) an inferior parietal lobule. The

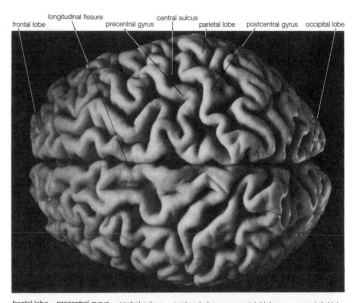

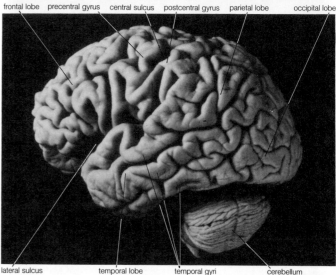

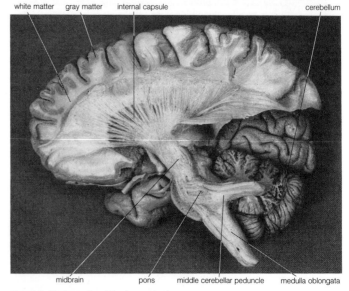

Figure 3: *Photographs of the human brain.*
(Top) Upper surface, showing division of the cerebrum into two hemispheres by the longitudinal fissure. (Centre) Left lateral surface, showing various lobes of the hemisphere. (Bottom) Dissection of the left hemisphere, showing internal capsule and middle cerebellar peduncle.

From (top and centre) N. Gluhbegovic and T.H. Williams, *The Human Brain: A Photographic Guide* (1980), J.B. Lippincott Co./Harper & Row; (bottom) original preparation by J. Klingler, Anatomical Museum, Basel, Switz.

postcentral gyrus receives sensory input, both superficial and deep, from the contralateral half of the body. The sequential representation is the same as in the primary motor area, with sensations from the head area being represented in inferior parts of the gyrus and impulses from the lower extremities represented above. Lesions in the postcentral gyrus result in impaired sensation from cutaneous (surface) and deep parts of the contralateral half of the body. The superior parietal lobule, located caudal to the postcentral gyrus, lies superior to the interparietal sulcus. This lobule is regarded as an association cortex, part of which may be concerned with motor function. The inferior parietal lobule (composed of the angular and supramarginal gyri) is a cortical region concerned with the integration of multiple sensory signals. Lesions in this lobule produce various syndromes of a devastating nature.

In the parietal and frontal lobes, each primary sensory or motor area is close to, or surrounded by, a smaller secondary area. The primary sensory area receives input only from relay nuclei in the thalamus, while the secondary sensory area receives input from the thalamus, the primary sensory area, or both. The motor regions receive input from the thalamus as well as the sensory areas of the cerebral cortex.

The temporal lobe, inferior to the lateral sulcus, fills the middle fossa of the skull. Near the margin of the lateral sulcus, two transverse temporal gyri constitute the primary auditory area of the brain. Audition is represented here in a tonotopic fashion—that is, with different frequencies represented on different parts of the area. The transverse gyri are surrounded by a less finely tuned secondary auditory area.

A medial, or inner, protrusion near the ventral surface of the temporal lobe, known as the uncus, constitutes a large part of the primary olfactory area. The outer surface of this lobe is an association area made up of the superior, middle, and inferior temporal gyri.

The occipital lobe lies caudal to (that is, below and behind) the parieto-occipital sulcus. As seen on the medial aspect of the hemisphere, this sulcus joins the calcarine sulcus in a Y-shaped formation. Cortex on both banks of the calcarine sulcus constitutes the primary visual area, which receives input from the contralateral visual field via the optic radiation. The visual field is represented near the calcarine sulcus in a retinotopic fashion—that is, with upper quadrants of the visual field laid out along the inferior bank of the sulcus and lower quadrants of the visual field represented on the upper bank. Central vision is represented most caudally and peripheral vision rostrally. Lesions in the calcarine cortex—or in the optic radiation, which projects to it—produce blindness in the contralateral visual field.

The insular, or central, lobe is an invaginated triangular area on the medial surface of the lateral sulcus; it can be seen in the intact brain only by separating the frontal and parietal lobes from the temporal lobe. Branches of the middle cerebral artery cover the surface of the insula.

The limbic lobe is a synthetic lobe on the medial margin (or limbus) of the hemisphere. Composed of adjacent portions of the frontal, parietal, and temporal lobes that surround the corpus callosum, it is concerned with visceral, autonomic, and related somatic behavioral activities. This region of the cerebral cortex receives inputs from thalamic nuclei that are connected with parts of the hypothalamus and with the hippocampal formation, a primitive cortical structure within the inferior horn of the lateral ventricle (see Figure 4).

White matter. Beneath the cerebral cortex is a mass of white matter, which is composed of nerve fibres projecting to and from the cerebral cortex, commissural systems connecting the two hemispheres via the corpus callosum, and association fibres connecting different regions of a single hemisphere. Myelinated fibres projecting to and from the cerebral cortex form a concentrated fan-shaped band, known as the internal capsule (see Figure 3). In horizontal sections of the brain (see Figure 5), the internal capsule can be seen to consist of two parts: (1) an anterior limb, between the caudate nucleus and the putamen; and (2) a larger posterior limb, running between the thalamus and

The internal capsule

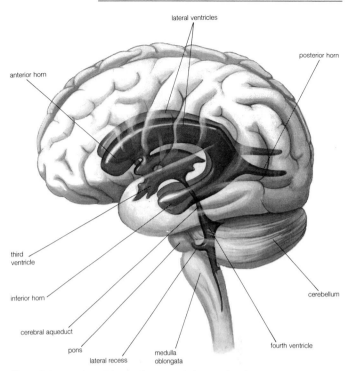

Figure 4: Lateral view of the cerebrum, cerebellum, and brain stem, highlighting features of the ventricular system.

the globus pallidus and putamen. These two limbs form an obtuse angle with the apex directed toward the centre of the brain; the junction is called the genu.

Ventricles. Deep within the white matter are fluid-filled cavities that form the ventricular system. These cavities include a pair of C-shaped lateral ventricles with anterior, inferior, and posterior "horns" protruding into the frontal, temporal, and occipital lobes, respectively (see Figure 4). Most of the cerebrospinal fluid is produced in the ventricles. About 70 percent of the fluid produced by the central nervous system is secreted by the choroid plexus, a collection of blood vessels in the walls of the lateral ventricles. The fluid drains via interventricular foramina, or openings, into a slitlike third ventricle, which, situated along the midline of the brain, separates the symmetrical halves of the thalamus and hypothalamus (see Figure 5). From there it passes through the cerebral aqueduct in the midbrain and into the fourth ventricle in the hindbrain. Openings in the fourth ventricle permit cerebrospinal fluid to enter so-called subarachnoid spaces surrounding both brain and spinal cord.

Basal ganglia. Deep within the cerebral hemispheres, large gray masses or nerve cells, called nuclei, form components of the basal ganglia. Four nuclei can be distinguished: (1) the caudate nucleus, (2) the putamen, (3) the globus pallidus, and (4) the amygdala. Phylogenetically, the amygdala is the oldest of the basal ganglia and is therefore often referred to as the archistriatum; the globus pallidus is known as the paleostriatum, and the caudate nucleus and putamen are together known as the neostriatum, or simply striatum. The putamen and the adjacent globus pallidus are referred to descriptively as the lentiform nucleus, while the caudate nucleus, putamen, and globus pallidus form the corpus striatum.

The caudate nucleus and the putamen are continuous rostrally and ventrally (see Figure 5), and they have similar cytology (cellular makeup), cytochemical features, and functions, but they also have slightly different connections. The putamen lies deep within the cortex of the insular lobe, while the caudate nucleus has a C-shaped configuration that parallels the lateral ventricle. The head of the caudate nucleus protrudes into the anterior horn of the lateral ventricle, the body lies above and lateral to the thalamus, and the tail is in the roof of the inferior horn of

The caudate nucleus and putamen

the lateral ventricle. The tail of the caudate nucleus ends in relationship to the amygdaloid nuclear complex, which lies in the temporal lobe beneath the cortex of the uncus.

There is an enormous number of neurons within the caudate nucleus and putamen; these are of two basic types, spiny and aspiny. Spiny striatal neurons are medium-size cells with radiating dendrites that are studded with spines. Axons of these cells project beyond the boundaries of the neostriatum. All afferent systems entering the neostriatum terminate upon the dendritic spines of spiny striatal neurons, and all output is via axons of the same neurons. Chemically, spiny striatal neurons are heterogeneous—that is, most contain more than one neurotransmitter. Neurotransmitters identified in spiny striatal neurons are gamma-aminobutyric acid (GABA), substance P, and enkephalin, with overwhelming dominance by GABA.

Aspiny striatal neurons have smooth dendrites and short axons confined to the caudate nucleus or putamen. Small aspiny striatal neurons secrete GABA, neuropeptide Y, somatostatin, or some combination of these. The largest aspiny striatal neurons are evenly distributed cholinergic neurons that play a crucial role in maintaining the balance of dopamine and GABA.

Because the caudate nucleus and putamen receive varied and diverse inputs from multiple sources that utilize different neurotransmitters, they are regarded as the receptive component of the corpus striatum. The most massive input originates from virtually all regions of the cerebral cortex, with the connecting corticostriate fibres containing the excitatory neurotransmitter glutamate. In addition, afferent fibres originating from the substantia nigra in the midbrain or from intralaminar thalamic nuclei in the diencephalon project to the caudate nucleus or the putamen. The neurotransmitter secreted by thalamostriate neurons has not been identified, while neurons from the substantia nigra synthesize dopamine. All striatal afferent systems terminate in patchy arrays referred to as strisomes; areas not receiving terminals are called the matrix. Striatal efferent systems—that is, spiny neurons containing GABA, substance P, and enkephalin—project in a specific pattern onto the globus pallidus and the substantia nigra; GABA, an inhibitory neurotransmitter, is dominant in all neostriatal projections.

The globus pallidus The globus pallidus, consisting of two cytologically similar wedge-shaped segments, the lateral and the medial, lies between the putamen and the internal capsule (see Figure 5). Fibres terminating on the pallidum arise mostly from the caudate nucleus and putamen; these so-called striatopallidal fibres converge on the globus pallidus like spokes of a wheel. Both segments of the pallidum receive GABAergic terminals, but in addition the medial segment receives substance P fibres, and the lateral segment receives enkephalinergic projections. The output of the entire corpus striatum (*i.e.*, the caudate nucleus, putamen, and globus pallidus together) arises from GABAergic cells in the medial pallidal segment and in the substantia nigra, both of which receive fibres from the striatum. GABAergic cells in the medial pallidal segment and the substantia nigra project to different nuclei in the thalamus; these in turn influence distinct regions of the cortex concerned with motor function. The lateral segment of the globus pallidus, on the other hand, projects almost exclusively to the subthalamic nucleus (in the ventral thalamus), from which it receives a reciprocal input. No part of the corpus striatum projects fibres to spinal levels.

Pathological processes involving the corpus striatum and related nuclei are associated with a variety of specific syndromes characterized by abnormal involuntary movements (collectively referred to as dyskinesia) and significant alterations of muscle tone. Parkinson's disease and Huntington's disease are among the more prevalent syndromes; each appears related to deficiencies in the synthesis of particular neurotransmitters.

The amygdala, located ventral to the corpus striatum in medial parts of the temporal lobe, is an almond-shaped nucleus underlying the uncus. Although it receives olfactory inputs, it plays no role in olfactory perception. This nucleus also has reciprocal connections with the hypothalamus, the basal forebrain, and multiple regions of the cere-

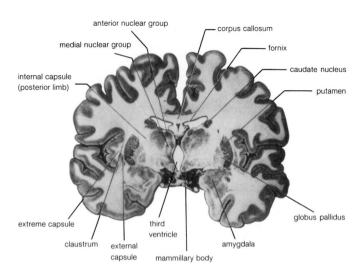
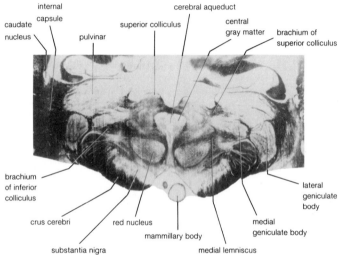
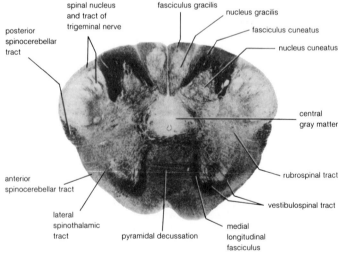

Figure 5: *Three cross sections of the brain.*
(Top) Frontal section through the thalamus, internal capsule, and basal ganglia. (Centre) Myelin-stained section through the midbrain and thalamus, showing the red nucleus, substantia nigra, and crus cerebri of the midbrain and the medial and lateral geniculate bodies of the thalamus. (Bottom) Myelin-stained section through the medulla oblongata, revealing the nuclei gracilis and cuneatus and the decussation of the corticospinal tract.
From M.B. Carpenter, *Core Text of Neuroanatomy*, 4th ed. (1991); Williams & Wilkins, Baltimore

bral cortex. It plays important roles in visceral, endocrine, and cognitive functions related to motivational behaviour.

Diencephalon. The diencephalon consists of a pair of egg-shaped nuclear masses that lie on each side of the third ventricle and medial to the posterior limb of the internal capsule (see Figure 5). Four subdivisions are recognized: (1) the epithalamus, (2) the thalamus, (3) the hypothalamus, and (4) the ventral thalamus, or subthalamus.

Epithalamus. The epithalamus is represented mainly by the pineal gland, which lies in the midline posterior and dorsal to the third ventricle. This gland synthesizes the hormone melatonin and enzymes sensitive to diurnal light. Rhythmic changes in its activity in response to cyclical photic input suggest that the pineal gland serves as the body's biological clock. With age it tends to accumulate calcium deposits.

Thalamus. The thalamus has long been regarded as the key to understanding the organization of the central nervous system. It is involved in the relay and distribution of most, but not all, sensory and motor signals to specific regions of the cerebral cortex. Sensory signals generated in all types of receptors are projected by complex pathways to specific relay nuclei in the thalamus, where they are segregated and systematically organized. The relay nuclei in turn supply the primary and secondary sensory areas of the cerebral cortex. Sensory input to thalamic nuclei is crossed for the somesthetic and visual systems, bilateral (but mainly crossed) for the auditory system, and ipsilateral for gustatory and olfactory sense.

The somesthetic relay nuclei of the thalamus, collectively known as the ventrobasal complex, receive input from the medial lemniscus (originating in the medulla), from spinothalamic tracts, and from the trigeminal nerve. Fibres within these ascending tracts that terminate in the central core of the ventrobasal complex receive input from deep sensory receptors, while fibres projecting onto the outer shell receive input from cutaneous receptors. This segregation of deep and superficial sensation is preserved in projections of the ventrobasal complex to the primary somesthetic (*i.e.,* sensory) area of the cerebral cortex.

The medial and lateral geniculate bodies form what is called the metathalamus. Fibres of the optic nerve end in the lateral geniculate body, which consists of six cellular laminae, or layers, folded into a horseshoe configuration. Each lamina represents a complete map of the contralateral visual hemifield, and all laminae are in perfect registration. Cells in all layers of the lateral geniculate body project via the optic radiation to the visual areas of the cerebral cortex. The medial geniculate body receives auditory impulses from the inferior colliculus of the midbrain and relays them to the auditory areas on the temporal lobe. Only the ventral nucleus of the medial geniculate body is laminated and tonotopically organized; this part projects to the primary auditory area and is finely tuned. Other subdivisions of the medial geniculate body project to the belt of secondary auditory cortex surrounding the primary area.

Major output from the cerebellum projects to specific thalamic relay nuclei in a pattern similar to that for somesthetic input. The thalamic relay nuclei in turn provide a major input to the primary motor area of the frontal lobe. This large system appears to provide coordinating and controlling influences that result in the appropriate force, sequence, and direction of voluntary motor activities. Output from the corpus striatum, on the other hand, is relayed by thalamic nuclei that have access to the supplementary and premotor areas. The supplementary motor area, located on the medial aspect of the hemisphere (see Figure 29), exerts modifying influences upon the primary motor area and appears to be involved in programming skilled motor sequences. The premotor area, rostral to the primary motor area, plays a role in sensorially guided movements.

Other major thalamic nuclei, besides those involved in relaying sensory impulses or controlling influences from the cerebellum and corpus striatum, include the anterior nuclear group, the mediodorsal nucleus, and the pulvinar. The anterior nuclear group receives input from the hypothalamus and projects upon parts of the limbic lobe (*i.e.,* the cingulate gyrus). The mediodorsal nucleus, part of the medial nuclear group, has reciprocal connections with large parts of the frontal lobe rostral to the motor areas. The pulvinar is a huge posterior nuclear complex

that, along with the mediodorsal nucleus, has projections to association areas of the cortex.

Output ascending from the reticular formation of the brain stem is relayed to the cerebral cortex by intralaminar thalamic nuclei, which lie in laminae separating the medial and ventrolateral thalamic nuclei. This ascending system is concerned with arousal mechanisms, maintaining alertness, and directing attention to sensory events.

Hypothalamus. The hypothalamus lies in the walls and floor of the third ventricle. It is divided into medial and lateral groups by fibres of the fornix, which originate in the hippocampal formation and adjacent subiculum and project to the mammillary body. Well-defined cell groups in the hypothalamus secrete hormones (*i.e.,* oxytocin and vasopressin) that are transported by nerve fibres to the neurohypophysis; other neurosecretory neurons convey hormone-releasing factors (*e.g.,* growth hormone, corticosteroids, thyrotropic hormone, and gonadotropic hormone) via a vascular portal system to the adenohypophysis. In this way the hypothalamus controls major endocrine functions; specific regions of the hypothalamus are also concerned with control of sympathetic and parasympathetic activities, temperature regulation, food intake, the reproductive cycle, and emotional expression and behaviour.

Ventral thalamus. The ventral thalamus is represented mainly by the subthalamic nucleus, a lens-shaped structure lying behind and to the sides of the hypothalamus and on the dorsal surface of the internal capsule. The subthalamic region is traversed by fibres related to the globus pallidus. Discrete lesions in the subthalamic nucleus produce hemiballism, the most violent form of dyskinesia known.

Midbrain and hindbrain. Below the diencephalon are the midbrain (or mesencephalon) and the hindbrain (or rhombencephalon). The hindbrain consists of the pons (or metencephalon) and the medulla oblongata (or myelencephalon). These parts of the brain stem are characterized by three main features: (1) a roof plate superior to the cerebral aqueduct and fourth ventricle; (2) a central core of gray matter, known as the reticular formation; and (3) a massive basal collection of fibres descending from the cerebral cortex to the brain stem and spinal cord.

The roof plate of the midbrain is formed by two paired rounded eminences, the superior and inferior colliculi. The superior colliculus receives input from the retina and the visual cortex and participates in a variety of visual reflexes, particularly the tracking of objects in the contralateral visual field. The inferior colliculus receives both crossed and uncrossed auditory fibres and projects upon the medial geniculate body, the auditory relay nucleus of the thalamus (see above *Diencephalon*). In the hindbrain the roof plate is formed by the cerebellum and a membrane containing the choroid plexus of the fourth ventricle.

The reticular formation contains a core collection of cells of various sizes that project to the thalamus, the cerebellum, and the spinal cord. Surrounding this core are long ascending and descending tracts in which various cranial nerve nuclei are embedded.

Fibres derived from the cerebral cortex lie on or near the ventral surface of the midbrain, pons, and medulla. At the midbrain they gather into two bundles called the crura cerebri; from there they descend into the pons, where most terminate upon cell nuclei that project into the cerebellum. These constitute the corticopontine tract. The other major tract, called the corticospinal tract, forms the medullary pyramids before descending to the spinal cord.

Midbrain. The midbrain contains the nuclear complex of the oculomotor nerve as well as the trochlear nucleus; these cranial nerves innervate muscles that move the eye and control the shape of the lens and the diameter of the pupil. In addition, between the midbrain reticular formation (known here as the tegmentum) and the crus cerebri is a large, pigmented structure called the substantia nigra (see Figure 5). This nucleus consists of two parts, the pars reticulata and the pars compacta. Cells of the pars compacta contain the black pigment melanin; these synthesize dopamine and project to cells of either the caudate nucleus or the putamen but not to both. By exercising an inhibitory action on large aspiny cholinergic neurons in

Relay functions of the thalamus

Secretion of hormones and hormone-releasing factors

The substantia nigra

the neostriatum, the dopaminergic cells of the pars compacta influence the output of the neurotransmitter GABA from spiny striatal neurons. These spiny neurons in turn project to cells of the pars reticulata, which, by projecting fibres to the thalamus, are in effect part of the output system of the corpus striatum.

At the caudal midbrain, crossed fibres of the superior cerebellar peduncle (the major output system of the cerebellum) surround and partially terminate in a large, centrally located structure known as the red nucleus. Most crossed ascending fibres of this bundle project to thalamic nuclei, which have access to the primary motor cortex. A smaller number of fibres synapse on large cells in caudal regions of the red nucleus; these give rise to the crossed fibres of the rubrospinal tract (see below *The spinal cord: Descending spinal tracts*).

Pons. The pons consists of two parts: the tegmentum, a phylogenetically older part that contains the reticular formation; and the pontine nuclei, a larger part composed of masses of neurons that lie among large bundles of longitudinal and transverse fibres.

Fibres originating from neurons in all major lobes of the cerebral cortex terminate upon the pontine nuclei, which in turn project to the opposite cerebellar hemisphere. These massive crossed fibres form the middle cerebellar peduncle (see Figures 3 and 6)—in effect serving as the bridge that connects each cerebral hemisphere with the opposite half of the cerebellum.

The reticular formation in the pontine tegmentum contains multiple cell groups that exert facilitating influences upon motor function. It also contains the nuclei of several cranial nerves. The facial nerve and the two components of the vestibulocochlear nerve, for example, emerge from and enter the brain stem at the junction of the pons, medulla, and cerebellum. Motor nuclei for the trigeminal nerve lie in the upper pons. Located on the periphery of the pons are long ascending and descending tracts that connect the brain to the spinal cord.

Medulla oblongata. The medulla, the most caudal segment of the brain stem, appears as a conical expansion of the spinal cord (see Figures 5 and 6). Both the pons and the medulla are separated from the overlying cerebellum by the fourth ventricle, and cerebrospinal fluid entering

From F.A. Mettler, *Neuroanatomy*, 2nd ed. (1948); The C.V. Mosby Co., St. Louis

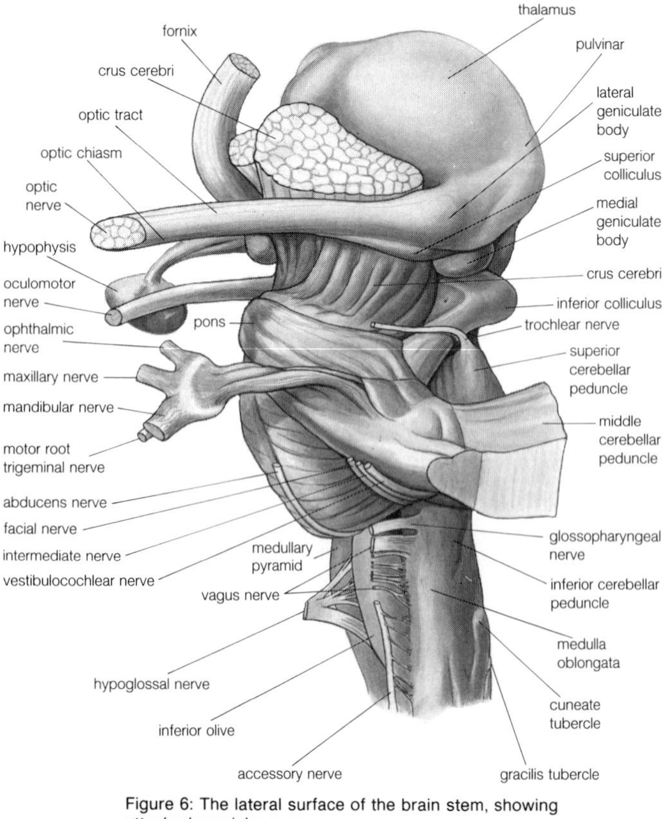

Figure 6: The lateral surface of the brain stem, showing attached cranial nerves.

the fourth ventricle from the cerebral aqueduct passes into the cisterna magna, a subarachnoid space surrounding the medulla and the cerebellum, via foramina in the lateral recesses and in the midline of the ventricle.

At the transition from the medulla to the spinal cord, there are two major decussations, or crossings, of nerve fibres. The corticospinal decussation is the site at which 90 percent of the fibres of the medullary pyramid cross and enter the dorsolateral funiculus of the spinal cord (see Figure 8). Signals conveyed by this tract provide the basis for voluntary motor function on the opposite side of the body (see below *The spinal cord: Descending spinal tracts*). In the other decussation, sensory fibres ascending in the fasciculus gracilis and fasciculus cuneatus of the spinal cord terminate upon large nuclear masses on the dorsal surface of the medulla. Known as the nuclei gracilis and cuneatus, these masses give rise to fibres that decussate above the corticospinal tract and form a major ascending sensory pathway known as the medial lemniscus. Present at all brain-stem levels, the medial lemniscus projects upon the somesthetic relay nuclei of the thalamus. **Decussation of nerve fibres**

The medulla contains nuclei associated with the hypoglossal, accessory, vagus, and glossopharyngeal cranial nerves. In addition, it contains portions of the vestibular nuclear complex, parts of the trigeminal nuclear complex concerned with pain and thermal sense, and solitary nuclei related to the vagus, glossopharyngeal, and facial nerves that subserve the sense of taste.

Of several medullary relay nuclei that project to the cerebellum via the inferior cerebellar peduncle, the largest is the inferior olive.

Cerebellum. The cerebellum overlies the posterior aspect of the pons and medulla and fills the greater part of the posterior fossa of the skull. This distinctive part of the brain is derived from the rhombic lips, thickenings along the margins of the embryonic hindbrain (see Figure 2). It consists of two paired lateral lobes, or hemispheres, and a midline portion known as the vermis. Cerebellar cortex appears very different from cerebral cortex in that it consists of small, leaflike laminae, referred to as folia (see Figure 3). Structurally the cerebellum consists of a three-layered, gray cellular mantle called the cerebellar cortex and a core of white matter containing four paired intrinsic (*i.e.,* deep) nuclei, the dentate, globose, emboliform, and fastigial. Three paired fibre bundles—the superior, middle, and inferior peduncles—connect the cerebellum with the midbrain, pons, and medulla, respectively (see Figure 6).

On an embryological basis the cerebellum can be divided into three parts: (1) the archicerebellum, related primarily to the vestibular system; (2) the paleocerebellum, or anterior lobe, concerned with control of muscle tone; and (3) the neocerebellum, known as the posterior lobe. Receiving input from the cerebral hemispheres via the middle cerebellar peduncle, the neocerebellum is the part most concerned with coordination of voluntary motor function.

The three layers of the cerebellar cortex are an outer synaptic layer (also called the molecular layer), an intermediate discharge layer (the Purkinje layer), and an inner receptive layer (the granular layer). Sensory input from all sorts of receptors are conveyed to specific regions of the receptive layer, which consists of enormous numbers of small nerve cells (hence the name granular) that project axons into the synaptic layer. There they excite the dendrites of the Purkinje cells, which in turn project axons to portions of the four intrinsic nuclei and upon dorsal portions of the lateral vestibular nucleus. Because most Purkinje cells are GABAergic and therefore exert strong inhibitory influences upon the cells that receive their terminals, all sensory input into the cerebellum results in inhibitory impulses being exerted upon the deep cerebellar nuclei and parts of the vestibular nucleus. Cells of all deep cerebellar nuclei, on the other hand, are excitatory (secreting the neurotransmitter glutamate) and project upon parts of the thalamus, red nucleus, vestibular nuclei, and reticular formation. **Layers of the cerebellar cortex**

The cerebellum thus functions as a kind of computer, providing a quick and clear response to any set of sensory signals. It plays no role in sensory perception, but it exerts profound influences upon equilibrium, muscle tone, and the coordination of voluntary motor function. Lesions of the cerebellum produce a constellation of disturbances, including intention tremor, ataxia, hypotonus, easy fatigability, and disturbances of speech.

THE SPINAL CORD

The spinal cord is an elongated cylindrical structure, about 45 centimetres (18 inches) long, that extends from the medulla oblongata of the hindbrain to a level between the first and second lumbar vertebrae of the backbone. The terminal part of the spinal cord is called the conus medullaris. Associated with local regions of the spinal cord and imposing upon it an external segmentation are 31 pairs of spinal nerves, each of which receives and furnishes one dorsal and one ventral root (see Figure 12). On this basis the spinal cord is divided into the following segments: 8 cervical (C), 12 thoracic (T), 5 lumbar (L), 5 sacral (S), and 1 coccygeal (Coc). Spinal nerve roots emerge via intervertebral foramina; lumbar and sacral spinal roots, descending for some distance within the subarachnoid space before reaching the appropriate foramina, produce a group of nerve roots about the conus medullaris known as the cauda equina. Two enlargements of the spinal cord are evident: (1) a cervical enlargment (C_5 through T_1), which provides innervation for the upper extremity, and (2) a lumbosacral enlargement (L_1 through S_2), which innervates the lower extremity.

Appearance in cross section

A cross section of the spinal cord reveals long tracts of myelinated nerve fibres (known as white matter) arranged around the periphery of a symmetrical, butterfly-shaped cellular matrix of gray matter (see Figure 7). The gray matter forms three pairs of horns throughout most of the spinal cord: (1) the dorsal horns, composed of sensory neurons; (2) the lateral horns, well defined in thoracic segments and composed of visceral neurons; and (3) the

ventral horns, especially large in the cord enlargements and composed of motor neurons. The white matter forming the ascending and descending spinal tracts falls in three paired funiculi, or sectors: the dorsal or posterior funiculi, lying between the dorsal horns; the lateral funiculi, lying on each side of the spinal cord between the dorsal-root entry zones and the emergence of the ventral roots; and the ventral funiculi, lying between the ventral median sulcus and each ventral-root zone.

Gray matter. The cellular gray matter has a "cytoarchitectural lamination" in which nine laminae are customarily indicated by Roman numerals (see Figure 7, bottom). Laminae I to V, forming the dorsal horns, receive sensory input. Lamina VII forms the intermediate zone at the base of all horns. Lamina IX is composed of clusters of large (alpha) motor neurons, whose axons innervate striated muscle, and small (gamma) motor neurons, which innervate contractile elements of the muscle spindle. Axons of both alpha and gamma motor neurons emerge via the ventral roots. Laminae VII and VIII have variable configurations, and lamina VI is present only in the cervical and lumbosacral enlargements. In addition, cells surrounding the central canal of the spinal cord form an area often referred to as lamina X.

All primary sensory neurons that enter the spinal cord originate in ganglia that are located in the intervertebral foramina. Peripheral processes of the nerve cells in these ganglia convey sensation from various receptors, and central processes of the same cells enter the spinal cord dorsolaterally as bundles of nerve filaments. Fibres conveying specific forms of sensation follow separate pathways. Impulses concerned with pain and noxious stimuli largely end upon cells in parts of laminae I and II, while impulses associated with tactile sense end in lamina IV or on processes of cells in that lamina. Signals from stretch receptors (i.e., muscle spindles and tendon organs) end upon cells in parts of laminae V, VI, and VII; collaterals of these fibres involved in the stretch reflex project into lamina IX.

Virtually all parts of the spinal gray contain interneurons, which connect various cell groups. Many interneurons have short axons distributed locally, but some have axons that extend for several spinal segments. Some interneurons may modulate or change the character of signals, while others play key roles in transmission and in patterned reflexes.

Ascending spinal tracts. Sensory tracts ascending in the white matter of the spinal cord arise either from cells of spinal ganglia or from intrinsic neurons within the gray matter that receive primary sensory input.

Dorsal column. The largest ascending tracts, the fasciculi gracilis and cuneatus, arise from spinal ganglion cells and ascend in the dorsal funiculus to the medulla. The fasciculus gracilis receives fibres from ganglia below thoracic 6, while spinal ganglia from higher segments of the spinal cord project fibres into the fasciculus cuneatus. The fasciculi terminate upon large nuclear masses (the nuclei gracilis and cuneatus) in the medulla. Cells of these nuclei give rise to fibres that cross completely and form the medial lemniscus; the medial lemniscus in turn projects to the ventrobasal nuclear complex of the thalamus. In this way, the dorsal column/medial lemniscal system conveys signals associated with tactile, pressure, and kinesthetic (or positional) sense to sensory areas of the cerebral cortex.

The fasciculi gracilis and cuneatus

Spinothalamic tracts. Fibres concerned with pain, thermal sense, and light touch enter the lateral-root entry zone and then ascend or descend near the periphery of the spinal cord before entering superficial laminae of the dorsal horn—largely parts of laminae I, IV, and V. Cells in these laminae then give rise to fibres of the two spinothalamic tracts. Those crossing in the ventral white commissure (ventral to the central canal) form the lateral spinothalamic tract, which, ascending in the ventral part of the lateral funiculus, conveys signals related to pain and thermal sense. The anterior spinothalamic tract arises from fibres that cross the midline in the same fashion but ascend more anteriorly in the spinal cord; these convey impulses related to light touch. At medullary levels the two spinothalamic tracts tend to merge and cannot be distinguished as separate entities. Many of the fibres,

From (top) D.E. Haines, *Neuroanatomy: An Atlas of Structures, Sections, and Systems*, 3rd ed. (1991), Urban & Schwarzenberg; (bottom) M.B. Carpenter and J. Sutin, *Human Neuroanatomy*, 8th ed. (1983), Williams & Wilkins, Baltimore

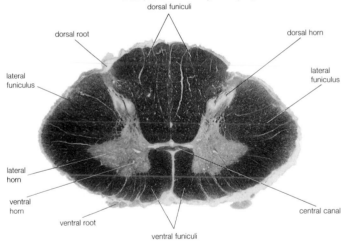

dorsal funiculi · dorsal root · dorsal horn · lateral funiculus · lateral funiculus · lateral horn · ventral horn · ventral root · central canal · ventral funiculi

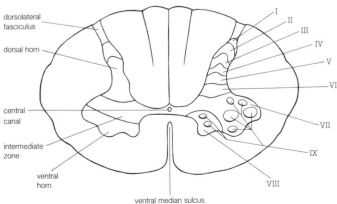

dorsolateral fasciculus · dorsal horn · central canal · intermediate zone · ventral horn · ventral median sulcus · I II III IV V VI VII IX VIII

Figure 7: *Lower cervical section of the spinal cord.*
(Top) Photograph of a cross section, with the white matter stained dark. (Bottom) Schematic drawing showing cytoarchitectural lamination.

or collaterals, of the spinothalamic tracts end upon cell groups in the reticular formation, while the principal tracts convey sensory impulses to relay nuclei in the thalamus.

Spinocerebellar tracts. Impulses from stretch receptors are carried by large-diameter fibres that synapse upon cells in deep laminae of the dorsal horn or in lamina VII. The posterior spinocerebellar tract arises from the dorsal nucleus of Clarke and ascends peripherally in the dorsal part of the lateral funiculus. The anterior spinocerebellar tract ascends on the ventral margin of the lateral funiculus. Both tracts transmit signals to portions of the anterior lobe of the cerebellum and are involved in mechanisms that automatically regulate muscle tone without reaching consciousness.

Descending spinal tracts. Tracts descending to the spinal cord are concerned with voluntary motor function, muscle tone, reflexes and equilibrium, visceral innervation, and modulation of ascending sensory signals. The largest and most important, the corticospinal tract, originates in broad regions of the cerebral cortex. Smaller descending tracts, which include the rubrospinal tract, the vestibulospinal tract, and the reticulospinal tract, originate in discrete and diffuse nuclei in the midbrain, pons, and medulla. Most of these brain-stem nuclei themselves receive input from the cerebral cortex, the cerebellar cortex, deep nuclei of the cerebellum, or some combination of these.

In addition, autonomic tracts, which descend from various nuclei in the brain stem to preganglionic sympathetic and parasympathetic neurons in the spinal cord, constitute a vital link between the centres that regulate visceral functions and the nerve cells that actually effect changes.

Corticospinal tract. Universally regarded as the single most important tract concerned with skilled voluntary activity, the corticospinal tract originates from pyramid-shaped cells in the premotor, primary motor, and primary sensory cortex. Containing about one million fibres, it forms a significant part of the posterior limb of the internal capsule and is a major constituent of the crus cerebri in the midbrain. As the fibres emerge from the pons, they form compact bundles on the ventral surface of the medulla, known as the medullary pyramids (see Figure 6). In the lower medulla about 90 percent of the fibres of the corticospinal tract decussate and descend in the dorsal part of the lateral funiculus of the spinal cord. Of the fibres that do not cross in the medulla, approximately 8 percent cross in cervical spinal segments (see Figure 8). As the tract descends, fibres and collaterals are given off at all segmental levels, synapsing upon interneurons in lamina VII and upon motor neurons in lamina IX. Approximately 50 percent of the corticospinal fibres terminate within cervical segments.

At birth, few of the fibres of the corticospinal tract are myelinated; myelination takes place during the first year after birth, parallel to the acquisition of motor skills. Because the tract passes through, or close to, nearly every major division of the neuraxis, it is vulnerable to vascular and other kinds of lesions. A relatively small lesion in the posterior limb of the internal capsule, for example, may result in contralateral hemiparesis, which is characterized by weakness, spasticity, greatly increased deep tendon reflexes, and certain abnormal reflexes.

Rubrospinal tract. The rubrospinal tract arises from cells in the caudal part of the red nucleus, an encapsulated cell group in the midbrain tegmentum (see Figure 5). Fibres of this tract decussate at midbrain levels, descend in the lateral funiculus of the spinal cord (overlapping ventral parts of the corticospinal tract), enter the spinal gray, and terminate on interneurons in lamina VII. Through these crossed rubrospinal projections, the red nucleus exerts a facilitating influence on flexor alpha motor neurons and a reciprocal inhibiting influence on extensor alpha motor neurons. Because cells of the red nucleus receive input from the motor cortex (via corticorubral projections) and from globose and emboliform nuclei of the cerebellum (via the superior cerebellar peduncle), the rubrospinal tract effectively brings flexor muscle tone under the control of these two regions of the brain.

Vestibulospinal tract. The vestibulospinal tract originates from cells of the lateral vestibular nucleus, which

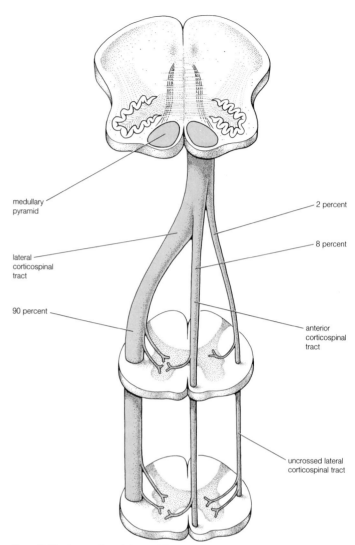

medullary pyramid

lateral corticospinal tract

90 percent

2 percent

8 percent

anterior corticospinal tract

uncrossed lateral corticospinal tract

Figure 8: The decussation of the medullary pyramids and the formation of the corticospinal system in the spinal cord.
From M.B. Carpenter, *Core Text of Neuroanatomy*, 4th ed. (1991); Williams & Wilkins, Baltimore

lies in the floor of the fourth ventricle. Fibres of this tract descend the length of the spinal cord in the ventral and lateral funiculi without crossing, enter laminae VIII and IX of the anterior horn, and end upon both alpha and gamma motor neurons, which innervate ordinary muscle fibres and fibres of the muscle spindle. Cells of the lateral vestibular nucleus receive facilitating impulses from labyrinthine receptors in the utricle and from fastigial nuclei in the cerebellum. In addition, inhibitory influences upon these cells are conveyed by direct projections from Purkinje cells in the anterior lobe of the cerebellum. Thus, the vestibulospinal tract mediates the influences of the vestibular end organ and the cerebellum upon extensor muscle tone.

A smaller number of vestibular projections, originating from the medial and inferior vestibular nuclei, descend ipsilaterally in the medial longitudinal fasciculus only to cervical levels. These fibres exert excitatory and inhibitory effects upon cervical motor neurons.

Reticulospinal tract. The reticulospinal tracts arise from relatively large but restricted regions of the reticular formation of the pons and medulla—the same cells that project ascending processes to intralaminar thalamic nuclei and play an important role in maintaining alertness and the conscious state. The pontine reticulospinal tract arises from aggregations of cells in the pontine reticular formation, descends ipsilaterally as the largest component of the medial longitudinal fasciculus, and terminates among cells in laminae VII and VIII. Fibres of this tract exert facilitating influences upon voluntary movements, muscle

Function in voluntary activity

Mediation of balance and coordination functions

tone, and a variety of spinal reflexes. The medullary reticulospinal tract, originating from reticular neurons on both sides of the median raphe, descends in the ventral part of the lateral funiculus and terminates at all spinal levels upon cells in laminae VII and IX. The medullary reticulospinal tract inhibits the same motor activities that are facilitated by the pontine reticulospinal tract. Both tracts receive input from regions of the motor cortex.

Autonomic pathways. Descending fibre systems concerned with visceral and autonomic activities emanate from collections of cells at various levels of the brain stem. For example, hypothalamic nuclei project to visceral nuclei in both the medulla and spinal cord; in the spinal cord these direct hypothalamospinal projections terminate upon cells of the intermediolateral cell column in thoracic, lumbar, and sacral segments. Preganglionic parasympathetic neurons originating in the oculomotor nuclear complex in the midbrain project not only to the ciliary ganglion but also directly to spinal levels. Some of these fibres reach lumbar segments of the spinal cord, most of them terminating in parts of laminae I and V. Pigmented cells in an area of the rostral pons known as the isthmus form a blackish blue collection visible in gross brain sections; known as the locus ceruleus, these cells are rich in norepinephrine and distribute this neurotransmitter widely to all regions of the brain and spinal cord. Fibres from the locus ceruleus descend to spinal levels without crossing and are distributed to terminals in the anterior horn, the intermediate zone, and the dorsal horn. Other noradrenergic cell groups in the pons, near the motor nucleus of the facial nerve, project uncrossed noradrenergic fibres that terminate in the intermediolateral cell column (that is, lamina VII of the lateral horn). Postganglionic sympathetic neurons associated with this system have direct effects upon the cardiovascular system. Cells in the nucleus of the solitary tract project crossed fibres to the phrenic nerve nucleus (in cervical segments 3 through 5), the intermediate zone, and the anterior horn at thoracic levels; these innervate respiratory muscles.

The peripheral nervous system

The peripheral nervous system is a channel for the relay of sensory and motor impulses between the central nervous system on the one hand and the body surface, skeletal muscles, and internal organs on the other hand. It is composed of (1) spinal nerves, (2) cranial nerves, and (3) certain parts of the autonomic nervous system. As in the central nervous system, peripheral nervous pathways are made up of neurons (that is, nerve cell bodies and their axons and dendrites) as well as the points at which one neuron communicates with the next (that is, the synapse). The structures commonly known as nerves (or by such names as roots, rami, trunks, and branches) are actually composed of orderly arrangements of the axonal and dendritic processes of many nerve cell bodies.

Ganglia   The cell bodies of peripheral neurons are often found grouped into clusters called ganglia. Based on the type of nerve cell bodies found in ganglia, they may be classified as either sensory or motor. Sensory ganglia are found as oval swellings on the dorsal roots of spinal nerves, and they are also found on the roots of certain cranial nerves. The sensory neurons making up these ganglia are unipolar. Shaped much like a golf ball on a tee, they have round or slightly oval cell bodies with concentrically located nuclei, and they give rise to a single fibre that undergoes a T-shaped bifurcation, one branch going to the periphery and the other entering the brain or spinal cord. There are no synaptic contacts between neurons in a sensory ganglion.

Motor ganglia are associated with neurons of the autonomic nervous system. Many of these are found in the sympathetic trunks, two long chains of ganglia lying along each side of the vertebral column from the base of the skull to the coccyx; these are referred to as paravertebral. Other motor ganglia (called prevertebral) are found near internal organs innervated by their projecting fibres, while still others (called terminal ganglia) are found on the surfaces or within the walls of the target organs themselves.

Motor ganglia contain multipolar cell bodies, which have irregular shapes and eccentrically located nuclei and which project several dendritic and axonal processes. Preganglionic fibres originating from the brain or spinal cord enter motor (autonomic) ganglia, where they synapse on multipolar cell bodies. These postganglionic cells, in turn, send their processes to visceral structures.

SPINAL NERVES

Sensory input from the body surface, from joint, tendon, and muscle receptors, and from internal organs passes centrally through the dorsal roots of the spinal cord. Fibres from motor cells in the spinal cord exit via the ventral roots and course to their peripheral targets (autonomic ganglia or skeletal muscle). The spinal nerve is formed by the joining of dorsal and ventral roots, and it is the basic structural and functional unit on which the peripheral nervous system is built.

Structure of the spinal nerve. In humans there are 31 pairs of spinal nerves. In descending order from the most rostral end of the spinal cord, there are 8 cervical (designated C_1–C_8), 12 thoracic (T_1–T_{12}), 5 lumbar (L_1–L_5), 5 sacral (S_1–S_5), and 1 coccygeal (Coc_1). Each spinal nerve exits the vertebral canal through an opening called the intervertebral foramen (see Figure 12). The first spinal nerve (C_1) exits between the skull and the first cervical vertebra; consequently, spinal nerves C_1–C_7 exit above the correspondingly numbered vertebrae. Spinal nerve C_8, however, exits between the 7th cervical and first thoracic vertebrae, so that, beginning with T_1, all other spinal nerves exit below their corresponding vertebrae.

Just outside the intervertebral foramen, two branches, known as the gray and white rami communicates, connect the spinal nerve with the sympathetic trunk. These rami, along with the sympathetic trunk and more distal ganglia, are concerned with the innervation of visceral structures. In addition, small meningeal branches leave the spinal nerve and gray ramus and reenter the vertebral canal, where they innervate dura and blood vessels.

More peripherally, the spinal nerve divides into ventral and dorsal rami (see Figure 9). All dorsal rami (with the exception of those from C_1, S_4, S_5, and Coc_1) have medial and lateral branches, which innervate deep back muscles and overlying skin. The medial and lateral branches of the dorsal rami of spinal nerves C_2–C_8 supply both muscles and skin of the neck. Those of T_1–T_6 are mostly cutaneous (that is, supplying only the skin), while those from T_7–T_{12} are mainly muscular. Dorsal rami from L_1–L_3 have both sensory and motor fibres, while those from L_4–L_5 are only muscular. Dorsal rami of S_1–S_3 may also be divided into

Ventral and dorsal rami

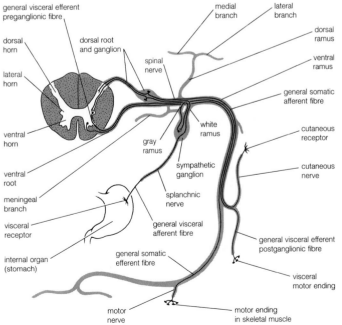

Figure 9: A typical spinal nerve.

medial and lateral branches, serving deep muscles of the lower back as well as cutaneous areas of the lower buttocks and perianal area. Undivided dorsal rami from S_4, S_5, and Coc_1 also send cutaneous branches to the gluteal and perianal regions.

Ventral rami of the spinal nerves carry sensory and motor fibres for the innervation of the muscles, joints, and skin of the lateral and ventral body walls and the extremities (see below *Plexuses of the ventral rami*). Both dorsal and ventral rami also contain autonomic fibres.

Functional components. Because spinal nerves contain both sensory fibres (from the dorsal roots) and motor fibres (from the ventral roots), they are known as mixed nerves. When individual fibres of a spinal nerve are identified by their specific function, they may be categorized as one of four types: (1) general somatic afferent, (2) general visceral afferent, (3) general somatic efferent, and (4) general visceral efferent. The term somatic refers to the body wall (broadly defined to include skeletal muscles as well as the surface of the skin), and visceral refers to structures composed of smooth muscle, cardiac muscle, or glandular epithelium (or a combination of these). Efferent fibres carry motor information to skeletal muscle and to autonomic ganglia (and then to visceral structures), and afferent fibres carry sensory information from them.

General somatic afferent receptors are sensitive to pain, thermal sensation, touch and pressure, and changes in the position of the body. (Pain and temperature sensation coming from the surface of the body are called exteroceptive, while sensory information arising from tendons, muscles, or joint capsules are called proprioceptive.) General visceral afferent receptors are found in organs of the thorax, abdomen, and pelvis; their fibres convey, for example, pain information from the digestive tract. Both types of afferent fibre project centrally from cell bodies in dorsal-root ganglia.

Carrying motor information

General somatic efferent fibres originate from large ventral-horn cells and distribute to skeletal muscles in the body wall and in the extremities. General visceral efferent fibres also arise from cell bodies located within the spinal cord, but they exit only at thoracic and upper lumbar levels or at sacral levels (more specifically, at levels T_1–L_2 and S_2–S_4). Fibres from T_1–L_2 enter the sympathetic trunk, where they either form synaptic contacts within a ganglion, ascend or descend within the trunk, or exit the trunk and proceed to ganglia situated closer to their target organs. Fibres from S_2–S_4, on the other hand, leave the cord as the pelvic nerve and proceed to terminal ganglia located in the target organs. Postganglionic fibres arising from ganglia in the sympathetic trunk rejoin the spinal nerves and distribute to blood vessels, sweat glands, and arrector pili muscles, while postganglionic fibres arising from prevertebral and terminal ganglia innervate viscera of the thorax, abdomen, and pelvis.

Plexuses of the ventral rami. All plexuses arising from the ventral rami of spinal nerves contain sensory, motor, and autonomic fibres. The plexuses are the cervical, brachial, lumbar, sacral, and coccygeal.

Cervical plexus. Cervical levels C_1–C_4 are the main contributors to the cervical plexus; in addition, small branches link C_1 and C_2 with the vagus nerve, C_1 and C_2 with the hypoglossal nerve, and C_2–C_4 with the accessory nerve. Sensory branches of the cervical plexus are the lesser occipital nerve (to scalp behind the ear), the great auricular nerve (to the ear and to the skin over the mastoid and parotid areas), transverse cervical cutaneous nerves (to lateral and ventral neck surfaces), and supraclavicular nerves (along the clavicle, shoulder, and upper chest). Motor branches serve muscles that stabilize and flex the neck, muscles that stabilize the hyoid bone (to assist in actions like swallowing), and muscles that elevate the upper ribs.

Originating from C_4, with small contributions from C_3 and C_5, are the phrenic nerves, which carry sensory information from parts of the pleura and pericardium and motor impulses to muscles of the diaphragm. Injury to the phrenic nerves would paralyze the diaphragm and render breathing difficult or impossible.

Brachial plexus. Cervical levels C_5–C_8 and thoracic level T_1 contribute to the formation of the brachial plexus;

small fascicles also arrive from C_4 and T_2 (see Figure 10A). Spinal nerves from these levels converge to form superior (C_5 and C_6), middle (C_7), and inferior (C_8 and T_1) trunks, which in turn split into anterior and posterior divisions. The divisions then form cords (posterior, lateral, and medial), which provide motor, sensory, and autonomic fibres to the shoulder and upper extremity.

Nerves to shoulder and pectoral muscles include the dorsal scapular (to the rhomboid muscles), suprascapular (to supraspinatus and infraspinatus), medial and lateral pectoral (to pectoralis minor and major), long thoracic (to serratus anterior), thoracodorsal (to latissimus dorsi), and

Innervation of the shoulder, arm, and hand

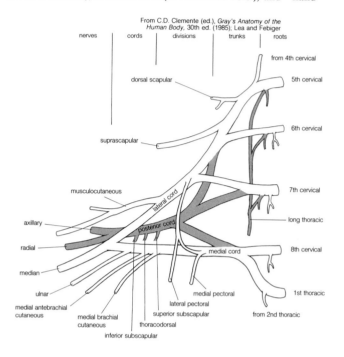

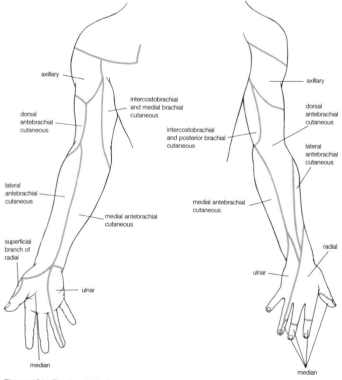

Figure 10A: *The brachial plexus.*
(Top) Formation from ventral rami of spinal nerves and branching into peripheral nerves; (bottom) anterior (left) and posterior (right) views of cutaneous sensory areas of the right arm supplied by the brachial plexus.

subscapular (to teres major and subscapular). The axillary nerve carries motor fibres to the deltoid and teres minor muscles as well as sensory fibres to the lateral surface of the shoulder and upper arm. The biceps, brachialis, and coracobrachialis muscles, as well as the lateral surface of the forearm, are served by the musculocutaneous nerve.

The three major nerves of the arm, forearm, and hand are the radial, median, and ulnar (see Figure 10B). The radial nerve innervates the triceps, anconeus, and brachioradialis muscles, eight extensors of the wrist and digits, and one abductor of the hand; it is also sensory to part of the hand. The median nerve branches in the forearm to serve the palmaris longus, two pronator muscles, four flexor muscles, thenar muscles, and lumbrical muscles; most of these serve the wrist and hand. The ulnar nerve serves two flexor muscles and a variety of small muscles of the wrist and hand.

Cutaneous innervation of the upper extremity originates, via the brachial plexus, from spinal cord levels C_3–T_2. The shoulder is served by supraclavicular branches (C_3, C_4) of the cervical plexus, while the anterior and lateral aspects of the arm and forearm have sensory innervation via the axillary (C_5, C_6), nerve as well as the dorsal (C_5, C_6), lateral (C_5, C_6), and medial (C_8, T_1) antebrachial cutaneous nerves. These same nerves have branches that wrap around to serve portions of the posterior and medial surfaces of the extremity. The palm of the hand is served by the median (C_6–C_8) and ulnar (C_8, T_1) nerves. The ulnar nerve also wraps around to serve medial areas of the dorsum, or back, of the hand. A line drawn down the midline of the ring finger represents the junction of the ulnar-radial distribution on the back of the hand and the ulnar-median distribution on the palm (see Figure 10A). A small part of the thumb and the distal thirds of the index, middle, and lateral surface of the ring finger are served by the median nerve. The inner aspect of the arm and adjacent armpit is served by intercostobrachial and posterior and medial brachial cutaneous nerves (T_1–T_2).

Lumbar plexus. Spinal nerves from lumbar levels L_1–L_4 contribute to the formation of the lumbar plexus, which, along with the sacral plexus, provides motor, sensory, and autonomic fibres to gluteal and inguinal regions and to the lower extremity. Lumbar roots are organized into dorsal and ventral divisions.

Minor cutaneous and muscular branches of the lumbar plexus include the iliohypogastric, genitofemoral, and ilioinguinal (projecting to the lower abdomen and to inguinal and genital regions) and the lateral femoral cutaneous nerve (to skin on the lateral thigh). Two major branches are the obturator and femoral nerves. The obturator enters the thigh through the obturator foramen; motor branches proceed to the obturator internus and gracilis muscles as well as the adductor muscles, while sensory branches supply the articular capsule of the knee joint. An accessory obturator nerve supplies the pectineus muscle of the thigh and is sensory to the hip joint.

The sartorius muscle and medial and anterior surfaces of the thigh are served by branches of the anterior division of the femoral nerve. The posterior division of the femoral nerve provides sensory fibres to the inner surface of the leg (saphenous nerve), to the quadriceps muscles (muscular branches), the hip and knee joints, and the articularis genu muscle.

Sacral plexus. The ventral rami of L_5 and S_1–S_3 form the sacral plexus, with contributions from L_4 and S_4. Branches from this plexus innervate gluteal muscles, muscles forming the internal surface of the pelvic basin (including those forming the levator ani), and muscles that run between the femur and pelvis to stabilize the hip joint (such as the obturator, piriformis, and quadratus femoris muscles). These muscles lend their names to the nerves that innervate them. Cutaneous branches from the plexus serve the buttocks, perineum, and posterior surface of the thigh.

The major nerve of the sacral plexus, and the largest in the body, is the sciatic (see Figure 10B). Formed by the joining of ventral and dorsal divisions of the plexus, it passes through the greater sciatic foramen and descends in back of the thigh. There, sciatic branches innervate the biceps femoris, semitendinosus and semimembranosus

Innervation of the leg and foot

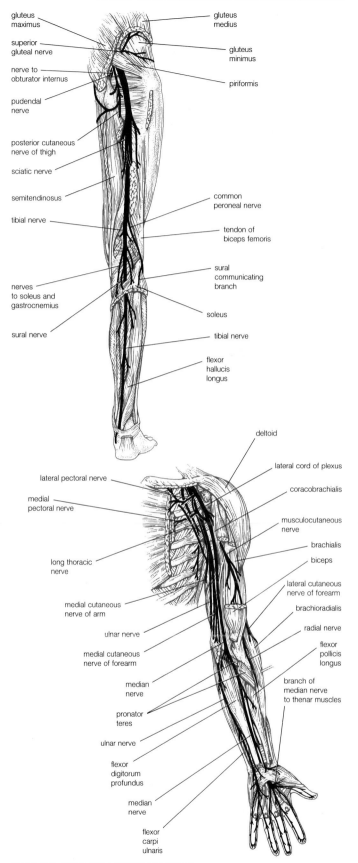

Figure 10B: *Nerves of the right leg and left arm.*
Posterior view of the leg showing the sciatic nerve and its branches, part of the sacral plexus. Anterior view of the arm showing the median, ulnar, and radial nerves and other branches of the brachial plexus.
From P.L. Williams *et al.*, *Gray's Anatomy*, 37th ed. (1989); Churchill Livingstone, Edinburgh

muscles, and part of the adductor magnus muscle. In the popliteal fossa (just above the knee) the sciatic nerve divides into the tibial nerve and the common fibular (or peroneal) nerve. The tibial nerve (from the dorsal division) continues distally in the calf and innervates the gastrocnemius muscle, deep leg muscles such as the popliteus, soleus, and tibialis posterior, and the flexor muscles, lumbrical muscles, and other muscles of the ankle and plantar aspects of the foot. The peroneal nerve, from the ventral division, passes to the anterior surface of the leg and innervates the tibialis anterior, the fibularis muscles, and extensor muscles that elevate the foot and fan the toes. Cutaneous branches from the tibial and common fibular nerves serve the outer sides of the leg and the top and bottom of the foot and toes.

Coccygeal plexus. The ventral rami of S_4, S_5, and Coc_1 form the coccygeal plexus, from which small anococcygeal nerves arise to innervate the skin over the coccyx (tailbone) and around the anus.

CRANIAL NERVES

Cranial nerves can be thought of as modified spinal nerves, since the "general" functional fibre types found in spinal nerves also are found in cranial nerves but are supplemented by "special" afferent or efferent fibres. Fibres conveying olfaction (in cranial nerve I) and taste (in cranial nerves VII, IX, and X) are classified as special visceral afferent, while the designation of special somatic afferent is applied to fibres conveying vision (cranial nerve II) and equilibrium and hearing (cranial nerve VIII). Skeletal muscles that arise from the branchial (pharyngeal) arches are innervated by fibres of cranial nerves V, VII, IX, and X; these are classified as special visceral efferent fibres.

The 12 pairs of cranial nerves are commonly identified either by name or by Roman or Arabic numeral.

Olfactory nerve (CN I or 1). Bipolar cells in the nasal mucosa give rise to axons that enter the cranial cavity through foramina in the cribriform plate of the ethmoid bone. These cells and their axons, totaling about 20–24 in number, make up the olfactory nerve. Once in the cranial cavity, the fibres terminate in a small oval structure resting on the cribriform plate called the olfactory bulb (see Figure 11). As stated above, the functional component of olfactory fibres is special visceral afferent. Injury or disease of the olfactory nerve may result in anosmia, an inability to detect odours; this may also dull the sense of taste.

Optic nerve (CN II or 2). Rods and cones in the retina of the eye receive information from the visual fields and, through intermediary cells, convey this input to retinal ganglion cells. Ganglion cell axons converge at the optic disc, pass through the sclera, and form the optic nerve. The optic nerve from each eye enters the skull via the optic foramen and joins its opposite to form the optic Crossing of chiasm. At the chiasm, fibres from the nasal halves of optic nerve each retina cross, while those from the temporal halves fibres remain uncrossed. In this way the optic tracts, which extend from the chiasm to the thalamus, contain fibres conveying information from both eyes. Injury to one optic nerve therefore results in total blindness in that eye, while damage to the optic tract on one side results in partial blindness in both eyes.

Optic fibres also participate in accommodation of the lens and in the pupillary light reflex. Since the subarachnoid space around the brain is continuous with that around the optic nerve, increases in intracranial pressure can result in papilledema, or damage to the optic nerve, as it exits the bulb of the eye.

Oculomotor nerve (CN III or 3). The oculomotor nerves arise from two nuclei in the rostral midbrain. These are (1) the oculomotor nucleus, the source of general somatic efferent fibres to superior, medial, and inferior recti muscles, to the inferior oblique muscle, and to the levator palpebrae superius muscle; and (2) the Edinger-Westphal nucleus, which projects general visceral efferent preganglionic fibres to the ciliary ganglion.

The oculomotor nerve exits the ventral midbrain, pierces the dura, courses through the lateral wall of the cavernous sinus, and exits the cranial cavity via the superior orbital fissure. Within the orbit it branches into a superior ramus (to the superior rectus and levator muscles) and an inferior ramus (to the medial and inferior rectus muscles,

the inferior oblique muscles, and the ciliary ganglion). Postganglionic fibres from the ciliary ganglion innervate the sphincter pupillae muscle of the iris as well as the ciliary muscle.

With the exception of the levator palpebrae superioris muscle, which is innervated bilaterally, oculomotor neurons project primarily to orbital muscles on the same side of the head. A lesion of the oculomotor nerve will result in paralysis of the three rectus muscles and the inferior oblique muscle (causing the eye to rotate downward and slightly outward), paralysis of the levator palpebrae superious muscle (drooping of the eyelids), and paralysis of the sphincter pupillae and ciliary muscles (so that the iris will remain dilated and the lens will not accommodate).

Trochlear nerve (CN IV or 4). The fourth cranial nerve is unique for three reasons. First, it is the only cranial nerve to exit the dorsal side of the brain stem. Second, fibres from the trochlear nucleus cross in the midbrain before they exit, so that trochlear neurons innervate the contralateral (opposite side) superior oblique muscle of the eye. Third, trochlear fibres have a long intracranial course before piercing the dura.

The trochlear nucleus is located in the caudal midbrain; the functional component of these cells is general somatic efferent. After exiting at the dorsal side of the midbrain, the trochlear nerve loops around the midbrain, pierces the dura, and passes through the lateral wall of the cavernous

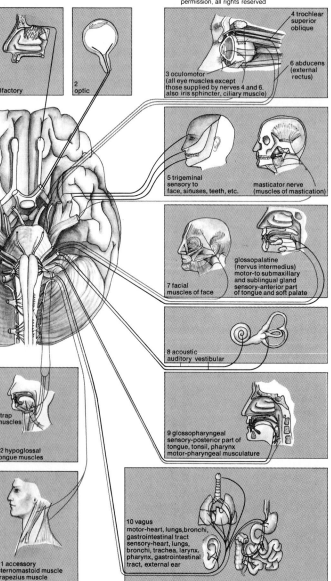

Figure 11: Cranial nerves.

sinus. It then enters the orbit through the superior orbital fissure and innervates only the superior oblique muscle, which rotates the eye downward and slightly outward. Damage to the trochlear nerve will result in a loss of this eye movement and may produce double vision (diplopia).

Trigeminal nerve (CN V or 5).   The trigeminal nerve is the largest of the cranial nerves. It has both motor and sensory components, the sensory fibres being general somatic afferent and the motor fibres being special visceral efferent. Most of the cell bodies of sensory fibres are located in the trigeminal ganglion, which is attached to the pons by the trigeminal root (see Figure 6). These convey pain and thermal sensations from the face, oral and nasal cavities, and parts of the dura and nasal sinuses, sensations of deep pressure, and information from sensory endings in muscles. Trigeminal motor fibres, projecting from nuclei in the pons, serve the muscles of mastication.

Lesions of the trigeminal nerve result in sensory losses over the face or in the oral cavity. Damage to motor fibres results in paralysis of the masticatory muscles; as a result, the jaw may hang open or deviate toward the uninjured side when opened. Trigeminal neuralgia, or tic douloureux, is an intense idiopathic pain originating mainly from areas supplied by sensory fibres of the maxillary and mandibular branches of this nerve.

Threefold division of the trigeminal nerve

The trigeminal ganglion gives rise to three large nerves, the ophthalmic, maxillary, and mandibular.

Ophthalmic nerve.   The ophthalmic nerve passes through the wall of the cavernous sinus and enters the orbit via the superior orbital fissure. Branches in the orbit are (1) the lacrimal nerve, serving the lacrimal gland, part of the upper eyelid, and the conjunctiva; (2) the nasociliary nerve, serving the mucosal lining of part of the nasal cavity, the tentorium cerebelli and some of the dura of the anterior cranial fossa, and skin on the dorsum and tip of the nose; and (3) the frontal nerve, serving the skin on the upper eyelid and the forehead and scalp above the eyes up to the vertex of the head.

Maxillary nerve.   The maxillary nerve courses through the cavernous sinus below the ophthalmic nerve and passes through the foramen rotundum into the orbital cavity. Branches of the maxillary nerve are (1) the meningeal branches, which serve the dura of the middle cranial fossa; (2) the alveolar nerves, serving the upper teeth and gingiva and the lining of the maxillary sinus; (3) the nasal and palatine nerves, which serve portions of the nasal cavity and the mucosa of the hard and soft palate; and (4) the infraorbital, zygomaticotemporal, and zygomaticofacial nerves, serving the upper lip, the lateral surfaces of the nose, the lower eyelid and conjunctiva, and skin on the cheek and the side of the head behind the eye.

Mandibular nerve.   The mandibular nerve exits the cranial cavity via the foramen ovale and serves (1) the meninges of middle and parts of the anterior cranial fossae (meningeal branches); (2) the temporomandibular joint, skin over part of the ear, and skin over the sides of the head above the ears (auriculotemporal nerve); (3) oral mucosa, the anterior two-thirds of the tongue, gingiva adjacent to the tongue, and the floor of the mouth (lingual nerve); and (4) the mandibular teeth (inferior alveolar nerve). Skin over the lateral and anterior surfaces of the mandible and the lower lip is served by cutaneous branches of the mandibular nerve.

Trigeminal motor fibres exit the cranial cavity via the foramen ovale along with the mandibular nerve. They serve the muscles of mastication (temporalis, masseter, medial and lateral pterygoid), three muscles involved in aspects of swallowing (anterior portions of the digastric muscle, the mylohyoid muscle, and the tensor veli palatini), and a muscle that has a damping effect on loud noises by stabilizing the tympanic membrane (tensor tympani).

Abducens nerve (CN VI or 6).   From its nucleus in the caudal pons, the abducens nerve exits the brain stem at the pons-medulla junction, pierces the dura, passes through the cavernous sinus close to the internal carotid artery, and exits the cranial vault via the superior orbital fissure. In the orbit the abducens nerve innervates the lateral rectus muscle, which turns the eye outward. Damage to the abducens nerve results in a tendency for the eye to deviate medially, or "cross." Double vision may result on attempted lateral gaze.

Facial nerve (CN VII or 7).   The facial nerve is composed of a large root that innervates facial muscles and a small root (known as the intermediate nerve) that contains sensory and autonomic fibres.

From the facial nucleus in the pons, facial motor fibres enter the internal auditory meatus, pass through the temporal bone, exit the skull via the stylomastoid foramen, and fan out over each side of the face forward of the ear. Fibres of the facial nerve are special visceral efferent; they innervate small muscles of the external ear, the platysma, the stapedius, the occipitofrontalis, the stylohyoid posterior belly of the digastric, the buccinator, and the muscles of facial expression.

The intermediate nerve

The intermediate nerve contains autonomic (parasympathetic) as well as general and special sensory fibres. Preganglionic autonomic fibres, classified as general visceral efferent, project from the superior salivatory nucleus in the pons. Exiting with the facial nerve, they pass to the pterygopalatine ganglion via the greater petrosal nerve (a branch of the facial nerve) and to the submandibular ganglion by way of the chorda tympani nerve (another branch of the facial nerve, which joins the lingual branch of the mandibular nerve). Postganglionic fibres from the pterygopalatine ganglion innervate nasal and palatine glands and the lacrimal gland, while those from the submandibular ganglion serve submandibular and sublingual salivary glands. Among the sensory components of the intermediate nerve, general somatic afferent fibres relay sensation from the caudal surface of the ear, while special visceral afferent fibres originate from taste buds in the anterior two-thirds of the tongue, course in the lingual branch of the mandibular nerve, and then join the facial nerve via the chorda tympani branch. Both somatic and visceral afferent fibres have cell bodies in the geniculate ganglion, which is located on the facial nerve as it passes through the facial canal in the temporal bone.

Injury to the facial nerve at the brain stem produces a paralysis of facial muscles known as Bell's palsy as well as a loss of taste sensation from the anterior two-thirds of the tongue. If damage occurs at the stylomastoid foramen, facial muscles will be paralyzed but taste will be intact.

Vestibulocochlear nerve (CN VIII or 8).   This cranial nerve has a vestibular part, which functions in balance, equilibrium, and orientation in three-dimensional space, and a cochlear part, which functions in hearing. The functional component of these fibres is special somatic afferent; they originate from receptors located in the temporal bone.

Vestibular receptors are located in the semicircular canals, which provide input on rotatory movements (angular acceleration), and in the utricle and saccule, which generate information on linear acceleration and the influence of gravitational pull. This information is relayed by the vestibular fibres, whose bipolar cell bodies are located in the vestibular (Scarpa's) ganglion. The central processes of these neurons exit the temporal bone via the internal acoustic meatus and enter the brain stem alongside the facial nerve.

Auditory receptors of the cochlear division are in the organ of Corti and follow the spiral shape (about 2.5 turns) of the cochlea. Air movement against the eardrum produces mechanical actions by the ossicles of the ear, which, in turn, cause movement of fluid in the spiral cochlea. This fluid movement is transduced by the organ of Corti into nerve impulses interpreted as auditory information. The bipolar cells of the spiral (Corti's) ganglion give rise to central processes that course with the vestibular nerve. At the brain stem, cochlear fibres separate from vestibular fibres to end in the dorsal and ventral cochlear nuclei.

Lesions of the vestibular root result in eye movement disorders (nystagmus), unsteady gait with a tendency to fall toward the side of the lesion, nausea, and vertigo. Damage to the cochlea or cochlear nerve results in complete deafness, ringing in the ear (tinnitus), or both.

Glossopharyngeal nerve (CN IX or 9).   The ninth cranial nerve, which exits the skull through the jugular foramen, has both motor and sensory components. Cell bodies of motor neurons, located in the nucleus ambiguus in the

Innervation of the pharynx and tongue

medulla, project as special visceral efferent fibres to the stylopharyngeal muscle. The action of the stylopharyngeus is to elevate the pharynx, as in gagging or swallowing. In addition, the inferior salivatory nucleus of the medulla sends general visceral efferent fibres to the otic ganglion via the lesser petrosal branch of the ninth nerve; postganglionic otic fibres distribute to the parotid salivary gland.

Among the sensory components, special visceral afferent fibres convey taste sensation from the back third of the tongue via lingual branches of the nerve. General visceral afferent fibres from the pharynx, the back of the tongue, parts of the soft palate and eustachian tube, and the carotid body and carotid sinus have their cell bodies in the superior and inferior ganglia, which are situated, respectively, within the jugular foramen and just outside the cranium. Sensory fibres in the carotid branch detect increased blood pressure in the carotid sinus and send impulses into the medulla that ultimately produce a reduction in heart rate and arterial pressure; this is known as the carotid sinus reflex.

Vagus nerve (CN X or 10). The vagus nerve has the most extensive distribution in the body of all the cranial nerves, innervating structures as diverse as the external surface of the eardrum and internal organs of the abdomen. The root of the nerve exits the cranial cavity via the jugular foramen. Within the foramen is the superior ganglion, containing cell bodies of general somatic afferent fibres, and just external to the foramen is the inferior ganglion, containing visceral afferent cells.

Pain and temperature sensations from the eardrum and external auditory canal, and pain fibres from the dura of the posterior cranial fossa, are conveyed on general somatic afferent fibres in the auricular and meningeal branches of the nerve. Taste buds on the root of the tongue and on the epiglottis contribute special visceral afferent fibres to the superior laryngeal branch. General visceral afferent fibres conveying sensation from the lower pharynx, larynx, trachea, esophagus, and organs of the thorax and abdomen to the left (splenic) flexure of the colon converge to form the posterior (or right) and anterior (or left) vagal nerves. Right and left vagal nerves are joined in the thorax by cardiac, pulmonary, and esophageal branches. In addition, general visceral afferent fibres from the larynx below the vocal folds join the vagus via the recurrent laryngeal nerves, while comparable input from the upper larynx and pharynx is relayed by the superior laryngeal nerves and by pharyngeal branches of the vagus. A vagal branch to the carotid body usually arises from the inferior ganglion.

Motor fibres of the vagus nerve include special visceral efferent fibres arising from the nucleus ambiguus of the medulla and innervating pharyngeal constrictor muscles and palatine muscles via pharyngeal branches of the vagus as well as the superior laryngeal nerve. All laryngeal musculature (excluding the cricothyroid but including the muscles of the vocal folds) are innervated by fibres arising in the nucleus ambiguus. Cells of the dorsal motor nucleus in the medulla distribute general visceral efferent fibres to plexuses or ganglia serving the pharynx, larynx, esophagus, and lungs. In addition, cardiac branches arise from plexuses in the lower neck and upper thorax, and, once in the abdomen, the vagus gives rise to gastric, coeliac, hepatic, renal, intestinal, and splenic branches or plexuses.

Damage to one vagus nerve results in hoarseness and difficulty in swallowing and speaking. Injury to both nerves results in increased heart rate, paralysis of pharyngeal and laryngeal musculature, atonia of the esophagus and intestinal musculature, vomiting, and loss of visceral reflexes. Such a lesion is usually life-threatening, as paralysis of laryngeal muscles can result in asphyxiation.

Accessory nerve (CN XI or 11). The accessory nerve is formed by fibres from the medulla (known as the cranial root) and by fibres from cervical levels C_1–C_4 (known as the spinal root). The cranial root originates from the nucleus ambiguus and exits the medulla below the vagus. Its fibres join the vagus and distribute to some muscles of the pharynx and larynx via pharyngeal and recurrent laryngeal branches of that nerve. For this reason, the cranial part of the accessory nerve is, for all practical purposes, part of the vagus nerve.

Fibres that arise from spinal levels exit the cord, coalesce and ascend as the spinal root of the accessory nerve, enter the cranial cavity through the foramen magnum, and then immediately leave through the jugular foramen. The accessory nerve then branches into the sternocleidomastoid muscle, which tilts the head toward one shoulder with an upward rotation of the face to the opposite side, and the trapezius muscle, which stabilizes and elevates (or shrugs) the shoulder.

Hypoglossal nerve (CN XII or 12). The hypoglossal nerve innervates certain muscles that control movement of the tongue. From the hypoglossal nucleus in the medulla, general somatic efferent fibres exit the cranial cavity through the hypoglossal canal and enter the neck in close proximity to the accessory and vagus nerves and the internal carotid artery. The nerve then loops down and forward into the floor of the mouth and branches into the tongue musculature from underneath. Hypoglossal fibres end in intrinsic tongue muscles, which modify the shape of the tongue (as in rolling the edges), as well as in extrinsic muscles that are responsible for changing its position in the mouth.

A lesion of the hypoglossal nerve on one side of the head would result in paralysis of intrinsic and extrinsic musculature on the same side. The tongue would atrophy and, on attempted protrusion, would deviate toward the side of the lesion.

The autonomic nervous system

The autonomic nervous system is a part of the peripheral nervous system that functions to regulate the basic visceral processes needed for the maintenance of normal bodily functions. It operates independently of voluntary control, although certain events, such as emotional stress, fear, sexual excitement, and alterations in the sleep-wakefulness cycle, change the level of autonomic activity.

The autonomic system is usually defined as a motor system that innervates three major types of tissue: cardiac muscle, smooth muscle, and glands. However, this definition needs to be expanded to encompass the fact that it also relays visceral sensory information into the central nervous system and processes it in such a way as to make alterations in the activity of specific autonomic motor outflows, such as those that control the heart, blood vessels, and other visceral organs. It also causes the release of certain hormones involved in energy metabolism (*e.g.,* insulin, glucagon, epinephrine) or cardiovascular functions (*e.g.,* renin, vasopressin). These integrated responses maintain the normal internal environment of the body in an equilibrium state called homeostasis.

The autonomic system consists of two major divisions: the sympathetic nervous system and the parasympathetic nervous system. These often function in antagonistic ways. The motor outflow of both systems is formed by two serially connected sets of neurons. The first set, called preganglionic neurons, originates in the brain stem or the spinal cord, and the second set, called ganglion cells or postganglionic neurons, lies outside the central nervous system in collections of nerve cells called autonomic ganglia. Parasympathetic ganglia tend to lie close to or within the organs or tissues that their neurons innervate, whereas sympathetic ganglia lie at a more distant site from their target organs. Both systems have associated sensory fibres that send feedback information into the central nervous system regarding the functional condition of target tissues.

A third division of the autonomic system, termed the enteric nervous system, consists of a collection of neurons embedded within the wall of the entire gastrointestinal tract and its derivatives. This system controls gastrointestinal motility and secretions.

SYMPATHETIC NERVOUS SYSTEM

Sympathetic preganglionic neurons originate in the lateral horns of the 12 thoracic and the first 2 or 3 lumbar segments of the spinal cord. (For this reason the sympathetic system is sometimes referred to as the thoracolumbar outflow.) The axons of these neurons exit the spinal cord in the ventral roots and then synapse on either sympathetic

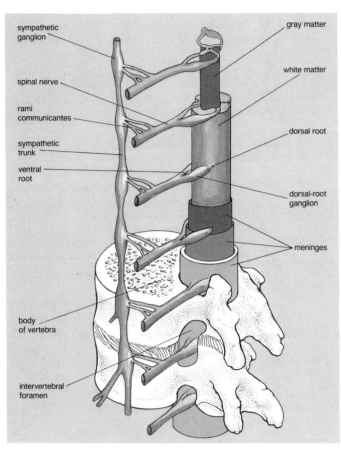

sympathetic
ganglion

gray matter

spinal nerve

white matter

rami
communicantes

sympathetic
trunk

dorsal root

ventral
root

dorsal-root
ganglion

meninges

body
of vertebra

intervertebral
foramen

Figure 12: Diagram of the spinal cord, vertebrae, and
sympathetic trunk (shown on one side only). Dorsal rami of
the spinal nerves are not shown.

From E. Gardner, *Fundamentals of Neurology*, 5th ed. (1968); W.B. Saunders Co.

Neurotransmitters and receptors. Upon reaching their
target organs by traveling with the blood vessels that supply them, sympathetic fibres terminate as a series of vari-
cosities close to the end organ. Because of this anatomical
arrangement, autonomic transmission takes place across a
junction rather than a synapse. "Presynaptic" sites can be
identified because they contain aggregations of synaptic
vesicles and membrane thickenings; postjunctional membranes, on the other hand, rarely possess morphological
specializations, but they do contain specific receptors for
various neurotransmitters. The distance between pre- and
postsynaptic elements can be quite large as compared to
typical synapses. For instance, the gap between cell membranes of a typical chemical synapse is 30–50 nanometres,
while in blood vessels the distance is often greater than
100 nanometres and, in some cases, 1–2 micrometres
(1,000–2,000 nanometres). Owing to these relatively large
gaps between autonomic nerve terminals and their effector cells, transmitters tend to act slowly; they become
inactivated rather slowly as well. To compensate for this
apparent inefficiency, many effector cells, such as those
in smooth and cardiac muscle, are connected by low-
resistance pathways that allow for electrotonic coupling of
the cells. In this way, if only one cell is activated, multiple
cells will respond and work as a group.

At a first approximation, chemical transmission in the
sympathetic system appears simple: preganglionic neurons
use acetylcholine as a neurotransmitter, whereas most
postganglionic neurons utilize norepinephrine (noradren-
aline)—with the major exception that postganglionic neurons innervating sweat glands use acetylcholine (see Figure
13). On closer inspection, however, neurotransmission is
seen to be more complex, because multiple chemicals are
released, and each functions as a specific chemical code
affecting different receptors on the target cell. In addition,
these chemical codes are self-regulatory, in that they act on
presynaptic receptors located on their own axon terminals.

Acetyl-
choline,
norepi-
nephrine,
and other
transmit-
ters

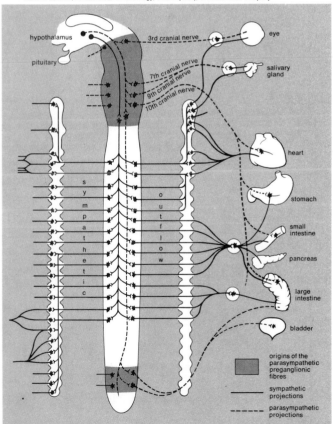

From E. Gardner, *Fundamentals of Neurology*, 5th ed. (1968); W.B. Saunders Company

Figure 13: Schematic representation of the general
arrangement of the autonomic nervous system. Autonomic
fibres to the organs of the head and trunk are shown on the
right side; the autonomic fibres on the left side represent
the sympathetic outflow to blood vessels, sweat glands, and
smooth muscle of hair follicles.

ganglion cells or specialized cells in the adrenal gland
called chromaffin cells.

Sympathetic ganglia. Sympathetic ganglia can be divided into two major groups, paravertebral and prevertе-
bral (or preaortic), on the basis of their location within
the body. Paravertebral ganglia generally lie on each side
of the vertebrae and are connected to form the sympathetic chain or trunk (see Figure 12). There are usually
21 or 22 pairs of these ganglia: 3 in the cervical region,
10 to 11 in the thoracic region, 4 in the lumbar region,
4 in the sacral region, and a single, unpaired ganglion
lying in front of the coccyx called the ganglion impar.
The three cervical sympathetic ganglia are the superior
cervical ganglion, the middle cervical ganglion, and the
cervicothoracic ganglion (also called the stellate ganglion).
The superior ganglion innervates viscera of the head; the
middle and stellate ganglia innervate viscera of the neck,
thorax (*i.e.*, the bronchi and heart), and upper limb. The
thoracic sympathetic ganglia innervate the trunk region,
and the lumbar and sacral sympathetic ganglia innervate
the pelvic floor and lower limb. All the paravertebral ganglia provide sympathetic innervation to blood vessels in
muscle and skin, arrector pili muscles attached to hairs,
and sweat glands (see Figure 13).

The three preaortic ganglia are the celiac, superior mesenteric, and inferior mesenteric. Lying on the anterior surface of the aorta, they provide axons that are distributed
with the three major gastrointestinal arteries arising from
the aorta. The three ganglia retain a pattern of innervation
that originates in the embryo. Thus, the celiac ganglion
innervates structures derived from the embryonic foregut,
including the stomach, liver, pancreas, duodenum, and
the first part of the small intestine; the superior mesenteric
ganglion innervates the small intestine, which is derived
from the embryonic midgut; and the inferior mesenteric
ganglion innervates embryonic hindgut derivatives, which
include the descending colon, sigmoid colon, rectum, urinary bladder, and sexual organs.

The sym-
pathetic
trunk

The chemical codes are specific to certain tissues. For example, most sympathetic neurons that innervate blood vessels secrete both norepinephrine and neuropeptide Y, sympathetic neurons that innervate the submucosal neural plexus of the gut contain both norepinephrine and somatostatin, and sympathetic neurons that innervate sweat glands contain calcitonin gene-related peptide, vasoactive intestinal polypeptide, and acetylcholine. In addition, other chemicals besides the neuropeptides mentioned above are released from autonomic neurons along with the so-called classical neurotransmitters, norepinephrine and acetylcholine. For instance, some neurons synthesize a gas, nitric oxide, that functions as a novel type of neuronal messenger molecule. Thus, neural transmission in the autonomic nervous systems involves the release of combinations of different neuroactive agents that affect both pre- and postsynaptic receptors.

Neurotransmitters released from nerve terminals bind to specific receptors, which are specialized macromolecules embedded in the cell membrane. The binding action initiates a series of specific biochemical reactions in the target cell that produce a physiological response. These effects can be modified by various drugs that act as agonists or antagonists. In the sympathetic nervous system, for example, there are five types of adrenergic receptors (receptors binding epinephrine): $\alpha_1, \alpha_2, \beta_1, \beta_2,$ and β_3. These are found in different combinations in various cells throughout the body. Activation of α_1 receptors in arterioles causes blood-vessel constriction, whereas stimulation of α_2 autoreceptors (receptors located in sympathetic presynaptic nerve endings) function to inhibit the release of norepinephrine. Other types of tissue have unique adrenergic receptors. Heart rate and myocardial contractility, for example, is controlled by β_1 receptors, bronchial smooth muscle relaxation is mediated by β_2 receptors, and lipolysis is controlled by β_3 receptors.

Cholinergic receptors (receptors binding acetylcholine) also are found in the sympathetic system (as well as the parasympathetic system). Nicotinic cholinergic receptors cause sympathetic postganglionic neurons, adrenal chromaffin cells, and parasympathetic postganglionic neurons to fire and release their chemicals. Muscarinic receptors are associated mainly with parasympathetic functions and are located in peripheral tissues (e.g., glands, smooth muscle). Peptidergic receptors exist in target cells as well.

The length of time that each type of chemical acts on its target cell is variable. As a rule, peptides cause slowly developing, long-lasting effects (one or more minutes), whereas the classical transmitters produce short-term effects (about 25 milliseconds).

The sympathetic nervous system normally functions to produce localized adjustments (such as sweating) and reflex adjustments of the cardiovascular system. Under conditions of stress, however, the entire sympathetic nervous system is activated, producing an immediate, widespread response that has been called the "fight or flight" response. This is characterized by the release of large quantities of epinephrine from the adrenal gland, an increase in heart rate, an increase in cardiac output, skeletal muscle vasodilation, cutaneous and gastrointestinal vasoconstriction, pupillary dilation, bronchial dilation, and piloerection. The overall effect is to prepare the individual for imminent danger.

The "fight or flight" response

PARASYMPATHETIC NERVOUS SYSTEM

The parasympathetic nervous system is organized in a manner similar to the sympathetic nervous system. Its motor component consists of a two-neuron system. The preganglionic neurons lie in specific cell groups (also called nuclei) in the brain stem or in the lateral horns of the spinal cord at sacral levels (segments $S_2–S_4$). Because parasympathetic fibres exit from these two sites, the system is sometimes referred to as the craniosacral outflow. Preganglionic axons emerging from the brain stem project to parasympathetic ganglia that are located in the head (ciliary, pterygopalatine [also called sphenopalatine], and otic ganglia) or near the heart (cardiac ganglia), embedded in the end organ itself (e.g., the trachea, bronchi, and gastrointestinal tract), or situated a short distance

from the urinary bladder (pelvic ganglion). Both pre- and postganglionic neurons secrete acetylcholine as a neurotransmitter, but, like sympathetic ganglion cells, they also contain other neuroactive chemical agents that function as cotransmitters.

The parasympathetic nervous system modulates mainly visceral organs such as glands. These are never activated en masse as in the "fight or flight" sympathetic response. While providing important control of many tissues, the parasympathetic system, unlike the sympathetic system, is not crucial for the maintenance of life.

The third cranial nerve (oculomotor nerve) contains parasympathetic nerve fibres that regulate the iris and lens of the eye. From their origin in the Edinger-Westphal nucleus of the midbrain, preganglionic axons travel to the orbit and synapse on the ciliary ganglion. The ciliary ganglion contains two types of postganglionic neurons: one innervates smooth muscle of the iris and is responsible for pupillary constriction, and the other innervates ciliary muscle and controls the curvature of the lens.

Various secretory glands located in the head are under parasympathetic control. These include the lacrimal gland, which supplies tears to the cornea of the eye; salivary glands (sublingual, submandibular, and parotid glands), which produce saliva; and nasal mucous glands, which secrete mucus throughout the nasal air passages. The parasympathetic preganglionic neurons that regulate these originate in the reticular formation of the medulla oblongata. One group belongs to the superior salivatory nucleus and lies in the rostral part of the medullary reticular formation. These neurons send axons out of the medulla in a separate part of the seventh cranial nerve (facial nerve) called the intermediate nerve. Some of the axons innervate the pterygopalatine ganglion, and others project to the submandibular ganglion. Pterygopalatine ganglion cells innervate the vasculature of the brain and eye as well as the lacrimal gland, nasal glands, and palatine glands, while neurons of the submandibular ganglion innervate the submandibular and sublingual salivary glands. A second group of parasympathetic preganglionic neurons belongs to the inferior salivatory nucleus, a group lying in the caudal part of the medullary reticular formation. Its neurons send axons out of the medulla in the ninth cranial (glossopharyngeal) nerve and to the otic ganglion. From this site, postganglionic fibres travel to and innervate the parotid salivary gland.

Preganglionic parasympathetic fibres of the tenth cranial nerve (vagus) arise from two different sites in the medulla. Neurons that slow heart rate arise from a part of the ventral medulla called the nucleus ambiguus, while those that control the gastrointestinal tract arise from the dorsal vagal nucleus. After exiting the medulla in the vagus nerve and traveling to their respective organs, the fibres synapse on ganglion cells embedded in the organs themselves. The vagus nerve also contains visceral afferent fibres that carry sensory information from organs of the neck (larynx, pharynx, and trachea), chest (heart and lungs), and gastrointestinal tract into a visceral sensory nucleus located in the medulla and called the solitary tract nucleus.

Parasympathetic components of the vagus nerve

ENTERIC NERVOUS SYSTEM

The enteric nervous system is made up of two plexuses, or networks of neurons, embedded in the wall of the gastrointestinal tract. The outermost collection, lying between the inner circular and outer longitudinal smooth-muscle layers of the gut, is called the myenteric (or Auerbach's) plexus. Neurons of this plexus regulate the peristaltic waves, consisting of polarized muscular activity, that move digestive products from oral to anal openings. In addition, myenteric neurons control local muscular contractions that are responsible for stationary mixing and churning. The innermost group of neurons is called the submucosal (or Meissner's) plexus. This group regulates the configuration of the luminal surface, controls glandular secretions, alters electrolyte and water transport, and regulates local blood flow.

Three functional classes of intrinsic enteric neurons are recognized: sensory neurons, interneurons, and motor neurons. Sensory neurons, activated by either mechanical or chemical stimulation of the innermost surface of the gut, transmit information to interneurons located within the myenteric and submucosal plexi, and the interneurons relay the information to motor neurons. Motor neurons in turn modulate the activity of a variety of target cells, including mucous glands, smooth muscle cells, endocrine cells, epithelial cells, and blood vessels.

Extrinsic neural pathways also are involved in the control of gastrointestinal functions. Three types exist: intestino-fugal, sensory, and motor. Intestinofugal neurons reside in the gut wall; they send their axons to the preaortic sympathetic ganglia and control reflex arcs that involve large portions of the gastrointestinal tract. Sensory neurons relay information regarding distention (pain) and acidity into the central nervous system. There are two types of sensory neurons: sympathetic neurons, which originate from dorsal-root ganglia found at the thoracic and lumbar levels; and parasympathetic neurons, which originate in the nodose ganglion of the tenth cranial nerve (vagus) or in dorsal-root ganglia at sacral levels S_2–S_4. The former innervate the entire gastrointestinal tract from the pharynx to the left colic flexure, and the latter innervate the distal colon and rectum. Each portion of the gastrointestinal tract receives a dual sensory innervation: pain sensations travel via sympathetic afferents, and information regarding the chemical milieu of the gut travels via parasympathetic fibres and is not consciously perceived.

The third extrinsic pathway, exercising motor control over the gut, arises from parasympathetic preganglionic neurons found in the dorsal vagal nucleus of the medulla and from sympathetic preganglionic neurons in the lateral horns of the spinal cord. These outflows provide modulatory commands to the intrinsic enteric motor system and are nonessential in that basic functions can be maintained in their absence.

Through the pathways described above, the parasympathetic system activates digestive processes while the sympathetic system inhibits them. The sympathetic system inhibits digestive processes by two mechanisms: (1) contraction of circular smooth muscle sphincters located in the distal portion of the stomach (pyloric sphincter), small intestine (ileo-cecal sphincter), and rectum (internal anal sphincter), which act as valves to prevent the oral-to-anal passage (as well as reverse passage) of digestive products; and (2) inhibition of motor neurons throughout the length of the gut. In contrast, the parasympathetic system provides messages only to myenteric motor neurons.

Motor innervation of the gut

DUANE E. HAINES. Professor and Chairman, Department of Anatomy, University of Mississippi School of Medicine, Jackson.

ARTHUR D. LOEWY. Professor of Neurobiology, Washington University Medical School, St. Louis, Mo.

CHARLES R. NOBACK. Emeritus Professor of Anatomy and Cell Biology, Columbia University College of Physicians and Surgeons, New York City.

America's Children:
Our Vision of the Future

by M. Joycelyn Elders, M.D.

If a society's reverence for its history is revealed by how it treats its elderly, then surely how we treat our children reveals our vision of the future. Our children are our link with the future. Through them we can see the 21st century. Indeed, the 21st century is being shaped today by the skills and values our children are learning. And while many children today are growing up healthy, too many are not.

Moments in America

It is startling to realize that in America:
- Every 35 seconds an infant is born into poverty.
- Every 2 minutes an infant is born at low birth weight.
- Every 11 minutes an infant is born at *very* low birth weight.
- Every 14 minutes an infant dies in the first year of life.
- Every 21 seconds a 15-to-19-year-old woman becomes sexually active for the first time.
- Every 32 seconds a 15-to-19-year-old woman becomes pregnant.
- Every 64 seconds an infant is born to a teenaged mother.
- Every 14 hours a child younger than 5 is murdered.
- Every 5 hours a 15-to-19-year-old is murdered.

Generational comparisons

Adolescence should be the healthiest time of life, and for most young people it is. Adolescents have fewer physician visits and occupy fewer hospital beds than any other age group. However, such standard mortality and morbidity data are being challenged as incomplete descriptors of child health. Comparative prevalences, population subgrouping, and trends over time are more enlightening.

Actually, for the first time in the history of this country, young people are less healthy and less prepared to take their places in society than were their parents. Consider these differences between the last two generations:
- In 1965, there were roughly 4 cases of gonorrhea and syphilis for every 1,000 American adolescents. In 1985, there were 12. The Centers for Disease Control and Prevention estimates that 2.5 million adolescents each year contract a sexually transmitted disease.
- In 1965, 16.7 out of every 1,000 unmarried teens aged 15–19 gave birth. In 1985, 31.6 out of every 1,000 did.
- In 1950, the rate of youths aged 14–17 who were arrested was 4 per 1,000. In 1985, the rate was 118 per 1,000.
- In 1950, fewer than 5% of youths experimented with an illicit drug before entering the 10th grade. In 1987, over 30% of youths had done so.
- In 1965, 9.8% of all children under 18 years lived in single-parent homes. In 1985, 21% did.

M. Joycelyn Elders, M.D., was Director, Arkansas Department of Health, when she received the prestigious Joseph W. Mountin Award for outstanding achievement in public health from the Centers for Disease Control and Prevention (CDC) in Atlanta, Georgia. Upon receipt of the award, in November 1991, she gave the Joseph W. Mountin Lecture, which the Annual's *editors are pleased to include in this volume. The lecture and award are named for the CDC's visionary founder, who in 1946 established what was then called the Communicable Disease Center. Elders' compelling message about the health and well-being of America's children is adapted with her permission and that of the CDC.*

213

• In 1960, 39% of mothers with school-age children worked outside the home. In 1987, 70% did.

Everywhere we look the statistics paint a dismal picture of how our children are doing:

• Every day 135,000 American students bring guns to school, and every day 30 children are wounded and 10 children die from guns.

• The homicide rate has doubled among 10-to-14-year-olds during the past 20 years, and homicide is the leading cause of death among black 15-to-19-year-olds.

• Over the past 20 years, the suicide rate has tripled among 10-to-14-year-olds and doubled among 15-to-19-year-olds.

• Abuse and neglect increased 74% during the past decade, and adolescents experience more abuse and neglect than younger children do. Every year over two million children and adolescents are reported abused or neglected, and hundreds of thousands more go unreported.

• Sexual activity is occurring at younger and younger ages, resulting in more than one million adolescents getting pregnant every year and an epidemic of sexually transmitted diseases, one of which is AIDS. Gonorrhea rates are actually higher among sexually active 15-to-19-year-olds than among 20-to-24-year-olds.

Racial and ethnic disparities

After steady advancements were made during the 1970s, progress on most key child health indicators stalled in the 1980s. And the differences in the status of children depending upon their race and ethnic background became more dramatic—underscoring the need for programs to respond to the diverse needs of racial and ethnic groups.

Poverty. Alarmingly, child poverty increased for all children during the 1980s. Today one of every five American children under 18 lives in poverty, and children from minority racial and ethnic backgrounds are overrepresented. Black children are the worst off, with 44% living in poverty, while Hispanic children are only slightly better off, with 38% in poverty.

Teenage sexuality. The U.S. surpasses all other Western developed nations in the rates of teenage pregnancy, abortion, and birth. Girls in the U.S. under age 15 are five times more likely to give birth than their counterparts in any other developed country for which data are available.

Blacks are much more likely than whites to be sexually active at younger ages. By age 15, black males are 3.5 times more likely than white males to have had intercourse. By age 15, black females are twice as likely as white females to have had intercourse. This tendency has been shown to correspond with other socioeconomic factors. Children who perceive they have poor prospects for the future and live in communities that are poor, segregated, and lack employment opportunities are more likely to initiate sex at an early age.

The number of births to unmarried teens also rose during the '80s to 8.2% in 1988. The percentage of out-of-wedlock teen births declined by 8% for blacks, while it rose by 25% for whites and 20% for Hispanics. However, the rate is still almost four times higher for black teens as compared with white teens, and nearly 40% of all black females become mothers before the age of 20.

Rates of gonorrhea among black adolescents are increasing, while overall rates are declining among other races and age-groups. Gonorrhea rates are more than seven times greater for nonwhite than white 15-to-19-year-old females. While black children under 15 represent 15% of the population, they represent 54% of the AIDS cases reported from 1981 to 1989.

Violent teen death. The chances that a teen will die a violent death—by either accident, suicide, or murder—increased for all teens during the 1980s. But there was a particularly dramatic shift in the danger of violent death for black teenagers. While white youths between 15 and 19 are three times more likely than blacks to die from motor vehicle injuries and twice as likely to die from suicide, black youths are five times more likely to die from homicide. Between 1984 and 1988, the black teen violent death rate increased 51%. By 1988, the black rate was 80 per 100,000 teens, far exceeding the white rate of 68 per 100,000.

The plight of young black males is especially precarious. They are dying disproportionately from homicide (their leading killer), suicide (tripled since 1960), and illicit drug abuse. Their risk-taking behavior often mimics reckless daredevils courting disaster. They are overrepresented among high school dropouts and underrepresented on college campuses. In Arkansas we have more young black men in prison than we have in college, and we are not unique.

Health insurance. In 1981, 18% of children 10 to 18 years old were not covered by health insurance; by 1986, the proportion of uninsured had risen to 21%. And while one in five American children has no public or private health coverage, one in four blacks and one in three Hispanics lack coverage.

Low birth weight. The overall percentage of babies born weighing less than 5.5 pounds increased slightly over the decade, but a black baby is more than twice as likely as a white or Hispanic baby to be born at low birth weight.

Infant mortality. Even though infant mortality rates did improve during the 1980s, a black baby is still twice as likely as a white baby to die during the first year of life.

Changes in American society

How did we get to this crisis? Well, we didn't arrive here overnight. Deep-rooted changes over the last several decades have fundamentally altered the future of our nation. We live in a society that at once denounces and glorifies sexual promiscuity and the use of illicit drugs, where children are taught to expect instant gratification without effort, instant solutions without sacrifice, and getting rather than giving. Family and community closeness has eroded, robbing our youth of guidance and support. Our society is more complex, more challenging, and more competitive than ever before.

A dramatic increase in poverty. The number of all children, irrespective of race or ethnic background, in poverty increased more than 20% from 1979 to 1986. Today 23% of children under age six live in poverty. Every

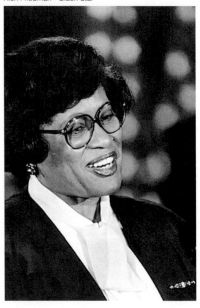

In mid-December 1992 U.S. President-elect Bill Clinton named M. Joycelyn Elders as his nominee for U.S. surgeon general. (The term of Surgeon General Antonia C. Novello expires in March 1994.) Throughout her professional life, Elders, a pediatric endocrinologist, has devoted herself to improving the lives of children, whom she considers "our link to the future."

Five years before selecting Elders for the nation's top health post, a youthful Governor Clinton chose her to run Arkansas's Department of Health. In describing his first meeting with the physician, Clinton said: "Now I know how Abraham Lincoln felt when he met Harriet Beecher Stowe. This is the little lady who started the great war." In Arkansas Elders earned a reputation for boldness, candor, and a willingness to confront controversy. Her approach to public health is a broad one—one that recognizes the important health impact of such factors as poverty, violence, and teenage sexuality.

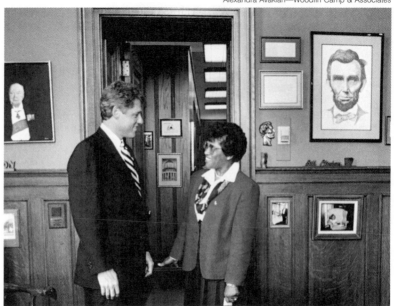

day in 3.4 million families with children, at least one parent goes to work, yet these families are still poor. There is no doubt that a life in poverty means poorer health, less medical care, inadequate housing, lower educational attainment, and more stress on families.

Drastic changes in family composition and stability. Divorce, remarriage, and a home with only one parent often create family instability, which affects healthy growth and development. One in four of our nation's youths lives with only one parent. However, among black families more than half of the young people do not have a father in the home.

Less contact between young people and adults. A University of Chicago study found that typical teenagers spend less than 40 minutes a day alone with their mothers and less than 5 minutes alone with their fathers. Society has become faster paced, more urbanized, more anonymous. Many families need two incomes. Single parents find it especially difficult to spend time with their children. Young people grow up more alone today.

Breakdown of traditional neighborhoods. Americans move frequently, making it difficult to make a strong commitment to their community. Extended family living nearby is a rarity. Children have become isolated.

Parents who do not act as parents. Some adults are not capable of being good parents—they are too young or distressed themselves. Others provide economic support but little emotional support. Still others are simply irresponsible.

Impact of television, radio, movies, and magazines. Children today are exposed to thousands of acts of violence, sex, greed, and substance abuse before they are able to understand the implications of such behavior. Many parents fail to help children recognize these negative messages for what they are.

Society's attitudes toward minorities. Racial and ethnic hostility and discrimination damage self-esteem and limit hope for many minority youths.

216

Inadequate housing and unsafe environments. Too many children grow up in impoverished environments with crime, violence, alcohol and drug abuse, teen pregnancy, spousal abuse, and other unhealthy behaviors—making them, too, likely to engage in such behavior.

By 1987, nearly half of the occupants of homeless shelters in New York City were children. Their average age was six years. Many of these children are growing up surrounded by diseases no longer seen in most developed nations. Whooping cough and tuberculosis, once considered archaic diseases, are now familiar in shelters.

The battle for America's future

These problems are inextricably linked with problems in the future. These children, on whom we will depend for decisions in the 21st century, face problems that threaten their ability to become healthy adults capable of leading full, productive lives. Business leaders and educators agree that the labor force of the future will need educated, healthy adults if the United States is to remain competitive in the global economy. Adolescents who are sick, hungry, or abused; who are distracted by family problems; who use alcohol or other drugs; or who feel they have no chance to succeed in this world are unlikely to attain the level of education required for success in the 21st century. Many will be only marginally employable.

We cannot afford to "write off" significant numbers of poor and minority citizens. By the year 2000, nearly one-third of the nation's 18-to-24-year-olds will be minorities, compared with fewer than one-quarter in 1980. In 2000, only one out of seven new workers will be a white male; some 43% will be from disadvantaged or minority backgrounds. We must ensure that all young people are prepared to be healthy, productive citizens.

All American children should enjoy access to good health care. A country that spends more per capita on personal health care than any other country, and perhaps leads the world in medical technology, has no acceptable excuse for the dismal state of our children. In response to a distant tyrant, this country sent hundreds of thousands of mothers and fathers, sons and daughters, husbands and wives, sisters and brothers to the Persian Gulf. No budget deficit or economic recession was allowed to stand in the way. How, then, can we reconcile failing to engage the enemies of poverty, violence, and family disintegration within our own country? In fact, America is engaged in a deadly battle over our children that poses as much of a threat to security and economic prosperity as any foreign enemy!

Americans must recognize the need to unite and work together to save our endangered future. Federal, state, and local governments and families all have key roles to play in our efforts to reverse these trends. This concept is exemplified by the success of immunization campaigns of the past. We have proved that total immunization can result in the eradication of a disease as prevalent as smallpox once was. To accomplish such a marvelous feat took the collaborative efforts of all the groups mentioned above.

One current barrier to successful cooperation is fragmentation. The profusion of problem-specific legislation at the state and federal level has resulted in a mishmash of regulations. In the long term this country must commit to providing adequate insurance coverage and the resources to develop services where they are needed. In the short run we must advocate additional federal funding for maternal and child health services through programs such as immunizations, Medicaid, WIC [Special Supplemental Food Program for Women, Infants, and Children], Title X family planning, the MCH [Maternal and Child Health] Block Grant, and Community and Migrant Health Centers. States should embrace Medicaid expansion options, establish state-funded insurance programs, provide state support for public health services, and implement methods for encouraging physicians to practice in medically underserved areas.

If we are to win the battle for the health of the next generation, it must also be waged at the community and neighborhood level. Communities are at the front line in providing services for children. They must be encouraged to structure their services so that they are accessible to adolescents. Access to and content of adolescent health services must remain priority issues. Services must be physically convenient and offered at convenient times. Services must be confidential. While parental involvement should be sought, it must not be allowed to prevent adolescents from obtaining services. Services must be comprehensive. While adolescents typically seek service because of one problem, they may have multiple problems and require a variety of services. Services must be age appropriate. Health providers must be sensitive to adolescents' desire to be treated as adults while still needing support in developing responsibility for their own health.

Businesses can play a key role in making health care more accessible and affordable for low-income working families. Private health professionals have a special responsibility to protect children's health by participating in publicly funded programs and serving the community. Families themselves must take responsibility for taking children to health care providers for preventive care, for providing safe environments, and for protecting their children's health to the best of their abilities.

Elders checks on a 15-year-old mother and her infant in a Little Rock hospital. High rates of teenage pregnancy were the number one problem that Arkansas's public health director set out to do something about. Nationwide, girls in the U.S. under age 15 are five times more likely to give birth than their counterparts in most other developed countries. In Elders' words, "All I want is every child born in America to be a planned, wanted child."

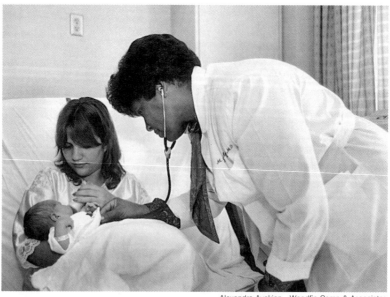

Alexandra Avakian—Woodfin Camp & Associates

Six prescriptions

As I have crisscrossed my state—and this nation—advocating for America's children, I have repeatedly offered my six prescriptions—strategies which, I believe, will secure an equal chance for our children.

1. Universal early childhood education to prepare our children to learn and achieve, removing some of the disadvantages that hold them back. At age four a child knows half as much as he will ever know. Why, then, are we waiting until kindergarten to intervene academically? Given the success of Head Start in improving school performance, there is no excuse for not making such resources available to all children who need them.

2. Comprehensive health and family life education should be taught to all children, starting in kindergarten and continuing through high school. Of course, this instruction should be appropriate to the child's ability to understand and need to know. But we must not be timid about facing our obligations even to the youngest children. After all, the messages they get from television and videos, from older siblings, and even from parents do not respect their ages. They need and should be encouraged to take responsibility for as much of their lives as they are capable. They need to know about human nutrition and physiology and the risks of substance abuse—tobacco, alcohol, all kinds of other drugs, and other dangerous substances that they may be offered by friends or strangers. In the same way, they need to be armed with knowledge about human reproductive biology and development. The risks of early and unprotected sexual activity are effectively learned in such a context. We must empower our children with useful facts and resources.

3. Parents need more support in nurturing, caring for, and teaching their children. So many of our social problems are worsened by parents' uninformed attitudes toward health and inappropriate behavior toward their children. Instruction, counsel, and peer discussion ought to be available. For our future parents—today's children—this can start in the comprehensive health and family life education mentioned above. For today's parents, accessible programs must be devised for their busy lives. Many resources can be tapped—churches, civic organizations, work sites, schools.

4. Male responsibility needs reinforcement. Family planning and sex education have traditionally focused on young females. This strategy appears to absolve young males of sexual responsibility. As with young females, many young males have few opportunities other than procreation to prove themselves. Accordingly, they must also be given opportunities for growth and self-expression in other arenas of life.

5. Comprehensive school-based clinics are needed to provide medical care to all teens. They are logical partners of comprehensive health and family life education. If children are taught health promotion and primary prevention, there will be demand for such services. Providing them in schools makes them nearly universally accessible.

6. Opportunities for higher education should be guaranteed. All children who make good grades, exhibit good citizenship, and have a low family income should be guaranteed assistance at state-supported colleges. Our society needs educated, critical minds, and our children need opportuni-

ties to develop fully. I am pleased to report that many states, including Arkansas, have recently taken steps toward filling these prescriptions.

Leadership is vital

But now you may ask, "What has this to do with me?" My challenge to each of you is to broaden your vision and become "leaders" in the battle to save our children. It is often hard to imagine ourselves as leaders. We view leaders as superpeople, able to keep going seemingly without limits of time or energy. Thus, people who lead ordinary lives with a job (or two or three), kids, aging parents, mortgages, plumbing that leaks, and a car that breaks down may be discouraged from ever trying to be a leader.

However, my personal experience has taught me that there is nothing mystical about being a leader. To begin with, it is hard work at best. Second, leaders take a lot of flak. Third, being a leader can be an isolating experience. But, I believe, to be effective in changing our nation as we know it, we must be leaders.

Lessons for the 1990s

As leaders, each of us shoulders tremendous responsibility. We must draw upon our life experiences to do what we know matters. We must remember the lessons of our generations. My friend, and another advocate for children, Marian Wright Edelman, president of Children's Defense Fund, has synthesized her experiences and submitted "Ten Lessons to Help Us Through the 1990s." They bear repeating.

Lesson 1: there is no free lunch. We must not feel entitled to anything we do not sweat and struggle for. Each of us must take the initiative to create opportunity. A people unable or unwilling to share, to juggle difficult, competing demands, or to make hard choices and sacrifices may be incapable of taking courageous action to rebuild our families and communities and to prepare for the future.

Lesson 2: set goals and work quietly and systematically toward them. We must resist quick-fix, simplistic answers. We must not talk big and act small. We cannot get bogged down in our ego needs. You can achieve a lot if you do not mind working hard and giving others the credit.

Lesson 3: assign yourself. Do not wait around for your boss or your friend to direct you to do what you are capable of figuring out and doing yourself. Do not do as little as you can to get by. If you see a need, do not ask, "Why doesn't somebody do something?" Ask, "Why don't I do something?"

Lesson 4: never work just for money. Do not confuse wealth or fame with character. Do not confuse legality with morality. Do not tolerate corruption. And demand that those who represent you do the same.

Lesson 5: do not be afraid of taking risks or being criticized. An anonymous sage said, "If you don't want to be criticized, don't say anything, do anything, or be anything." It does not matter how many times you fall down, it is how many times you get up.

Lesson 6: take parenting and family life seriously. Our leaders mouth family values we do not practice. Seventy nations provide medical care

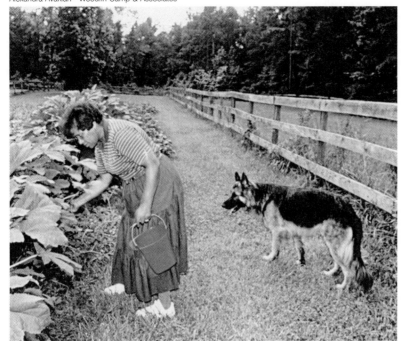

In what little leisure time she has, Elders, the daughter of Arkansas sharecroppers, tends the sprawling garden at her home outside Little Rock.

and financial assistance to all pregnant women; we are not one of them. Seventeen industrialized nations have paid maternity leave programs; we are not one of them.

Lesson 7: remember and help America remember that the fellowship of human beings is more important than the fellowship of race and class and gender in a democratic society. We must realize that our country's ability to compete and lead in the new century is as inextricably intertwined with our poor and nonwhite children as with white privileged ones.

Lesson 8: do not confuse style with substance or political charm with decency or sound policy. Words alone will not meet the children's or the nation's needs. Leadership and different priorities will.

Lesson 9: listen for the sound of the genuine within yourself. There are so many competing demands in our lives that many of us never learn to be quiet enough to hear the sound of the genuine within ourselves or other people.

Lesson 10: never think life is not worth living or that you cannot make a difference. In other words, never give up. I know how discouraging it can be to struggle year after year with the same issues. But we have to realize that it is not necessary to "win" immediately in order to make a difference.

Sojourner Truth, an illiterate slave woman who hated slavery and the second-class treatment of women, was heckled one day by an old white man. "Old woman, do you think that your talk about slavery does any good? Why, I don't care any more for your talk than I do for the bite of a flea." "Perhaps not," Sojourner rejoined, "but the Lord willing, I'll keep you scratching."

Enough committed fleas can make even the biggest dog uncomfortable and transform even the biggest nation.

WORLD OF MEDICINE

A review of
recent developments

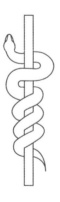

Aging

The health of older persons is becoming a dominant public health issue. In part, this dominance stems from the demographic imperative. Elderly people represent a growing proportion of the population in the industrialized countries. In Japan, for example, the elderly constituted only 4.9% of the population in 1950; by 1990 the proportion that was aged 65 and over was 11.7%; it is expected to double—to 23.9%—by 2025.

In the United States there were 31.8 million persons aged 65 and over in 1991, representing 12.6% of the total population. That number is expected to grow to 39.4 million by 2010, and the over-65 age group is expected to number 65.6 million, representing 21.8% of the population, by 2030. Although this overall increase in the number of older persons anticipated over the next half century in the U.S. is notable, several other projections are even more compelling. First, the older population itself is getting older, and the 85-and-older group, in particular, is the fastest growing segment. Second, an especially dramatic increase in the number of older persons will occur between the years 2010 and 2030 as the baby-boom generation reaches age 65. Third, disproportionate growth in the minority elderly population is expected; although minority members counted for 14% of older U.S. residents in 1990, by the year 2030 these groups will represent 25% of the elderly.

The implications of this major demographic shift on health and health care utilization are striking. Most older persons have at least one chronic medical condition, and many have multiple conditions that may interact. The most common conditions of older persons are arthritis (affecting 47%), hypertension (37%), and hearing impairments (32%). The repercussions of these and other medical conditions can be profound. For example, surveys have indicated that older Americans are restricted in their usual activities owing to illness or injury approximately one month (31 days) of every year. Although older persons represent less than 13% of the present U.S. population, this group accounts for 34% of all hospitalizations and 36% of the total health care expenditures.

Nevertheless, most older Americans continue to rate their health as good or excellent, and almost 12% continue to work, either full- or part-time. Moreover, this pattern is expected to become much more common. In a recent survey conducted by the Alliance for Aging Research, 26% of currently working respondents reported that they plan to retire *after* the age of 65 and 12% that they plan to *never* retire.

Five health-related subjects that are especially relevant to the rapidly aging population are addressed below: older drivers, incontinence, menopause, aggressive treatments and limitations of care, and Parkinson's disease. Each of these has been the focus of recent research, and several have been at the center of controversy, at a societal level as well as within the medical community.

Older drivers: safety questions

Most older drivers can, and do, drive safely. In fact, one small study of healthy older persons demonstrated that they committed fewer errors on a standardized road test than did younger drivers. Other studies, however, have shown that elderly motorists as a group commit some types of minor moving vio-

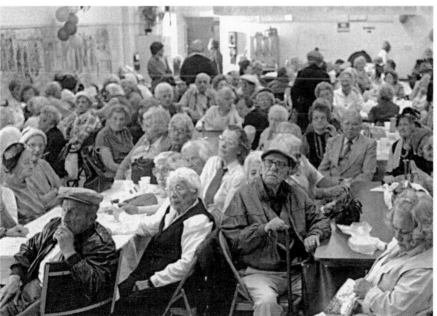

Bill Aron—Photo Edit

The elderly constitute the most rapidly growing segment of the U.S. population. The over-65 age group is expected to number nearly 40 million by the year 2010 and nearly 66 million—representing approximately 22% of the total population—by 2030. Because older people utilize a far greater proportion of health care services than younger people, establishing the medical priorities of society's senior members has become a dominant public health issue.

lations more than any other age group. Moreover, in the U.S. motor vehicle crashes are the leading cause of accidental death in persons aged 65 to 74 and are second only to falls as a cause of accidental death in persons over 75.

Although older drivers have lower overall crash rates, after adjustments for the total distance (number of miles) driven have been made, they have higher crash rates than any other age group except teenage drivers. The reasons for this apparent contradiction are several. Older drivers tend to drive shorter distances (fewer total miles), and some groups of older drivers have extremely high crash rates. Older persons with neurological impairments such as dementia, for example, are at much higher risk of being involved in motor vehicle crashes. Other conditions, such as decreased vision and diabetes, which become increasingly prevalent with advancing age, may also contribute to the higher crash rates in this age group. Additionally, elderly people commonly take medications that are sedating or may interfere with vision; these side effects can compound their medical problems and increase the risk of unsafe driving.

Unfortunately, no method that is currently available can reliably distinguish the unsafe from the safe older driver. The role of physicians and other health professionals is to identify medical conditions that may impair safe driving, determine the need for continued driving, explore alternatives to driving, and treat medical and functional conditions that might contraindicate

An 86-year-old widow from Kansas who had to give up her driver's license owing to failing vision and knee problems finds it hard adjusting to being "grounded" and accepting "that you have to stop doing some of the things you've always done."

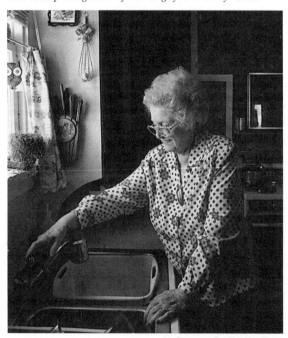

Ian Doremus—The New York Times

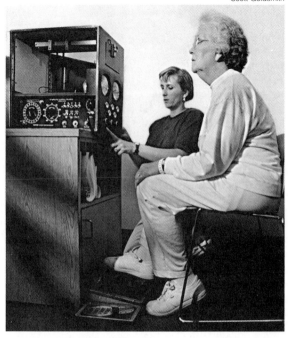

After having suffered a stroke, an older driver tests her reflexes to see if she is still capable of operating a motor vehicle safely. Many conditions associated with advancing age put elderly drivers at risk of being involved in crashes.

operating a motor vehicle. Governmental agencies, however, establish rules governing licensure to operate a motor vehicle and are responsible for issuance and revocation of licenses under these guidelines. With respect to the licensing of drivers with medical conditions, they are assisted by medical advisory boards comprising physicians and other health professionals. This idea of shared responsibility for the older driver between the health care system and governmental agencies works best when there is mutual cooperation and when each body respects the complementary role of the other.

One example of how this cooperation can work effectively is the approach recently taken in the state of California. As mentioned previously, the risk of unsafe driving is markedly increased among older drivers with dementia (*e.g.,* Alzheimer's disease). Many of the cognitive and perceptual deficits associated with dementia are likely to interfere with the ability to operate a motor vehicle. To arrive at an approach that was both uniform and fair, the California Department of Motor Vehicles Drivers Control Policy Division convened a panel of diverse experts, including physicians with expertise in evaluating and treating dementia, driver safety officers, and consumer groups. The panel developed a protocol that recognizes the very high risk of driving with moderate or severe dementia; the state now revokes the licenses of these persons. Yet it allows older drivers who have only mild dementia to be evaluated by their physicians and the licensing bureau to determine whether they are still capable of driving safely. Such an evaluation includes a medical examination by their doctors, a driving-knowledge test, a vision test, and a road test.

In some other states older persons are required to undergo more frequent, and often more thorough, testing than younger drivers. Although some senior citizens regard such rules as age discrimination, such testing often provides peace of mind for drivers and their families about the older person's "fitness" to drive and his or her likely safety on the road.

Urinary incontinence: effective treatments

The involuntary loss of urine is not a normal consequence of aging. It is, however, a common and expensive health problem that primarily affects older persons. Urinary incontinence (UI) can range from an occasional or slight loss of urine to frequent bed-wetting to major disability. UI is about twice as common in women as in men. Anatomic differences account for much of this difference. In females the muscles that support the bladder may be weakened following pregnancy, or hormonal deficiency associated with menopause can predispose to the development of stress incontinence. In males UI may occur as the result of an enlarged prostate, which blocks the flow of urine from the bladder.

In the U.S. the cost of managing this problem in nursing home residents and community-dwelling older persons is estimated to be $10 billion annually. The prevalence among those residing in nursing homes is 50% or higher, accounting for close to 10% of the costs of nursing home care. Despite its prevalence and high cost, UI is widely underdiagnosed and often goes untreated. This is particularly unfortunate because the problem *can* be effectively treated and often cured.

Because UI takes such a huge toll on the physical and psychological health of the older population, and because there was an urgent need to educate health professionals and the public alike about it, the Agency for Health Care Policy and Research of the U.S. Department of Health and Human Services recently convened an interdisciplinary panel, comprising physicians, nurses, gerontologists, allied health professionals, and consumers, to address the issue of appropriate and effective care of urinary incontinence in adults. The agency then issued clinical practice guidelines in March 1992 based on the panel's recommendations.

In general, urinary incontinence can be classified into two types: acute and persistent. The former is attributable to an acute medical illness that may or may not be localized to the urinary tract. It commonly occurs in hospital settings. For example, an older person who develops pneumonia may become confused (delirious) and as part of that delirium may develop urinary incontinence. Generally, such acute UI can be evaluated with simple diagnostic tests (*e.g.,* a blood test or urine culture to determine whether the person has a bacterial infection or diabetes) and effectively managed by treatment (*e.g.,* with antibiotics or insulin) of the underlying cause.

In some cases acute, or transient, UI is caused by medications the older person takes. Benzodiazepines such as flurazepam and diazepam may accumulate in the body, causing confusion and secondary incontinence. Alcohol, frequently used as a sedative, can also have this effect. Diuretics used in the treatment of hypertension may overwhelm bladder capacity and precipitate incontinence, especially in frail elderly persons. The problem is usually alleviated by withdrawal of the culprit medication.

In contrast, persistent urinary incontinence is usually present for months or years before it is evaluated and managed. There are four basic types of persistent incontinence.

Stress incontinence usually occurs in women and is characterized by the loss of urine with increased abdominal pressure (*e.g.,* from coughing, sneezing, or laughing). This type of incontinence is generally caused by increased mobility of the urethra (through which urine is excreted from the body), which may occur after pregnancy or abdominal surgery or perhaps as the result of hormonal changes.

Urge incontinence is the most common type of UI in persons aged 75 and over and in those who reside in nursing homes. This type results from inappropriate contraction of the muscles of the bladder, causing it to empty uncontrollably, which generally occurs when the bladder is irritated (*e.g.,* by a urinary tract infection) or when there is a dysfunction in the central nervous system. Sometimes, however, the underlying cause cannot be found, and the bladder muscles simply contract involuntarily before the bladder has filled with urine.

In *overflow incontinence* the bladder fills beyond capacity, causing it to leak small amounts day and night. This type usually occurs because there is an obstruction in the urinary tract system (*e.g.,* enlarged prostate) or damage to the nerves that are responsible for bladder contraction (*e.g.,* as a complication of diabetes).

Finally, *functional incontinence* has no direct physiological cause but occurs when a person whose urinary tract is functioning normally is either unable or unwilling to use the toilet appropriately. This may be due to medical conditions that restrict mobility (*e.g.,* arthritis) or, in nursing home residents, to use of physical restraints. It may also occur in conditions associated with declining mental function, such as dementia.

Within these four basic categories are several subgroups with multiple causes. Moreover, some patients

Stress incontinence treatments: typical outcomes				
	percentage affected			
outcome	pelvic muscle exercises	bladder training	alpha-agonist drugs	various surgical procedures
cured	12	16	0–14	78–84
improved	75	54	19–60	4–5
side effects	0	0	0–20	not applicable
complications	0	0	5–33	20

Source: *Urinary Incontinence in Adults: Clinical Practice Guideline,* Agency for Health Care Policy and Research, March 1992

may have "mixed incontinence," in which more than one of these types are present simultaneously. A number of tests may be done to determine the specific nature of the problem. These include (1) urinalysis to examine for signs of infection, blood, blood sugar, and other abnormalities; (2) blood tests to determine blood levels of various chemicals; (3) postvoid residual measurement, which measures urine in the bladder after urination; (4) a stress test that checks for urine loss when stress is put on bladder muscles (usually by coughing or lifting); (5) so-called urodynamic tests to examine bladder and urethral sphincter function (which may involve inserting a small tube and taking X-rays of the bladder); and (6) cystoscopy, which involves the insertion of a small tube into the bladder through which the doctor looks for abnormalities in the bladder or urinary tract.

Treatment of urinary incontinence depends upon the specific type of incontinence. For example, women who have stress incontinence may benefit from behavioral techniques that enable them to regain control of bladder function. These include scheduled toileting and pelvic muscle exercises (known as Kegel exercises) that help strengthen weak muscles around the bladder. Estrogen or other medications (*e.g.,* antispasmodics that eliminate abnormal contractions of the bladder muscles) may be beneficial in some cases. Severe stress incontinence, however, may require surgical treatment to restore a normal urinary tract anatomy (*e.g.,* returning the bladder neck to its proper position). Urge incontinence also may respond well to bladder-training techniques as well as bladder-relaxant medications (*e.g.,* propantheline or oxybutynin). When overflow incontinence is due to obstruction, surgical intervention to relieve the obstruction (*e.g.,* prostatectomy) may cure the incontinence. In other cases, particularly when the problem is due to nerve dysfunction, the treatment may be more difficult. Occasionally, a permanent indwelling catheter may be necessary to keep the person dry. Functional incontinence is usually best managed with scheduled

toileting or "prompted" urination; both of these techniques require a caregiver who is willing to work with the patient extensively.

Menopause and hormone therapy

As women born in the baby-boom generation are entering their fifth and sixth decades, menopause has emerged as a prominent issue in aging research and clinical medicine. With menopause, ovarian estrogen production ceases, which may be associated with hot flushes, dryness of the vagina and painful intercourse, loss of sexual desire, and mood disturbances. In addition, the drop in estrogen production is associated with longer-term consequences such as loss of bone mass (osteoporosis), increased risk of heart disease, and possibly urinary incontinence. Thus, this natural transition of aging may have adverse health consequences that are at least partially preventable with adequate hormone replacement therapy.

While some of the physiological changes (*e.g.,* decreases in circulating estrogen hormones) have been well described, and some of the clinical manifestations of menopause are well recognized (*e.g.,* hot flushes), other physiological aspects (*e.g.,* changes in androgen, or "male hormones") and more subtle clinical symptoms (*e.g.,* thinking and sleeping difficulties) are less well understood. Furthermore, the symptoms of menopause have been hard to characterize because of wide individual variability among women, even with respect to a particular symptom. For example, in some women hot flushes may be associated with profuse perspiration, whereas other women perspire only minimally.

The treatment of menopause-related symptoms is also complicated. Estrogen replacement therapy usually alleviates most symptoms of menopause and may prevent some of its long-term complications such as osteoporosis and coronary heart disease. A number of studies have suggested that taking postmenopausal estrogen reduces the risk of hip fracture by approximately 50%. Studies have also shown that estrogen reduces the risk of coronary heart disease and cardiovascular death in women by as much as 50%.

On the other hand, hormone replacement therapy is not free from side effects. Many studies indicate that taking estrogen alone is associated with increased risk of cancer of the endometrium, the lining of the uterus. Yearly monitoring with an endometrial biopsy, a procedure that can be done in a physician's office, or combining a progesterone hormone with estrogen therapy can reduce this risk.

Regardless of the choice of hormone therapy, most women who are receiving hormone replacement and have not had a prior hysterectomy will have some vaginal bleeding. A relationship between long-term estrogen therapy and cancer of the breast has been speculated but not proved. Furthermore, there are women, such as those who previously have had cancers of the breast or uterus, for whom estrogen therapy is contraindicated. For women who have other conditions (*e.g.,* gallstones, migraine headaches), estrogen therapy may have other risks.

Guidelines on long-term hormone replacement were issued in late 1992 by the American College of Physicians. On the basis of available evidence, the College recommended that all postmenopausal women be considered candidates for hormone therapy but that before starting estrogen replacement every woman discuss the specific benefits and risks with her doctor. The best method of treating the symptoms of menopause and preventing the outcomes of osteoporosis, coronary heart disease, and other disorders for women who cannot take estrogen is still unknown.

Recently the National Institute on Aging held a workshop to identify research priorities for menopause. Some of the issues identified as targets for research in the coming decade include the effects of menopause on more subtle clinical symptoms such as changes in mood and cognitive function as well as the effects of estrogen therapy on the urinary tract.

Aggressive treatments: an age bias?

As noted earlier, older persons consume health care disproportionately to their representation in the population. Moreover, this utilization of health care is not equally distributed over the group aged 65 and over. For example, fewer than 20% of older persons in the United States who are eligible for Medicare account for 80% of the total program payments. Adding to this conundrum is the fact that older persons frequently are denied access to effective treatments on the basis of age alone. Finally, there are many unresolved questions about whether older persons can tolerate certain aggressive treatments that are likely to be effective for younger persons. For example, some chemotherapy regimens are effective at full doses in younger persons but have intolerable toxicity in older persons; reduction in the dose of these agents renders them less effective.

Recently, investigators examined the value of a number of preventive and therapeutic modalities from a cost-effectiveness perspective. In these analyses the anticipated life-span was considered, as were the expected benefits of treatment and the costs associated with treatment. For some, including mammography, the results suggest that there should be no upper age limit for screening otherwise healthy older persons. Similarly, new data indicate that treatment of hypertension, both systolic-diastolic (high and low numbers are both elevated) and isolated systolic (only the high number is elevated), is beneficial even in persons aged 80 years and older.

Furthermore, therapy that was once considered "too aggressive" for older persons is now becoming

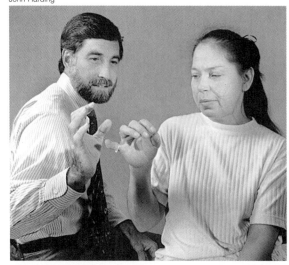

A patient who suffered from a severe Parkinson-like condition demonstrates the manual dexterity she regained after undergoing a highly experimental fetal brain tissue transplant performed by a team of Swedish physicians.

standard treatment. Notably, thrombolytic therapy, in which blood clots in coronary arteries that are responsible for a heart attack are dissolved with drugs, has generally been withheld from older persons. However, when critically reviewing the studies regarding its effectiveness in older persons, researchers concluded that this therapy should not be withheld on the basis of age alone.

Surgical procedures, too, including coronary artery bypass, heart valve replacement, orthopedic joint replacement, and cancer surgery, are being increasingly performed on older persons. A recent study indicated that two-thirds of persons aged 80 years and older experienced no complications following major surgery requiring general anesthesia even though almost half of these procedures had been conducted on an emergency basis.

Nevertheless, there are situations and points in the treatment course when aggressive and expensive therapy will improve neither survival nor the quality of life of a patient. In these situations it becomes the responsibility of the physician, the elderly patient, and the family to establish goals that are palliative rather than curative and recognize that further aggressive treatment is futile.

Alleviating symptoms of Parkinson's disease

Parkinson's disease, a neurodegenerative disease of unknown origin, has been the subject of intensive research over the past several years. The most common clinical findings in Parkinson's disease are slowness in initiating movement, reduced speed of movements (bradykinesia), increased motor tone (rigidity), and resting tremor. Other features include shuffling gait,

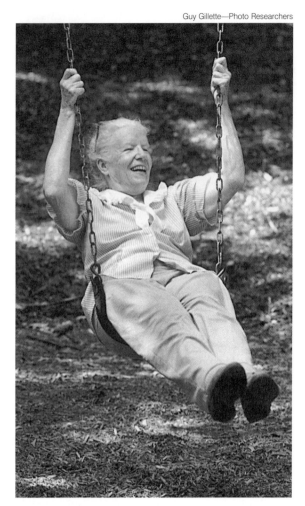

Guy Gillette—Photo Researchers

The U.S. has established an agenda for aging research to ensure that the future health needs of the elderly are met. Reducing or preventing functional disabilities could help many older people lead more independent and productive lives.

softening of the voice, dementia, depression, constipation, and salivary drooling. Parkinson's disease affects an estimated 500,000 to one million older men and women in the United States, and about 50,000 new patients are diagnosed each year.

The primary disorder in Parkinson's disease is a deficiency of dopamine, a neurotransmitter. Although the drug levodopa (L-dopa), combined with carbidopa, has been used therapeutically for years to replace a precursor of dopamine, psychiatric and cardiac side effects and often severe movement disorders limit the effectiveness of this treatment. More recently, another drug, selegiline (formerly called deprenyl), an inhibitor of the brain chemical monoamine oxidase type B, has been shown to be effective in early Parkinson's disease, prolonging the time until treatment with levodopa or other more toxic medications becomes necessary. Other newer medications that also increase dopamine effect, such as bromocriptine and pergolide, have

been increasingly utilized, thereby sparing the need for high dosages of levodopa and perhaps providing some protection for surviving neurons (nerve cells) that produce dopamine. Other drugs that may be used to control some symptoms include anticholinergics such as benztropine and trihexyphenidyl (especially for drooling and tremor), the antiviral amantadine, and antidepressants.

Recent reports have described the benefits of transplantation of fetal brain tissue for the treatment of severe Parkinson's disease. The number of persons who have received these transplants is still very small, and a variety of techniques have been used. Therefore, it is difficult to make general statements about the effectiveness of this form of therapy. Nevertheless, some symptoms have improved in some patients, although it is unknown how long the benefits of these grafts will be maintained. Early in his administration U.S. Pres. Bill Clinton lifted a ban on the use of federal funds for fetal tissue research that had been in place since 1988, which means that the potential of this therapy will be more fully explored in the future. Presently, however, fetal cell implants for Parkinson's disease are not widely available and are being carried out at only a few specialized research centers.

A national agenda for research on aging

In June 1991 the Institute of Medicine of the National Academy of Sciences released a report that outlined an agenda for research on aging in the United States. Fifteen high-priority research areas were identified within five broad categories: basic biomedical research, clinical research, behavioral and social research, research on the delivery of health services, and research into biomedical-ethical issues.

Among the specific areas to be investigated in the near future are the causes (*e.g.,* falls), prevention (*e.g.,* exercise programs), and management (*e.g.,* rehabilitation) of functional disability in older persons. The report also emphasized the need for research on the treatment of certain geriatric syndromes (*e.g.,* urinary incontinence, acute confusional states, and mismanagement of medications). Investigation of the basic social and psychological processes of aging was also designated as a priority area, as were long-term care and continuity of care. Biomedical-ethics research will emphasize quality-of-life issues and particularly decisions regarding life-sustaining treatments in older persons.

In addition to increased funding from the National Institutes of Health, the report recommended the establishment of additional centers for teaching and research (such as the Claude D. Pepper Older American Independence Centers). Additional training of geriatrics faculty will help ensure that this important research is conducted.

—*David B. Reuben, M.D.*

228

Special Report
Mind, Mood, and Medication in Later Life

by Miriam Cohen, Ph.D.

In the 3rd century BC, Aristotle thought that the aging process involved a loss of "inward heat." The 2nd-century Greek physician Galen recommended the generous ingestion of wine for the disequilibrium that people sometimes encounter in old age. Today, at the end of the 20th century, physicians frequently prescribe drugs for older patients to help restore functions of the body and mind that sometimes fail, in part, owing to aging.

The drugs that are used are largely those that act on the central nervous system, collectively called "psychoactive" drugs. These include medications that induce sleep, antianxiety agents, antidepressants, antipsychotics, and drugs for pain (narcotics). The appropriate and rational use of *all* medications in the elderly—and particularly of psychoactive drugs— is a matter of growing medical and social concern. Older people are quite sensitive to both the therapeutic and the toxic effects of drugs in general; doses of medications that are effective in younger adults are often toxic in the elderly. This is due partly to physical changes associated with aging and partly to the fact that older people often take many drugs for many different conditions. When psychoactive drugs are prescribed, the unique dimensions of the clinical problems that older people present as well as the age-related changes in their biology that will affect their ability to absorb, metabolize, distribute, and excrete drugs must be considered. Coexisting medical illnesses and concomitant medications are additional factors that affect both the potential benefits and the risks of psychoactive drugs. The older the patient, the greater the need for vigilance.

One reason that the use of these drugs is of concern is that prescriptions for them are dispensed disproportionately to older people—for problems that develop during their later years as well as for lifelong problems. Primary care physicians, psychiatrists, and geriatric specialists who may be but are not necessarily psychiatrists all frequently prescribe psychoactive drugs for elderly patients. Primary care physicians are most likely to treat the more common problems for which the drugs are useful, such as sleep disorders, anxiety, and alcohol and drug abuse. Both primary care physicians and psychiatrists see older patients with depression—a prevalent disorder in this age group— and may give antidepressant medications, but there is a general consensus that depression in older people is underdiagnosed and undertreated by primary care physicians. Psychiatrists are more likely than other medical specialists to treat schizophrenia in older patients. Geriatricians are the most likely to see patients with dementing disorders, such as Alzheimer's disease, and may prescribe psychoactive drugs for some of the symptoms. Similar illnesses in elderly patients, however, are sometimes diagnosed and treated differently by these three groups of physicians.

All of the aging-associated problems just mentioned—sleep disturbances, anxiety, depression, dementia, schizophrenia, and alcohol and drug abuse— can be, and often are, effectively treated with psychoactive medication. Moreover, if these problems remain untreated, they may limit the quality and even the length of life.

Sleep and aging

Sleep disturbances cause human misery and ill health at any age; among the elderly these disturbances are commonplace. The quality and quantity of sleep, the maintenance and depth of sleep, and the ability to sleep in a consolidated fashion all diminish with age. Older people may complain about difficulty in falling asleep or staying asleep, not getting enough sleep, waking up too early, or getting too much sleep. These sleep problems can lead to daytime fatigue, daytime napping, or excessive daytime sleeping.

The age-related changes in sleep in many cases are independent of any medical or psychiatric disorders. In addition, sleep disorders in the elderly may be caused by transient illnesses, poor sleep habits, pain, chronic illness, dementia, affective disorders or milder mood disturbances, breathing problems during sleep (*e.g.,* apnea and snoring), prescribed and over-the-counter drugs (including appetite suppressants, antihistamines, corticosteroids, cardiovascular drugs, hormones, and even certain vitamins and herbal medicines), and periodic leg jerks (nocturnal myoclonus).

Benzodiazepines are the most widely prescribed group of sedative-hypnotic drugs for sleep disorders; in 1985 over 20 million prescriptions in the U.S. were written—the most frequently prescribed being flurazepam (Dalmane), temazepam (Restoril), triazolam (Halcion), and lorazepam (Ativan). Their rapid seda-

229

tive action (meaning the person falls asleep sooner) and rapid elimination from the body (meaning the person does not suffer day-after "hangover" effects, or prolonged sedation) are two reasons for the popularity of these particular benzodiazepines. The 20 million benzodiazepine prescriptions written in 1985 represented a 38% increase in prescriptions over the number prescribed in 1980. Sixty-year-old patients received 66% more prescriptions for these sedative-hypnotic agents than did those aged 40 to 59 years. Although adults aged 65 years and older constitute only 12% of the population, 25–40% of the benzodiazepine prescriptions are written for them.

The benzodiazepines are generally effective and safe and preferable to other medications that are commonly used to aid sleep. However, they can cause sensory-motor impairments. Driving or operating any machinery when taking such a medication should be avoided. Excessive doses decrease energy, clear thinking, libido, and sexual performance. When the benzodiazepines are used for an extended period of time, dependence can occur and the potential for abuse develops (i.e., the person takes more than the prescribed dose). Dependence manifests itself most acutely when the elderly person *stops* taking the drug; he or she experiences withdrawal symptoms, which include anxiety, agitation, and the desire to relieve these symptoms by resuming drug ingestion. If the physician gradually reduces the dose over a period of several weeks, however, such withdrawal symptoms are minimized.

A physician faced with a distraught older patient who complains about insomnia and other sleep problems is often tempted to prescribe a drug, but most geriatric specialists agree that the use of sedative-hypnotic agents for chronic sleep disturbances should be postponed until other measures have been tried. Such other measures include: increasing daytime activities; regularizing and curtailing the number of hours spent in bed; assuring that the environment for sleep is optimal in terms of noise, light, temperature, and bedding; using the bedroom exclusively for sleeping—not for watching television, working, solving problems, or worrying; avoiding coffee, tea, nicotine, alcohol, and certain over-the-counter medications that contain substances with stimulating effects; and determining whether diet and prescription medications for other conditions are contributing to sleep problems.

Since biblical times warm milk, which contains the amino acid l-tryptophan, has been recognized as a "natural sedative." Alcohol is frequently used by elderly people to facilitate sleep, and some doctors may recommend a glass of wine or a shot of brandy before bedtime. In general, however, alcohol is a relatively poor sedative-hypnotic; it sometimes deepens sleep for the first few hours but then disrupts it later in the night.

Over-the-counter sleeping aids are generally not a good choice for older people. The active agent in most such medications (e.g., Sominex, Nytol, Compōz) is an antihistamine. Antihistamines may put the older patient at risk for delirium, and sleeping aids generally do not include special usage and dosage instructions for the elderly.

If a sedative-hypnotic is prescribed, the continuing need for it should be reassessed at frequent intervals. If daytime sedation or confusion develops with the dose of medication that is being taken, that is a clue that the dose is too high.

Anxiety disorders

Anxiety is a subjective feeling of fear and uneasy anticipation. Physical manifestations include breathlessness, choking sensations, palpitations, restlessness, increased muscular tension, tightness in the chest, giddiness, trembling, sweating, and flushing. These symptoms, when they are not based on an objective fear and persist for a long time, are the basis for a diagnosis of anxiety disorder. Like sleep disorders, anxiety disorders in the elderly are usually treated with benzodiazepines, and the benefits and risks associated with such treatment are similar.

One of the newer drugs used in the treatment of anxiety disorders is buspirone (BuSpar), which is not a benzodiazepine. Its advantages are that it does not cause sedation or functional impairment and it has little potential for abuse. On the other hand, buspirone has two main disadvantages: it must be taken frequently—usually three times per day—and it takes a few weeks before it is effective.

Many older people have symptoms of both anxiety and depression. This will affect which specific category or categories of drugs are used. The physician will decide in the case of each individual patient whether to use anxiolytics (drugs used to relieve anxiety), antidepressants, or a combination of both groups of drugs to treat these coexisting problems.

Depression in later life

One's ability to think, feel, socialize, experience gratification or a sense of purpose, and care for others and/or for oneself is impaired when one suffers from depression. As already noted, depression in the elderly is often underdiagnosed and undertreated. Too often caregivers, family members, and the person who is suffering assume that depression is an inevitable part of the aging process. The unwitting acceptance by society of depression as "natural" to aging closes the door to effective intervention; particularly, it may prevent the older person who is suffering from seeking help. Failure to realize that the older person's despair is an illness deprives the person of not only insight into his or her condition but, more important, relief from it.

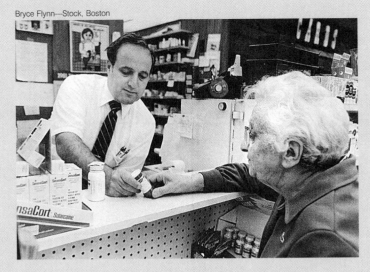

Psychoactive medications for sleep problems, anxiety, depressive and psychotic disorders, pain, and some of the symptoms associated with dementia are prescribed disproportionately for older individuals. Precautions are needed to ensure the appropriate use of such drugs—and of all medications—among elderly patients; the older the patient, the greater the need for vigilance. Owing to physical changes associated with aging, the older person's ability to absorb, metabolize, and excrete drugs may be affected; thus, dosages that may be safe and effective in younger adults are often toxic in the elderly.

In the elderly, depressive symptoms may include mood disturbance, loss of appetite, sleeplessness, lack of energy, and a loss of interest in and enjoyment of the normal pursuit of life. Depression in later life frequently coexists with changing life roles, important losses of social and emotional support, and chronic diseases and disabilities such as cancer, cardiovascular disease, neurological disorders, various metabolic disturbances, arthritis, and loss of sensory functions. Estimates of the prevalence of depression among the elderly vary widely, depending on the definition of depression that is used, the criteria considered for a diagnosis, and the setting (*e.g.,* whether the person resides in the community or in a nursing home). Recent studies have documented higher rates of depression in the institutionalized elderly compared with those living in the community. In 1991 researchers from Johns Hopkins University School of Medicine, Baltimore, Md., reported that depression in residents of eight Baltimore nursing homes not only was prevalent but was associated with increased mortality.

Because there is no specific diagnostic test for depression, the physician's attentive and focused clinical assessment is essential for diagnosis. Moreover, the elderly often do not present themselves for evaluation; their depressive symptoms often are not typical; and depression may be masked by other illnesses. Atypical manifestation and the presence of coexisting illness, however, do not mean that the depression cannot be treated.

Therapeutic pessimism based on age is unwarranted in the treatment of depression. Biological therapies for depression include antidepressant drugs and electroconvulsive therapy (ECT), in which electrodes send small charges of electricity through select portions of the brain. Psychosocial treatments include cognitive therapy (which involves focusing on correcting negative thought processes) and interpersonal psychotherapy ("talk" therapy). Adults over the age of 60 are the ones most likely to receive ECT, and when other treatments have failed, ECT should be considered. The evidence for short-term efficacy is very strong. Studies have shown up to a 90% response rate. Moreover, ECT has the advantage of not having the side effects in older patients that antidepressant drugs often have. ECT has been largely misunderstood; its potential benefits are greater than most people generally believe.

Since the 1950s, antidepressant drugs have constituted the major method of treating depression. Although antidepressant action usually occurs in two to three weeks in younger people, it can take longer in the elderly. Compliance with the medication regimen is essential. Several different types of antidepressant drugs are thought to be equally effective; the drugs, however, have different side effects, which are more or less acceptable to different individuals, depending on their medical problems as well as their personal coping capacities.

Physicians have had the most experience with tricyclic antidepressants (*tricyclic* refers to the drugs' chemical structure). Nortriptyline (Pamelor), desipramine (Norpramin), amitriptyline (Elavil), and imipramine (Tofranil) are examples. Among the common side effects are sedation, postural hypotension (*i.e.,* the dizziness and light-headedness experienced when a person changes from the sitting to the standing position), and so-called anticholinergic effects: dry mouth, constipation, urinary retention, and blurred vision. Elderly patients are particularly sensitive to these latter effects, which may produce confusion or delirium if drug doses are too high. Many drugs in addition to antidepressants have anticholinergic effects, and since elderly people often take more than one drug, care must be taken that the anticholinergic effects of multiple drugs do not result in a confusional state.

In overdose, tricyclic antidepressants are potentially lethal. The most common manifestations of overdose

231

Side effects of selected antidepressants

drug	sedative effect	anticholinergic effect	typical dose (mg) adults/elderly
amitryptyline	+++++	++++	150–200/100
trimipramine	++++	+++	150–200/100
doxepin	++++	+++	150–250/100
imipramine	+++	+++++	150–200/100
clomipramine	+++++	+++++	150–200/100
nortriptyline	++	+++	75–100/100
desipramine	+	+	150–250/100
maprotiline	++++	++	200–250/150
trazodone	++++	++	150–400/100
fluoxitine	+/-	+	20–40/10

Source: Joel Eisen et al., "Psychotropic Drugs and Sleep," British Medical Journal, vol. 306 (May 15, 1993), pp. 1331–34

are a rapid heartbeat and hypotension (low blood pressure). Life-threatening cardiac arrhythmias can also occur. These serious cardiovascular complications are dose related and are usually clinically evident within 24 hours after an overdose.

Other antidepressants that have been available for several decades are the monoamine oxidase (MAO) inhibitors. These include isocarboxazid (Marplan), phenelzine (Nardil), and tranylcypromine (Parnate). These antidepressants block the action of the brain enzyme monoamine oxidase and may be particularly effective in those who have not responded to other drugs or those who have atypical depressive symptoms. MAO inhibitors are not prescribed as frequently as the other antidepressants, however, because severe hypotension and hypertensive crises can occur if foods containing tyramine (e.g., some cheeses, aged or fermented foods, fava beans, chicken livers, wines, and some other alcoholic beverages) are not scrupulously avoided.

In addition to manifesting depressive symptoms, patients with bipolar disorder (manic-depression) become hyperactive, impulsive, and aggressive and experience sleep disturbances when they are in the manic phase. Bipolar disorder occurs less frequently than unipolar disorders. Lithium salts, which must be monitored regularly for potential toxicity, are the most commonly used drugs to treat manic-depression.

The newest class of antidepressants available is referred to as the selective serotonin reuptake inhibitors (so called because of their hypothesized mechanism of action—inhibiting activity of the neurotransmitter serotonin). Drugs available in the U.S. in this group

include sertraline (Zoloft), fluoxetine (Prozac), and paroxitine (Paxil). Because these drugs are new, physicians have not had as much experience using them as they have with tricyclics. However, a large body of knowledge has cumulated in a relatively short time because the selective serotonin reuptake inhibitors have been widely prescribed over the last few years. Fluoxetine became the most commonly prescribed antidepressant in the U.S. soon after it was first marketed in 1987. The major side effects are nausea, diarrhea, agitation, and sexual dysfunction, but the potential for orthostatic hypotension is low. Claims have been made that fluoxetine gives rise to suicidal ideation and violent behavior, but these have not been substantiated.

Other antidepressants that cannot be grouped into a single class include trazodone (Desyrel), buproprion (Wellbutrin), amoxapine (Asendin), and maprotoline (Ludiomil). They have varying side effects but are not considered to be more or less effective than the other groups of antidepressants.

Elderly people receiving drug treatment for depression should be treated with sufficient doses for a sufficient length of time to maximize the likelihood of recovery. Maintenance therapy should be continued with the same doses that produced remission of the acute depressive episode. Families and primary care physicians play an important part in recognizing depression in the elderly; special efforts are needed to locate and identify elderly people who live alone to ensure that they are treated if they suffer from depression and that the care they receive is relevant to their needs.

Alzheimer's disease

Alzheimer's disease, a debilitating illness resulting in progressive dementia, affects approximately 10% of individuals aged 65 or older. In the 85-and-older group the likelihood of Alzheimer's disease is 50%. Men and women are affected in equal numbers. Approximately 1.6 million Americans suffer from severe dementia, and an additional one million to 5 million suffer from mild to moderate dementia. Approximately one-half of all nursing-home beds in the U.S. are occupied by patients with Alzheimer's disease.

It is now recognized that a significant decline in cognitive function is not an inevitable part of aging; rather it is the result of disease. Forgetfulness is the first symptom of Alzheimer's disease. First, short-term memory and immediate recall are impaired. As the illness progresses, more and more cognitive and functional abilities are affected. Mood becomes unstable—patients tend to become irritable and more sensitive to stress, and they may become intermittently angry, anxious, or depressed. Finally, memory loss is very severe. The rate of decline in intellect, personality, and neuropsychological functioning, however, is quite variable, and the area of greatest decline in individual patients also varies widely. In some patients psychotic symptoms (*i.e.*, delusions and hallucinations); restlessness; wandering, which often occurs at night (known as "sundowner's syndrome"); agitation; assaultiveness; and uncontrolled, socially inappropriate behavior often accompany the memory failure.

Drugs to treat Alzheimer's disease are being tested, but none is yet known to be effective; in 1993 tacrine (Cognex) was the first pharmacological agent being considered for approval. It can improve cognitive functioning in some patients but is potentially toxic to the liver. Currently, treatment mainly involves general support and provision of a safe and comfortable environment for the patient and counseling and support for the patient's family. Antipsychotic, or neuroleptic, drugs (particularly thioridazine and haloperidol), however, are frequently used to control the psychotic symptoms and the more profound behavioral disturbances. The same group of drugs, described below, is also used to treat schizophrenia.

Schizophrenia in the elderly

Schizophrenia is characterized by an overwhelming lack of will, drive, enthusiasm, and assertiveness and disturbances in mood, thinking, and behavior. The illness has an insidious onset, usually becoming manifest in early adulthood. The onset of schizophrenia in old age is rare. However, schizophrenia is a chronic illness, and patients are treated for a lifetime with drugs to control psychotic symptoms and prevent relapse.

Since the 1950s neuroleptic drugs have been the mainstay of treatment. They do not cure the illness, but they provide relief from the most disturbing symptoms (delusions and hallucinations). Neuroleptics that have been used for many years include chlorpromazine (Thorazine), trifluoperazine (Stelazine), perphenazine (Trilafon), fluphenazine (Prolixin), thioridazine (Mellaril), mesoridazine (Serentil), thiothixene (Navane), molindone (Moban), loxapine (Loxitane), and haloperidol (Haldol).

The side effects of neuroleptics are similar. The most common are neurological syndromes, to which the elderly are very prone. Such syndromes are manifest by rigidity, tremors, involuntary movements, a slowing and reduction of volitional movements, and a reduction in facial expression. These side effects are similar to the symptoms observed in patients with Parkinson's disease. The flat facial expression and retarded movements are sometimes mistaken for signs of depression. Akathisia, a subjective feeling of severe restlessness, is another neurological side effect that can be very distressing to the patient, who feels compelled to be in constant movement. Tardive dyskinesia, a movement disorder, occurs frequently in the elderly who have been taking neuroleptics for some time. "Tardive" refers to the fact that the movement disorder occurs late during the course of treatment. Tardive dyskinesia is characterized by stereotyped involuntary movements, most often consisting of sucking and smacking of the lips, lateral jaw movements, and a darting movement of the tongue. There may also be quick movement of the extremities. It is not known whether the parkinson-like symptoms disappear when neuroleptic medication is discontinued or how long it takes for them to disappear.

Other side effects of neuroleptics include sedation, orthostatic hypotension, and anticholinergic effects (*i.e.*, dry mouth, blurred vision, constipation, and urinary retention). When the drugs cause sedation, this often leads to unhealthy inactivity and may compromise cognitive functioning. Orthostatic hypotension may lead to falls that could prove fatal. Anticholinergic effects may lead to aggravation of glaucoma, urinary disorders, or bowel obstruction.

Because the side effects of neuroleptics can be so profound, compliance with therapy is often a problem. Many of the neuroleptics have an injectable form, which is administered every two to four weeks and permits caregivers and schizophrenic patients to avoid the issue of daily compliance. This method of administration of the neuroleptics is not generally used in patients with Alzheimer's disease.

For many years the drugs that were available to treat schizophrenia were limited to the group of similar drugs just described, but now there is a new medication available that has different benefits and risks. In 1989 the U.S. Food and Drug Administration approved the use of clozapine (Clozaril) for treatment-resistant schizophrenia. Clozapine is often effective in treating schizophrenics who have not responded to other neuroleptics. It does not have the neurological side effects associated with the neuroleptics described above; it has, however, been found to cause agranulocytosis (destruction of infection-fighting white blood cells), which can be life threatening in 1–2% of patients who take it. Frequent monitoring of the blood is necessary to reduce the risks associated with this side effect.

Psychoactive drug use in nursing homes

Psychoactive drug use in nursing homes should be justified in the same way that the prescribing of these medications is justified in any treatment setting. The prescription must be based on a clear diagnosis, and it must be suitable for treating the condition for which it is used. The lowest possible effective dose of the drug in question should be used for the shortest possible period of time. Unfortunately, the unnecessary use of psychoactive drugs in nursing homes has been a common practice. Such unnecessary use involves giving excessive doses for excessive periods of time without a diagnosis or justification and without adequate monitoring.

The motivation for excessive use of drugs is often the desire to keep nursing home residents sedated and calm, which may minimize the amount of care they need. In the United States, since 1990, there have been federal regulations governing the use of psychoactive drugs in all Medicare- and Medicaid-certified nursing homes.

Alcohol and drug dependence in the elderly

Alcohol and drug addiction are chronic, progressive, relapsing disorders that require continuous treatment for maintaining remission. The dependence syndromes associated with alcohol and drug abuse include a preoccupation with the substance, compulsive use of it despite adverse consequences, and a tendency to relapse (manifested by an inability to reduce or abstain from the use of the substance despite recurrent adverse effects). Addiction, unfortunately, is an underrecognized, underdiagnosed, and undertreated problem among elderly people.

Addiction is generally defined in terms of both tolerance and dependence. Tolerance is the loss of an effect at a particular dose or the need to increase the dose to maintain the same effect. Dependence is characterized by the onset of stereotypical and predictable signs and symptoms on cessation of alcohol or drugs. One can become addicted to drugs prescribed by physicians or to illicit (*i.e.,* "street") drugs. Prescription drugs to which many elderly people become addicted include the benzodiazepines, which, as described previously, are commonly used to treat sleep disorders and anxiety; the barbiturates—another group of hypnotic drugs sometimes prescribed for sleep, although the barbiturates are prescribed much less frequently today than they were in the past; and narcotics (potent analgesics that are prescribed for pain). Elderly patients are less likely to have access to illicit drugs such as amphetamines and cocaine—both stimulants—and narcotics such as heroin.

Denial of the addiction is common in addicted individuals. Difficulties with interpersonal relationships such as dependency conflicts, isolation, and social withdrawal are cardinal manifestations of alcohol and drug dependence. However, these same conflicts are also common accompaniments of the aging process and can be manifest even without alcohol and drug dependence. Psychiatric and medical problems—anxiety, depression, insomnia, and occasionally dementia—are the most frequent complications of such dependence in the elderly, whereas the threat of job loss and disruption of family are more common complications in younger people. One of the reasons for continued use of the drugs and alcohol is that the substances transiently relieve the symptoms.

During intoxication and withdrawal, depressants (alcohol, benzodiazepines, and narcotics) and stimulants, in both acute and chronic use, may produce psychotic symptoms such as delusions and hallucinations. The substances can also produce a dementia or delirium syndrome; compromised cognition is always a risk; and intentional and accidental suicide are not uncommon with alcohol and drug dependence.

The symptoms of alcoholism and drug dependence among older people are often confused with other psychiatric disorders. Anxiety symptoms typically improve within weeks of cessation of alcohol and drug use, although withdrawal symptoms after the cessation of benzodiazepine use may be prolonged. Alcohol- and drug-induced hallucinations and delusions typically resolve shortly after the cessation of the substance's use. The dementia syndrome that sometimes occurs in alcoholics may resolve only after years of abstinence.

Some drugs accumulate in fat and muscle and are released into the bloodstream slowly over time. Consequently, their effects on cognition, memory, and mood may be experienced for weeks to months after the person has stopped ingesting them. The complete withdrawal from alcohol and drugs may take weeks to months in the aged, compared with days or weeks in younger individuals, and cognitive improvement and reduction in anxiety, depression, chronic pain, and insomnia originating from substance dependence may resolve in older people only over a prolonged period of time, making compliance with abstinence otherwise difficult.

When addiction problems are recognized in the elderly, physicians may prescribe benzodiazepines, which are useful in the treatment of withdrawal signs and symptoms. The doses of benzodiazepines required for suppressing the signs and symptoms of withdrawal in older people are usually one-half to one-third the doses required for middle-aged adults.

Psychoactive drugs in the 21st century

The many biological, psychiatric, and pharmacological developments that have been converging over the last decade, and are continuing to converge, have resulted in substantial advances in understanding of the mechanisms of action of psychoactive drugs. Development of new psychoactive agents is now progressing at a rapid rate. These drugs may have greater benefits and fewer risks.

Moreover, pharmacological and psychological approaches to psychiatric problems and behavioral disturbances are no longer viewed as competitive. Thus, it is becoming an increasingly common practice to prescribe psychoactive drugs to reduce patients' vulnerability, which then enhances the role of psychosocial treatments that help people gain coping skills. Ultimately, this progress means that greater numbers of elderly as well as younger people will be able to overcome disorders that cause so much pain and suffering.

AIDS

The Ninth International Conference on AIDS, convened in Berlin in June 1993, offered little hope that the AIDS pandemic, now well into its second decade, would be brought under control anytime soon. Only minute progress was reported by scientists in the more than 5,500 presentations made at the conference. Hope appeared dim that a vaccine against the human immunodeficiency virus (HIV), the virus that causes AIDS, would be available in the forseeable future, and the effectiveness of some anti-HIV drugs already in use was in question. Meanwhile, the disease continued to take its relentless toll, and the number of persons infected continued to grow. In the United States the number of reported cases is now expected to rise substantially, in part because of an expanded definition by the Centers for Disease Control and Prevention (CDC) of what constitutes the disease.

Scope of the pandemic

The Global AIDS Policy Coalition (an international group of AIDS researchers), which estimated that approximately 12 million adults worldwide were infected with HIV in 1992, projected that the number would rise to about 17 million in 1995. In addition, 2.3 million children worldwide were expected to be infected with the virus. The coalition described its estimates as "refined guesses" based upon expert opinion. Like all global health statistics, however, these estimates are just that—estimates. The World Health Organization (WHO) reported lower numbers, but these were based upon official reports from the governments of member nations; because they are influenced by political considerations, such reports are considered not wholly reliable.

Regardless of the source, however, the numbers are overwhelming, particularly in less developed countries, which are hit proportionately harder by all diseases than are industrialized countries. The coalition estimates that by the year 2000, sub-Saharan Africa may have experienced 21 million to 34 million cases of HIV infection in adults. Southeast Asia could surpass that number, with an estimated 11 million–45 million HIV-infected adults. Predictions for the United States and Canada are two million–eight million cases; Latin America, two million–nine million; and Western Europe, one million–two million. Other smaller regions bring the upper, or worst-case, estimate to 109 million adults infected. Of the more than two million children expected to have become infected with HIV by 1995, 90% will be in sub-Saharan Africa.

The epidemic in the U.S.

Adolescent and young adult HIV transmission guarantees the continuation of the AIDS/HIV epidemic, barring a substantially expanded national prevention effort. . . . The health crisis of

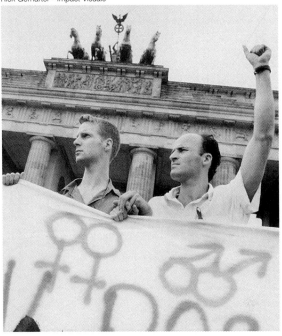

Subdued demonstrations reflected the overall atmosphere at the June 1993 Ninth International Conference on AIDS in Berlin, where scientists and activists alike seemed more daunted than in previous years by the formidable nature of the disease.

AIDS/HIV is of immense significance in the United States and will remain so beyond this millennium.
—*Journal of the American Medical Association,* June 1993

Because of the CDC's revised case definition of AIDS, the actual number of reported cases in the U.S. was expected to rise by 75% in 1993, the first full year the new definition was in effect. Earlier the CDC had projected a lower rate of increase in the number of AIDS cases, possibly reaching a plateau between 1993 and 1995. The arrival of that plateau now has been delayed. In addition to adding several diseases to the list of so-called AIDS-defining disorders, the revised definition stipulates that an HIV-infected person may be classified as having AIDS even without clinical symptoms of the characteristic opportunistic infections of AIDS—such as pneumonia and tuberculosis—if that person has a low level of the white blood cells called CD4 T lymphocytes (or CD4 cells). These lymphocytes are vital to the immune process.

The CDC reported rapid increases during 1992 in the number of AIDS cases among women, infants, adolescents, minorities, and heterosexuals. Overall, populations that previously had experienced a lower rate of infection showed larger increases than groups that had previously had a larger proportion of cases. Thus, although only 771 new AIDS cases in children were reported in 1992, this represented an increase of 11% over the previous year. Women accounted for

235

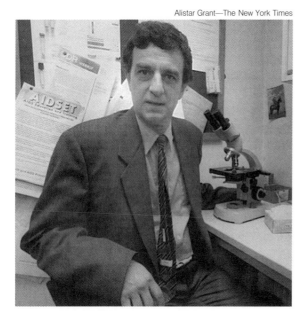

Ian Weller, who led the British arm of the Anglo-French Concorde study, shares the unanticipated finding of the three-year-long trial that starting the drug AZT soon after infection with HIV fails to prolong patients' lives.

6,645 new cases, only 14% of the total but a 10% increase. Two trends noted in previous years continued: an increasing number of cases among minorities and an increase in the number of cases connected directly or indirectly to intravenous (IV) drug use. Included in the latter category were heterosexual partners of IV drug users and children born to mothers who became infected with HIV through shared needles or sex with an infected drug user.

Most of the AIDS cases reported in the U.S. in 1992—51%—occurred among homosexual men. That number, however, represented a 1% decrease from the number of new AIDS cases reported in this group in 1991. On the other hand, cases attributed to intravenous drug use rose 1%, accounting for 24% of new cases. Heterosexual transmission accounted for 9% of the total cases reported in 1992, but this category increased by 17%.

A particularly sobering development in the U.S. was the CDC's July 1993 announcement that HIV infection had become the second-leading cause of death among young men aged 25–44. (Unintentional injury was first.) In many cities and states, AIDS was already the number one killer in this age group. Data from the National Center for Health Statistics showed HIV infection to be the leading cause of death among young men in five states—New York, New Jersey, California, Florida, and Massachusetts—and 64 cities. In three states, HIV infection had become the second-leading cause of death for young women.

The CDC also reported that 7,000 AIDS cases of "undetermined" cause were under investigation.

These are cases where no identifiable risk has yet been pinpointed.

Treatment: little progress to report

Another troubling development of 1993 was the finding that antiviral drugs that had initially provided reason for optimism were proving to be less effective than early studies had showed. Scientists have given up hope of developing a single, universally effective drug—a "magic bullet" that would vanquish the virus. In fact, what they have found is that HIV is becoming resistant to the available drugs, resulting in a disease that is increasingly complex to treat.

AZT's limited benefits. The most significant of the new reports, published in April 1993 in the British journal *The Lancet*, called into question the effectiveness of AZT (zidovudine; Retrovir), which was first licensed for use in 1987 and had been considered the most promising anti-HIV drug. That promise was clouded by the results of the largest AIDS treatment trial to date, known as the Concorde study. Concorde, a collaborative effort of the British Medical Research Council and the French National AIDS Research Agency, lasted three years and involved 1,749 participants. It not only examined how the patients with AIDS fared but also monitored those infected with HIV before they showed symptoms of AIDS.

Although there had been intimations that AZT was not as effective as its proponents had originally claimed, the medical community was unprepared for the findings; 79 AIDS-related deaths occurred in the group receiving AZT, compared with only 67 in a control group taking a placebo. Moreover, those taking AZT developed more side effects than those on the placebo. The study results also raised questions about the method of assessing immune function, the CD4 and T4 cell counts. These immune system cells are targeted by the virus, and their levels drop as the disease progresses. While patients given AZT early in the Concorde trial did show increased levels of CD4 and T4 cells, supposedly a sign of enhanced immunity, these patients did not live longer than those in the control group. The conclusion was that AZT does benefit some patients seriously ill with AIDS, but starting the drug soon after a positive test for HIV does not prolong survival. Researchers now are looking more intensely at treatment regimens using combinations of AZT and other anti-HIV agents.

New treatment guidelines. Two weeks after the Berlin conference, the National Institutes of Health (NIH), Bethesda, Md., convened a three-day conference of an independent panel of experts and issued major revisions in the recommendations for the treatment of HIV and AIDS. The new guidelines, providing greater flexibility than previous ones, emphasize that patients and their physicians should decide jointly when and how HIV should be treated. The guidelines also stress that all primary care physicians can provide appropriate care for patients in the early stages of HIV infection.

The most radical shift in the treatment guidelines is that treatment with AZT is no longer necessarily recommended for HIV-infected individuals with low CD4 counts. Healthy people have CD4 blood counts of 800 to 1,200 cells per microliter. The NIH guidelines recommend starting AZT in patients with counts between 200 and 500. However, the guidelines state that an equally valid option in such cases is to carefully monitor patients and defer drug treatment until such time as their condition changes for the worse or laboratory tests indicate a deterioration in immune function. The panel continued to recommend AZT as the drug of first choice against HIV but suggested that its use be reserved for later stages of the disease than previously recommended. The experts also suggested that those patients who do not improve with AZT treatment be switched to the anti-HIV drug ddI (didanosine; Videx).

While warning that studies have not shown conclusively that combinations of anti-HIV drugs, either together or in sequence, have any benefit, the panel cautiously supported combination therapy as a treatment option. While these guidelines have no regulatory authority, they are nonetheless expected to have wide impact because of the prestige and expertise of the panel members.

Kemron controversy. Although the scientific establishment has put little credence in reports from Kenya and from some practicing physicians in the U.S. that alpha interferon (also called Kemron) benefits people with AIDS, the NIH agreed in 1993 to sponsor clinical trials of low oral doses of the drug. Alpha interferon is a protein that is produced by the human immune system and enhances the body's ability to fight infection. Currently it is used, with Food and Drug Administration (FDA) approval, as intravenous therapy to treat several types of cancer, including Kaposi's sarcoma, an often fatal opportunistic disease common in AIDS patients.

In 1990 Davy K. Koech of the Kenya Medical Research Institute touted Kemron as a "cure" for AIDS. The scientific establishment viewed the drug as another krebiozen or laetrile, agents that were promoted in the 1950s and '60s as cancer cures but eventually proved worthless. Moreover, Koech's research has been criticized because the patients in his study who were treated with Kemron were not compared with a group who went untreated or received a placebo.

Proponents of the drug argue that even if oral interferon does not kill HIV or restore lost immune cells, it does restore patients' energy and increase their appetite, thereby making them feel better. As happened with other anti-HIV drugs prior to FDA approval, an underground distribution system developed to provide Kemron to those who sought it.

Many doctors who treat HIV-positive African-Americans report that Kemron appears to alleviate the symptoms of AIDS even if it does not cure the disease, and pressure for clinical trials has mounted, notably from the National Medical Association, the largest organization of black U.S. doctors. Controlled studies to be carried out under the auspices of the NIH will match groups of patients who receive Kemron and those who receive a placebo. This provision should furnish objective evidence as to whether Kemron really improves the quality of life of people with AIDS even if it does not cure the disease.

A new class of drugs. One of the few positive reports that emerged from the Berlin conference came from the drug manufacturer Hoffman-LaRoche, Inc., of Nutley, N.J., announcing that a new class of drugs, called protease inhibitors, shows some promise in helping to overcome AIDS. Initial studies of the protease inhibitor called Ro 31-8959 showed beneficial, albeit transient, antiviral and immune system effects when combined with AZT. Nationwide trials of Ro 31-8959 were scheduled to begin in the near future at 19 U.S. medical centers.

Gene therapy. The rapidly evolving advances in genetic engineering are now thought to offer one of the most promising avenues of research in the worldwide effort to conquer AIDS. The potential of gene therapy was recognized in 1993 when the NIH approved two preliminary studies involving the transfer of genes into HIV-infected people. Although neither of these procedures is expected to provide a cure, both might help scientists better understand the behavior of the virus and thus lead to effective therapies.

One of the studies, to be conducted by scientists in Los Angeles, will evaluate the safety of transferring DNA that presumably will cause the recipient's cells to make certain HIV proteins. These, in turn, are expected to activate the body's immune response and slow the progression of the disease. The second trial, which will be carried out by investigators at the University of Michigan, will involve a small group of AIDS patients who are already receiving AZT. The researchers will separate and grow T lymphocytes from each patient's blood. Some of these cells then will be altered genetically to produce a mutated form of an HIV protein called *rev*, which inhibits viral replication and is expected to prolong the life of the cells. An inactivated form of the same gene will be given to other cells so they will *not* produce *rev*. The altered cells then will be reinfused into the volunteers' bloodstreams, and the scientists will compare the survival of the two groups of cells to determine the protective effects of the *rev* protein.

New and intriguing questions

Another part of the complex puzzle of AIDS that has not been solved is why it affects people so differently—why some die quickly after being infected while others live for many years. Many investigators are probing this question in hopes that they may find a key to long-term survival that could be used to fashion an effective therapy. At the Berlin conference Nancy Hessol of the San Francisco Health Department reported on a study of genetic factors in 593 long-term survivors of HIV infection. She and her colleagues identified genes responsible for an improved outcome and, for the first time, isolated the type of immune response shared by these survivors. In this all-male group, 12% had developed AIDS 5 years after HIV infection; 51% had become ill after 10 years; and 68% were sick by the 14th year after infection. Of the remaining 32%, categorized as long-term survivors, 42 showed no symptoms of illness and had vigorous, although slightly compromised, immunity. The long-term survivors were found to have certain genes that encode special antiviral immune defense molecules.

Similar research was under way at Northwestern University Medical School in Chicago, where three groups of HIV-infected homosexual men have been monitored for eight years to follow the progress of their disease. Northwestern researcher John Phair reported in Berlin that while the CD4 cell counts in two groups have declined in varying degrees, this indicator has remained stable in one group of 56 men. And, in stark contrast to the other two patient cohorts, none in the third group has died.

Equally intriguing was a report from researchers at the University of Manitoba, who found that 29 female prostitutes in Nairobi, Kenya, showed no signs of HIV infection despite having had unprotected sexual intercourse with HIV-positive men an average of 32 times a year for as long as eight years. The Canadian researchers are trying to determine what in the genetic and immunologic makeup of these women may protect them from HIV infection.

Vaccine research

Some hope was engendered in Berlin by early reports of the effectiveness of vaccines to mobilize the immune systems of people who have never been infected with HIV. Anthony Fauci, head of the U.S. National Institute of Allergy and Infectious Diseases, reported that more than 10,000 healthy volunteers are participating in clinical trials of various vaccines. So far the vaccines have shown that they can stimulate an immune response in uninfected persons and are safe. Other researchers, however, do not share even the cautious optimism expressed by Fauci; they cite the lack of progress so far despite the fact that intensive work on AIDS vaccines has been under way for a decade in nine European and six U.S. laboratories.

The development of an AIDS vaccine is more complicated than that of vaccines for other viral diseases, such as influenza, because HIV is far more complex than many other viruses. At least 30 subtypes of HIV-1—the most common form of HIV in the U.S. and

Europe—have been identified. HIV-2 is the primary cause of AIDS in Africa and some other parts of the world. Moreover, the virus continues to evolve, producing other subtypes. It is therefore unlikely that any one vaccine will be effective against both forms of HIV and all of their subtypes.

Efforts to develop an effective vaccine have been further stymied by the fact that no suitable animal model exists for the study of HIV. The closest parallel is simian immunodeficiency virus (SIV), which causes an AIDS-like illness in monkeys. Scientists have found that rhesus monkeys can be protected temporarily from SIV infection through vaccination with deactivated HIV. However, they still do not know the extent and duration of protection.

One study with macaque monkeys has shown that a vaccine derived from SIV can prevent infection in female animals exposed vaginally to the virus. This finding is of potentially great importance, given that, worldwide, heterosexual intercourse is the primary means of transmission of HIV. However, scientists point out that years of additional research will be required before a similar human AIDS vaccine can be developed, if this is possible at all.

The NIH agreed in 1993 to back a controversial congressional order to begin the first large-scale clinical trial of therapeutic vaccines—i.e., those designed to bolster the immune systems of people with HIV. These vaccines are in contrast to preventive AIDS vaccines, which are intended to protect those who have not yet been infected. The NIH advisory committee recommended the trial on the basis of preliminary medical evidence of the vaccines' effectiveness and the urgency of the AIDS epidemic. The therapeutic vaccines to be tested contain proteins called gp120 and gp160, which are cloned from the outer shell of HIV. Many small, independent clinical studies have suggested that these vaccines might slow or stop the progress of HIV in persons already infected.

The controversy arose when Congress intervened—in the wake of heavy lobbying by MicroGeneSys, the Connecticut biotechnology company that developed gp160—and ordered that gp160 be tested even though data supporting its efficacy are questionable. Congress allocated $20 million to the Department of Defense for the purpose of conducting the trial. Federal scientists protested, arguing that scientists, not politicians, should set the AIDS research agenda. The dispute was resolved when an agreement was reached to transfer the money to the NIH for testing of not only gp160 but gp120 as well. The tests were not expected to begin before the end of 1994.

The NIH had already begun the first test of three experimental therapeutic vaccines for HIV-infected children. Ninety children around the country, aged one month to 12 years, who are infected but have not developed symptoms will be involved in the trial, which is designed to compare the safety of the vaccines. HIV-infected children develop the disease more rapidly than adults, making all the more crucial the development of a pediatric vaccine that could stave off symptoms. The trial is designed to determine whether the experimental vaccines, which are made with HIV proteins that have been genetically engineered to contain only a piece, or subunit, of the virus, can increase existing HIV-specific immune responses in the immature immune system and stimulate new ones. In small, ongoing trials in HIV-infected adults, these so-called subunit vaccines so far have been found to be well tolerated.

Another therapeutic vaccine, produced by Jonas Salk, developer of the first polio vaccine, yielded disappointing results, according to a report at the Berlin conference. Salk's long-awaited data showed that his vaccine was only moderately effective in boosting the immune systems of persons already infected with HIV.

Just before his death in 1993 one of the nation's most eminent scientists, Albert Sabin, expressed doubt that an effective AIDS vaccine ever can be developed. Sabin, who developed the oral polio vaccine, observed that "the available data provide no basis for testing any experimental vaccine in human beings or for expecting that any HIV vaccine could be effective in human beings." Other scientists privately agreed with this position. Sabin's view was based on the fact that vaccines are successful against polio and measles because these diseases are caused by viruses that are "free," whereas HIV attaches itself to living cells. HIV vaccines will not work, in Sabin's opinion, because HIV has the ability to "hide" inside cells. Sabin said that scientists should work instead on developing a way to target and kill the cells that harbor viral genes, suggesting that one tactic would be to search for a "repressor" protein that the virus must produce in order to remain dormant inside cells. The protein could then be used as a marker to identify infected cells. Drugs to kill the cells would seek out the protein.

The costs: pay now or pay later?

As the AIDS epidemic has continued unabated, the frustration of research scientists, clinicians, and AIDS activists has intensified, as has their anger at the seeming indifference of public officials. No one disagrees that there is a limit on the amount of money that can be spent beneficially in seeking effective treatments or a cure for AIDS. However, scientists and activists alike agree that for the moment, and probably for several years to come, the answer lies in prevention—and efforts in this regard have been inadequate, many say.

WHO officials at the Berlin conference predicted that without significant increases in funding for prevention programs, the number of AIDS case will more than triple by the year 2000. Michael Merson, director

While volunteers like these Massachusetts teenagers work to educate their peers about AIDS, the U.S. government has so far been reluctant to support the kind of prevention programs that would have a real impact on the spread of the disease.

of WHO's Global AIDS Program, said that an annual increase of $2.9 billion in health care budgets worldwide—less than 1% of the $90 billion spent worldwide on health care—would cut by half the number of expected new infections. "It would," Merson said, "take just a fraction of the cost of Operation Desert Storm or the cost of one Coke for every person in the world to save millions of lives."

In the U.S. especially, political considerations have prevented such measures as sex education for the young and condom-distribution and needle-exchange programs for drug users, actions that would effectively retard the spread of HIV. Merson said governments must be convinced on economic grounds of the wisdom of prevention. They can, he added, "pay now or pay a much higher price later," the greater cost being the loss of economically productive lives.

By coincidence, just days after the NIH issued its revised recommendations for treatment of AIDS, the National Commission on AIDS officially ended its task, issuing a final report repeating its plea for the federal government to devise a national plan to combat the epidemic. As they wound up their work, members of the commission lauded Pres. Bill Clinton for his appointment of Kristine M. Gebbie as White House AIDS coordinator to guide the administration's efforts to defeat the disease. They also applauded Clinton's request for a substantial increase in funds for the effort—from $2.1 billion to $2.7 billion, the largest increase requested by any U.S. president—and characterized the attitude of Pres. George Bush's administration to its recommendations as "complacent unresponsiveness." The commission reiterated its recommendations of two years ago, most of which have been ignored, including proposals that the government devise a single plan to combat AIDS, that treatment for drug abuse be made available to all who need it, that laws preventing drug users from getting clean needles be abolished, and that medical coverage be provided for all HIV-infected persons, including the cost of medications.

Among the commission's earlier recommendations that *have* been put into effect is the redefinition of what constitutes full-blown AIDS to include people previously classified only as being HIV infected. The group's final report concluded, "Our nation has continued on its shortsighted course. Sadly, we must continue to report that America is still doing poorly."
—*Charles-Gene McDaniel, M.S.J.*

Alternative Medicine

Alternative medicine is often defined in terms of what it is *not:* not approved by the medical mainstream, not widely taught in medical schools, not generally available in most hospitals. In more positive terms, alternative medicine can be distinguished by its adherence to the ancient Hippocratic dictum that above all, the physician should do no harm. While some alternative treatments have turned out to have unwanted side effects, most are utilized precisely because they do *not* have the adverse effects that can be associated with many conventional treatments.

"Alternative therapies" are not easily defined, in part because they do not constitute a single entity; rather, such treatments encompass a wide range of ideas, theories, and practices. Some treatments derive from old medical systems that have been largely ignored or neglected in the course of medical progress, such as homeopathy, chiropractic, and traditional Chinese and Indian Ayurvedic systems based on herbs and other natural products. Some are based on remedies discovered by indigenous peoples in the local flora—*e.g.,* the wee-dee plant, a member of the nutmeg family found in South American rain forests (for fungal infections), and echinacea, or purple cone flower, a popular Native American treatment (for colds and flu). Still others rely on synthetic chemicals that have not undergone formal routes of testing to establish their safety and efficacy but have been adopted by the alternative medicine community because they are

thought to have important therapeutic effects—*e.g.,* hydrazine sulfate (for cachexia, or wasting associated with chronic illness); DMSO, or dimethyl sulfoxide (for muscle injuries); and EDTA (ethylenediamine-tetraacetic acid) chelation (for atherosclerosis). Alternative therapies also include some practices, such as radionics or psychic surgery, whose rationale eludes even staunch defenders of the unconventional.

There is hardly a medical condition—from dire illnesses such as AIDS and cancer to the common cold—that has not been approached through the use of alternative therapies. The field is large and growing, and its practitioners include thousands of chiropractors, naturopaths, homeopaths, herbalists, acupuncturists, doctors of osteopathy, and even M.D.'s who have had traditional medical education and training. In the United States there is hardly a town that does not have an alternative practitioner or a "health food" emporium doing a brisk business in natural foods, nutritional supplements, vitamins, minerals, herbs, and a variety of other remedies—this despite perennial raids by the Food and Drug Administration (FDA), condemnation by orthodox medical authorities, confrontations with state licensing authorities, and malpractice lawsuits.

The struggle between orthodox and alternative medicine exists in many countries but is fiercest in the United States. In many other countries traditional folk forms of medicine have remained viable and have been integrated into the mainstream. In China, for instance, acupuncture, moxibustion, herbal medicines, body manipulation, and other approaches are practiced alongside Western scientific medicine, sometimes in the same clinic or hospital. In Japan there is widespread interest in so-called Kampo treatments (complex herbal recipes), and scientists there are vigorously pursuing the healing potential of substances such as polysaccharides found in many traditional Asian foods (*e.g.,* mushrooms, seaweed, and green tea). In India thousands of practitioners today continue to practice the ancient medical art of Ayurveda. In fact, the World Health Organization has adopted resolutions calling on its member states to give "adequate importance to the utilization of their traditional systems of medicine."

In Germany, Austria, and Switzerland *Naturheilkunde* ("natural healing") is increasingly popular. In 1992 the German government established a center, based at the Berlin-Steglitz university clinic, to document at least 250 such therapies. In the early 1980s the Dutch government was among the first in Europe to establish a commission to promote tolerance of alternative practices. In England "complementary" medicine, including homeopathy, acupuncture, iridology, reflexology, and yoga, among others, has a growing list of adherents. A survey in the United Kingdom in 1989 found that 74% of adults wished to see some form of complementary medicine introduced into the National Health Service. Interest in alternatives is also quite high among British general practitioners. In 1992 the University of Exeter was the first in Britain to establish both a Centre for Complementary Health Studies and an endowed chair in complementary medicine.

Deep-seated opposition to the unconventional

In the U.S., however, scientific medicine has long been entrenched. In part this is because folk and other unconventional practices have often been associated with socially disadvantaged groups (Native Americans, black slaves, women, and immigrants). Moreover, many valid folk traditions have fallen into sharp disfavor because *some* degenerated into the dubious "snake oil" treatments of the frontier "medicine show."

It is noteworthy that almost from the start American medicine defined itself in opposition to the unconventional. One of the earliest attempts to legally license the medical profession (in Connecticut in 1763) was justified by a need "to Distinguish between the Honest and Ingenious Physician and the Quack or Empirical Pretender." When the American Medical Association (AMA) was founded in 1847, it refused to allow its members to make referrals to "irregular" practitioners, such as homeopaths, whose treatments were based on minute doses of drugs. The motive is said to have been economic. According to the contemporary medical historian Paul Starr, "Monopoly was doubtless the intent of the AMA's program."

In evaluating current controversies it is important to bear in mind that many now-orthodox procedures were themselves once regarded as quackery. The 19th-century Hungarian obstetrician Ignaz Semmelweis, a pioneer of antisepsis, went mad trying to get fellow doctors simply to wash their hands before examining patients. Ether anesthesia emerged as a carnival attraction. Hypnosis was a drawing-room sensation. Even radiation and cancer chemotherapy were regarded as unwarranted departures from "sound" medicine early in this century.

This does not mean, of course, that every unconventional idea is correct. Some indeed have proved to be erroneous or even mad delusions. Nonetheless, orthodoxy has a habit of forgetting its unconventional roots. Throughout the 20th century the battle between mainstream and "fringe" medicine has been both bitter and destructive. For years the AMA maintained a Committee on Quackery until it was successfully challenged in federal courts by the chiropractic profession. In November 1990 the U.S. Supreme Court ruled that the AMA had maintained "a lengthy, systematic, unsuccessful, and unlawful boycott" of chiropractors. This decision supported an appeals court decision in February of that year that had ruled that the AMA's House of Delegates, by branding chiropractic an "unscientific cult" in 1965, had attempted to "destroy a

An herbal "pharmacy" in California attracts a growing clientele seeking alternatives to drugs that often have unwanted side effects. Proponents claim that herbal remedies are as effective as Western drugs but less likely to do harm.

competitor." The American Cancer Society continues to maintain an aggressive committee on "questionable" or "unproven" treatments, and orthodoxy has won most of its battles against unorthodox cancer therapies (*e.g.,* krebiozen and laetrile). Although such evaluations may aim at protecting patients from worthless or harmful therapies, these attacks may also have had the effect of alienating a good many patients from the medical establishment as a whole.

Growing momentum for alternatives

Despite—or possibly because of—the passionate opposition of orthodox medicine, alternative medicine continues to grow. A report in the Jan. 28, 1993, issue of the *New England Journal of Medicine* looked at the prevalence, costs, and patterns of use of unconventional therapies in the U.S. A survey conducted in 1990 revealed that one in three Americans had used such therapies in the previous year. The treatments were most often used by patients with cancer, AIDS, arthritis, chronic back pain, gastrointestinal problems, chronic renal failure, and eating disorders. They spent a total of $13.7 billion on 425 million office visits to unconventional practitioners, a number that "exceeds the number of visits to all U.S. primary care physicians," including general and family practitioners, pediatricians, and specialists in internal medicine. A 1991 *Time* magazine/CNN poll revealed that the satisfaction level of patients who seek unconventional treatments is very high; 84% said they would go to an alternative doctor again or recommend such treatment approaches to others.

These trends notwithstanding, most observers were unprepared for the dramatic way alternative medicine burst onto the American scene in 1992–93. In quick succession, numerous articles and radio and television programs indicated that U.S. patients were, in the words of the *New York Times,* "rushing to alternatives." Among the most popular media presentations was the Public Broadcasting System's five-part series "Healing and the Mind," moderated by Bill Moyers, which explored alternative healing methods ranging from ancient Chinese practices to the emerging new field of psychoneuroimmunology.

Gaining respectability: government office opened

The "coming of age" of alternative medicine in the U.S. can be said to have actually begun on Nov. 22, 1991, when a bill establishing an Office of Alternative Medicine (OAM) within the office of the director of the National Institutes of Health (NIH) was passed by the U.S. Congress. This was a major step because, as the *New York Times* put it, the NIH is not just the "country's pocketbook for biomedical research" but "a stern protector of the most rigorous brand of science."

The OAM was largely the brainchild of Berkley Bedell, a six-term Democratic representative from Iowa,

Seeking unconventional treatments	
therapy	used by U.S. adults (percentage)
relaxation techniques	13
chiropractic	10
massage	7
imagery	4
spiritual healing	4
commercial weight-loss programs	4
lifestyle diets (*e.g.,* macrobiotics)	4
herbal medicine	3
megavitamin therapy	2
self-help groups	2
energy healing	1
biofeedback	1
hypnosis	1
homeopathy	1
acupuncture	<1
folk remedies	<1
exercise	26
prayer	25

Adapted from David M. Eisenberg, M.D., *et al.,* "Unconventional Medicine in the United States," *New England Journal of Medicine,* vol. 328, no. 4 (Jan. 28, 1993), pp. 246–252

who convinced his fellow Iowan U.S. Sen. Tom Harkin of the need for such an agency. Bedell himself had developed prostate cancer after retiring from Congress in 1986 and had been treated both conventionally and with an unconventional medicine called 714-X. Bedell attributed his continuing good health to this nitrogen-and-camphor treatment and impressed upon Harkin the need to seriously consider such controversial treatments. Bedell teamed up with Frank Wiewel of the Otho, Iowa-based organization People Against Cancer. Wiewel was the relative of a patient who received treatment at the Immunology Researching Center of Lawrence Burton in Freeport, The Bahamas. The center specializes in immunoaugmentative therapy (IAT), based on the use of products obtained from pooled human blood that are injected into patients with cancer. In July 1985, Bahamian authorities, at the behest of the U.S. government, had padlocked the facility because sera used in the treatment of patients were alleged to be contaminated by bacteria, hepatitis B, and the human immunodeficiency virus (HIV), the virus that causes AIDS. As president of the IAT patients association, Wiewel led a protest in Washington, D.C. There cancer patients found many government representatives who not only feared cancer themselves but were impatient with the slow progress of the official "war on cancer." Through congressional efforts, the Freeport clinic was reopened in 1986. (No patients had been found to have developed AIDS or any other of the alleged infections.)

That same year, at the urging of pro-IAT patients, Rep. Guy V. Molinari (Rep., N.Y.), Rep. John Dingell (Dem., Mich.), and 41 other members of Congress asked the Office of Technology Assessment (OTA) for a study of this and other unconventional cancer treatments. For the next four years, the OTA investigation was the focus of a fierce struggle between the medical establishment and the alternative cancer therapy movement. "Sides are closely drawn, and the rhetoric is often bitter," the OTA complained. Nonetheless, in 1990 it recommended a demonstration project "for evaluating unconventional cancer treatments," funded by either the National Cancer Institute (NCI) or another office. The NCI drew up some guidelines but, in effect, nothing happened. According to Harkin, the congressional committee was "not satisfied that the conventional medical community as symbolized by NIH [had] fully explored the potential that exists in unconventional medical practices." In 1991 the senator, as chairman of the appropriations subcommittee that finances health research, acted on Bedell's proposal to allocate $2 million for a new office, which would "fully investigate and validate these practices" and "convene and establish an advisory panel to screen and select the procedures for investigation."

Reluctantly at first, the NIH began to organize a rapprochement between the alternative and conventional scientific communities, and in June 1992 a two-day conference was held at the NIH campus in Bethesda, Md. As the *Washington Post* reported, "Hundreds of men and women—kindred health-care professionals— have found each other. There is no turning back." The June meeting was a prelude to an even more enthusiastic conclave in September 1992, attended by more than 100 leaders of the alternative medicine community. A number of important decisions were then made. The NIH declared that "not all alternative medical practices are amenable to traditional scientific evaluation, and some may require development of new methods to evaluate their efficacy and safety." In other words, the double-blind, placebo-controlled clinical trial, once the sine qua non of all clinical research, was no longer considered the obligatory way of assessing all therapies.

After the euphoria of these meetings came the difficult task of deciding which of hundreds of competing methods should be chosen for investigation. Various panels were established to consider alternative approaches, which include:

• diet-, nutrition-, and lifestyle-related therapies (*e.g.,* macrobiotics and the so-called Gerson diet, promoted by the Gerson Institute, Bonita, Calif., an organization devoted to the nutritional management of disease)

• mind/body control (including art therapy, biofeedback, guided imagery, and hypnotherapy)

• traditional therapies and ethnomedicine (*e.g.,* acupuncture, Ayurvedic systems, homeopathy, and Native American and Oriental healing methods)

• structural and energetic therapies (*e.g.,* acupressure, chiropractic, massage therapy, reflexology, rolfing, and "therapeutic touch")

• pharmacological and biological treatments (*e.g.,* antioxidants and oxidizing agents, cellular and metabolic therapies, chelation, and others)

• electromagnetic applications (*e.g.,* electromagnetic bone repair, transcutaneous electrical nerve stimulation [TENS], and electroacupuncture)

All of the panels made recommendations to the OAM, which since October 1992 has been headed by Joseph J. Jacobs. Jacobs is a Native American physician who trained in pediatrics at Yale University School of Medicine, New Haven, Conn., and Dartmouth Medical School, Hanover, N.H., and received a Master of Business Administration degree from Wharton School at the University of Pennsylvania. Jacobs became familiar with traditional Native American practices as a child and later worked as a pediatrician on a Navajo reservation. The OAM's deputy director is Daniel Eskinazi, a dentist and an expert on homeopathy.

In Jacobs' words, the new office is like "Star Ship Enterprise," aiming "to look at those things on the fringe and give them a rigorous review." By mid-1993, however, there was still considerable controversy over the basic direction the office would take. One ap-

A patient receives an Ayurvedic treatment in which warm, herb-infused oils are dripped on the forehead to relieve such ailments as insomnia, hypertension, and indigestion. Therapies based on this ancient Indian system are among the unconventional practices that will be evaluated by the new U.S. government-sanctioned Office of Alternative Medicine.

proach thus far has been for the office to put out requests for grant applications from interested scientists seeking funding for studying specific alternative methods. Beginning in March 1993, the office began holding seminars to instruct unconventional scientists about the process of applying for government-sponsored biomedical research grants. This is being done to ensure that the research will be of very high academic standards, although some unconventional medicine adherents believe that the process may in fact dilute the relevance of some of the work.

Congress' main intent in funding the office was to evaluate existing controversial treatments, especially for major killer diseases, such as cancer and AIDS, and chronic degenerative conditions like arthritis and other autoimmune disorders, for which there are few if any beneficial standard treatments. Even some of those who are deeply skeptical of such treatments favor this strategy, believing it could put to rest the belief in useless or even dangerous treatments. This

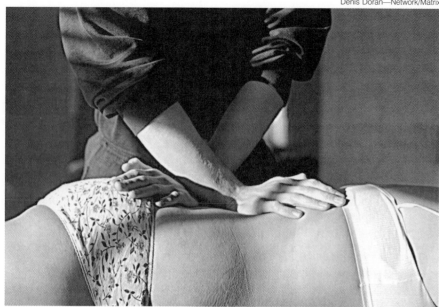

Denis Doran—Network/Matrix

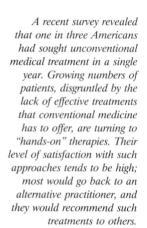

A recent survey revealed that one in three Americans had sought unconventional medical treatment in a single year. Growing numbers of patients, disgruntled by the lack of effective treatments that conventional medicine has to offer, are turning to "hands-on" therapies. Their level of satisfaction with such approaches tends to be high; most would go back to an alternative practitioner, and they would recommend such treatments to others.

could be done by means of "patient outcomes research" that would reveal how sick people fare when they undergo a particular treatment. This is an approach that has been utilized by the Agency for Health Care Policy and Research, which was established in 1989 to "enhance the quality, appropriateness, and effectiveness of health care services," especially for medical conditions affecting large numbers of people but where there is uncertainty of the benefits of specific forms of treatment.

Leaders of the OAM have begun to visit a few select unorthodox practitioners to explore setting up such studies. In January 1993 Jacobs, Eskinazi, and OAM adviser Wiewel traveled to Houston, Texas, to examine case histories of cancer and AIDS patients treated by Stanislaw Burzynski with "antineoplaston" peptides, compounds originally isolated from human urine, which purportedly cause cancer cells to stop dividing and prevent HIV from progressing. In March 1993 the two OAM officers and this author visited Charles Simone, a cancer specialist in Lawrenceville, N.J., to discuss setting up a trial with shark cartilage, a proposed unconventional treatment for cancer and arthritis. A cartilage product is now widely sold in health food stores and has been the subject of clinical trial in Cuba, which was reported on the television program "60 Minutes" (Feb. 28, 1992). The same team also met with Emanuel Revici, a 96-year-old practitioner in New York City, who has been using lipids and other nontoxic substances in the treatment of cancer since the 1920s.

Crisis in American medicine

Today it is generally recognized that not only is orthodox medicine in the United States in a state of profound crisis, but the crisis has led the country into an economic impasse. Legislators in particular are alarmed by the soaring costs of high-technology medicine. According to a study conducted by researchers from Tufts University, Medford, Mass., it now costs over $231 million to develop a new drug in the U.S. This fact alone guarantees that new medicines are expensive and that strong patents on synthetic therapeutic agents are necessary for pharmaceutical companies to recoup their investments. Alternative treatments, being generally nonpatented and/or natural, tend to be, by comparison, considerably less costly. Most vitamins, minerals, and herbs cost pennies, and in 1990 the average charge for a visit to an alternative practitioner was only $28.

Alternative treatments are not just economical but, at their best, adhere to a new paradigm of health care—one in which patients themselves take responsibility for their own health. Most alternatives are holistic—that is, they focus not only on the ailment but on the whole individual. Today there is a heavy emphasis on prevention and wellness, as opposed to the symptomatic, treatment-oriented approach of most fee-for-service medicine. This, too, should make alternative approaches attractive to legislators.

Antibiotics, early diagnosis, chemotherapy that cures childhood cancers—the products of orthodox medicine—are undeniable triumphs. Nonetheless, as a comprehensive approach to health, mainstream U.S. medicine has serious deficiencies and is, to a large extent, failing its patients. For counteracting the emotional chill at the heart of contemporary scientific medicine, a dose of alternative medicine may be "just what the doctor ordered."

—*Ralph W. Moss, Ph.D.*

244

Editors' Choice
A Cartoon a Day . . .

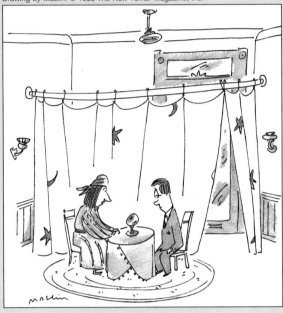

"According to an article in the upcoming issue of 'The New England Journal of Medicine,' all your fears are well founded."

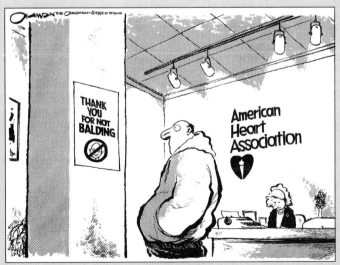

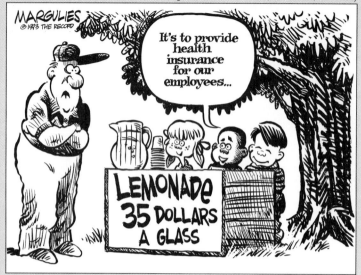

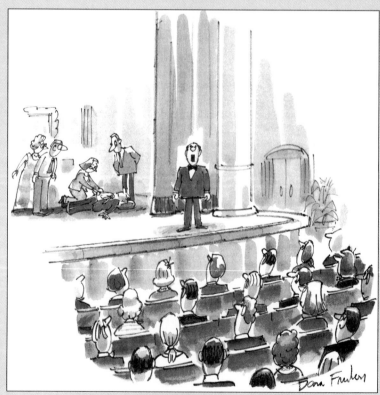

"Are there several doctors in the house, so we can have a little managed competition?"

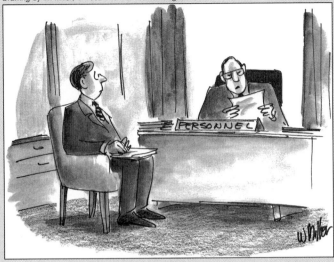

"Of course, with the position that has the benefits—medical, dental, et cetera—there is no salary."

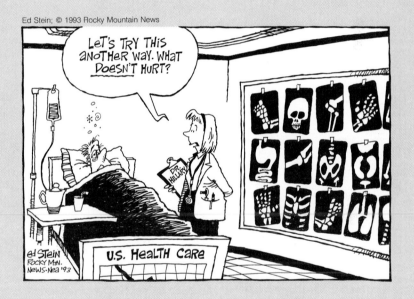

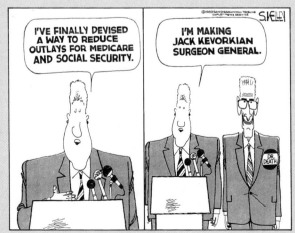

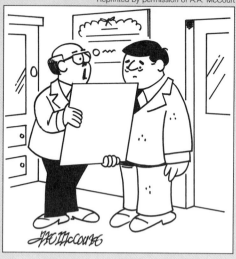

*"Here's your problem . . . You've been
reading the Food Pyramid upside down."*

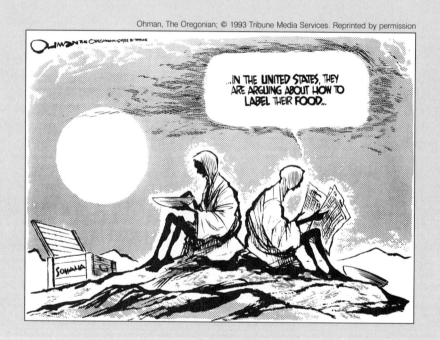

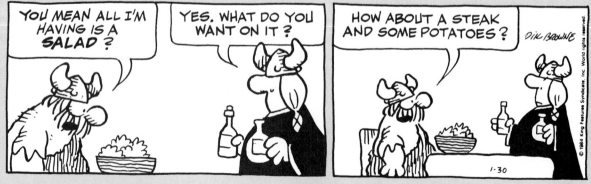

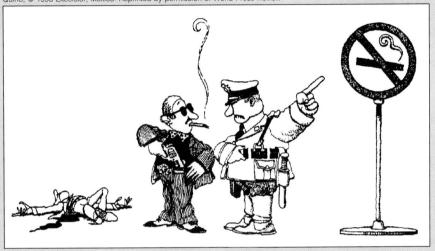

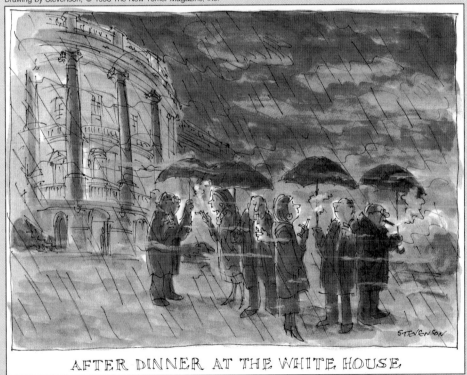

AFTER DINNER AT THE WHITE HOUSE

Cancer

Cancer is an ancient disease; it was described by Hippocrates and Galen under different names. At the end of the 19th century, physicians for the first time could diagnose cancer in medical terms. However, only in 1915, after two Japanese researchers, K. Yamagiwa and K. Ichikawa, had shown that continuous application of coal tar to rabbits' skin produced malignancy, were experimental studies on cancer initiated.

For the most part, however, cancer research was not active at the beginning of this century—probably because the mortality rate was not very high. In 1900 cancer was only the ninth leading cause of death in the United States. However, by the 1950s the mortality rate had doubled, and cancer emerged as the second leading cause of death. Certain types of cancer, such as lung cancer, were increasing steadily. Even as recently as the 1960s, the causes of lung cancer had not been unraveled. Epidemiologists had gathered data and formulated theories that purported to connect cancer of the lungs to cigarette smoking, but they were not taken seriously.

In the past several decades cancer research has come a long way—mainly owing to rapid developments in molecular biology and heightened understanding of genetics at the cellular level, which have disclosed many of the causes of cancer and its mode of propagation. Cancer, as medical scientists' present information reveals, causes cellular anarchy; cells that have become cancerous lose their normal growth-control mechanism, resulting in an inability to respond to signals that normally regulate their functions. This diverse disarray in the functioning of the internal cellular machinery can be brought about in different ways. Cancer is not, therefore, a single or a simple disease. Cancer in one organ is different in both its rate of growth and its aggressiveness from that in another, and even in the same organ there may be different types of cancers, depending on the nature of the cells involved. More than 250 different kinds of cancers with different causes, symptoms, and degrees of lethality have been discovered.

Although there are many theories regarding the causes of cancer, the fundamental idea underlying these theories is that the genetic material, the DNA of the cell, has been changed; the various theories attempt to explain how this change was brought about. The DNA of a cancer cell is slightly different from that of a normal cell. This means that the sequence of the bases—adenine (A), guanine (G), thymine (T), and cytosine (C)—in a given strand of DNA is not the same. These sequences dictate the sequence of the transcribed messenger RNA, which in turn specifies the kinds of proteins to be synthesized in a cell. The change in the DNA sequence in the cancer cells results in abnormal proteins. These new proteins influence the mechanism of growth control in such a way that cell division continues indefinitely.

One of the important characteristics of a cancer cell is its lack of "contact inhibition." Normal cells reproduce by dividing, but they stop dividing when the number of cells reaches a certain point. Precise control of cell division is a basic function of all multicellular organisms. The growth-control signal is transmitted by various proteins that interact with the cell-surface protein receptors.

Insights into cancer's causes

The basic change in the DNA, known as mutation, can be caused by many factors, such as ultraviolet (UV) and ionizing radiation, chemicals, so-called free radicals, and viruses. Mutation does not necessarily cause cancer; this occurs only if proteins that result from mutation affect cellular growth-control mechanisms.

Radiation damage of DNA. The relationship between radiation and DNA damage has been the focus of considerable study. The process is very complex. Absorption of short-wave UV radiation by DNA causes breakage in its strand, the opening of the rings of its bases, and the formation of thymine dimers (*i.e.,* compounds formed by the union of two thymine bases).

Ultraviolet radiation from sunlight is the main cause of skin cancer. Increased UV-radiation exposure—much of it caused by sunbathing or tanning under a UV lamp—is the main contributing factor to skin cancer, the incidence of which is rising rapidly worldwide. Of the three types of UV radiation—UV-A, UV-B, and UV-C—UV-B is the most harmful. Recent extensive animal experiments suggest that UV-A may also cause skin cancer.

UV-B is attenuated by the Earth's ozone layer. Several other factors modulate the amount of UV radiation to which people are exposed: time of day, season, humidity, and distance from the equator. Skin cancer risk also depends on the skin type; fair skin that freckles or burns easily is more at risk than very dark-pigmented skin. People who live in sunny climates and have red or blond hair and blue or light-colored eyes are at especially high risk. Among the photochemical reactions that take place when UV-B penetrates the skin is mutation of the DNA in skin cells. Humans have repair enzymes that can correct this damage, but as the person ages, depending on his or her lifestyle, the mutations accumulate, and the repair system will eventually be overtaxed, leading to skin cancer. The damage begins accumulating early—in childhood; by young adulthood about 50% of lifetime sunlight exposure has already accumulated.

Scientists have not known the precise genomic location of the damage from UV radiation that results in skin cancer. Recently, however, cancer researcher Douglas E. Brash and his colleagues of Yale University discovered that in certain skin cancer patients—

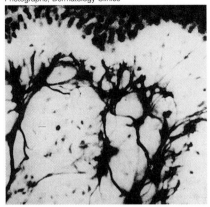

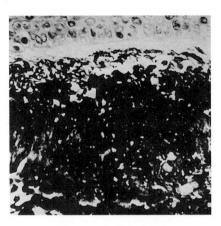

Protecting the skin from the sun's harmful rays is the best way to prevent skin cancer. Skin that has been overexposed to sunlight over many years (left) has suffered severe ultraviolet radiation damage. By contrast, older skin that has been protected (far left) has retained its elastic fibers (dark network). Because damage is cumulative, precautions against excessive exposure should be taken from an early age.

those with squamous cell carcinoma—UV radiation caused mutation of the p53 gene (on chromosome 17) by converting its two contiguous cytosines (C-C) into thymines (T-T). This T-T pair is more prone to UV-directed dimer formation. Squamous cell carcinoma is the second most common form of skin cancer, following basal cell carcinoma. Both types originate in the epidermal (outer) skin layer. Squamous cell skin cancer is not very aggressive, though early treatment is crucial to prevent fatality. Now that a specific defect has been located, it may be possible to develop DNA-directed "gene therapy" for such skin cancer.

The researchers at Yale are now investigating whether UV-B can also produce melanoma—a highly malignant metastatic skin cancer that originates in the melanocytes (pigment-containing skin cells). Because it spreads so rapidly, it is almost always fatal. Although several highly experimental treatments have been tried, none has proved to be effective for any substantial length of time.

Proto-oncogenes and oncogenes. In the search for the cause of cancer, researchers discovered that the human genome itself carries the seeds of cancer—proto-ocogenes, specific genes that can be modified in various ways to become cancer-causing oncogenes. Since the early 1970s researchers have isolated over 100 such oncogenes with fundamental roles in cell growth and differentiation.

When mutated or overproduced, these genes cause cancer. The names that were given to oncogenes when they were originally discovered are associated with particular types of cancer; for example, the *ras* gene was found in rat sarcoma, although subsequently it was found to be involved in human bladder, lung, colon, and many other forms of cancer. Generally speaking, the same gene product can cause various types of cancer by independent mechanisms involving various metabolic effects. Even though considerable information has been gathered about oncogenes in the last several years, the precise biochemical mechanisms in the transformation of a normal cell to a cancer cell still are not well documented.

Tumor suppressor genes. Another type of gene, referred to as a "tumor suppressor gene," has received extensive attention since the early 1980s. Scientists believe that the expression of such genes is necessary for normal growth and division of a cell and that the absence and/or inactivation of these genes will cause abnormal growth. Evidence of tumor suppressor genes was first observed in so-called hybrid cells, which form when a normal cell is fused with a tumor cell. It was observed that if these laboratory-produced hybrid cells were allowed to divide and multiply in a cell culture, nontumorogenic hybrid cells developed, indicating that the normal cell was contributing something that suppressed the expression of the tumor cell's characteristics. In other words, the tumor cells did not have certain genetic information. This shortage of information led them to be cancerous. In 1986 Robert Weinberg at the Massachusetts Institute of Technology, along with Stephen Friend of Harvard Medical School, cloned the retinoblastoma (RB) gene and demonstrated that the absence of the RB gene led to retinoblastoma, a rare type of eye cancer. Subsequently Wen-Hwa Lee at the University of California at San Diego showed that when the RB gene was inserted into tumor cells, the cells lost their tumor-forming capacity.

In multicellular organisms interaction between cells is crucial in maintaining the structural and functional integrity of the organism. The interaction between cells depends on two types of signals—growth stimulating and growth inhibiting. Recent research has shown that tumor suppressor genes can inhibit cell growth in three possible ways: (1) cells may not enter the DNA synthesis phase and, thus, cell division does not occur; (2) cells may divide but at the end of division will differentiate and will not divide again (called terminal differentiation); or (3), the most dramatic, the cell goes through apoptosis, or programmed cell death.

To date, several of the suppressor genes have been identified, and mutation or lack of their presence is thought to be responsible for colorectal cancer, retinoblastoma, neurofibromatosis (soft tumors associated with pigmentation and affecting the entire body), Wilms' tumor (a type of kidney cancer), and possibly others. The p53 gene is one of the tumor suppressor genes. It seems to be very essential for normal cells and has been found to be involved in many of the different tumor cells that have been investigated.

Since an inactive tumor suppressor gene acts in a recessive manner and can be transferred to offspring in a mutant form, genetic diagnostic tests may signal its presence. This will enable the identification of individuals with predispositions to many types of cancer. For families with RB this type of genetic diagnosis is already available. In the future it may also be possible to insert functional suppressor genes into tumor cells that lack them. Such experiments are already under way in many research laboratories.

Viral causes of cancer. Viruses could be another factor leading to cancer. This idea arose from the observation that certain kinds of viruses, when injected into animals, produced tumors. In humans it is difficult to prove that the virus is the direct cause of cancer. Infection may remain latent for years or decades before there is any expression of malignancy. However, over the years certain DNA viruses have been linked to certain human cancers—e.g., the hepatitis virus (liver cancer), papillomavirus (cervical and skin cancers), Epstein-Barr virus (lymphoma and nasopharyngeal carcinoma), and herpes simplex virus (cervical cancer).

Even if they are not directly involved in malignancy, viruses may activate a proto-oncogene to become an oncogene. A recent finding is that viruses can also indirectly lead to cancer by suppressing the immune system. For this reason those infected by the human immunodeficiency virus (HIV), the virus that causes AIDS, are at risk of developing Kaposi's sarcoma and B-cell lymphoma.

Chemical carcinogens. Most carcinogens—agents that cause cancer—act by altering the DNA molecule and causing mutation; they are therefore known as "mutagens." Some chemicals by themselves are not carcinogens, and their conversion is usually not a single step or simple process. When they enter the living cells, they are converted to potent mutagens by a membranous structure in the cell ("microsome"), which contains various kinds of enzymes. The microsomal enzymes detoxify drugs and convert other unwanted compounds into more soluble, excretable products. In some people the presence of various levels of inherited microsomal enzymes may limit their degree of susceptibility to the carcinogenic effect of chemicals.

The human race lives in an era in which new synthetic chemicals—most of which make life on Earth better—are created virtually every day. Some, however, can be lethal. The availability of diagnostic tests to determine chemical carcinogenicity has made a

significant difference in the management of cancers that result from chemicals. For instance, the Ames test, developed by Bruce Ames of the University of California at Berkeley, allows scientists to identify the carcinogenic chemicals in the environment in a quick, reliable, and inexpensive way. A bacterium such as salmonella is cultured in the presence of the chemical; if the chemical causes genetic changes in the bacteria, there is a significant probability it can cause cancer in humans.

At present there is a long but by no means exhaustive list of agents that can cause cancer. Several that have been identified in the past few years are: (2,4-dichlorophenoxy) acetic acid (2,4D), an herbicide; DDE, a breakdown product of DDT; hexachlorocyclohexane, an insecticide; and tetrachlorodibenzo-p-dioxin (TCDD), a by-product of the manufacture of herbicides, disinfectants, and other chemicals. As scientists improve their understanding of how this complicated disease progresses, more new mechanisms underlying carcinogensis become known.

A multistage disease

Recent insights have helped clarify the various steps involved in carcinogenesis, or malignant tumor formation. Cancer is a cumulative and progressive disease following a multistage process. Exposure to cancer-causing agents does not result immediately in cancer. There are three major steps in carcinogenesis: initiation, promotion, and progression. The primary, and essential, step in the formation of a malignant tumor is initiation, the irreversible chemical change in the gene, or the DNA. In humans there are corrective enzymes that can repair certain damage and reverse the adverse effect. Initiators can also produce transformed cells that can persist for the life-span of an individual without producing cancer. In such a case the damaged gene in the transformed cells remains recessive because the damaged gene is not expressing an abnormal protein.

The second step, promotion, activates the gene to synthesize the abnormal protein. Some chemicals act as both initiators and promoters. Benzo[a]pyrene, a product of incomplete combustion of carbonaceous material—e.g., fossil fuels from automobiles, industry, and refuse burning—is such a chemical. In small doses it initiates genetic damage, and in higher or repeated doses a promotion reaction ensues.

The agents that are involved in the onset of promotion cause cancer not by themselves but only in an initiated cell. Phorbol esters in cottonseed oil and the artificial sweetener saccharin are both examples of promoters. Promotion is gradual; moreover, some of the earlier steps are reversible. In the promotion stage, abnormal proliferation of the affected cell occurs, presumably owing to a high concentration of growth factors or modified cell-surface receptors. If the damage to the gene is not drastic, most of the normal components of the cell will be produced and will be responsive to normal growth-inhibiting factors. Animal experiments suggest that the time lapse between initiation and promotion is not critical. During the later stage of promotion, however, cumulative genetic changes take place, culminating in totally irreversible neoplastic transformation.

Once a cell has been irreversibly modified, a cancer cell is born. Then it multiplies to produce a large number of cancer cells that form tumors. The third stage, progression, is now beginning to set in. Some of these cells will eventually travel to other tissues—the process known as metastasis.

Metastasis: why does cancer spread?

The most fearsome aspect of cancer is the spread of malignant cells from the primary site to other parts of the body. This process of metastasis is the primary cause for the failure of treatment in cancer patients. Tumor metastasis is not a random process, nor is it a simple one. The physiological condition of the host will determine how extensive the dissemination of the malignant cells will be. The same type of cancer may metastasize diffusively at a very early stage in one patient, whereas it may become a large tumor without invading other tissues in another.

During metastasis continuous changes take place in the tumor, and the function and behavior of the tumor cells in the late stage are quite different from those in the early stage. The late stage of the disease is characterized by invasive activity and the appearance of a variety of cancer cell types. Some of the cells, which have the inherent ability to detach from the primary site, will eventually travel via the blood or lymph to start a secondary tumor in another site. Most frequently the location of metastasis is in the organ or organs that are served by blood vessels from the original cancer site. For example, lung cancer most commonly spreads to the brain, while colorectal cancer spreads to the liver.

Growth and survival of a tumor require nourishment, which is provided by new blood vessels near the tumor site. Development of these new blood vessels is called angiogenesis. Rarely can any metastasis occur before angiogenesis has taken place. Today scientists are gaining better understanding of angiogenesis and many other aspects of the metastatic process. Understanding how and why tumors spread has led to better treatment and prevention strategies.

New methods for detecting cancer

Since certain stages of cancer are reversible and in many cases there is no specific symptom until the tumor has developed to an advanced stage (ovarian cancer is one such example), early diagnosis plays an important part in prognosis. For early detection

sensitive, specific, and relatively inexpensive screening methods are needed. Many such methods are now available thanks to recent advances in technology. In the last decade or so, a great number of old techniques have been improved and new ones developed. Sophisticated imaging techniques such as magnetic resonance imaging (MRI) and safer and less costly mammograms are the results of such technological advances.

Active research is now under way on so-called tumor markers that can be employed to test for the presence of cancer in a blood sample. Tumor markers, or biomarkers, are specific protein molecules (antigens) secreted by tumors or present on the surface of tumor cells. These tumor-specific antigens stimulate antibody production and can interact with antibodies developed specifically to test for their presence. A few such antigen tests are already available. One of these is CA 125 for ovarian cancer, a test that has proved valuable for gauging the success of therapy and for monitoring women with a family history of ovarian cancer but is not sensitive enough to be widely used for detecting early tumors. Prostate specific antigen (PSA), on the other hand, can signal the presence of a prostate tumor before it is detectable by other means and before it produces symptoms.

A further type of biomarker is produced by repair

Leading cancers: 1993 estimates of incidence*	
male	female
prostate 165,000	breast 182,000
lung 100,000	colon and rectum 75,000
colon and rectum 77,000	lung 70,000
bladder 39,000	uterus 44,500
lymphoma 28,500	lymphoma 22,400
oral 20,300	ovary 22,000
melanoma 17,000	melanoma 15,000
kidney 16,800	pancreas 14,200
leukemia 16,700	bladder 13,300
stomach 14,800	leukemia 12,600
pancreas 13,500	kidney 10,400
larynx 10,000	oral 9,500
all sites 600,000	all sites 570,000

*excluding basal and squamous cell skin cancer and carcinoma *in situ*
Source: American Cancer Society, *1993 Cancer Facts and Figures*

enzymes. Recently Japanese researchers reported the usefulness of the enzyme glutathione-S-transferase-pai (GST-pai) as a tumor marker in patients with oral cancer. Increased levels of this enzyme were found in the blood of patients whose cancers recurred after surgery but were not yet clinically detectable. Blood levels of GST-pai also dropped markedly in patients who responded to chemotherapy.

In all tests based on tumor markers thus far developed, sometimes normal (noncancerous) cells may also show up as cancerous (a false-positive result). Therefore, tumor-marker technology has not yet reached the stage of maturity for early detection of most cancers or for widespread cancer screening.

Statistically, 80% of cancers are caused by environmental agents; the rest are genetically transmitted. These genetic defects can be detected in the DNA obtained from blood samples. In inherited colorectal cancer, for example, some patients are prone to develop polyps that are benign at the beginning but can develop into malignant tumors in the course of time, known as familial adenomatus polyposis. Recently, Bert Vogelstein and Kenneth Kinzler of the Johns Hopkins University School of Medicine, Baltimore, Md., Yusuke Nakamura of the Tokyo Cancer Institute, and Ray White of the University of Utah identified the gene responsible for this colorectal cancer in a discrete portion of chromosome 5, which is mutated in patients who are found to have inherited this disease.

In May 1993 an international team of scientists headed by Vogelstein in the U.S. and Albert de la Chapelle at the University of Helsinki, Fin., provided evidence of the presence of a gene located on chromosome 2 that could carry the inherited susceptibility to a much more common form of colon cancer in which there is no development of polyps. These patients have what is known as hereditary nonpolyposis colorectal cancer (HNPCC) and are also prone to develop other malignancies such as cancer of the ovary, uterine lining, and kidney. The scientists selected two large families—one from Canada and the other from New Zealand—in whom they focused on "microsatellite DNAs"—short repetitive DNA sequences interspersed throughout the genome. These sequences are highly informative because their length (hence their nucleotide sequence) varies from one person to another. They checked 345 microsatellite DNAs and eventually determined that one of the loci, on the short arm of chromosome 2 (2p15-16), is implicated in HNPCC.

The scientists found that the microsatellite DNA varied in length from tumor to tumor, indicating that a DNA replication error had taken place—i.e., nucleotide repeat fragments were either deleted or inserted. They also found that about 13% of "sporadic" colorectal tumors—i.e., those in patients with no family history of colon cancer—also had abnormalities in the specific

satellite DNA length. The most surprising observation, however, was the presence of nonrandomly distributed similar-size alterations in microsatellite DNA at many other chromosomal sites in most of the HNPCC-related tumors. The scientists speculate that the HNPCC gene may be the one producing replication errors in both sporadic and familial cases.

Although colorectal cancer is very common, its cause has been difficult to determine. Now the chromosome 2 satellite DNA could be used as a marker and a simple blood test developed to identify high-risk individuals. Once a person has been identified as a carrier, preventive measures can be taken, and the individual can be closely monitored for the first sign of malignancy.

With today's sophisticated molecular technology it is now possible to detect and diagnose more and more abnormalities in the DNA of cancer patients. This technology can even be used in healthy individuals genetically predisposed to cancer.

New horizons in treatment: biological therapy

Recently acquired knowledge of carcinogenesis is helping to improve therapeutic modalities. Besides surgery, radiation, and chemotherapy, researchers are developing the new mode of therapy known as "biological therapy," which is designed to be more selective than previous modalities in that it destroys the cancer cells but not the surrounding normal cells. Radiation and chemotherapy, on the other hand, cannot distinguish between normal and cancerous cells.

The human immune system offers a powerful deterrent to cancer growth. Because the immune system does not function at its maximum capacity in cancer patients, it cannot destroy malignant cells. Scientists are therefore attempting to stimulate immune responses in a number of ways in order to contain the growth of cancer cells. In one such approach known as "immunotherapy," cytokines (nonantibody proteins synthesized by immune system cells in response to antigens) are administered to patients to stimulate immunity. Interferons, naturally occurring antiviral substances, and interleukin-2 (IL-2), a product of immune system cells known as T lymphocytes, are among the cytokines that are being used in various trials in patients with advanced cancers that are resistant to other therapies (e.g., malignant melanoma, renal-cell cancer, colorectal cancer, non-Hodgkin's lymphoma, and adenocarcinoma of the lung). In a few cases a dramatic response has been reported. In most cases, however, although survival has been prolonged, patients are not "cured," and tumors later recur.

An even newer strategy is to use "vaccination" to stimulate immunity. Generation of a vaccine requires an immunogenic protein, a cancer-specific antigen. Thus far, all tumor antigens have been found to be very weak immunogens that cannot elicit strong immune

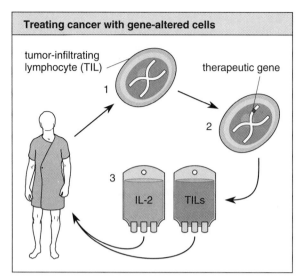

Treating cancer with gene-altered cells

tumor-infiltrating
lymphocyte (TIL)

therapeutic gene

1

2

3

IL-2

TILs

Several new cancer therapies are based on the genetic engineering of a patient's own cells. In one strategy, immune cells called tumor-infiltrating lymphocytes (TILs) are taken from the patient's tumor (1) and given a gene for tumor necrosis factor, a natural toxin that finds and destroys tumor cells (2). The altered TILs are then returned to the patient along with interleukin-2 (IL-2), a protein normally made by immune cells, which stimulates the TILs to multiply (3).

responses. Therefore, an alternative is to produce a "virus construct"—that is, to combine the tumor antigen with a highly immunogenic, unrelated virus strain such as vaccinia (closely related to the smallpox virus). This "recombinant" virus is then administered to immunize against cancer. At present, the aim of such vaccines is not to prevent cancer from arising in the first place but to arrest the progress of cancer in patients with tumors that would otherwise follow a rapidly lethal course. In the future, however, such vaccines could conceivably be developed to prevent primary tumors. In 1992 scientists at Stanford University successfully boosted the immunity of nine patients with B-cell lymphoma, a cancer that affects 20,000 Americans each year. The therapeutic vaccine was custom made from each patient's own tumor cells.

Another exciting recent development in cancer therapy is "gene therapy," where a specific gene can be introduced into immune system cells, which are first removed from the patients, then genetically modified and reintroduced into the immune system so that these new cells will destroy the cancer cells. In early 1993 more than 10 trials of gene therapies for various advanced cancers—including malignant melanoma, neuroblastoma, brain tumor, and kidney, lung, and ovarian cancers—were under way internationally in selected patients in highly experimental protocols.

Other biological therapies are still in very preliminary stages of development but hold promise. One is the use of genetically engineered cells (tumor-infiltrating

lymphocytes) to secrete a biological poison (tumor necrosis factor) at the tumor site. This "immunotoxin" will then destroy the tumor without producing systemic toxicity. Monoclonal antibodies—bioengineered antibodies specifically targeted to deliver powerful anticancer drugs or radioactive substances directly to the tumor site so as not to destroy the normal, healthy surrounding cells—are also being developed.

"Differentiation therapy" is another biological therapy. Under normal conditions cells undergo division, multiplication, and differentiation in a "coupled" and integrated manner. In cancer cells the proliferation and differentiation steps are not integrated, and overproduction of abnormal cells follows. The basic idea underlying this new therapy is to induce production of the normal component of a cell that will enable the cancer cell to normalize its function—*i.e.,* to couple proliferation and differentiation. At present the most promising differentiation inducer is retinoic acid, a derivative of vitamin A, and its analogues. Already this treatment has been observed to be remarkably effective in the form of blood cancer known as acute promyelocytic leukemia.

New and better drugs

Cancer-fighting drugs are potent, and they cannot distinguish between healthy and malignant cells. Researchers are always looking for naturally occurring drugs with tolerable side effects. In recent years taxol, derived from the bark of special yew trees, has caught the attention of scientists. Even though it was discovered in the early 1960s (by chemists Monroe E. Wall and Mansukhlal C. Wani of Research Triangle Institute in North Carolina), because of its short supply and insolubility in water, clinical trials were delayed. However, in 1989 William McGuire and his associates from the Johns Hopkins School of Medicine reported a significant improvement in patients with advanced, refractory ovarian cancer who were treated with taxol. In 1992 the FDA approved the use of taxol (paclitaxel; Taxol) for ovarian cancer; patients with many other forms of the disease, such as breast and lung cancers, are also receiving the drug in clinical trials.

Since there is enormous interest in taxol and the supply is scanty, researchers are looking for alternate analogues. The structure of taxol is very complex for chemical synthesis. Rhône-Poulenc Rorer, a pharmaceutical company in France, has developed a compound called taxotere that is very similar to taxol in structure and is produced semisynthetically from a precursor of taxol, isolated from yew needles, which are abundant. Scientists are also trying to develop water-soluble inactive taxol "prodrugs" that could be easily delivered to patients and would be converted to the active drug within the body. Recently, in collaboration with scientists from the University of Turin, Italy, Young Hoon Park and his colleagues from the State

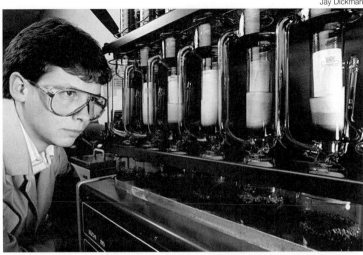

Raw taxol from Pacific yew trees is processed and purified in a chemical laboratory. In 1992 the U.S. Food and Drug Administration approved the use of taxol for ovarian cancer; the drug also shows potential as a treatment for advanced breast and lung cancers. Because of its limited supply, cancer researchers around the world are actively investigating a number of taxol analogues. A recently discovered fungus in yew bark may prove to be an important source of the drug in the future.

University of New York at Stony Brook discovered a promising new family of analogues of taxol and taxotere in the yew needles.

More exciting news for taxol researchers came in April 1993 when plant pathologist Gary Strobel of Montana State University and his colleagues reported the presence of a fungus, given the name *Taxomyces andreanae,* in yew bark, which can produce taxol even when removed from the tree and grown in the laboratory. Although the actual amount of taxol produced by this fungus is very low, the investigators believe that modification of culturing techniques and the use of genetic engineering procedures may improve the yield of this fungal form of taxol.

Synthesis of drugs with anticancer potency is also active on many other fronts. Kyriacos C. Nicolaou and his colleagues at the Scripps Research Institute and the University of California at San Diego recently reported the synthesis of several organic compounds that have anticancer potency much greater than the drugs cisplatin and doxorubicin, which have been widely used in cancer therapies for years. The design of these new synthetic agents was based on the structure of the natural compound dynemicin A, an anticancer antibiotic containing enediyne (two double-bonded carbons flanked by two pairs of triple-bonded carbons). Dynemicin A was discovered in the late 1980s at a Bristol-Myers laboratory in Japan. The California researchers believe that unlike many anticancer drugs, these new "designed enediynes" can be structurally modified in such a way that they could distinguish between a healthy cell and a cancerous one. The altered chemistry of cancer cells may also preferentially activate these agents.

Another drug, carboxamide-amino-imidazole (CAI), the first antimetastatic and antiproliferatic drug, was approved by the U.S. Food and Drug Administration (FDA) in January 1992 for clinical trial. Elise Kohn at the NCI discovered that this synthetic compound interferes with tumor spread. In preclinical studies involving human cancer cells, CAI was found to block growth of over 20 different types of cancers, including those of the colon, breast, prostate, and ovary.

The drug cladribine (Leustatin) was recently approved by the FDA for hairy cell leukemia, a rare and often fatal blood and bone marrow cancer. The advantage of this drug is that it is administered only once in one continuous treatment over a seven-day period. Because only one treatment is required, patients may not experience some of the recurrent side effects frequently associated with multiple treatments, such as nausea, vomiting, headache, and rashes.

Aldesleukin recently became the first FDA-approved drug treatment specifically for kidney cancer. Derived from genetically engineered bacteria, aldesleukin is an analogue of human IL-2, a lymphokine that has a central role in regulating immune responses. Use of this drug represents one of the first successful attempts to combat cancer by stimulating the body's own immune system. However, this treatment causes severe side effects; therefore, the FDA suggests that the drug be administered only in a hospital setting under proper supervision.

Suramin, a polysulfonated drug, has a broad range of biological activity and in the laboratory has been found to be effective against a variety of solid tumor cell lines. In clinical studies using the drug in patients with advanced, hormone-refractory prostate cancer, NCI researchers found that the compound was of significant benefit. Neurotoxicity, however, is a dose-limiting problem.

Toxicity is a frequent problem in cancer chemotherapy. The NCI's Dvorit Samid observed that phenylacetic acid, a naturally occurring nontoxic agent, exerted anticancer activity by arresting the growth of human tumor cells rather than killing them. On the basis of her work, the Elan Pharmaceutical Research Corp. has produced a drug, EL530, which is being tested to determine its safe and effective dosage for the treatment of cancer.

Failure to achieve the optimal therapeutic effect varies in different types of cancer and among individual patients. Understanding such failure is necessary to the design of proper and effective therapies. Resistance to drugs, known as multiple drug resistance (MDR), has long posed a significant problem in chemotherapy. (MDR also occurs in some forms of the new biological therapies.) Recently researchers have discovered that a specific glycoprotein (p-gp) in the cell membrane in cancer patients actively pumps drugs out of the cells, thus reducing their level in the cell. When a specific pathway of resistance like this is known, then agents that are more likely to have maximum efficacy can be developed.

Prevention: a powerful weapon against cancer

All in all, dedicated research has improved the life expectancy and quality of life of many cancer patients, and yet no universal cure for cancer has been found. Because about 80% of cancers arise from nongenetic causes, researchers are now increasingly shifting their strategy from cure to prevention.

Epidemiological studies suggest that lifestyles can affect the incidence of many cancers enormously. Lung cancer is the most obvious example. For several decades it has been known that smoking is a major cause of lung cancer; within the past year or two it has also become well established that nonsmokers who are exposed to secondhand smoke are also at high risk of developing lung cancer. It has been widely documented that giving up smoking reduces lung cancer death rates, and that not smoking in the first place is an even more effective strategy. Exposure to sunlight is a major cause of skin cancer. Simple preventive measures against sun damage could reduce the high incidence of such cancers. These include using effective sunscreen, wearing protective clothing, avoiding

direct sun exposure between 10 AM and 2 PM, and refraining from using tanning devices. These measures should be begun at a very early age because the damage from the sun is cumulative.

Choice of food varies widely among racial and ethnic groups in different parts of the world. The incidence of cancer also varies from nation to nation and from region to region within countries. All natural food products contain chemicals, some of which can cause cancer while others may prevent it. Some chemicals present in plants (phytochemicals) can stimulate the synthesis of various enzymes that promote detoxification of cancer-causing chemicals. Recently Paul Talalay, Gary H. Posner, and their co-workers at Johns Hopkins identified a specific chemical, sulforaphane, in cruciferous vegetables such as broccoli that can selectively stimulate the synthesis of a specific detoxifying enzyme. Phenols and indoles present in many vegetables can also have the same effect.

Chemicals can also act as antioxidants, preventing harmful effects of active free radicals (unstable molecules that cause damage to DNA) and reducing cancer risk. Vitamins C and E and beta-carotene present in many fruits and vegetables are all potent antioxidants. By selecting diets that emphasize foods with such anticarcinogenic properties, one can increase the content of "good" chemicals that will counteract some of the effects of "bad" chemicals. The fact that natural chemicals present in food can affect enzyme activity and counteract oxidative damage has opened up a vast new vista of research on the strategy known as "chemoprevention." The NCI is presently devoting research efforts to identifying beneficial chemicals in foodstuffs. A goal of such research is to create "designer foods" that will help prevent cancer.

It has also been shown that there is a relationship between a low-fiber diet and the development of colorectal cancer—the third leading cause of cancer deaths in both men and women in the United States.

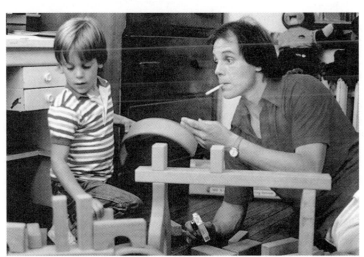

In the past several years, a number of major studies have confirmed that secondhand smoke causes lung damage in nonsmokers. Children who are exposed to parents' cigarette smoking are especially vulnerable. In December 1992 the U.S. Environmental Protection Agency released the most condemning report to date, which concluded that environmental tobacco smoke is a human lung carcinogen and that in the United States alone it is responsible for more than 3,000 lung cancer deaths in nonsmokers annually.

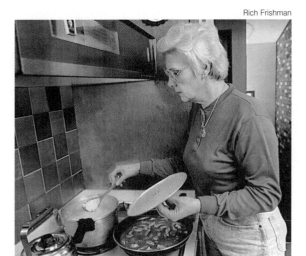

A woman taking part in a cancer-prevention study prepares a low-fat meal. Dietary fat is known or believed to increase the risk of a number of cancer types. One theory is that a high-fat diet suppresses immune defenses that destroy cancerous cells.

The composition of natural fiber is very complex. Fiber provides bulk in the diet; it can also absorb potent carcinogens, decreasing their effective concentration and reducing their transit time through the digestive tract, thereby shortening the amount of contact between tissues and carcinogens.

Fat that makes food delicious can increase the risk of certain types of cancer such as large bowel, hepatic, and pancreatic cancers. Although the mechanism involved is not well understood, scientists are beginning to offer some explanations. One of these is that an excess of certain fatty acids in foods may alter the membrane structure, thus affecting intercellular communication. It is also known that fat can be oxidized in the body into the mutagen hydrogen peroxide. Fat present in meat is known to produce potent carcinogens when grilled on a charcoal fire. Recently it has been suggested that a high-fat diet may suppress the immune defenses that are necessary to destroy cancer cells, and research is under way to determine more precisely how this might occur.

Investigators have suggested for many years that women who lower their fat intake and also increase dietary fiber might reduce their risk of breast cancer. Recently a large trial run by Walter C. Willett of Harvard Medical School offered the most convincing evidence to date that dietary fat and fiber do *not* contribute to breast cancer development. No apparent link was seen in nearly 90,000 women, aged 34 to 59, who were followed for eight years. Other researchers still believe the fat and breast cancer link may be important and deserves further investigation.

Prevention of some cancers seems to work in animals. However, extending animal experiments to hu-

mans cannot always be undertaken with a high level of confidence. In 1992 the NCI, using the antiestrogen tamoxifen, launched a massive breast cancer preventive trial among women at high risk. The NCI estimates that over the next decade some 1.5 million women in the U.S. will be diagnosed with breast cancer and that about 500,000 will die of the disease. Research has suggested that tamoxifen may reduce the mortality by a third. Women over age 60 are considered at high risk. Factors that determine risk in younger women (aged 35–59) are: the number of first-degree relatives (mother, daughters, sisters) who have had breast cancer; whether a woman has had children (the highest risk being for those with no children); age at first delivery (the older the age, the higher the risk); the number of times breast lumps have been found; and whether a noninvasive breast tumor has ever been diagnosed. Other preventive trials, using retinoids for lung, breast, cervical, and skin cancers, are also under way.

Impressive gains have been made in reducing the death rate from heart disease by modifying lifestyle (stopping smoking, eating a low-fat diet, maintaining a healthy weight, and exercising). It may be possible that cancer incidence, too, can be cut by strict adherence to preventive measures. Many of these have been well elucidated. Unfortunately, too many people are not properly motivated to make changes. Studies have shown that primary care physicians could have a significant influence on their patients' behaviors but that they generally underestimate their ability to effect behavior changes. However, if more doctors concerned themselves with their patients' lifestyles, the grim cancer statistics might be altered.

—*Mukti H. Sarma, Ph.D.*

Child Care

As the 21st century approaches, currents of social change have swept millions of mothers of young children into the U.S. workforce. And even more women workers will be needed to meet the nation's employment needs during the coming century. Although mothers of young children return to work for a variety of reasons, the most common motivation is financial necessity. Today only one job in five will adequately support a family of four; thus, many families find that they need two wage earners if they are to maintain a middle-class standard of living. Moreover, an increasing proportion of children live in single-parent households headed predominantly by women, who must work to support them.

In 1991, of the approximately 60 million American children under age 18, about 60% (37 million) had two working parents (or one working parent in the case of single-parent families). The proportion of working mothers with children under age six increased from 32% in 1970 to 58% in 1990. Even more dramatic has been the increase in the number of women in the labor force who have infants younger than one year old—in 1991 more than 50% of such women were employed. The Children's Defense Fund, a national nonprofit child advocacy organization, projects that by 1995 over two-thirds of all preschool-age children and over three-fourths of all school-age children—a total of 49 million children—will have mothers employed outside the home.

Regulation and responsibility: a historical view

Day care—group care of infants and young children outside the home—is by no means a recent innovation. The day nurseries of foundling hospitals and orphanages date back at least as far as the Middle Ages. In the U.S. records of day nurseries date from the early 19th century. These first programs typically were run by charitable organizations, which had sole responsibility for their operation. By the mid-19th century day nurseries in New York City were being regulated by the sanitary code of the municipal health department. When the city's Bureau of Child Hygiene was established in 1908, it assumed responsibility for regulation of child-care facilities. In time, most states passed their own legislation to govern child-care programs. In Kansas, for example, day nurseries were specifically included under the state's child-care-licensing act passed in 1919. Earlier, state investigators had found that infants in the day nurseries of Kansas orphanages were at risk of death from infections and marasmus (chronic undernourishment).

Private nursery schools became popular among middle-class families in the earlier part of the 20th century as a means of enhancing the socialization process and providing an opportunity for preschool education. It was not until the Depression era, however, that publicly run facilities were established for working families needing full-time child care. The widening employment of women during World War II gave further impetus to full-time programs; the Lanham Act appropriated federal funds to provide day care for women assisting in the war effort. Although the act was repealed after the war, the need for child care persisted, and during the 1950s private child-care centers and care in family homes emerged to replace publicly operated programs.

In 1950 a group of educators, legislators, and public health officials met in Washington, D.C., for the Mid-Century White House Conference on Children and Youth. They adopted a recommendation calling upon "appropriate public bodies" to establish minimum standards for the licensing of all child-care and preschool groups. Ten years passed, and at the 1960 White House Conference on Children and Youth, the call for action took on greater substance and urgency. This time the assembled experts called upon the government to assist and support "the establishment

and/or expansion of day care services for children of working mothers."

Notable expansion of federal support for child care did take place in the '60s and '70s. Included were such initiatives as the Head Start program for disadvantaged preschool-age youngsters, a child-care food program, a child-care tax credit, tax incentives for employers who established day-care programs, and government funding of child-care services for poor families. Head Start was an especially notable achievement in that it provided much more than the custodial care that had been traditional in programs serving poor children.

A wide-ranging, $2 billion child-care bill passed by Congress in 1971 was vetoed by Pres. Richard Nixon because of its high price tag and "family-weakening implications." However, the Title XX program, a social-service grant to the states enacted in the 1960s, provided federal funding of child care for the poor, and under this program a set of federal standards for child care was established. Although these regulations served as a model for some states to upgrade their child-care requirements, they were never fully implemented, as many states did not have the resources to comply. Moreover, these standards were repealed in 1981, when federal responsibility for children's social services was transferred to the states. During the past decade, in the absence of a federal code, some states have modeled their standards for child-care facilities after guidelines issued by national professional organizations such as the Child Welfare League of America and the National Association for the Education of Young Children (NAEYC).

Today's options

What kinds of child-care options are available for today's working parents? Whereas in the past much care was provided by relatives, this practice is declining now that more and more family members of all generations are employed outside the home. By 1990, in fact, fewer than 20% of families relied on care by a relative, and more than half of all child care was being provided by unrelated persons—usually outside the child's home. Not only are qualified nannies difficult to find (witness the dilemma of Zoë Baird, Pres. Bill Clinton's ill-fated nominee for attorney general), but with the cost ranging from $11,000 to $18,000 per year, full-time care at home remains an option only for high-income parents.

The category of family care includes a variety of different arrangements—care by parents with staggered working hours, care by a relative in either the child's or a relative's home, and care of younger children by an older sibling. Unfortunately, many children, some as young as preschool age, are in so-called self-care—commonly known as latchkey children. On the basis of interviews with more than 4,000 parents, the National Child Care Survey of 1990 estimated that 3.4

Who's watching the children?		
child-care arrangement	number of children (percentage)*	
licensed day-care center	3.8 million	(38)
relative	2.7 million	(27)
family day-care home	2 million	(20)
other	910,000	(9.1)
unrelated caregiver in child's home	560,000	(5.6)

*U.S. children under age five cared for by someone other than a parent, 1990
Source: Children's Defense Fund

million children aged 5–12 (12% of this age group) and 71,000 children younger than 5 (1.4%) regularly looked after themselves at least some time during a typical week. These numbers are probably low, as parents may be reluctant to admit to an interviewer that their children are being left alone. A 1990 report by the National Research Council may be closer to the truth—it estimated that as many as 15 million young children are on their own during some part of the day.

The type of out-of-home child care chosen by parents varies with the age of the child. In families with working mothers, care in family homes in the community seems to be preferred for children under three, whereas day-care centers are chosen for children three to four years of age; self-care predominates for children 5 to 12 years of age. A third of families in which the mother is *not* employed also choose day-care centers on a part-time basis for their three- to four-year-olds because they think the experience is important developmentally.

The major change in child-care arrangements in the last 10 years has been the shift from in-home care to care in other families' homes and day-care centers. These facilities generally include: small family homes, usually caring for six or fewer children; larger family homes caring for 7 to 12 children, usually with two adults in attendance; and child-care centers in nonresidential settings. The latter category includes full-time day-care programs for 13 or more children; preschools; Head Start programs; after-school programs; infant-toddler care; care of children with special needs; and "mother's day out" programs.

Costs

In the U.S. the cost of child care in state-regulated centers and homes varies with the age of the child, the nature of the facility, and the area of the country. For example, in 1990 the average annual cost for full-time day care of a four-year-old in a licensed child-care center ranged from $3,120 in Orlando, Fla., to $7,176 in Boston, according to the periodical *Child Care Information Exchange.* The 1990 National Child Care Survey found that low-income parents of preschool-age children may spend as much as one-fourth of their income on child care. "High-quality" programs such as those accredited by the NAEYC tend to be more expensive. The U.S. General Accounting Office reported in 1990 that the average annual cost of these better-quality programs for four-year-olds was $4,797 nationwide.

Despite the high costs of child care, the staffs of these facilities earn among the lowest wages of all U.S. workers, averaging, according to 1990 figures, about $9,000 per year. The highest-paid teachers in child-care centers, most of whom have college-level training, make around $15,000 a year, according to figures released in 1993 by the Child Care Employee Project, an Oakland, Calif.-based research group. (By comparison, the average annual salary of a high-school graduate in the U.S. is $19,309.) If child-care professionals had comparable salaries to others whose jobs demand similar levels of education

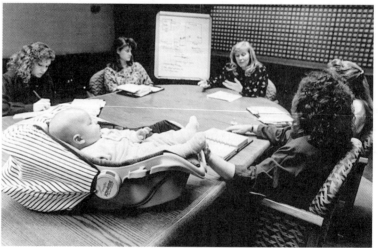

An accountant for a Kansas engineering firm keeps a watchful eye on her five-month-old while she attends a business meeting. Not only has the proportion of working mothers increased over the past 30 years, the number of women in the labor force with infants under one year of age has also risen dramatically—in 1991 more than 50% of such women were employed.

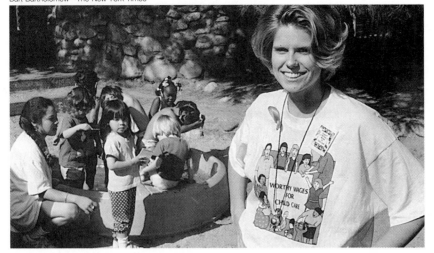

A Pasadena, Calif., preschool teacher proclaims her support for "worthy wages"—adequate pay for child-care workers, who are among the lowest paid in the U.S. Currently, the highest-paid employees in child-care centers—most of whom have college-level training—make less than the wage of an average high school graduate. Low wages are a major factor in the high turnover rate of child-care workers.

and responsibility, the annual cost of child care in an accredited center, according to the NAEYC, would be almost double what it is now. Obviously, child-care workers, through their low salaries, involuntarily subsidize the U.S. child-care system. These low wages certainly explain the high turnover of child-care staff, which, according to a 1989 study by the Child Care Employee Project, was 41% in 1988. This high turnover rate adversely affects quality of care, has a harmful effect on the children's language and social development, and could even jeopardize their emotional well-being, as it makes for repeated separation from adults who are important to them.

The issue of quality

In the absence of national health, safety, and program standards for child care, there is a great deal of state-by-state variation in it's regulation. Some states, for example, exempt church-operated centers, programs that operate less than four hours a day, or small family day-care homes with six or fewer children. Throughout the country unregulated care typically costs less, as unregulated facilities are free to accept more children for each adult caregiver, which, in turn, usually translates into poorer care. Even when state laws require licensing of care in family homes for small numbers of children, there is a large "underground" segment. While the actual number is not known, some studies suggest that between 50 and 75% of family homes that provide care are outside of state regulatory systems. This situation places an added responsibility on parents to thoroughly assess the health and safety aspects of the facility and the quality of the program. Moreover, even where states do have regulatory codes, the standards may not be the highest. In 1990, for example, 19 states permitted the care of five or more infants by one adult, despite recommendations by many child-development experts of a ratio of one adult to every three or four infants.

Over the past decade the supply of state-regulated centers and homes in the U.S. has not kept pace with the number of children in need of out-of-home care. This shortage could lead to an increasing number of children being tended by fewer adults, with the potential for lowering the quality of care and increasing both the extent of unregulated care and the number of children in self-care. A 1990 study by an independent policy research organization found that the majority of U.S. child-care centers were at 93% capacity, with particular shortages of space for infants and toddlers. Some states have made a concerted effort to keep pace with the growing demand. In Kansas, for example, where there were 5,831 regulated child-care programs in 1984 serving an estimated 70,000 children, by 1993 there were 10,180 such programs serving approximately 120,000 children.

Safeguarding children: what parents can do

In order to protect children who receive out-of-home care by nonrelatives, states have enacted laws for the licensing or registration of these facilities. Most states assign this responsibility to social service agencies, although in a few states this role is fulfilled by public health agencies. Almost all states regulate full-time day-care centers, as well as family homes that serve 7 to 12 children. Facilities are inspected annually to see that they meet certain basic standards. A number of states have developed procedures whereby providers can attest that they meet basic standards, and then either they are not inspected unless there are complaints or a sample of a state's facilities (perhaps 20%) are inspected in any given year.

Parents can play a key role in ensuring that the care they select for their children is safe, is healthful, and promotes optimal growth and development. It is important for them to become familiar with the law in their state and the state's basic standards for day-care facilities. They should find out whether the facility they

261

are considering is inspected regularly and whether it complies with child-care standards and health and safety codes.

The first step for a parent seeking a quality child-care program is to call the local social child-care agency (*e.g.,* human services department, children and family services agency) or health department for the name of a child-care resource and referral agency in the community. These agencies maintain a listing of the regulated family homes and child-care centers in the community and can provide parents with pertinent facts about them—for example, their location, whether they are regulated by state law, whether they have met the state's minimal standards for health and safety, and whether the provider has had child-care training.

The next step is for the parent to visit the provider and ask some questions. A partial list might include:
• How many children are in care, and what is the ratio of adults to children?
• What experience does the caregiver have?
• Can the caregiver provide the names of some satisfied parents as references?
• Are parents welcome to visit the home or center unannounced at any time?
• What kinds of books and educational toys are present?
• Does the daily schedule include activities and experiences that the parent thinks are important and beneficial?
• How much time, if any, do the children spend watching television?
• Does the building have functioning smoke detectors, and is an emergency plan in place for evacuation in case of fire?
• Are medications, household cleaning agents, and other toxic substances stored out of reach of the children? Are electrical outlets covered with safety protectors? Are windows and stairways safeguarded to prevent falls?
• If there is a swimming pool or body of water nearby, are children protected from potential mishaps?
• Are the children ever left in the care of the provider's own older children?
• If children are transported for outings, are there safety restraints in the vehicle?
• Will children be provided with nutritious meals and snacks?
• Is outdoor play equipment safe? Is the playground secured by a fence with a working gate?
• Are staff and children required to have had a recent health appraisal and to be up to date on immunizations?

Despite the shortage of affordable, good-quality child-care facilities in the U.S., there are indications that most state-regulated child care meets health and safety standards and provides sound developmental experiences. A recent review of childhood injuries and deaths from fire, poisoning, drowning, and gunshots found that regulated child-care programs actually have a far lower incidence than occurs among children in their own homes. Another positive sign: 95% of children in day care have been immunized, compared with fewer than 50% of "stay-at-home" children.

Potential health and safety risks

Early in the 1980s the national news media, from the *Wall Street Journal* to numerous weekly magazines, focused public attention on problems occurring in day-care programs. These ranged from unsanitary conditions and outbreaks of infectious diseases to child abuse and neglect. Public health authorities have now begun to address these concerns, and considerable progress has been made. In 1984 a national conference on infectious disease was held in Minneapolis,

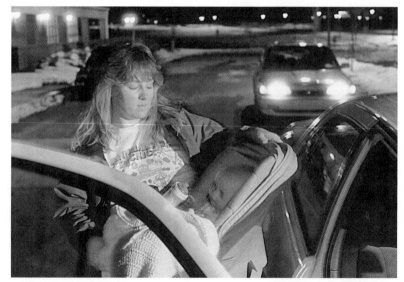

After finishing her shift at 3 AM, an employee of Toyota Motor Manufacturing, U.S.A., in Kentucky calls for her baby at a round-the-clock company-run child-care center. Recognizing the need of workers for safe and reliable child care, a growing number of businesses in the U.S. are starting their own programs or taking an active part in helping parents make satisfactory child-care arrangements.

Keith Williams—The New York Times

Minn., attended by a broad representation of physicians, nurses, social workers, day-care providers, researchers, mental health workers, and parents. The conferees considered recent reports by the Centers for Disease Control and Prevention (CDC) and various state and local health departments, which had found that infectious disease outbreaks in day-care facilities were occurring primarily in centers caring for infants and toddlers in diapers. When investigated, many of these centers were found to be overcrowded, to practice questionable hygiene, and to have an insufficient number of adults to provide proper care. The Minneapolis meeting spawned a number of initiatives, such as the publication by the CDC of an information packet entitled "What to Do to Stop Disease in Child Day Care Centers." It also stimulated state and local health departments to issue various protocols and manuals on child health and infectious diseases. The major recommendations of the conference called for improving environmental and staffing standards, establishing basic hygiene measures, and training child-care providers in principles of disease transmission.

In the same year, concerns about child abuse, to some extent fueled by widespread coverage of sensational cases in California, Minnesota, and New York City, led to the enactment of Public Law 98-473, which made federal funds available to states for training programs on the prevention of child abuse in child-care settings. Another provision required states to establish procedures for checking of the employment and criminal record history of all operators and employees of child-care facilities. Staff supervision, probation periods for new staff members, and parental access to facilities were also addressed in this legislation.

In addition to states' setting basic requirements for and conducting regular inspection of child-care facilities, legal intervention is occasionally necessary to safeguard children. In the state of Kansas, for example, the Department of Health and Environment, which is responsible for licensing child-care facilities, reported that legal action—in the form of either closure or fines—was taken with regard to 112 child-care programs during the five-year period 1980–84; this represented only about 2% of the state's regulated homes and centers. The small number is a tribute to the effectiveness of the standard setting, regular inspection, and health education and consultations required by Kansas state law.

Overall, where sound licensing and inspection programs are in place, the potential benefits to younger children of good-quality child care appear to outweigh any health and safety risks. The positive aspects of care include the promotion of preventive health services, including immunizations and early medical intervention; provision of nutrition programs and dental education; prevention of injuries; and exposure to stimulating growth and developmental activities.

Toward national standards

In the absence of federally mandated health and safety standards for child-care facilities, the states have developed their own. In 1988, in an effort to obtain some uniformity, the U.S. Department of Health and Human Services awarded a grant to the American Public Health Association and the American Academy of Pediatrics to develop national health and safety guidelines. The result was a 450-page document, *Caring for Our Children: National Health and Safety Performance Standards: Guidelines for Out-of-Home Child Care Programs.* Issued in 1992, it was developed over a four-year period by 11 technical panels of experts.

This publication is a comprehensive source for information on the development and evaluation of health and safety aspects of child-care facilities. The guidelines address the needs of children ranging from infancy to 12 years of age. They provide a rationale for each standard and set performance requirements for each of the following groups:

• regulatory agencies seeking national guidelines to upgrade state and local child-care-licensing requirements
• child-care providers, early childhood educators, public health professionals, pediatricians, and officials of accreditation and credentialing agencies
• parents of children enrolled in care

The areas addressed by the standards include environmental quality, prevention and control of infectious diseases, injury prevention and control, general health, nutrition, prevention of child abuse, staff health, children with special needs, health concerns related to social environment and child development, and health and safety organization and administration.

The movement for national standards is gaining momentum. In 1992 grants were awarded by the federal Maternal and Child Health Bureau to upgrade child-care standards in 10 states. In 1993 a national resource center for health and safety in child care was established at Georgetown University, Washington, D.C., by the U.S. government.

Slowly but surely, a national child-care policy is emerging in the U.S. In 1990 Congress enacted the Child Care Development Block Grant for states, a program to provide assistance for low-income families in obtaining child care, as well as funds to increase the number and kinds of facilities available and upgrade the quality of care. The Family and Medical Leave Act, passed in 1992, assures job security and health insurance to workers taking up to 12 weeks of unpaid leave to care for new infants and seriously ill family members. Other federal programs include Head Start; the supplemental food program, which provides meals in publicly run child-care facilities; the Family Support Act programs, which enable parents participating in job training to obtain child care while they are learning new skills; block grants for care of school-age children

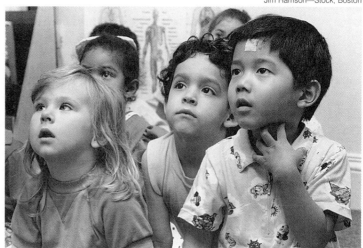

There is a pressing need for child care in the U.S.—and this exists for families at virtually all socioeconomic levels. Not surprisingly, there is wide public support for provisions that meet the needs of all *parents, and many are hopeful that a comprehensive national child-care policy will be developed for the 21st century.*

of working parents; and a tax credit for some of the money paid out by working families for care of their dependent children. Taken together, these initiatives add up to a significant federal commitment. Other positive signs are the growing number of businesses taking an active part in helping employees obtain care for their children and the development of school-based preschool programs in the nation's public schools.

European "models"

As the U.S. moves toward a comprehensive child-care policy, increasing interest has focused on the policies and programs of other countries, especially those of other industrialized nations. In contrast to the U.S., where child care is primarily privately run or proprietary, most European nations have well-subsidized programs and operate them largely within the public sector. In France, Sweden, and Italy, for example, programs for 2½- to 6-year-olds are free or charge only a modest, income-related fee and operate during regular school hours.

European child-care policy has moved to institute universal preschool education from age 2½ to the age at which compulsory schooling begins; the goal has been to establish preschool programs as a legal right, or entitlement, of all families. Children attend these programs regardless of parental employment status, family income, or cultural background. Preschool programs are viewed as beneficial for all children in preparing them for primary school. Participation is close to 90% in most countries—compared with less than 70% in the U.S.

The cost for families is also quite different; U.S. families pay about 90% of child-care costs, while European parents pay no more than 5–15%. Another major difference is that most European countries provide fully paid maternity or family leave for six months to one year, and in some countries employers pay a partial salary to a stay-at-home parent until the

child reaches two years of age. Most countries link their preschool programs to the schools; Sweden and Finland, however, have freestanding institutions under the auspices of social welfare agencies.

By combining the best features of the European programs with already existing U.S. initiatives, a comprehensive child-care policy can be developed for the U.S. First and foremost in importance is the adoption of federal and state standards to ensure the health and safety of children in out-of-home care. The next most pressing need is for the development of child-care systems in local communities, providing quality programs for families of all economic levels. Networks of day-care centers and family-care homes could be developed through the public schools or other community systems. These facilities could be organized so that families with both preschool- and school-age children would have a single neighborhood source of care. Expanding funding of the Child Care Development Block Grant to the states would assist in developing additional day-care facilities, providing financial assistance to more low-income families, and improving the quality of care, in part by upgrading the salaries of child-care workers. An extension of the dependent-child-care tax credit from the current $700 a year to $3,000 or more is another possibility.

The care of infants and toddlers presents perhaps the most difficult problems. Currently there simply are not enough places to accommodate these very young children, and there are too few adults to supervise their care. One proposal is that the government provide a yearly allowance of up to $5,000 to families with infants and toddlers so that parents could have the choice of remaining at home or purchasing quality care if they want or need to work. There are, at least, hopeful signs that a national child-care policy can be developed for the 21st century, one that will meet the needs of children, families, and the nation as a whole.

—*Patricia T. Schloesser, M.D.*

Special Report
Dental Implants: On the Cutting Edge
by Robert A. Goepp, D.D.S., Ph.D.

The proper function and good appearance of teeth are important for virtually everyone. In recent years remarkable progress has been made in building and placing artificial dental implants to replace missing teeth. Efforts to replace natural teeth are hardly new, as evidence in the annals of antiquity testifies. The ancient Egyptians tried to implant teeth by drilling a hole in the jawbone or using the hole from a recent extraction and placing a donor tooth in the site. The new tooth was fixed to adjacent teeth with fine gold wire. Egyptian dental practitioners may have found that if the donor tooth came from the recipient or an identical twin, the chance for success was improved. Even so, they did not understand why such an implant, which was located partially inside and partially outside the body, would likely cause infection. These implants must have provided only short-term satisfaction before they became intolerable because of infection or the inflammation associated with immune rejection.

The Egyptians were superb technologists, but their biological knowledge was understandably limited. In fact, only in the past few decades has the necessary knowledge of biology and materials sciences for predictably successful implants come to light. In modern times dental implant techniques have used biologically inert materials and advanced methods to prevent or treat infection, and they have commonly involved the anchoring of metal implants either under the gum and on the jawbone (subperiosteal implants) or in holes drilled in the bone (endosseous implants). Generally such implants have given service ranging from a few years to more than a decade. Nevertheless, the wide range of useful life reveals a need for improved consistency and predictability in the outcome of implants, issues that research continues to address.

Osseointegration: a breakthrough

A singular advance in placing implants into bone was made in the 1970s by Per-Ingvar Brånemark, a Swedish orthopedic surgeon. Brånemark used an inert material, the metal titanium, in the form of an anchoring fixture that could be screwed into a drilled hole in the jawbone under precise, controlled conditions. These conditions encouraged new bone to grow around the fixture and bond to it, resulting in intimate contact between the bone and the titanium surface.

Brånemark termed this benign and intimate contact between bone and implant material osseointegration. He reasoned that such an anchorage should be stable, and indeed it proved to be so over many years of studies. Titanium had been tried previously as an implant material with mixed results, but the key to consistent success lay in Brånemark's procedural innovations, which essentially consisted of precise methods of handling the metal fixture, cutting the bone, and placing the fixture in the bone under the most germ-free conditions possible. His technique included completely burying the implanted fixture; that is, closing the gum tissue over the implant so that it had no contact with the oral environment. This diminished the chances that infection would be established during healing, which takes several months. Moreover, burying the implant prevented outside forces—for example, from chewing—from acting on it during healing. Such forces would cause the implant to move, thereby provoking the formation of soft, capsulelike tissue between implant and bone and making the implant unstable. When the bone healed and X-ray examinations showed the implant to be well established, the gum could be opened, an abutment attached that extended above the gum surface, and the working part, *i.e.*, the toothlike crown, connected to the abutment.

The technique developed by Brånemark markedly enhanced the success rate for dental implants and encouraged many more dentists in the 1980s and early '90s to provide implant services for their patients. According to a survey reported in 1993 in the *Journal of the American Dental Association,* the number of dental implants done in the U.S. nearly quadrupled between 1986 and 1990, from 116,148 to 435,685. During the same period, the number of dentists providing implant services increased from 6,244 to 9,794.

Although most individuals who receive implants benefit from improved chewing ability and cosmetic appearance, there still are difficulties. First, not all tooth areas have a bone configuration suitable for implant placement. Second, the site at which the implant passes through the gum surface remains a possible route for bacteria to enter the body. Third, biting and chewing forces on the crowns of teeth are considerable and can come from unfavorable directions, causing eventual loosening of the implant or the surrounding natural teeth. It should be pointed out that whereas the surgical placement of a fixture in bone is of great importance to long-term success, so is the construction of a crown and an abutment with the ability to correctly distribute incoming forces.

Natural teeth: a tough act to follow

Brånemark's work not only was a substantial advancement in implant technology but also gave research workers a more organized way to think about the capabilities and limitations of implants and about how to improve them. A good way to begin to explore those aspects is to examine the unique and remarkable biology of the natural tooth.

Human teeth arise from two of the three basic tissues that form all human tissues. These are the epithelium, mesenchyme, and endothelium. The epithelium covers external body surfaces and lines such body parts as the intestines, lungs, and sinus cavities in the upper jaw. The mesenchyme gives rise to connective tissue, which is basically the structural framework of the body. The endothelium gives rise to internal lining tissue for such structures as blood vessel walls.

In most nonmammalian animals, teeth or toothlike structures form mainly from epithelium through a calcification process. Such teeth can be very strong and sharp—sharks' teeth are an example—but they can only cut; they cannot grind or mash. Human teeth form from both epithelium and mesenchyme, creating a sophisticated biological structure that fills several needs. Human teeth provide sensory information; cut large chunks of food into chewable pieces; prepare a mixed diet of plant and animal matter for digestion by chopping, mashing, and grinding; resist the ravages of wear and disease; and have an aesthetic value.

Filling all of these needs seems a large-enough order for an artificial implant, but there are still other requirements. Natural teeth are not fixed rock hard in the jawbone but allow some movement. Further, though they emerge from bone through the gum, that arrangement is normally quite adequate for preventing infectious agents from entering the body. Finally, natural teeth are not rejected as foreign materials by the body's defense mechanism.

Movement and stability: ongoing concerns

The movement of individual natural teeth can be beneficial or detrimental. Some movement is good for the health of a tooth, and even a certain amount of force in "wrong" directions can be accommodated. Excessive movement, however, particularly in wrong directions, can be destructive. A natural tooth is not welded to the jawbone. Instead, it is physically connected through a joint called a gomphosis, a sliding suture joint like those between the skull bones. This joint allows for tooth movement, which in turn promotes strong, healthy bone around the tooth root and strong, healthy cementum, the bonelike tissue that covers the surface of the root. Connecting the bone and cemen-

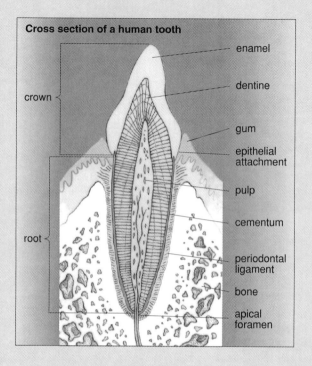

Cross section of a human tooth

- enamel
- dentine
- crown
- gum
- epithelial attachment
- pulp
- cementum
- root
- periodontal ligament
- bone
- apical foramen

tum together and thus holding the tooth in place is a soft-tissue ligament, the periodontal ligament. The fibers of this ligament are arranged in such a way that forces, such as those produced by chewing, on the crown of a tooth actually create pulling forces on the bone—somewhat the way the weight of a body in a hammock pulls on the supporting posts. This relationship is crucial, for if strong forces could not be dissipated, the less elastic bone or tooth would break. Whereas pushing forces on bone cause the bone to resorb, or melt away, pulling forces on bone stimulate it to grow and strengthen through mineralization.

The artificial tooth implants now in use do not provide for an elastic absorber and stimulator between the implant and the bone. This deficiency would be expected to lead to instances of small but discernible bone fractures and, indeed, in rare cases these have been observed. More likely and insidious, however, are clinically nondetectable, repeated, microscopic fractures. The significance of microscopic fractures is not known. In some cases they may heal without lasting change to the implant-bone relationship. In others repeated fractures over time may denature enough body proteins in the area (*i.e.,* deprive them of normal activity through structural changes) such that they are recognized as foreign material. This would provoke the body's immune system, resulting in low-grade inflammation, the production of fibrous tissue, or both. The presence of such processes over time might compromise the integrity of the implant.

The long-term stability of a dental implant depends a great deal on the strength of the bone in which it is placed. Bones are strongest, that is, most densely mineralized, at their surface, which is called the cortex. The interior of bone primarily comprises soft marrow tissue embedded with a lacy pattern of thin, mineralized walls. Bone marrow provides little or no support for the stability of an implant. In humans the lower jaw, or mandible, has a very dense lower border. Thus, dentists usually plan, if possible, to have the implant extend into the lower border to take advantage of the stability offered by that part of the bone. Indeed, implants placed in the mandible have a somewhat higher success rate than those placed in the upper jaw, or maxilla. Nevertheless, the long-term success rate of osseointegrated implants overall is quite good, ranging from 78 to 99% according to one large study.

The maxilla consists of bones that have relatively thin cortical surfaces and that contain internal spaces, or sinuses. Dentists have been imaginative in anchoring implants in the few locations in the maxilla where dense bone can be found, including the base of the nose, sites under the cheekbones, and portions of the hard palate. They have also developed techniques to raise the floor of the sinus located just above the back teeth area and replace the space so created with a bone material. Researchers are also looking for ways to initiate the production of bone or cementum in the bone marrow around the implant, a process that occurs around natural teeth.

Controlling inflammation and infection

The natural tooth possesses a barrier that prevents entry of bacteria and other foreign material. How the barrier works is not completely understood, but it appears to involve a gluing of the gum to the tooth surface, possibly similar to the attachment of cuticle to the top surface of a fingernail. With effort, cuticle can be lifted from the nail, and similarly the gum can be separated from the tooth. For teeth such a separation is usually associated with acute injury or the chronic buildup of debris—food particles and bacteria—around teeth. The debris is an irritant, provoking gum inflammation (gingivitis), and allows a low-grade chronic infection to ensue. This slowly progressing process, called periodontal disease, ultimately destroys the attachment of the tooth to the gum and bone.

The same process can also occur at the site of an implant, which is probably more vulnerable to periodontal disease than the natural tooth. Consequently, the oral part of the implant must be kept scrupulously clean. Ceramic materials are being studied as a way of improving the interface between gum and implant surface as well as between implant and bone.

When implants are suitable

What kind of tooth-replacement needs can be handled by implants? What are the advantages and disadvan-

In a typical single-tooth implant procedure (top), an anchoring titanium fixture is placed into a precisely drilled hole in the jawbone. The gum is then closed over the fixture and left to heal. Months later, after bone has bonded to the fixture, the gum is reopened, an abutment attached to the fixture, and an artificial crown secured to the abutment. Replacing more than one tooth in the same area (bottom) calls for a bridge that is secured to two or more implanted fixtures.

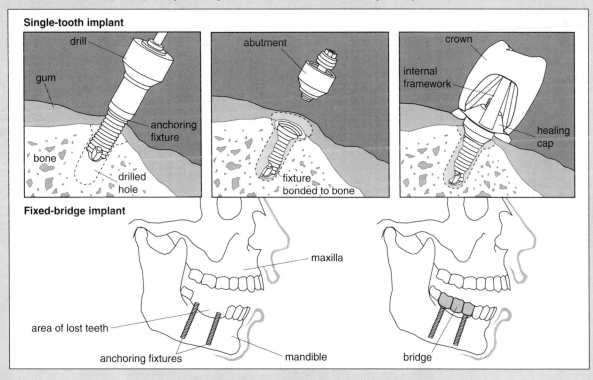

tages of implants? What are the requirements and commitments for having an implant done?

Most lost-tooth problems, whether they involve the absence of one tooth or of all the natural teeth, can probably be solved with implants. In fact, the use of implants to replace one tooth or a few missing teeth in one area spares the cutting of adjacent, presumably healthy teeth in order to anchor a fixed bridge. To replace lost teeth in several places in the same arch—either upper or lower—traditional dentistry often calls for a removable partial denture. Such an appliance must anchor or clamp to some natural teeth, and over time those anchor teeth may become damaged. By contrast, a fixed appliance anchored solely to a number of implanted fixtures is not likely to affect the status of natural teeth. In a completely toothless mouth, as few as four implanted fixtures can be used to anchor a complete set of artificial teeth.

For patients who have lost some teeth but have adjacent healthy teeth, fixed bridges are the closest to natural teeth in comfort, function, and appearance. Implants provide the same benefits. In both cases, however, conscientious personal and professional care is necessary to keep the artificial-tooth sites clean. In cases of total tooth replacements, care of the implant sites is just as crucial.

The big drawback of an implant procedure is its greater complexity compared with other methods of replacing teeth. For example, a fixed bridge of any extent may require a few weeks from start to finish. An implant procedure requires from three to six months or more. Implant materials are necessarily more precise and are made of expensive, exotic substances. There is a substantial increase in the time of direct professional contact, which adds to cost. The above-gum, working part of the implant must be meticulously designed and fabricated to compensate as much as possible for the lack of the shock-absorber mechanism associated with the roots of natural teeth. Care must be taken in design to prevent maldirected or excessive chewing forces on the artificial crowns. Thus, the cost of an implant procedure is many times that of a comparable fixed-bridge procedure—and many times more again than the cost of a removable appliance for the same problem.

The long-term success of an implant depends on good materials and good techniques, but it also requires comprehensive planning. The dentist must make an assessment of the candidate's general health, abilities, and level of commitment. Chronic diseases (*e.g.,* certain kinds of leukemia, anemia, or immunodeficiency) that weaken the body's resistance to infection or retard healing make implant placement inadvisable, as do metabolic diseases that soften or demineralize bone. Radiation treatment of the jaws, especially the lower jaw, for cancer seriously hampers the jawbone's ability to resist infection or heal from implant surgery. Some persons may have insufficient or unsuitably shaped bone. Children before their mid-teens are usually not considered suitable candidates for implant replacement of permanent teeth because their jawbones are still growing. Finally, the candidate must possess both an ability and a willingness to endure the long, complicated process of implant placement and to maintain meticulous care of the implant-anchored teeth.

As described above, the long-term stability of an implant depends on taking as much advantage as possible of sites of dense bone. Evaluation of bone is thus crucial and presently can be done only through X-ray examination. The common dental X-ray, while yielding exceptionally clear detail, cannot cover the entire bone area. Moreover, it often has geometric distortion and can show the bone in only one direction. The panoramic dental X-ray displays the entire jawbone, but it lacks good detail, has distortion, and shows the bone only from one direction. Sophisticated X-ray techniques such as tomography are necessary to evaluate bone to the desired level of detail from many different directions with geometric fidelity.

In choosing an implant dentist, the prospective patient would be wise to inquire about the dentist's training and experience. Beyond some fundamental experience, the number of implants that a dentist has done is not necessarily important. More important is that he or she can demonstrate an up-to-date knowledge of implant technology and an understanding of the biology associated with implant placement. If possible, the prospective patient should talk with some of the dentist's prior implant patients. A single dentist may do both the construction and the placement of the implant, but it is more common to find the two tasks handled by separate professionals.

The future

The remarkable advances of recent years in the technology of dental implants have enabled dentists to provide a service, with a high degree of success, to patients for the replacement of lost teeth. Researchers will continue to fine-tune and improve present technology to increase both the success rate and the longevity of implants. The number of lost-tooth problems has decreased in recent decades because of public education about oral health, more conscientious use of techniques to maintain oral health, and better management of the prevention and treatment of oral diseases. Yet the need to replace missing teeth will remain if only because of trauma. The ultimate replacement tooth may well be one that is "grown" directly in the recipient by means of advanced biotechnological techniques. Some fundamental steps in this direction, such as the cloning of the genes that make dental enamel, have already been done and suggest yet another new advance to come for implant dentistry.

Diet and Nutrition

Following a delay caused by a disagreement between two Cabinet-level offices—the U.S. Department of Agriculture (USDA) and the Department of Health and Human Services (HHS)—the most comprehensive set of food-labeling regulations compiled to date was finally published on Jan. 6, 1993. The regulations, mandated by the Nutrition Labeling and Education Act of 1990, were intended to make nutrition information on food packages more truthful and more readily accessible to the consumer. By mid-1994 nutrition labels on all processed foods and most meat and poultry products produced in the U.S. will carry detailed information about the food's nutrient content as well as its place in a healthy diet.

The labeling saga

The new labeling regulations were mired for a time in a bureaucratic dispute between the Food and Drug Administration (FDA), a division of HHS, and the USDA's Food Safety and Inspection Service (FSIS). Initially the FDA proposed that the new label list the amounts of each nutrient in grams and as a percentage of the "daily value"—that is, the percentage of a day's worth of the nutrient, based on a reference diet of 2,000 calories per day. Thus, the label on a 1¾-oz bag of potato chips not only would state that it contains 18 g of fat—as had been the practice under the old labeling standards—but also would indicate that this amount represents 28% of the daily value for fat. (The calories derived from fat should be no more than 30%. Since each gram of fat represents 9 calories, in the 2,000-calorie diet a maximum of 65 g—or 585 calories—should come from fat.)

The FSIS argued that the caloric prescription of this reference diet was in fact too low for many people, suggesting instead that the reference diet be based on 2,500 calories. The FDA defended its choice, explaining that it had selected the lower figure because the recommended dietary intakes for most women and children are between 1,900 and 2,200 calories, whereas the value of 2,500 calories is more appropriate for men and very active women. Therefore, the FDA felt that increasing the caloric value of the reference diet would effectively increase the recommended daily amount of dietary fat, potentially putting some people at risk of exceeding recommended limits on fat consumption.

Under compromise rules developed following intervention by then president George Bush and the White House staff, it was agreed that the labels would list nutrient amounts in grams and as percentages of the daily value based on a 2,000-calorie diet but would also include a footnote giving the daily values for both a 2,000- and a 2,500-calorie diet. The new regulations also standardize serving sizes and specify which in-formation about dietary components must appear on the label and in what order it must be listed.

Label information: facts only. The sample label shown on this page shows the proposed format of the new "Nutrition Facts" label. This type of label will appear on almost all packaged foods. Every label will include a footnote explaining that the percentages of daily values have been calculated on the basis of a 2,000-calorie diet and stating, "Your daily values may be higher or lower depending on your calorie needs."

Foods containing insignificant amounts of seven or more of the nutrients that must be listed may use a simplified label format. Nevertheless, information on total calories, total fat, and carbohydrate, protein, and sodium must be listed even if the amounts present are insignificant. Other nutrients must also be listed if present in more than insignificant amounts.

Among foods exempted from mandatory nutrition labeling are foods sold by small businesses (*e.g.,* homemade cakes, cookies, chocolates, and the like sold in small quantities), foods sold in restaurants and fast-food outlets and intended for immediate consumption, and ready-to-eat foods such as take-out sandwiches and salads prepared on site in delicatessens

Nutrition Facts

Serving Size ½ cup (114g)
Servings Per Container 4

Amount Per Serving

Calories 90   Calories from Fat 30

	% Daily Value*
Total Fat 3g	**5%**
Saturated Fat 0g	**0%**
Cholesterol 0mg	**0%**
Sodium 300mg	**13%**
Total Carbohydrate 13g	**4%**
Dietary Fiber 3g	**12%**
Sugars 3g	
Protein 3g	

Vitamin A	80%	•	Vitamin C	60%
Calcium	4%	•	Iron	4%

* Percent Daily Values are based on a 2,000 calorie diet. Your daily values may be higher or lower depending on your calorie needs:

	Calories	2,000	2,500
Total Fat	Less than	65g	80g
Sat Fat	Less than	20g	25g
Cholesterol	Less than	300mg	300mg
Sodium	Less than	2,400mg	2,400mg
Total Carbohydrate		300g	375g
Fiber		25g	30g

Calories per gram:
Fat 9   •   Carbohydrate 4   •   Protein 4

Food and Drug Administration, 1993

Diet and nutrition

and convenience stores. Also exempt are foods of no nutritional significance such as coffee and tea, foods for infants and children less than two years of age, medical foods, custom-processed fish and game, and donated foods.

Fresh fruits and vegetables and fresh fish need not carry nutrition labels. However, nutrition information on the 20 most frequently consumed foods in each of these categories is to be displayed in food stores under a voluntary compliance program. Furthermore, if nutrition-related health claims are made for selected foods, produce, or items on restaurant menus, nutrition labeling becomes mandatory, and the FDA criteria governing health claims apply.

Standardization of terms. The new regulations set strict guidelines for the use of such words as *free, low,* and *reduced* to describe the nutrient or caloric content of foods. For example, to use the descriptor *low-fat,* a serving or 50 g of food (whichever is greater) must contain no more than 3 g of fat. The terms *less* and *reduced* have been made synonymous, and the manufacturer can make the claim only if the product contains at least 25% less of the nutrient (or calories) than is present in a comparable reference food. Thus, a company that makes regular chicken-noodle soup with 1,000 mg of sodium per serving must reduce that number to 750 mg in order to label its product as "reduced sodium." The actual percentage of the reduction also has to be included on the label.

The agency also defined and specified conditions for the use of such terms as *fresh, natural, organic, lean, extra lean,* and *good source.* For example, foods listed as a "good source" of a specific nutrient must contain 10–19% of the daily value of that nutrient per serving. According to this definition, however, a candy bar containing 16 g of fat could, in theory, be labeled as a "good source" of fat. Moreover, because the regulations were primarily concerned with accurate labeling of the fat content of foods, there is room for other unexpected applications. For example, the proposed definition of the term *healthy* requires foods to be low in total fat and low in saturated fat. Jelly beans qualify as "healthy" under this definition.

Health claims: allowed but restricted. For the first time, claims about the relationship between a food or nutrient and the risk of chronic disease will be permitted on food labels. Following an exhaustive FDA review of data from clinical trials and epidemiological studies linking diet and chronic disease, seven areas for health claims will be allowed. These include:

• fiber-containing fruits, vegetables, and grain products and reduced cancer risk
• fiber-containing fruits, vegetables, and grain products and reduced risk of coronary heart disease
• fruits and vegetables and reduced cancer risk
• saturated fat and cholesterol and increased risk of coronary heart disease

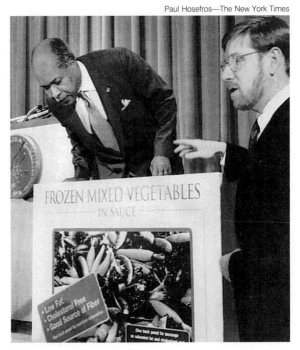

Secretary of Health and Human Services Louis W. Sullivan (left) and FDA Commissioner David A. Kessler introduce new U.S. labeling rules in December 1992—Sullivan proclaiming, "The Tower of Babel in food labels has come down."

• fat and increased cancer risk
• calcium and reduced risk of osteoporosis
• sodium and increased risk of hypertension (high blood pressure)

Even though there have been studies suggesting specific health benefits from certain nutrients in foods, at present no other health claims are allowed. The FDA disallowed claims that linked specific levels of dietary fiber intake with reduced risk of cancer and coronary heart disease. Also disallowed were health claims relating so-called omega-3 fatty acids and reduced risk of coronary heart disease; zinc and enhanced immune function in the elderly; folic acid and reduced risk of neural tube defects; and antioxidant vitamins and reduced cancer risk. The FDA will reevaluate the latter two issues at a later date.

The new regulations are an important step in the continuing federal effort to promote the nutritional health and welfare of the public. Providing consumers with detailed information about the nutrient content of foods and the role of various foods in a healthy diet is expected to lead to better food choices and improved eating habits. The emphasis on the accurate labeling of the fat content of foods and the allowing of health claims linking the consumption of grains, vegetables, and fruits to lower risk of cancer and heart disease will strengthen the efforts of nutrition professionals to implement the dietary guidelines for the American public, especially the admonition to eat less fat.

270

Dietary fat, heredity, and obesity

Unfortunately, giving up fat may not be an easy matter. The typical American diet derives the bulk of its calories from only two ingredients, sugar and fat. According to nutritional surveys, fat accounts for 37% of total daily calories, while sugars, both natural and added, contribute another 22%. Diets that are rich in fats and low in complex carbohydrates have been linked to an increased risk of chronic disease, including coronary heart disease and some forms of cancer. Moreover, the increasing popularity of such diets around the world has also been associated with an increased prevalence of obesity. A recent survey found that more than 60% of Americans are overweight.

Relationship of dietary fat and body fat. By all accounts, obesity was uncommon in traditional societies whose diets were largely based on roots and grains that could be gathered in the wild or raised in small garden plots. The introduction of field agriculture replaced such dietary staples as tubers and starchy roots with cultivated grasses, including maize, oats, and barley, and the major food crops rice and wheat. The diets of preindustrial peoples were invariably high in carbohydrates but low in oils and fat. For example, until fairly recently the typical Japanese diet derived less than 10% of its energy (calories) from fat.

Ironically, in the Western world it was economic prosperity that brought about increased meat consumption and, in turn, selective breeding of livestock for the maximum fat content. Indeed, historians have long used meat consumption as an index of the prosperity of an era or an indication of membership in a given social class. A study of the diets and economies of 85 nations conducted in the 1960s by the Food and Agriculture Organization in Rome showed a direct relationship between the size of a country's per capita gross domestic product and the availability of fats and sugars in its food supply. A more recent illustration is provided by the changing nutritional profile of increasingly affluent industrialized Asian nations, where the traditional rice-based diet is gradually being replaced by Western-style eating habits. The proportion of fat in the Japanese diet has more than doubled over the past 25 years. At the same time, childhood obesity is rapidly becoming a major public health problem in Japan.

Numerous clinical and epidemiological studies have emphasized the role of dietary fat in human obesity. In the past some of these surveys have reported a puzzling finding, an inverse correlation between overeating and overweight—that is, obese subjects seemingly ate less than their lean counterparts. Today, however, it is widely believed that these findings are the result of poor methodology, particularly in the gathering of data on the amount of food consumed. The conventional methods of assessing the dietary intake of obese persons—primarily, the keeping of food diaries—are suspected of being highly unreliable.

The inaccuracy of such data has been amply demonstrated by recent controlled studies of so-called diet-resistant individuals (those who report that they fail to lose weight on a diet of fewer than 1,200 calories a day). This research indicates that such individuals typically underreport by 20–25% the amount they have eaten. In one such investigation at the Obesity Research Center at New York City's St. Luke's-Roosevelt Hospital, a group of diet-resistant patients failed a "food recall" test in which they were asked what foods they had eaten in a hospital lunch the previous day. The patients remembered eating only

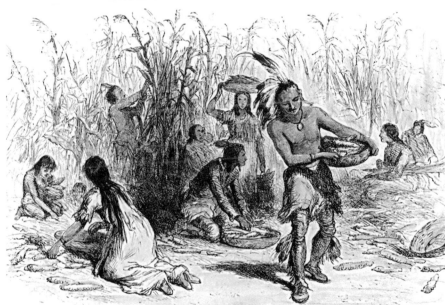

North Wind Picture Archives

By all accounts, obesity was not a problem among preindustrial peoples, whose diets were invariably high in complex carbohydrates and low in oils and fat. Some authorities speculate that such diets simply were not palatable enough to tempt people to overeat.

80% of their actual intake, while members of a control group were able to recall much more accurately what they had consumed. Using more precise ways of measuring energy expenditure, such as the method that employs water labeled with radioactive isotopes, scientists who study obesity have shown conclusively that overweight individuals actually expend more energy than do lean control subjects. Given that the weight of the obese subjects remains stable, this finding indicates that they must be taking in more calories than they are reporting.

Dietary surveys have also reported that obese people eat more fat and less carbohydrate than do their lean counterparts. Some studies have found that the proportion of fat calories in a person's diet is directly related to the percentage of body fat. In other studies obesity has been linked to an elevated proportion of fat in the diet and a lower dietary carbohydrate-to-fat ratio. In one investigation conducted over a three-year period, elevated intake of dietary fats was linked with greater gain in body weight. All of this evidence points to the same conclusion: fat in the diet ultimately manifests itself as body fat.

Biochemical studies have now shown that a fat-rich diet may actually promote the deposition of body fat. Thus, while excess carbohydrate calories tend to be dissipated by the body as heat, excess fat calories are far more likely to be stored in adipose (fat) tissue. Fat-rich diets may therefore be more fattening than diets that contain the same number of calories but are low in fat. Some investigators have also noted that repeated cycles of weight loss and regain—so-called yo-yo dieting—may lead to increased metabolic efficiency and increased deposition of body fat, much like the body's response to famine situations, where metabolic slowdown allows more efficient utilization and storage of fat over time.

Conversely, reducing the proportion of fat calories in the diet may bring about weight loss, even without restrictions on the quantities of food consumed. In one study that tested this hypothesis, subjects adhering to a low-fat diet for two weeks lost an average of 0.4 kg (one kilogram = 2.2 lb); in another, 11-week study, participants lost 2.5 kg. However, in both cases only low-fat foods were permitted. A recent women's health intervention trial showed that the women who followed a diet providing only 20% of calories from fat for up to two years (current guidelines call for a limit of 30%) lost an average of 3.1 kg, compared with 0.4 kg in the control group.

The contribution of genetics. Dietary fat is only part of the story, however. The development of obesity is thought to be determined at least partly by genetic vulnerability and partly by consumption of a calorie-rich diet. As long as the diet remains low in both energy and fat, the population stays lean. However, a substantial change in the proportion of fat in the diet may trigger obesity-promoting genes in some people.

Evidence for a genetic component in obesity is largely based on adoption and twin studies, which attempt to distinguish between the influences of heredity and environment. This research reveals that biological children of obese parents are themselves likely to be obese. Studies of obese twins have shown that identical twins resemble each other closely in body build, distribution of body fat, and metabolic response to overfeeding. Even in twins, however, the extent of obesity seems to be determined by their choice of diet.

Forgoing fat: why so difficult?

The question arises whether individual vulnerability to the effects of diet can be mediated through the sensory pleasure response to fats. People like the taste of fat-containing foods and are reluctant to give them up. Poor compliance with very low-fat diets is a well-known problem in the dietary management of elevated cholesterol levels, and the craving for fat-rich desserts is commonly blamed for failed attempts at weight reduction. Most people find that using little or no fat to flavor their food is among the most difficult health habits to sustain. Others who are attempting to modify their diets report particular problems avoiding tempting desserts and table fats (butter, margarine) and limiting meat consumption. Even heart-attack survivors, who are among the most highly motivated dieters, prove resistant to diets consisting entirely of grains, vegetables, and fruits.

Why are fat-containing foods so difficult to pass up? One reason is that fats, because they serve as a concentrated source of energy, are able to reduce hunger more effectively than other foods. Young children readily acquire preferences for flavors associated with high fat content, the taste of chocolate being a prime example. In addition, the sensory properties of fats make a diet flavorful, varied, and rich. Fats are responsible for the texture ("mouth feel") and aroma of many foods and make a major contribution to the palatability of the diet. Some authorities have suggested that people in traditional societies do not habitually overeat because the foods available to them—grains, beans, and the like—simply are not especially tasty. These theorists reason that obesity becomes a problem only when people have access to fatty, more highly flavorful foods. In short, the amount of fat that people consume appears to be influenced more strongly by the sensory qualities of fat than by energy needs or health concerns.

Studies of taste preferences and food choices have thus assumed a new importance in obesity research. The sense of taste, in particular, seems to mediate the link between the central nervous system and food-related behaviors. Clinical research has demonstrated that the preference for sweet high-fat foods, such as milk shakes, cake frostings, and ice cream, is influenced by the individual's degree of overweight. In one study women who were obese selected drinks that were rich in fat, while emaciated, anorectic women preferred intensely sweet liquids but showed a dislike for, if not an aversion to, fatty preparations. In another investigation normal-weight subjects were asked to taste a variety of foods with varying fat content. The investigators observed a positive relationship between the fat levels people preferred and their percentage of body fat. There is also some evidence that sensory preferences for fat in foods are linked to fluctuations in body weight. Researchers found that obese yo-yo dieters liked cake frostings and ice creams more than obese women whose body weight was stable.

It may be that sensory preferences for fat in foods are influenced by physiological events in the brain. Among the biochemical substances that have been advanced as potential triggers of food cravings among women are the neurotransmitters serotonin and galanin and the endogenous opioids. The possible connection with the latter, the natural opiates produced by the body, is particularly interesting since these molecules mediate the body's response to pleasure and pain and are involved in drug addiction. "Food addicts" may be affected as well. In clinical studies of obese and bulimic women, intravenous infusions of the opioid antagonist drug naloxone reduced the pleasure response to sweetened dairy products and selectively diminished the consumption of snack foods that were either sweet, rich in fat, or both.

However, the sensory pleasure response does not always predict food consumption, and opioid imbalance is not likely to be the explanation for the problem of obesity. Because learning and past experience play a major role in food selection, each person's food preferences are different. There are also male-female differences. A recent study of food preferences of several hundred overweight patients showed that obese men typically listed as most irresistible steaks and roasts, hamburgers, french fries, pizza, and ice cream. In contrast, obese women tended to list starchy foods such as bread, as well as cakes, cookies, ice cream, chocolate, pies, and other desserts. Although overweight people are sometimes reported to be "carbohydrate addicts," the researchers observed a marked preference for foods that were high in fat, especially sweet, fat-rich desserts. The "fat tooth" rather than the proverbial "sweet tooth" may be a characteristic feature of human obesity.

The logical conclusion from the research to date is that strategies for reducing fat consumption must be very carefully designed. If preferences and "cravings" for high-fat foods are ruled by physiological as well as behavioral factors, then merely telling people to eat less fat is not likely to work, especially given that low-fat diets tend to be unpalatable. An alternative would be to promote the consumption of fats that make for a good-tasting and satisfying diet but have minimal adverse effects on blood cholesterol levels and overall health.

The Mediterranean diet myth

Some nutritionists believe that olive oil is just such an "ideal" fat. Rich in oleic acid, which is a mono-unsaturated fatty acid, olive oil does not raise low-density lipoproteins (LDL)—the "bad" cholesterol—as

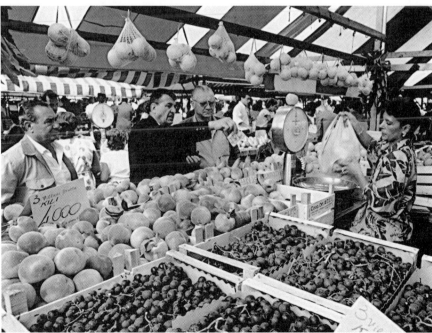

Shoppers at a market in Italy choose from a profusion of fresh fruits. While the so-called Mediterranean diet may be largely mythical, people in this part of the world do eat more fresh produce, less red meat and saturated fats, fewer eggs, and more whole grains than most Americans. They also have much lower rates of death from heart disease.

Tompix/Peter Arnold, Inc.

do butter and some types of margarine. Moreover, its vitamin E content may block the oxidation of cholesterol and thereby help prevent development of fatty, artery-blocking deposits. A centuries-old mainstay of the Mediterranean diet, olive oil has been widely promoted as a healthy alternative to animal fats.

Clearly, olive oil owes some of its appeal to the romance of the Mediterranean. The classic Mediterranean table is reputed to offer an abundance of vegetables and fruits and a variety of starches—breads, pasta, couscous, rice—as well as ample wine, but only a limited amount of fat-containing dairy products, poultry, and fish. Olive oil is the principal fat in Mediterranean cuisine, while red meat is consumed only a few times per month. In truth, this picture of the Mediterranean diet owes more to fantasy than to the available data. For one thing, there really is no such diet; food-consumption patterns of countries from Morocco to Greece show little or no uniformity. There are significant differences between Mediterranean countries in the consumption of olive oil, wine, grains, meat, and fish; these variations are due partly to cultural and religious differences and partly to patterns of economic development. Thus, the diet of urban, industrialized northern Italy is lower in bread and vegetables than the diet of the still-rural southern Mezzogiorno region but is predictably higher in milk, meat, and sugar. For another thing, the fantasy of wholesome and abundant Mediterranean fare falls far short of the reality. The typical supper of a family in rural Greece would seem Spartan and unsatisfying by American standards and probably would not meet the current dietary guidelines for many nutrients known to be essential to good health. Certainly it would bear no resemblance to the meals served in certain trendy, chic eateries that purport to offer "authentic Mediterranean cuisine."

While the positive value of olive oil should not be underestimated, the idealized Mediterranean diet, high in complex carbohydrates and very limited in animal proteins and fats, is in fact essentially a diet of poverty. People who ordinarily eat this way do not do so by choice. While very high-carbohydrate diets may provide a healthy alternative in a culture of dietary excess, they are abandoned at the first opportunity by the very people who, out of necessity, have consumed them for centuries.

The French paradox

The French diet is famous for favoring taste over health. The high consumption of red meat, butter, eggs, cheese, and wine that is characteristic of French eating habits, coupled with a high prevalence of cigarette smoking, does not amount to a particularly healthy way of living, yet the incidence of coronary heart disease in France is substantially lower than in other Western countries.

American nutritionists have struggled to come to terms with this so-called French paradox since it defies the conventional wisdom. One proffered explanation for the unexpectedly low rate of heart disease in France is the use of olive oil as the primary source of fat in the French diet. Statistics show, however, that olive oil is the main source of fat only in the southern region of France, while the rest of the country relies, as it always has, on the two "unhealthiest" fats, butter and lard. Claims have also been made for the therapeutic value of foie gras (the fatty liver of force-fed geese and ducks) and for its reputed effect on the longevity of the population of southwestern France. But even in this region, where it is produced, foie gras is a luxury product and is eaten relatively rarely. Another explanation holds that the French pattern of calorie consumption—with the main meal being eaten at midday—has a favorable impact on cholesterol levels.

Of all the theories that have been advanced to explain the French paradox, however, claims regarding the beneficial effects of wine are among the most popular ones. Red wine (and, some argue, *French* red wine) contains compounds that may be effective antioxidant agents, delaying the oxidation of LDL-cholesterol. The proponents of this view ignore the fact that the amount of wine that is drunk in France has plummeted in past years, as has the consumption of complex carbohydrates. In contrast, the consumption of sugar and fat is still on the rise, evidence that the economy of the country—if not its physical health—is steadily improving.

Some nutritionists have posited that the French diet, like the traditional Japanese diet, was once high in complex carbohydrates and only recently became rich in fat. Adverse health effects, the theory goes, have merely been postponed, and a major increase in coronary heart disease will be observed in 20 to 30 years' time. This argument is rejected, with some indignation, by French nutritionists, who point to a centuries-old culinary tradition of high-fat foods. Michel Montignac, a former drug company executive and self-styled diet expert, has garnered an enormous amount of publicity by advocating a weight-loss regime based on precisely these foods. Montignac claims that conventional diets, which emphasize calorie counting, actually make people fat, and he cites the parallel increases in dieting and obesity in the U.S. as confirmation of his theory.

In 1893 in an "Address on Dietetics," the U.S. physician Ephraim Cutter wrote:

Patients, cooks and almost all the laity are not willing to deny their appetites and had rather eat and die than eat to live. They will not give up what they like to eat on the principle that the French now lay down . . . that any agreeable food [is] nutritious.

Apparently, little has changed in the past 100 years!

—*Adam Drewnowski, Ph.D.*

Special Report
Cholesterol Counts
by James I. Cleeman, M.D., and Claude Lenfant, M.D.

The year 1993 was marked by two important milestones in the effort to control high blood cholesterol in the United States. The first was the announcement of results from the third National Health and Nutrition Examination Survey (NHANES III) showing what had happened to cholesterol levels among U.S. adults in the 12 years from 1978 to 1990. The second was the release of updated cholesterol-treatment guidelines for adults, developed by the National Cholesterol Education Program (NCEP) second Adult Treatment Panel (ATP II), whose report covers the major controversial issues concerning cholesterol that have recently come to the fore.

Declining cholesterol levels

The NHANES III results show that blood cholesterol levels in the U.S. declined substantially in the 12-year period. That is noteworthy progress toward a chief aim of the NCEP. Since its inception in 1985, the NCEP has sought to heighten the attention paid to cholesterol by the public and health professionals. Two basic strategies for lowering the cholesterol levels of Americans have been used: (1) a clinical strategy that detects and treats individuals at high risk for coronary heart disease (CHD) and (2) a public health strategy that attempts to shift the cholesterol levels of the entire population to a lower range, chiefly through dietary changes.

From 1978 to 1990 the average total cholesterol level in U.S. adults declined from 213 to 205 mg/dL (milligrams per deciliter; see Table 1). The decline was evident for women and men of all ages and for blacks as well as whites. This drop is due to a decline in low-density lipoprotein (LDL), or "bad," cholesterol from 136 to 128 mg/dL; levels of high-density lipoprotein (HDL), or "good," cholesterol were virtually unchanged. The fall in average cholesterol levels is the result of a downward shift across the entire range of cholesterol values. The proportion of adults with desirable cholesterol levels (less than 200 mg/dL) rose from 44 to 49%. The proportion with high cholesterol levels (240 mg/dL or above) fell from 26 to 20%, thereby achieving—ahead of time—the prevention goal that had been set for the year 2000 with respect to reducing high levels. The proportion with borderline-high cholesterol (200–239 mg/dL) was virtually unchanged during this period. Thus, there has been a movement of individuals from the high into the borderline-high category and from the borderline-high into the desirable category.

A reduction from 1978 to 1990 is also seen in the proportion of adults who, according to the guidelines, need dietary therapy to lower their high blood cholesterol. In 1978 the proportion who would have required dietary therapy was 36%; in 1990 it was 29%. So whether one looks at average cholesterol levels, the distribution of cholesterol values, or the prevalence of high blood cholesterol requiring dietary therapy, the picture is the same: cholesterol levels have moved significantly downward.

Why the decline?

There are many factors that may have contributed to this decline. The fall in cholesterol levels goes back 30 years, and over those three decades the changing eating patterns of the American public, including reduced intakes of saturated fat, total fat, and cholesterol, are likely to have played an important role. More than half of the decline occurred in the latter 12 years. Thus, cholesterol levels of the American public have recently been moving faster in the right direction. This occurred at a time when a markedly increased amount of cholesterol information was being directed to professionals and to the public. Within a relatively short span of time: the results of the Coronary Primary Prevention Trial, proving the bene-

Table 1. Cholesterol profile of Americans		
	1978	1990
	levels (mg/dL)	
average total cholesterol	213	205
average LDL-cholesterol	136	128
	percentage	
have high total cholesterol ($\geq$ 240 mg/dL)	26	20
have desirable total cholesterol (< 200 mg/dL)	44	49
require dietary therapy	36	29

Source: NHANES III

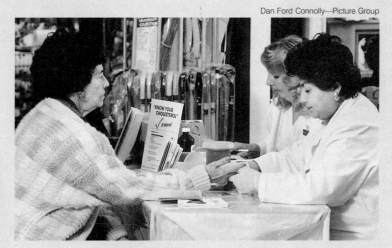

A woman shopping in Clearlake, Texas, stops to have her cholesterol checked. Declining cholesterol levels of Americans over the past decade in part reflect the success of screening programs that make cholesterol measurement readily accessible to the public. Between 1983 and 1990 the proportion of Americans who had had their cholesterol levels checked rose from 35 to 65%.

fits of cholesterol lowering, were announced (1984); a consensus-development conference concluded that lowering high blood cholesterol would reduce the risk of heart attack and lent its support to creation of a National Cholesterol Education Program (1984); the NCEP was launched (1985); and the first Adult Treatment Panel (ATP I) guidelines were released (1987) and published by the NCEP (1988).

Several other indicators of the knowledge, attitudes, and practices of professionals and the public suggest that these cholesterol education efforts have had an effect. Surveys conducted in 1983 and 1990 showed that there was a sharp increase (from 39 to 69%) in the proportion of physicians who believed that reducing high cholesterol would have a large effect on CHD. At the same time, the cholesterol values at which physicians reported initiating diet and drug therapy fell markedly to levels approximating the NCEP recommendations. Among the public, the proportion who ever had their cholesterol checked nearly doubled (from 35 to 65%). Finally, patient visits for high blood cholesterol, after rising slowly from 1983 to 1986, leaped dramatically, beginning in 1987, so that by 1990 the level was 11 times as high as in 1983.

Taken together, all of these indicators suggest that the combined clinical and public health strategies recommended by the NCEP and many cooperating organizations have made a substantial contribution to the decline in cholesterol levels of the population as a whole and in the percentage of individuals with especially high levels. Indeed, guidelines and educational programs aimed at reducing high cholesterol levels appear to be working.

ATP II: the new guidelines

It is important to bear in mind that despite the good news, 29% of American adults, or 52 million individuals, still need dietary therapy for high blood cholesterol. So there remains a huge challenge to be met. The updated ATP II guidelines were formulated to ad-

dress that challenge. These guidelines stand squarely on the shoulders of ATP I; the basic principles are the same, and ATP II is an evolutionary development from the first guidelines. The second set of guidelines, like the first, regards a high level of LDL as the main target of therapy; it still advocates dietary therapy as the first-line and principal treatment; and it maintains a cautious approach to drug treatment, reserving it for high-risk patients. Nonetheless, as would be expected, there are some important new features in the ATP II report, and these make the new guidelines an even better tool to help professionals and the public deal effectively with high cholesterol levels.

Specific issues addressed by ATP II and considered below are:
- patients with existing CHD
- age
- young adults, women, and the elderly
- HDL-cholesterol
- dietary therapy, weight loss, and physical activity
- cholesterol lowering and prolongation of life
- cost-effectiveness

Patients with existing CHD. ATP II recommends a more aggressive approach to lowering cholesterol levels in patients with existing CHD or other atherosclerotic disease. These patients have the highest risk of having a heart attack or dying from heart disease in the near future. Fortunately for them, it is not too late. Cholesterol lowering in CHD patients has the greatest potential to prevent heart attacks and heart attack deaths and will almost certainly prolong life. Yet most CHD patients are not getting the cholesterol-lowering treatment that is needed. This is a very important missed opportunity. ATP II recommends lowering LDL in these high-risk patients to a level of 100 mg/dL or lower, if feasible. That corresponds to a total cholesterol level of about 160 mg/dL. ATP I recommended lowering LDL in these patients to a level below 130 mg/dL, corresponding to a total cholesterol level of about 200 mg/dL.

The general principle of the ATP II guidelines is that a patient's overall risk for CHD should be used in deciding how aggressively to try to lower a high cholesterol level; patients with a higher risk for developing problems from CHD in the near future should receive more aggressive treatment. There are three general categories of CHD risk: (1) those patients at highest risk because of existing CHD or other atherosclerotic disease, (2) patients without evident CHD who are at high risk because of high blood cholesterol together with multiple other risk factors for CHD, and (3) patients who have high blood cholesterol but are at low risk otherwise. This last group includes young adult men (under 35 years of age) and premenopausal women.

Age. The ATP II guidelines recognize that CHD risk increases with age. An older person's risk of developing CHD in the near future is much higher than that of a young person, even when their cholesterol levels are the same. For this reason age has been added to the list of major risk factors that physicians should consider in choosing a cholesterol-lowering therapy. For men age becomes a risk factor at 45 years; for most women it begins to figure significantly at 55 years.

Young adults, women, and the elderly. ATP II deals explicitly with cholesterol lowering in all three of these groups. The new guidelines specify that cholesterol lowering is important for reducing the risk of CHD in each of the groups, with dietary therapy as the mainstay of treatment.

In young men (under 35 years of age) and premenopausal women, high levels of total cholesterol and LDL-cholesterol predict an increased risk of CHD decades into the future. For this reason, it is important to measure cholesterol levels in young adults, both to identify the minority of individuals who need medical advice and to encourage the vast majority to make changes in eating patterns and other lifestyle habits to promote improved health in the long run. Nevertheless, compared with older adults, younger persons have a much lower risk of CHD in the next 10 to 20 years, even if their cholesterol levels are high. Therefore, diet modification should be used to lower a high cholesterol level in a young adult, but drug treatment in most cases should be delayed. An exception to the delay of drug treatment should be considered if a young adult also has multiple other CHD risk factors or if the individual has very high cholesterol levels (*i.e.,* an LDL of 220 mg/dL or greater, corresponding to a total cholesterol of 300 mg/dL or above).

High blood cholesterol increases the risk for CHD in women. In general, women are at lower risk for CHD than are men of the same age. As mentioned previously, premenopausal women are at low risk, but after menopause the risk rises progressively, so that there are as many women who die of CHD annually as there are men. Therefore, women with high cholesterol levels should use dietary therapy; weight loss for overweight women and increased physical activity are also important treatment strategies, but drugs should be used more cautiously in women than in men of the same age.

Postmenopausal women with very high cholesterol levels or multiple other risk factors can be considered

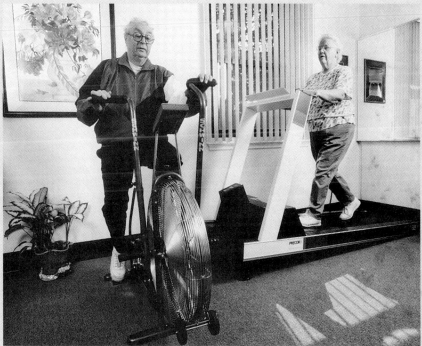

C.C. Duncan—Medical Images, Inc.

Updated cholesterol-management guidelines issued in 1993 for U.S. adults emphasize that those in the over-65 age group can significantly reduce their coronary heart disease (CHD) risk and improve their quality of life by lowering cholesterol. For the majority of elderly persons, the mainstays of treatment are increased physical activity, weight loss for those who are overweight, and a diet that is reduced in saturated fat, total fat, and cholesterol. Older people with existing CHD or multiple risk factors may need drug treatment as well.

for drug treatment. However, many postmenopausal women with high cholesterol may be able to effectively reduce their risk for CHD through estrogen replacement therapy rather than by using a cholesterol-lowering drug. Because the benefits of estrogen replacement therapy have not been conclusively established, the decision as to its appropriateness should be made jointly by the physician and the individual patient after a full discussion of the probable benefits and risks in her particular circumstances.

Rates of CHD are much higher in elderly people (those aged 65 and over) than in younger groups. As a result, even though a high cholesterol level may be a stronger risk factor in the middle aged, it leads to a greater number of heart attacks and other CHD problems in the elderly. Studies show that even advanced disease of the coronary arteries responds to cholesterol-lowering treatment. It is reasonable to predict that the elderly can achieve substantial benefit in reducing their risk for CHD through cholesterol lowering, and elderly persons who are otherwise in good health should not be excluded from cholesterol-lowering strategies. Prudent treatment with diet, physical activity, and weight loss when appropriate should be the mainstay of therapy; elderly patients with existing CHD or multiple risk factors may need drug treatment in addition. There are, however, certain elderly patients who are not suitable candidates for aggressive treatment; this group includes those who are in otherwise poor health.

HDL-cholesterol. ATP II reaffirms ATP I's recommendation that a low HDL—under 35 mg/dL—should be regarded as a major independent risk factor for CHD. However, the new guidelines recommend in addition that HDL be measured together with total cholesterol at initial testing in the health care setting if an accurate HDL reading can be obtained. ATP II also newly establishes a high HDL—60 mg/dL or above—as a "negative" risk factor, one that reduces the risk for CHD and lessens the need for aggressive treatment. Nonetheless, LDL remains the major target of treatment because there is stronger evidence from clinical trials that the risk for CHD is effectively reduced by lowering LDL rather than raising HDL. In patients in whom a low HDL is found, exercise, weight loss for the overweight, and smoking cessation may help raise the level. If drug treatment is needed to lower a high LDL in a patient who also has a low HDL, a drug that both lowers LDL and raises HDL should be considered.

Dietary therapy, weight loss, and physical activity. ATP II emphasizes dietary therapy using a diet reduced in saturated fat, total fat, and cholesterol, as did ATP I, but the new guidelines provide additional help, such as a tool to assess a patient's current eating patterns. ATP II also gives increased emphasis to weight loss and physical activity as elements of dietary therapy.

Evidence has been mounting that weight reduction in overweight patients and increased physical activity can enhance the effects of dietary therapy, enabling patients to achieve average cholesterol reductions of 10% or more. In addition, weight reduction and physical activity not only promote reductions in LDL-cholesterol and total cholesterol levels but reduce the risk for CHD in several other ways, such as raising HDL, reducing high blood pressure, and decreasing the risk for diabetes. For all these reasons, obesity and physical inactivity should be considered important targets for treatment.

Cholesterol lowering and prolongation of life. ATP II considers from two perspectives the question of whether cholesterol lowering prolongs life. First, the report examines whether low cholesterol levels could carry an increased risk of certain diseases. Observational studies show that individuals with the lowest naturally occurring cholesterol levels may be at increased risk in subsequent years for death from suicide, cancer of the lung and liver, digestive diseases, noncancerous lung disease, and intracranial hemorrhage. The study that provides the best data suggests that these increased rates of certain noncoronary conditions are seen only at cholesterol levels below 140 mg/dL, which represents less than 5% of the U.S. population. There is no proof that low cholesterol causes any of these particular conditions, and most experts believe that the most likely explanation is the opposite: that the disease itself leads to a low level of cholesterol even before that disease is fully apparent. In some cases other factors—*e.g.,* smoking, alcohol consumption, and weight loss—which are known to lead to low cholesterol levels, may be associated with such noncoronary conditions.

The second perspective on the question of whether cholesterol lowering prolongs life is provided by the results of clinical trials. Such trials have established that cholesterol lowering reduces the incidence of new heart attacks and heart attack deaths. Several lines of evidence show that dietary therapy improves health and reduces CHD risk. In patients with existing CHD, cholesterol lowering with drugs not only reduces the risk for future heart attacks but almost certainly prolongs life. However, the question has arisen as to whether cholesterol lowering with drugs prolongs life in patients *without* CHD. Clinical trials have not shown a reduction in "total mortality"—that is, the sum of deaths from CHD and all other causes—for these patients. So far, clinical trials have not been large enough or lasted long enough to answer this question. Some of these trials have raised the possibility that drugs may increase deaths from causes other than CHD. The causes of non-CHD death have varied from accidents and violence in some cases to malignancies in others. It is not known whether these increases are due to drug therapy or to chance.

278

A definite answer will not be available until a large clinical trial that is now being planned has investigated this issue. Until then, drug treatment for patients without CHD should be reserved for those at high risk for CHD. As already indicated, those most likely to benefit from drug therapy are patients having high cholesterol levels together with multiple other risk factors. Dietary therapy is safer and should be the major form of treatment for most persons.

It is important to bear in mind that the goal of lowering a high cholesterol level is not only to reduce the risk of death but also to improve the *quality of life*. Lowering high cholesterol reduces the toll exacted by CHD. People will live better because they suffer less angina and fewer heart attacks, are less likely to be hospitalized or need treatment in a coronary care unit, require fewer cardiovascular procedures such as angioplasty and coronary artery bypass surgery, and have less disability and less interference with their normal pattern of living.

Cost-effectiveness. Is cholesterol lowering worth what it costs? ATP II uses the lessons from "cost-effectiveness analysis"—that is, weighing the costs against the improvements in health—to help answer this question. The aggregate cost of CHD in the United States is enormous, estimated at $50 billion to $100 billion annually for medical treatment and lost wages. Prevention of CHD could greatly reduce this economic toll.

The most cost-effective form of prevention would be through a public health approach. Such an approach targets the entire population for reductions in the major risk factors for CHD, especially smoking, high blood cholesterol, and high blood pressure. It involves public education and a commitment from governments and the private sector.

Since treatment of high cholesterol uses the health care system, it carries costs for detection, therapy, and long-term monitoring of patients. Currently, the greatest costs are associated with drug treatment. It is expected, however, that drug costs will decline in coming years as the number of new drugs increases and as other drugs become available in generic form.

In patients with existing CHD, drug treatment to lower cholesterol actually saves money. For patients without existing CHD, ATP II recommends reserving drug treatment for use only in those at high risk. For these patients drug treatment *is* likely to be cost-effective. For the vast majority of patients without existing CHD, though, the guidelines recommend relying on less expensive dietary therapy.

Essence of ATP II recommendations

ATP II identifies and defines the following risk factors that lower the target goal for cholesterol reduction:
 • age (45 years or older in men and 55 years or older in women)
 • a family history of early CHD

Table 2. Cholesterol evaluation and treatment: who requires what?

	percentage of adults requiring action
nonfasting total and HDL-cholesterol measurement	100
fasting lipoprotein analysis	40
dietary therapy	29
drug treatment	7

Source: Second Report of the NCEP Expert Panel on Detection, Evaluation, and Treatment of High Blood Cholesterol in Adults, 1993

 • cigarette smoking
 • high blood pressure
 • low levels of HDL (less than 35 mg/dL)
 • diabetes

As noted above, high HDL (60 mg/dL or above) is considered a negative risk factor; if the patient has a high HDL, one risk factor is subtracted. In addition, obesity and physical inactivity are important CHD risk factors that should be treated.

In a nutshell, the thrust of the ATP II recommendations can be stated as follows: All adults 20 years of age and older who do not have CHD should have their total cholesterol and HDL-cholesterol measured. Those results, together with other coronary risk factors, will determine who needs a measurement of LDL-cholesterol—a lipoprotein analysis after fasting 9–12 hours. Patients with CHD, on the other hand, should go straight to a fasting LDL determination. The LDL-cholesterol level, together with other risk factors, will determine who needs dietary therapy to lower the LDL. Drugs are to be reserved for high-risk patients.

The philosophy of the ATP II guidelines is to target cholesterol-lowering strategies to those who are most likely to benefit from them (*see* Table 2). All adults should have their total and HDL-cholesterol measured, but this need not mean a special trip to the doctor. Rather, at a person's next visit to the doctor, he or she should have cholesterol tested if it has not already been done.

On the basis of the cholesterol tests, 40% would require a further fasting lipoprotein analysis to determine the LDL level. On the basis of the LDL measurement, about 29% of adults would require dietary therapy to lower their high blood cholesterol. After an adequate trial of dietary therapy, and assuming that diet would lower LDL levels by about 10%, about 7% of adults might be candidates for drug treatment. About one-third of this group would be patients with existing CHD. These descending percentages reflect the intent of the guidelines to identify those patients who are most likely to benefit from cholesterol-lowering therapy, to

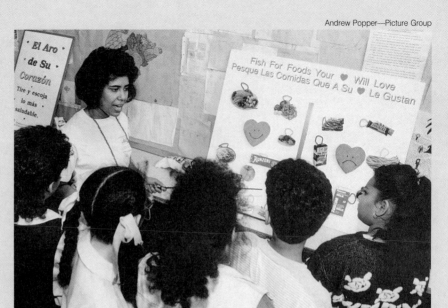

A community health worker leads New York City schoolchildren in the "fishing game" to teach them about choosing foods that are good for their hearts. Because lifestyle habits that increase the risk of developing coronary heart disease in adulthood often begin early in life, an important public health strategy is to encourage the population at large to adopt heart-healthy eating habits.

rely on dietary therapy as the mainstay in most cases, and to take a cautious approach to drug treatment, reserving it for patients at high risk for CHD.

ATP II recommends that individuals who need to lower cholesterol be started on the Step I diet, which calls for a reduction in saturated fat intake to 8–10% of total calories, total fat to 30% or less of total calories, and dietary cholesterol to less than 300 mg a day (*see* Table 3). These reductions can be achieved by an emphasis on foods such as grains, pasta, bread, fruits and vegetables, low-fat milk products, poultry, fish, and lean cuts of meats. In addition to changes in the diet, ATP II also recommends increased physical activity and weight loss when appropriate—changes that can substantially enhance the degree of cholesterol lowering and reduce the risk for CHD in a variety of ways.

If the Step I diet does not produce adequate cholesterol lowering, the Step II diet should be tried. The Step II diet further reduces saturated fat intake to less than 7% of total calories and cholesterol to less than 200 mg a day. The involvement of a registered dietitian can be very helpful for an individual who needs to follow the Step II diet.

For most people dietary therapy will be their main treatment. The Step I and II diets should be given a chance to succeed and should not be abandoned prematurely. Three out of four individuals who need to lower their cholesterol levels will be able to use dietary therapy and not have to go on to drug treatment. However, if after an adequate trial of intensive dietary therapy, generally lasting about six months, the cholesterol level remains significantly elevated, then drug treatment should be considered.

Table 3. Dietary therapy for high blood cholesterol

nutrient*	Step I diet	recommended intake (% of total calories)	Step II diet
total fat	30% or less		30% or less
saturated fatty acids	8–10%		less than 7%
polyunsaturated fatty acids	up to 10%		up to 10%
monounsaturated fatty acids	up to 15%		up to 15%
carbohydrates	55% or more		55% or more
protein	approximately 15%		approximately 15%
		recommended intake	
cholesterol	less than 300 mg/day		less than 200 mg/day
total calories	to achieve and maintain desired weight		to achieve and maintain desired weight

*calories from alcohol not included

ATP II classifies cholesterol-lowering drugs into two categories: "major" drugs and "other" drugs. The major drugs include bile acid sequestrants (cholestyramine and colestipol), nicotinic acid, and statins (lovastatin, pravastatin, simvastatin). Other drugs include fibric acids (*e.g.*, gemfibrozil) and probucol. The decision about which drug to use is best made on an individual basis after a thorough discussion between the patient and the doctor.

Implications for cholesterol education

The gratifying results of the NHANES III and ATP II reports have several specific implications for educating both health professionals and the U.S. public. The NCEP will play a particularly important role in promoting these strategies. First, the NCEP will continue to pursue a combination of public health and clinical strategies for lowering high cholesterol levels. This combination appears to be succeeding, as witnessed by the decline both in average cholesterol levels and in the percentage of individuals with high blood cholesterol requiring therapy. Moreover, both strategies are still needed, as evidenced by the fact that average cholesterol levels are still over 200 mg/dL and 29% of adults still need dietary therapy. The NCEP and its many partner organizations will continue to encourage the general population to adopt heart-healthy eating habits and will continue to encourage adults to have their blood cholesterol checked, know their cholesterol numbers, and lower high blood cholesterol to reduce their risk for CHD.

These themes will be incorporated in the NCEP's public service advertising campaigns. These campaigns, which have been conducted since 1986, have used print, television, and radio public service announcements to help promote the public health strategies as well as to encourage clinical strategies for lowering cholesterol.

Second, the NCEP will promote the implementation of the ATP II guidelines on a nationwide basis. The ATP II report has been approved by representatives of the more than 40 organizations on the NCEP Coordinating Committee. The report itself, which was prepared by 25 panel members, is thus not simply an expression of *their* views but has a broad consensus supporting it. These organizations will in turn conduct educational activities to help their constituencies carry out the guidelines. Further, the NCEP will ensure that the ATP II report is widely disseminated to health professionals. At the same time, the NCEP's information center will make available updated patient education booklets that incorporate the ATP II recommendations.

Third, the NCEP will encourage physicians and other health professionals to use the new guidelines to target CHD patients and others at high risk for CHD for aggressive treatment. The patient with CHD has much to gain from cholesterol lowering. Yet, as

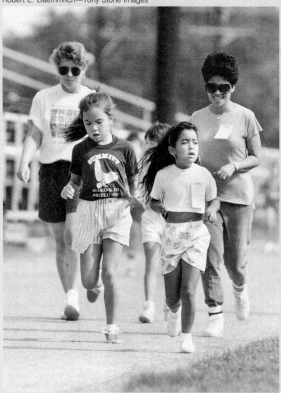

The impressive population-wide gains in lowered cholesterol levels realized over the past decades are likely to reduce future heart disease rates, reflecting an important improvement in the overall health and well-being of the American public.

previously noted, most CHD patients are not getting the cholesterol-lowering treatment they need. Patients with existing CHD will account for almost half of future heart attacks; aggressive cholesterol lowering would do much to reduce this toll.

Prospects for the future

Together the recently released NHANES III and ATP II reports provide a solid basis for looking ahead with optimism. According to various estimates, the 6 to 8% decline in cholesterol levels over the last 30 years might itself be expected to produce a 12 to 32% decline in rates of coronary disease. A 54% reduction in death rates from CHD has already occurred over the last 30 years, and lower cholesterol levels have made a substantial contribution to this reduction.

Through sustained application of the population-directed and clinical strategies, it should be possible to lower average American cholesterol levels to 200 mg/dL to meet the established goal for the year 2000. It should also be possible to reduce further the prevalence of high blood cholesterol and to contribute to a continued decline in the rates of illness and death from coronary disease and to a continued improvement in the health and well-being of the American public.

Disease Eradication

After smallpox became the first disease of humans to be eradicated from the world in 1977, public health experts hesitated before agreeing on other candidates for eradication. A reason for their hesitancy was the abandonment in 1969 of the expensive earlier attempt to eradicate malaria. Two other diseases, poliomyelitis and dracunculiasis (guinea worm disease), are now slated to be eradicated before the end of the 20th century, and preparations are under way for attacking more diseases in this way. Eradication is defined as a state of zero incidence of a disease or condition such that further control measures are unnecessary.

Candidates for conquest

Between 1989 and 1992 the International Task Force for Disease Eradication, comprising a group of public health scientists working with a secretariat established at the Carter Center in Atlanta, Ga., with assistance from staff of the Centers for Disease Control and Prevention (CDC) and other expert consultants, systematically reviewed candidate diseases to evaluate their potential eradicability. After preliminary consideration of about 80 infectious diseases, the task force reviewed 29 of them in depth, as well as one noninfectious condition, iodine deficiency. Criteria used in the evaluation process included the scientific feasibility of eradication, based on characteristics of the particular disease in question, and the available means to prevent or otherwise control it. Other considerations were the burden of the disease, the expected cost of eliminating it, and the existence of or potential for public and financial support for the eradication effort.

The task force concluded that six of the diseases they reviewed were potentially eradicable. Two were poliomyelitis and dracunculiasis—both of which had already been targeted for eradication by the World Health Organization (WHO). Two other viral diseases were targeted: mumps and rubella (German, or three-day measles), both of which occur worldwide and most often affect children.

Rubella causes a minor illness in children and a somewhat more troublesome illness in adults. It can be serious, however, when it affects a woman in the early months of pregnancy, causing severe birth defects in her fetus. Vaccination of infants provides long-lasting immunity to the illness, as does early infection with the illness. The global toll is not known.

The global toll of mumps is not known either; in rare cases the disease can be fatal. Mumps causes fever and swelling of salivary glands. Uncommon but severe complications include orchitis (inflammation of the testes), which can lead to sterility; meningitis, which can lead to deafness; and encephalitis (swelling of the brain). There are mumps epidemics every two to three years; the virus spreads readily, in the same manner as rubella, by respiratory droplet infection.

Most likely, eradication of mumps and rubella will entail the mass immunization of young children with the combined measles/mumps/rubella (MMR) vaccine. Immunization against mumps and rubella is increasing in some countries but is still far from the level that will be needed to eradicate either disease.

Two parasitic infections were also selected for eradication: lymphatic filariasis and cysticercosis. Lymphatic filariasis affects some 80 million persons worldwide but is most common in Asia: in India, China, Indonesia, and some Pacific islands. Filariasis infection can be severely debilitating and disfiguring but usually is not fatal. It is spread by repeated bites of mosquitoes; the main parasite, *Wuchereria bancrofti,* is usually spread by *Culex* mosquitoes. Associated disfigurement and crippling are a result of inflamma-

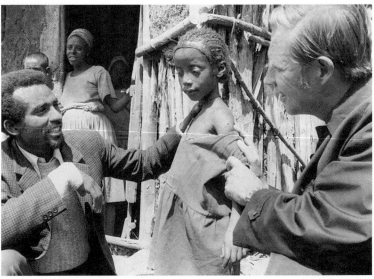

Donald A. Henderson (far right), leader of the World Health Organization's smallpox eradication campaign, checks an Ethiopian child's vaccination scar during a village-by-village search for cases. In 1977 smallpox became the first disease of humans to be officially eradicated from the face of the globe.

tion and scarring in the lymph passages, which can lead to grotesque swelling of limbs (elephantiasis) or genital organs. The approach to eradication is to reduce opportunities for mosquitoes to bite humans and to treat infected persons with drugs.

Cysticercosis, or pork tapeworm infection, is primarily found in rural areas of Latin America, Asia, and Africa; in the United States it occurs occasionally among migrant workers and recent immigrants from Central and South America. The infection is acquired through the eating of inadequately cooked contaminated pork and is manifested by numerous cysts in internal organs, including the brain. When the brain is infected, it causes epilepsy and seizure disorders (neurocysticercosis). Cysticercosis affects about 50 million persons each year, of whom about 50,000 die. Diagnosis and destruction of infected swine, proper disposal of human feces, and thorough cooking of all pork before it is eaten are the main control measures. Global efforts to control filariasis and cysticercosis are still in the early stages, and no target dates have been set for their eradication.

Unlikely candidates

The task force concluded that it could *not* support two recent resolutions by WHO that call for the global elimination of neonatal tetanus by 1995 (*see* below) and for the elimination of leprosy (defined as reduction of incidence to less than one case per 10,000 persons) by 2000. Eradicating leprosy would require overcoming strong social stigma, having better diagnostic and therapeutic tools than are currently available, and addressing the possibility that a reservoir of infection exists in armadillos. The task force also concluded that measles could not be eradicated in the near future (*see* below).

Other diseases that were considered for eradication—for example, Chagas' disease, tuberculosis, hepatitis B, cholera, schistosomiasis, ascariasis, and hook worm disease—were judged not to be eradicable in the foreseeable future with the weapons that are now available. In some instances, however, the task force noted that key manifestations of certain diseases, such as blindness caused by trachoma or onchocerciasis (river blindness); rabies in urban areas; and goiter caused by clinical iodine deficiency could conceivably be controlled without eradication of the underlying condition or infection altogether. Further transmission of a microbe in human populations (such as the spirochete *Treponema pertenue*, which causes yaws) might also be prevented without total eradication.

Global efforts toward the eradication of polio and dracunculiasis are presently well under way; each of these is considered in more detail below. For most of the other diseases just mentioned, there has been little action taken in pursuit of eradication up to now. In

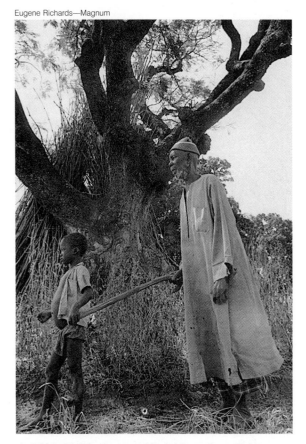

Eugene Richards—Magnum

A child in Mali leads a man blinded by onchocerciasis, a scourge that affects some 17 million people in the tropics. Eradication of onchocerciasis is not presently feasible, but the use of insecticide in rivers where the black flies that transmit the disease breed has greatly reduced its incidence, and a drug can now prevent its most devastating symptoms.

drawing attention for the first time to the *potential* eradicability of mumps, rubella, cysticercosis, and filariasis and by highlighting key technological obstacles to eradicating some of the other diseases it considered, the International Task Force for Disease Eradication may have inspired future efforts toward the conquest of a number of diseases that still take a huge toll in the world. Such efforts will gain added impetus if the campaigns to eradicate dracunculiasis and polio are successful.

Guinea worm: an end in sight

In 1986 WHO first officially targeted the parasitic disease dracunculiasis for eradication, and in 1991 it set the target date of 1995 for achieving eradication. This disease, which still affects up to two million to three million persons in parts of India, Pakistan, and 16 African countries, is transmitted by contaminated drinking water from stagnant ponds or open wells that harbor the *Cyclops,* a tiny water flea containing the embryonic guinea worm parasite. The water fleas are killed by digestive juices in the person's stomach, thus releasing the worm larvae, which penetrate the stomach or intestine and migrate into the tissues of the abdomen. In a few months the worms mate; then the male worms die. The female migrates, usually to the victim's lower leg or sometimes to the breast, scalp, tongue, scrotum, or uterus, where it emerges as a slender 60–90-cm (2–3-ft)-long adult worm about 12 months after the infective water fleas were swallowed. When a person with an emerging worm enters a body of water, the female worm releases hundreds of thousands of larvae into the water, where they may be eaten by *Cyclops* to begin the vicious cycle again.

People who are infected experience no symptoms until the adult female worm is ready to emerge. The worm secretes a toxin that causes a painful blister to appear on the skin. Half or more of the victims may be temporarily incapacitated for periods of one to three months. A small number of victims are permanently crippled by scarring from secondary infections. No matter how often they are infected, people do not become immune. Modern medicine offers no cure or vaccine for dracunculiasis. Palliative drugs (such as aspirin for pain and antiseptic ointments and liquid dressings for inflamed blisters) can help relieve the pain and minimize secondary infections, but once persons have been infected, they must await the worm's emergence, then begin winding it carefully around a stick.

Recently an Indian practitioner of Ayurvedic medicine began popularizing a method for surgical removal of worms just before they emerge naturally. Used properly, this technique can reduce the compli-

cations and disability that are often associated with emergence of the worm and reduce the potential for recontamination of ponds. However, practical constraints (logistics, scarcity of medical personnel and supplies in remote rural areas) limit the utility of surgical extraction as a public health intervention in Africa to the end stage of eradication programs, when numbers of cases are low and strict containment of each case is required.

Fortunately, however, dracunculiasis can be prevented. Filtering drinking water through a fine cloth or boiling the water, providing safe sources of drinking water such as a protected well, educating populations to avoid entering water sources when the adult worms are emerging from their bodies, and applying a chemical to kill the immature worms in contaminated ponds are ways to achieve this.

Substantial progress has been made in the fight against guinea worm disease. It already is on the verge of being eradicated from Asia. Pakistan reported only 23 cases in 1992, while India, which had had over 44,000 cases 10 years earlier, found only 1,081 cases in 1992.

In Africa, now the major battleground, more than 70% of the 23,000 villages where dracunculiasis is known to still occur have begun measures to get rid of it. Two of the most highly endemic countries, Ghana and Nigeria, reduced their combined total of cases by approximately 70% in just three years: from about 820,000 cases in 1989 to about 250,000 cases in 1992. Cameroon, with 127 cases in 1992, is close to achieving eradication. Of the four remaining African countries where the full extent of the disease has not

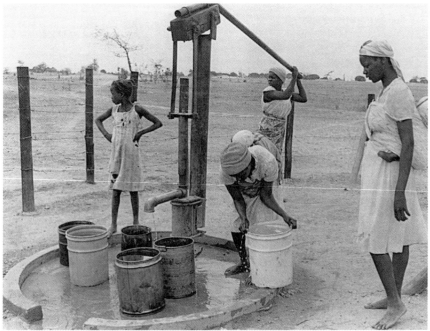

A newly installed borehole well provides safe drinking water for Nigerian villagers. The installation of such wells is one of the keys to eradicating dracunculiasisis (guinea worm disease) from the world by 1995. Other important eradication measures are the use of larvicide in stagnant ponds and open wells where the water fleas (Cyclops) that harbor the guinea worm breed and the education of those who live in endemic areas so that they learn to filter or boil their drinking water in order to eliminate the tiny fleas that transmit infection.

yet been ascertained, only one, Kenya, has not yet begun a nationwide, village-by-village search for cases.

Former U.S. president Jimmy Carter, who actively joined the fight against dracunculiasis in 1986, has continued his efforts to mobilize national leaders and health ministers in affected countries to support their national guinea-worm-eradication programs. During a visit to five French-speaking countries in West Africa in 1992, Carter persuaded a former head of state and brigadier general in Mali to lead the fight against dracunculiasis in that country. Carter planned to make a similar visit to East Africa in 1993. Through the Carter Center the former president has also raised funds from major donors, such as the king of Saudi Arabia, who recently pledged $1.9 million annually for the next four years for dracunculiasis-eradication efforts.

The most serious remaining threat to eradicating guinea worm disease by the target date of December 1995 is the civil war that rages in The Sudan. Continued fighting prevents epidemiological surveys from being carried out and appropriate control measures from being implemented, particularly in the eastern equatorial region of southern Sudan, which is suspected of being one of the most highly endemic areas of the country and which borders known endemic areas of Uganda, Kenya, and Ethiopia. About $48 million of the $68 million estimated cost of dracunculiasis eradication (not including the costs for the provision of safe water supplies) is already available, but additional support and funding are still needed. Most indications are, however, that guinea worm will soon be a thing of the past.

Polio: major progress against a costly crippler

Two years after it targeted dracunculiasis for global extinction, in 1988 WHO set the goal of eradicating polio from the world by the year 2000. Unlike dracunculiasis, however, polio occurs worldwide, and most persons who are infected show no sign of the infection. In serious cases, however, it attacks the brain and spinal cord and may lead to extensive paralysis, including paralysis of the muscles involved in breathing. It spreads mostly by respiratory droplets from infected persons. Polio can be prevented by a series of three or four injections (the "Salk" vaccine) or oral doses of the "Sabin" vaccine.

Since effective vaccines became available in the 1950s, polio has been virtually eliminated from North America and most developed countries, although cases still occur among those who have not been vaccinated. Interest in the possible eradication of polio globally received a vital boost in 1985, when the director of the Pan American Health Organization (PAHO) courageously announced a campaign to eliminate the disease from Central and South America by 1990. Rapid progress toward accomplishing that goal generated much of the momentum for the global effort that

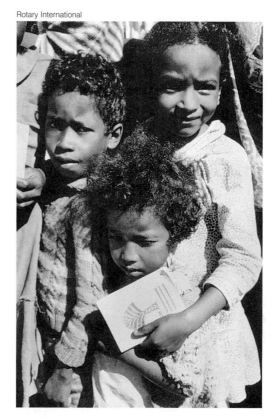

Children in Madagascar line up for polio vaccination. If the goal of eradicating polio is achieved, the world will realize annual savings of about $500 million—not to mention the vast reduction of human suffering.

is now under way. Although PAHO did not quite make its 1990 target, it came close; the last indigenous wild poliovirus detected in the Americas was found in Peru in August 1991.

Of the 14,128 cases of polio worldwide that were reported to WHO in 1991, over half were from India and China, another 1,147 were from Pakistan, and a total of 2,393 cases were reported from three African countries: Kenya, Nigeria, and Egypt. (WHO estimates that only about 10% of polio cases are reported in most areas. Moreover, for each actual case, about 1,000 other persons are infected but do not develop symptoms.) In the decade since 1981, however, East and South Asia reduced the reported incidence of polio by 70 and 87%, respectively. That dramatic decline is due to increasing immunization as a part of the effort led by the United Nations to attain "universal child immunization" against six major childhood diseases, including polio, by the end of 1990. Globally, this effort increased the average immunization level of infants against polio to 85% in 1990 from only about 20% 10 years earlier.

The nations of the western Pacific, including China, have now set themselves the goal of eradicating polio by 1995. One potential obstacle facing the region

Disease eradication

is a lack of funds to purchase vaccine and conduct eradication activities. Already some mass immunization campaigns in China have been hampered by an inadequate supply of vaccine.

Europe, too, has set a 1995 eradication target date. In Sweden the spread of wild poliovirus was halted as long ago as 1962. In The Netherlands, however, where the spread of indigenous polio was also eliminated for several years by high immunization levels, an outbreak of 68 cases, including 2 deaths, occurred in 1992. The outbreak was caused by an imported case that rapidly spread among a poorly immunized religious minority whose members oppose vaccination. This episode demonstrated again the continued potential vulnerability of polio-free countries as long as the disease still occurs anywhere. A similar outbreak had occurred among members of the same religious group in the same country in 1978.

The most difficult challenge to the eradication of polio is in sub-Saharan Africa, where average immunization rates of infants against polio were still under 60% in 1991. This region also recorded a decline of only 4% in reported cases of polio between 1981 and 1989, the smallest such reduction in incidence of all the regions of the world in that period. A few African countries, such as Botswana, Zimbabwe, Algeria, and Morocco, are all on the verge of eliminating polio, but in the African region as a whole, much remains to be done to improve reporting of cases, ensure routine administration of immunizations, and limit the spread of outbreaks and cases that are discovered.

Eradicating polio will cost an estimated $1.4 billion over the decade of the 1990s. As was the case with smallpox eradication, however, the world will recover the costs of the achievement—in fact, much more—if the campaign is successful. WHO estimates that if progress continues at the present rate, the savings from polio eradication will be about $500 million per year by the year 2000; the savings by 2015 will have increased to $3 billion per year.

Efforts to control neonatal tetanus

Tetanus is transmitted when spores of the bacterium contaminate wounds. Such spores are found widely in the environment, being common in the feces of grazing animals such as horses and cattle. The stump of the umbilical cord of newborn infants is particularly prone to developing this infection if it becomes contaminated by unsterile methods used to cut the cord at birth or by unsterile materials applied to the stump, such as cow dung. Once it has developed, tetanus is difficult to treat successfully, and most victims die as a result of the severe muscle spasms that develop and prevent normal breathing.

As noted above, in 1989 WHO set the goal of eliminating neonatal tetanus by 1995, despite the fact that tetanus has an inexhaustible environmental reservoir.

World Health Organization

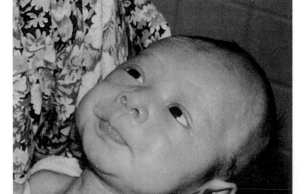

Victims of neonatal tetanus die when severe muscle spasms prevent normal breathing. Infection occurs mainly in poor nations where birthing practices are unsanitary. Vaccinating mothers is the way to prevent it.

The recommended strategy calls for immunization of women of childbearing age with two or more doses of tetanus toxoid vaccine and for promotion of clean childbirth practices. An adequately immunized pregnant woman passes enough antibodies to her infant before birth to protect it against tetanus in the newborn period, even if the infant's cord becomes contaminated at or after delivery.

WHO estimated that the death toll from neonatal tetanus in 1991 was 434,000, of which 212,000 occurred in Southeast Asia and 127,000 in Africa, the two areas where newborns are most at risk. About four-fifths of the total reported deaths were in six countries of Asia and seven in Africa. Most of these countries have prepared plans of action for eliminating the disease. But as of 1990 only about 58% of females of childbearing age worldwide had received the two injections required for protecting their infants. In the poorest countries that percentage was about 43%.

Much thus remains to be done, and time is running out for achieving the established objective on time. Because of the ubiquity of the tetanus organism in the environment, it will not be possible to ever truly eradicate neonatal tetanus; control measures will always be needed to prevent infection of newborns.

Elimination of measles: still elusive

Measles still kills over one million children each year, a toll that is greatly reduced from former years, thanks to increasingly widespread immunization against this highly infectious disease. Owing to its rapid, easy spread, virtually every unprotected child will contract

286

the disease, which is most likely to be fatal in children in poor nations, who may already be weakened by malnutrition, chronic diarrhea, or other infections.

Although this is a very serious disease with a high mortality rate, especially in less developed countries, and has long been considered a potential target for eradication, its rapid spread and the fact that the vaccine used against it is not effective in newborns up to nine months of age have made the eradication of measles a difficult, if not elusive, task. The United States, which set out in 1977 to stop indigenous spread of measles by 1982, reduced the number of reported cases to fewer than 3,000 per year for a short time (from prevaccine era levels of 400,000 to 500,000 cases reported per year) only to see the disease increase again to more than 27,000 cases in 1990.

WHO and UNICEF have set the goal of reducing measles incidence worldwide by 90% and measles deaths by 95% from prevaccine levels, with a target date of 1995. Czechoslovakia, Sweden, and Finland eliminated or nearly eliminated indigenous measles in the 1980s, while Cuba, which aimed to eliminate it by 1990, now reports fewer than a dozen confirmed cases each year. The English-speaking island nations of the Caribbean are working to eliminate measles by 1995. Europe has set itself a similar target for the year 2000.

Achievement of unprecedentedly high levels of measles immunization in less developed countries as part of WHO's Expanded Program on Immunization has helped build momentum toward such goals. But global immunization coverage has already slipped by 2% since 1990. Measles eradication is thus unlikely to be achieved before the next century. If measles is eventually eradicated, however, all countries will realize great savings in terms of deaths prevented and a much-reduced burden of serious illness. These savings will be similar to those that are anticipated for polio eradication and those that the world already enjoys from the eradication of smallpox.

—*Donald R. Hopkins, M.D., M.P.H.*

Environmental Health

During the past few years, environmental agencies across the U.S. have been reviewing their attempts to protect the nation's environmental health, reexamining both progress and priorities. While many regions have noted improvement in areas such as air and water quality, scientific scrutiny has also indicated that some of the most serious environmental health threats are receiving far less attention and fewer resources than others that, in the opinion of many authorities, pose less risk.

Many of the recent reviews were sparked by the groundbreaking report *Reducing Risk,* which was issued in 1990 by the U.S. Environmental Protection

Agency (EPA). This report stressed that efforts to clean up hazardous-waste sites were receiving far greater resources than were programs to handle more significant problems, such as air pollution resulting from industrial emissions and auto exhaust. The EPA document also noted that although indoor pollution—from tobacco smoke and toxic substances in consumer products—may pose a relatively significant health risk because of the large number of people affected, it receives comparatively little attention from most state and federal agencies. Further, owing to the weak state of the U.S. economy, the cost-effectiveness of programs for reducing environmental health threats is now coming under scrutiny. The EPA and many in the field question whether environmental dollars might be spent more effectively than they have been in the past. Finally, important questions are being asked about whether environmental protection initiatives have been targeted fairly, with some alleging that minority and low-income neighborhoods have shouldered a disproportionate share of environmental hazards.

Along with this reevaluation of the country's environmental agenda, there have been a number of noteworthy scientific developments in environmental health. Four areas that have been the subject of recent assessment and research are: the safety of drinking water, the true nature of the dioxin hazard, the pressing need for solutions to the problem of disposal of radioactive waste, and the ongoing controversy over the health effects of electromagnetic fields.

Is it safe to drink the water?

Two events that took place in April 1993 shook the confidence of Americans in the safety of their drinking water. First, in Milwaukee, Wis., and surrounding communities, a parasite in the local water supply caused an estimated 200,000 people to become sick with a stomach ailment. Subsequently, a few who had been suffering from preexisting chronic diseases died. The cryptosporidium organism, which is present in the intestinal tracts of animals and had previously been known to cause human disease, was believed to have entered the water supply via runoff from agricultural land into Lake Michigan. Cryptosporidia are resistant to chlorine but can be removed from the water with high-performance filtration. The presence of cryptosporidia would probably have gone unnoticed by inspectors because the Milwaukee facility—like others in the U.S.—does not routinely test for the presence of these organisms.

In the wake of this outbreak, the General Accounting Office released a report showing that states are failing to meet federal standards for inspection of water systems. According to the report, inspections, when made at all, are likely to be haphazard, and state water-quality agencies do not follow up to see that problems are corrected once they have been identified. Further, the report found that most state water inspectors are inadequately trained.

Recent studies have focused on the consequences of low levels of certain additives and contaminants common in U.S. water supplies. One additive that has come under scrutiny is fluoride. The addition of fluoride to drinking water reduces the incidence of dental caries (tooth decay) in children, and the fluoridation of community water supplies is one factor credited with having improved overall dental health in the U.S. Concern was raised by new data that suggested a possible link between fluoride and osteosarcoma, a bone cancer that had been found to occur in laboratory tests in rodents. However, in one study of human exposure to fluoride, researchers at the New York State Department of Health and the State University of New York at Albany found that the rates of bone cancer in New York state residents living in communities with artificially fluoridated water supplies were not significantly different from those in communities without fluoridation.

Fluoride is known also to have an effect on bone growth and is sometimes prescribed (as sodium fluoride) along with calcium to restore bone lost in osteoporosis, the thinning and weakening of the bones that often comes with aging. But because the new bone stimulated by fluoride may be unusually brittle, there has been concern that fluoridated water might contribute to osteoporosis. Several research teams have been investigating this question. A study that examined hip fracture rates in Utah's elderly population between 1984 and 1990 found that the risk of fracture in both men and women was 25–50% greater for those exposed to artificially fluoridated water. Investigators from the University of Michigan studying three rural Iowa communities found that over a five-year period postmenopausal women who drank water containing naturally occurring fluoride at the EPA's maximum allowable fluoride level (four parts per million) had twice the fracture risk of their counterparts in a community with lower levels of fluoride added through fluoridation. On the other hand, Canadian researchers who compared the rate of hospitalization for hip fracture in two cities, Edmonton, which has fluoridation, and Calgary, where no fluoride is added to drinking water, found no statistical difference in fracture rates. The Canadian investigators concluded that fluoride has no impact on the risk of fracture.

Adding chlorine to water supplies, a routine approach to reducing bacterial contamination, may also create health problems. When added to drinking water, chlorine interacts with trace chemicals in the water to form cancer-causing by-products. Previous studies comparing the cancer rates of populations with and without chlorination have had equivocal results. However, in July 1992 the *American Journal of Public Health* published the results of a new statistical analy-

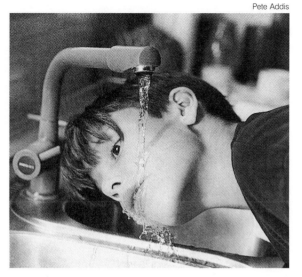

Lead in drinking water is an important source of environmental lead exposure in the U.S. Recent data suggest that such exposure can have an adverse effect on cognitive functioning in young children.

sis of a series of studies from the 1970s that had explored the association between cancer and chlorinated drinking water. On the basis of this statistical appraisal, or meta-analysis, the researchers found significantly increased risks of rectal and bladder cancer in people who drank chlorinated water. Some scientists question the validity of meta-analysis, but others are sufficiently impressed with the findings that they are now calling for alternative means of disinfecting drinking water. Still others believe that the benefits of chlorination far outweigh any risks.

With mounting evidence of the adverse effects of lead exposure on growth and learning aptitude in children, the EPA in 1991 announced tighter rules for the amount of lead in drinking water. Under the new action level (*i.e.,* the level at which water purveyors are required by law to fix the problem), lead levels in household water must not exceed 15 ppb (parts per billion) in 90% of those households surveyed. (The old standard had allowed an average of 50 ppb.) The principal sources of lead in tap water are lead pipes used in older plumbing systems and lead solder used to join more modern copper pipes. Nationwide tests conducted by Consumers Union, published in 1993 in *Consumer Reports,* revealed that levels in household water in many cities were above the mandated 15 ppb. An EPA report released in May 1993 said that more than 800 U.S. water systems it surveyed—serving 30 million people—had excessive lead levels.

Natural contaminants in drinking water have also come under scrutiny. One study conducted at Taipei, Taiwan, examined the association of cancer mortality and contamination with arsenic, which comes from the Earth's crust. The investigators found increased rates of a variety of cancers in populations served by groundwater containing arsenic. California regulators consequently suggested a reduction in the allowable amount of arsenic (now set at 50 ppb) in drinking water to better protect the public.

Dioxin reevaluated

Dioxin, long considered one of the most potent carcinogens, has been the subject of considerable research, speculation, and regulatory controversy ever since it was first identified in the 1950s. Dioxin, or 2,3,7,8-tetrachlorodibenzo-*p*-dioxin, is ubiquitous in the environment worldwide; trace amounts are formed during many types of combustion and as a by-product of wood, paper, and herbicide production. Because of dioxin's ability to cause cancer in laboratory animals, the presence of even trace amounts of the chemical in proximity to humans has been considered sufficient reason for strict regulation. In 1982–83 the U.S. government relocated an entire population of more than 2,000 people in Times Beach, Mo., after it was revealed that dioxin-containing oil sprayed on local roads had contaminated the soil. Scientists, however, have noted that incidents in which many people were exposed to dioxin—for example, an industrial accident in 1976 in Seveso, Italy; the spraying in Times Beach; the exposure of U.S. troops in Vietnam to Agent Orange, a dioxin-contaminated herbicide—have not resulted in consistent outbreaks of cancer, although some studies have noted increased cancer rates among people who were exposed. Further, some studies have documented increased cancer rates among workers occupationally exposed to dioxin in chemical and pesticide

plants. These inconsistencies have led to a reexamination of dioxin's toxicity and carcinogenic potential. In August 1991 some federal health officials went so far as to suggest that the stringent standards imposed on dioxin were too restrictive and that the evacuation of Times Beach may have been "an overreaction."

In fact, as they have studied the mechanisms by which dioxin may cause cancer, scientists have discovered that the chemical acts in subtle ways to alter normal physiological processes—in much the same way as do naturally occurring hormones. For this reason, dioxin is now sometimes referred to as an "environmental hormone." Its ability to disrupt certain vital functions—for example, immune responses—is seen as possibly even more of a health hazard than its cancer-causing potential. Understanding dioxin's role as a hormone may explain the discrepancies in the findings of the human cancer studies. Scientists believe that by mimicking the action of natural hormones, this one chemical is capable of giving rise to many different cancers and to many different sensitivities in different animals. And because dioxin acts like a hormone, the physiological response of a given species to dioxin exposure may be due, in part, to that species' (or even an individual's) hormonal balance and the ability of the body to compensate for exposure to the chemical. Researchers have therefore begun constructing models of how dioxin works at the molecular level. Some scientists have suggested that there may be a human threshold for dioxin exposure— a level of exposure below which no adverse health effects are found. If this were confirmed, it would have far-reaching implications for regulators and industry,

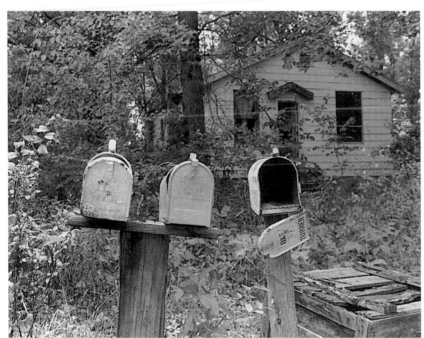

Bill Stover—The New York Times

Abandoned homes on overgrown lots are sharp reminders of the alarm raised over dioxin contamination of the town of Times Beach, Mo., a little over a decade ago, which led the federal government to evacuate more than 2,000 residents. In recent years scientists have been reevaluating the toxicity and cancer-causing potential of this chemical, once considered one of the most dangerous of all substances known to humans. Some authorities have now concluded that the dramatic evacuation of Times Beach might have been unnecessary.

Environmental health

leading to a relaxation of environmental standards for dioxin contamination. However, most of the accumulated data from laboratory studies still leave many questions unanswered. For the time being, exposure to even the smallest amount of dioxin is thought to increase an individual's risk of disease.

Getting rid of radioactive wastes

The end of the cold war has forced the U.S. to grapple with the legacy remaining from 50 years of building nuclear weapons. Federal facilities in 13 states spanning thousands of square kilometers now pose a monumental environmental quandary. The full extent of contamination on site, as well as in surrounding areas, still is not well understood. The extent, if any, of health risks to those who worked at these sites or live near them is also poorly understood.

A 1991 report by the National Academy of Sciences concluded that cleanup of hazardous-waste sites is hampered by the inability of authorities to determine which sites pose a threat to human health. Nuclear weapons facilities are even more difficult to characterize, as they contain large amounts of mixtures of hazardous and nuclear wastes. Moreover, studies of plant workers have had conflicting results. For example, a 1991 study of the Oak Ridge, Tenn., facility found higher than normal rates of cancers such as leukemia in those who worked at the facility between 1943 and 1972, a finding that contradicted the results of earlier investigations.

Meanwhile, researchers continued to sift through many years of data covering sites regulated by the Department of Energy (DOE) in hopes of reconstructing the doses that surrounding communities might have received over the years. A 1992 DOE report chronicling four decades of accidents at the Hanford, Wash., nuclear plant did little to calm the fears of those who live nearby. While some scientists caution that the impact on residents' health is likely to be minimal and that there is no immediate danger, others fear that the millions of cubic meters of radioactive wastes that have been dumped into rivers or on land may be extremely hazardous. There is particular concern about certain populations—*e.g.,* Native Americans who consume fish from rivers in the Northwest as a substantial part of their diet. Unfortunately, at least with currently available technology, environmental restoration of some sites may be impossible.

As the United States moves to reduce its nuclear arsenal, scientists must also continue to explore ways to safely recycle, reuse, or destroy weapons materials in the missiles that were built at these facilities. In addition, nuclear waste has been stockpiled at federal facilities and stored at nuclear power plants (another major source of nuclear waste), where they await permanent disposal. The DOE is exploring whether nuclear waste can be stored in rock formations at

Yucca Mountain, Nevada, in order to isolate the waste from both people and the environment for thousands of years. A 1992 National Academy of Sciences report refuted the contention of opponents of the project who suggested that an earthquake could raise the water table in the area, thus releasing the waste to the environment.

While the debate about the safe disposal of high-level nuclear waste continues, the states are mandated to seek secure disposal sites for low-level radioactive waste from nuclear power plants, hospitals, medical laboratories, and manufacturers of such items as smoke alarms. Although most experts contend that establishing disposal facilities for these wastes is safer than leaving them at the facilities where they are generated, community opposition to waste sites in many states is slowing the disposal process.

Electromagnetic fields: still a charged issue

The controversy continues over the health effects of exposure to electromagnetic fields (EMFs), the magnetic and electric fields generated by electric-power-distribution systems (including high-voltage transmission lines, transformer stations, and local electric lines) as well as certain home appliances and office equipment. In the past, several studies have suggested that the risks of leukemia and brain cancer are elevated in people who are exposed to high levels of EMFs. Some studies suggest that breast cancer and reproductive

A worker dons protective garb for a cleanup project at the Hanford, Wash., nuclear plant. The extent of contamination— on site and in adjacent areas—at this and other former weapons-production facilities remains unclear.

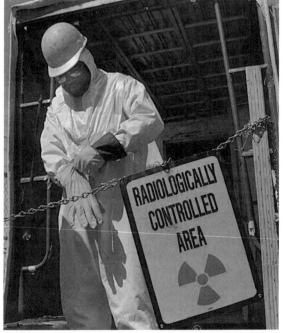

Jeff Green—The New York Times

290

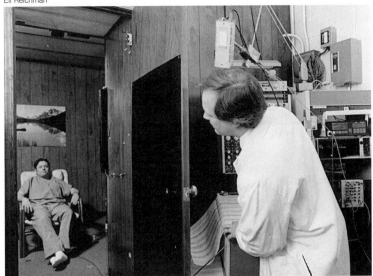

Eli Reichman

An investigator at the Kansas City, Mo., Midwest Research Institute prepares to expose a volunteer to the type of electromagnetic field produced by power lines. The health consequences of such exposure continue to be a subject of intense controversy.

problems also may be linked to magnetic fields. One perplexing aspect of these investigations is that their results have been inconsistent—some studies finding a relationship, some not. Moreover, closer correlations between cancer rates and EMFs were found when crude measures of exposure were used than have been demonstrated recently by more precise measurements. Another puzzling feature of this research is that scientists still do not know if EMFs are capable of causing the cellular changes associated with cancer.

In a study published in November 1991 in the *American Journal of Epidemiology,* researchers from the University of Southern California showed that small increases in the rates of childhood cancers were associated with living in close proximity to major overhead power lines. However, no correlation between cancer risk and actual EMF measurements made at each home was found.

Two Swedish studies released in 1992, one residential and one occupational, seemed to support the notion that EMFs may cause cancer. In the first, investigators from the Karolinska Institute in Stockholm gathered data on cancer rates among people living within 300 m (990 ft) of high-voltage electrical lines. They determined the magnitude of exposure by evaluating the size of the power lines adjacent to the subjects' homes and calculating past patterns of electricity transmission over each line (using historical data compiled by the Swedish government). They found that people exposed to higher magnetic fields were at elevated risk of developing leukemia but not other, more common cancers. The risk was two to four times higher than normal for children and up to two times higher for adults. However, the researchers did not find a correlation between leukemia cases and current EMF measurements. In the second study, conducted by an epidemiologist at the National Institute of Occu-

pational Health in Solna, increased rates of leukemia were found among men whose past employment (as determined by their job descriptions) suggested relatively high EMF exposure. Results of a similar survey of brain cancer and occupational exposure, however, were equivocal.

Additional occupational studies conducted in the U.S. and elsewhere examined rates of breast cancer, leukemia, and brain cancer among workers exposed to EMFs. Because the investigators could not exclude the possibility that the diseases were due to other job-related factors, the results were viewed as suggestive rather than conclusive. A 1992 report concluded that there was no association between birth defects and the use of electric blankets and heated water beds, both of which generate low-level magnetic fields.

Finally, health concerns have arisen recently in connection with cellular phones, which emit another form of nonionizing electromagnetic radiation. While little study on human health effects has been conducted to date, the industry has said it will fund a major epidemiological investigation.

Establishing priorities

As the ability to detect environmental contaminants is refined and expanded, the pressure to set national—and global—environmental priorities will undoubtedly increase. For example, if EMF exposure does elevate cancer rates, how much, if anything, would consumers be willing to pay to reduce their risk? And would the health of the public be better served by investing in primary health care, cleaning up abandoned hazardous-waste sites, or putting all electrical wires underground? It is unlikely that science alone can provide the answers to these difficult questions.

—*Daniel Wartenberg, Ph.D.,
and Caron Chess*

291

Special Report
Health Care Reform in Eurasia: The Next Revolution

by George A. Gellert, M.D., M.P.H., M.P.A.

The newly emerged states of the former Soviet Union and the newly freed nations of eastern Europe are confronted by profound problems that originated in decades of social, political, and economic domination by a harsh totalitarian center. Daily these new nations struggle to envision anew and reshape the very fabric of their societies. The dissolution of the Soviet empire has created a new openness and candor regarding the excesses of the past, the failures of the present, and the threats the future may portend. Nowhere is this more evident than in the area of health. While there is considerable variation from nation to nation and from Eurasia to eastern Europe, there are many commonalities underlying the health "crisis" in this vast region of the world. These include public health and environmental problems, deficiencies in the health care systems, and obstacles that must be overcome in order for there to be successful health care reform. ("Eurasia" is used here to refer to all 15 republics of the former Soviet Union, including the Russian Federation and its autonomous regions, the western frontier, the Baltics, Transcaucasia, and Central Asia.)

The health picture: rapidly deteriorating

Eurasian and eastern European nations are regressing rapidly with respect to leading health indicators. Public health improvements have slowed and in many cases reversed over recent decades. Eurasian life ex-

pectancy is five years shorter at birth and two years shorter at age 65 than in the United States. While nations of the industrialized West have experienced significant gains in life expectancy over the past three decades, Eurasia has seen a decline of two years in male life expectancy and only minimal progress for females. The infant mortality rate is two and one-half times the U.S. rate, and maternal mortality is six times that in the U.S. Eurasians are twice as likely as Americans to die from infectious and circulatory diseases, injury, and poisoning. Similar figures could be cited for eastern European nations.

Eurasian levels of immunization are falling, largely because single-use syringes are in short supply. Hepatitis B viral infection is endemic throughout Eurasia, and there is bubonic plague in Central Asia. Diphtheria, an acute infection that has been virtually eliminated in the West, has spread rapidly in Russia and Ukraine. By the end of 1992 there were an estimated 4,000 cases and, by some reports, as many as 100 deaths in Russia.

Lack of readily available contraceptives is a serious public health problem, and a heavy reliance on abortion results in the average Eurasian woman's having from three to five registered abortions during her reproductive years. (By comparison, in the U.S. the average number of abortions is one for every other woman of childbearing age.) Official statistics report

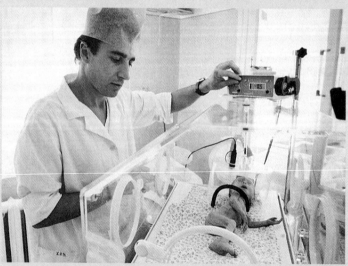

An obstetrician checks on a baby born prematurely and kept alive in an incubator in a hospital in Magnitogorsk, Russia. In many parts of Eurasia leading health indicators have declined rapidly, and infants are especially at risk. The infant mortality rate in the former Soviet Union is about two and one-half times the U.S. rate and more than three times higher than in many western European countries.

Itar—Tass/Sovfoto

6.2 million legally induced abortions a year in Eurasia, a figure that exceeds the number of live births. It is estimated that for every registered abortion there are at least one and possibly three unreported procedures.

Heavy abuse of tobacco and alcohol plagues many Eurasian societies. In the former Soviet Union, despite the campaign against alcohol launched in 1985 by Mikhail Gorbachev, alcoholism remains a pernicious and pervasive problem. In 1990, eight million people in the U.S.S.R. were apprehended by authorities for drunkenness, and 15% of the adult population was treated in detoxification centers. Other mental health problems abound; *Meditsinskaya Gazeta,* a Russian medical weekly, reports that up to 50% of all patients who consult a doctor are in need of counseling, psychotherapy, or medications, yet few Soviet physicians were given any psychological training.

The states of the former Soviet Union, with a collective population of almost 300 million, represent the largest group still presumed to be largely uninfected with the human immunodeficiency virus (HIV). As recently as 1988, the Soviet Union did not recognize AIDS as a national concern. (In Russia the official number of HIV carriers in 1992 was 566; however, a group of independent specialists estimated that the actual number was upwards of 20,000.) Although studies indicate a relatively low penetration of the virus into Eurasian and eastern European populations, behaviors that carry high risk of HIV infection, including unprotected sex, are common. Outbreaks of hospital-acquired HIV infection have resulted from the repeated use of inadequately sterilized hypodermic syringes. Drug abuse, which increases the risk for HIV infection, is common in certain subgroups, such as veterans of the Afghanistan war. Meanwhile, efforts to educate high-risk populations about AIDS prevention have been limited. Although condoms are now openly for sale in Eurasia, the numbers either produced locally or imported amount to only five or six per mature male per year. With political liberalization over the next decade and increasing international movement to and from Eurasia (including tourism and commercial exchanges), the threat of HIV transmission will become very real. Czech and Slovak experts predict increasing rates of HIV infection as a consequence of rising tourism, prostitution, and illicit drug importation. Unless widespread programs of HIV prevention are launched without delay, a Eurasian/eastern European HIV epidemic may be in the making; once missed, the opportunity to slow the spread of AIDS will never return.

Recent public health assessments have been conducted in the Russian Federation by the aid organization CARE and the U.S. Centers for Disease Control and Prevention (CDC). These surveys documented that vaccine-preventable diseases such as measles and pertussis had increased dramatically from 1990

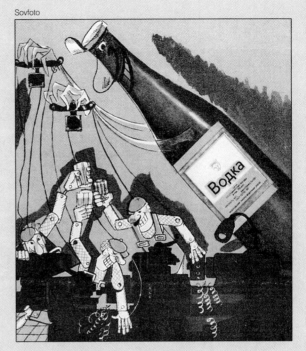

Drinkers are depicted as puppets in the hands of vodka in a Russian cartoon. Alcoholism is a problem that plagues many Eurasian societies.

to 1991. Gastroenteric infections had increased as a result of problems in maintaining water-purification systems. And greater numbers of women and children were found to suffer from anemia and critical nutritional deficiencies. In much of Eurasia food costs have become prohibitive, and food shortages are common. Expenditures on food have increased from 40 to 90% of income in many cases. The elderly were found to have high rates of chronic diseases and dental problems that interfered with eating.

In rural areas 27% of hospitals have no sewerage systems, and 17% lack running water. Shortages of essential medical supplies and drugs are common. Pharmaceuticals are in short supply, and drug costs have skyrocketed. In the former U.S.S.R. pharmaceutical production has dropped to below 5% of the 1990 level. A particularly acute crisis in pharmaceutical supplies has been reported in the three Baltic states, and many traditional sources of medical supplies to Eurasia have been cut off.

In light of such a widespread public health crisis, the CARE and CDC assessment teams recommended that assistance be targeted at providing vaccines against childhood diseases (such as measles), support for water-purification plants, and provision of essential and lifesaving drugs and other basic medical supplies. The team also underscored the need for international food assistance, especially for the elderly and the young, who are at heightened risk for problems associated with poor nutrition.

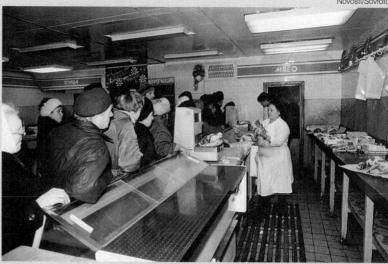

Muscovites wait in line in a butcher shop in hopes of getting some of the meager meat supplies available. Because food shortages are common in parts of Eurasia, both the young and the elderly in particular are often at risk for diseases associated with poor nutrition.

Environmental degradation

The environment in the former Soviet Union is emerging as one of globally unprecedented disaster, and health effects are only starting to be assessed. Pollution of lakes, rivers, and soil represents a particularly serious problem. Environmental specialists Murray Feshbach and Alfred Friendly, Jr., of Georgetown University, Washington, D.C., have described the environmental crisis in Eurasia by noting that "no other great industrial civilization so systematically and so long poisoned its air, land, water, and people. None so loudly proclaiming its efforts to improve public health and protect nature so degraded both." Over two mil-

A child in Ukraine tests the atmosphere for radioactivity. Millions of Ukrainians and Belorussians live in areas highly contaminated by fallout from the 1986 accident at the Chernobyl nuclear power station.

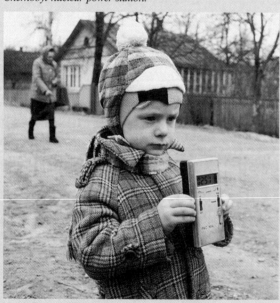

lion Ukrainians and Belorussians need to be relocated from areas affected by the loss of radioactive containment at Chernobyl; 70% of the total radioactive fallout from the world's worst nuclear catastrophe landed on Belarus, and 3 million of its 10 million people still live in contaminated areas. Researchers from Belarus have reported a dramatic increase in childhood thyroid cancer (from an average of 4 cases a year before the Chernobyl fallout to about 60 afterward). In the city of Gomel alone, the thyroid cancer rate is now about 80 times the world average.

Eurasian and eastern European environmental decay stem from a history of forced industrialization that espoused a philosophy of growth at any cost. Production was long emphasized over efficiency; centrally planned and controlled industries were shielded from competition and felt no need to improve efficiency or to adopt cleaner modern technologies. The Czech Republic has some of the highest levels of air pollution in all of Europe; the government estimates that 60% (six million) of its people live in highly polluted areas. An estimated 35% of the Russian population living in 103 cities is exposed to air-pollution levels that are five times the allowable limits in most industrialized nations. Eurasia, with only one-tenth the number of automobiles, has two-thirds the amount of U.S. pollution from autos.

The Baltic Sea is dying from chemical and heavy metal pollution. The 3,530 km (2,200 mi) of the Volga River constituted the heart of the Soviet military-industrial complex, and dams, hydroelectric plants, and 3,000 factories spewing waste are destroying its ecology. The radioactively contaminated Techa River is considered by ecologists to be one of the deadliest rivers on Earth. In the town of Muslimovo, Russia, on the banks on the river, high rates of tumors, stillbirths, and anemia are reported, which the local people call "the river disease." The Siberian forests are disappearing at a rate that may pose a greater threat to the global environment than the destruction of the Brazilian rain forests. Roughly 900,000 bbl of oil, or one in 10, produced daily in Russia are spilled—equivalent to a single *Exxon Valdez* spill every six hours!

Eurasian nations are too poor to rebuild their economies and, at the same time, repair ecological damage. This situation is compounded by the lack of an ecologically sensitive culture and by a history of social fatalism.

Populations on the move

A disintegrating public health system will add incentives for Eurasians and eastern Europeans to emigrate as a way to escape the many ills of their societies. In 1993 more than 600,000 former Soviet citizens were on the move within Eurasia, and up to three million may move to other nations in the next few years. Internal migration will increase as 25 million ethnic Russians living in other former Soviet republics seek security within Russia or beyond Eurasia (this figure represents just one group among the 60 million Eurasians living outside their homelands). The demobilization of four million troops will add to the problem, overburdening an already-taxed civilian health system.

Among the threats posed by migration are: an increased incidence of disease through dislocation, exposure to new agents of disease, and breakdown of access to health services and good nutrition. With economic declines of 20% or higher expected for each of the coming years, the creation in Eurasia of economic as well as ecological refugees is probable. The Organization for Economic Cooperation and Development has warned, however, that the industrialized nations will be unable to absorb a vast number of immigrants from the former Soviet Union over a short time.

Crumbling health care infrastructure

The infrastructure for health in Eurasia and eastern Europe is in decay. While the numbers of physicians and hospital beds in Eurasia are comparable to those in western Europe, Eurasian health care relies excessively on the hospital as a provider of primary services. A fundamental reorienting of health care systems is needed to shift from hospital-centered services to community-based primary care and prevention. A major danger is that existing health- and social-protection systems may be overwhelmed by fiscal pressures and new shortages in supply.

With the fall of the centralized Ministry of Health of the U.S.S.R., the future of medical and public health research, education, and norms of practice in Eurasia is in question. The former Soviet Union once could boast of having the world's largest workforce of trained scientists (twice that of the United States), but a "brain drain" is occurring because of harsh economic conditions and the inability of laboratories to meet payrolls. Eurasian physicians are struggling to redefine their professional roles after decades during which the public at large lacked faith in the medical profession. Because there are few general practitioners, medical practice is dominated by excessive specialization. Official neglect of, or only rhetorical support for, preventive health care is a legacy of communism. Health care personnel need to be retrained to provide more prevention-oriented and primary care services. Eurasian sources state that many primary care physicians are poorly trained, and a collaborative mission of the United Nations Children's Fund and the World Health Organization to Central Asia in February 1992 found that many outdated and questionable clinical practices were common (such as giving the average child about 40 injections per year—many of which are

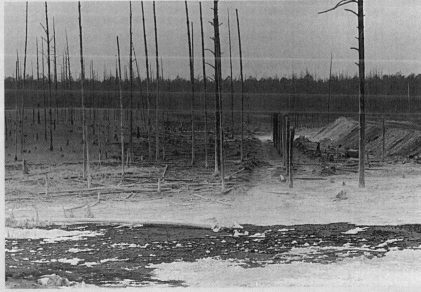

Foam from a chemical plant has killed the trees of this Siberian forest. In the former Soviet Union, industrial pollution, especially from chemicals and heavy metals, has damaged great stretches of land and water and caused severe health problems for many people.

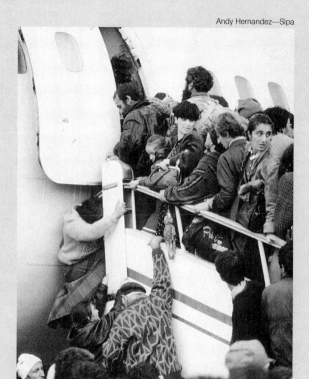

Georgians seeking refuge from their country's continuing turmoil crowd aboard a flight. Vast internal migration is already placing heavy burdens on overstrained Eurasian health systems, and migration in coming years is expected to rise.

for the most trivial ailments). Minor illnesses among the populations often result in hospital admissions, which in itself has associated infection risks. Eurasian physicians now will have to earn the public's trust in their abilities as well as improve their expertise as health care providers.

Although there are numerous hospitals, they and other health care facilities are very unevenly distributed, and many are inadequate. Inefficiency and inequity pervade the health care system, and there is a deep public distrust of government central planning and paternalism. The Soviet Union spent one-eighth the amount the U.S. does on centrally planned health services and less than half the average of what the industrialized nations spend. Current spending is 3–4% of gross domestic product (GDP), compared with 6.5% in the United Kingdom and 13% in the U.S. A number of Eurasia's and eastern Europe's public health problems are caused by the erosion of hard-currency income; this is occurring largely as a result of spiraling inflation and the removal of restrictions on retail prices for basic commodities. Health services have been financed from central government revenues, but a large black-market economy exists with extensive use of tips and gifts to health care providers (who have been historically underpaid), which contribute up to 30% of their total salaries.

Centralized Soviet assets used in health research and practice have been nationalized by each new Eurasian state. However, the process of nationalization has not occurred equitably, leaving some former republics relatively well endowed and others (particularly in Central Asia and autonomous areas of the Far East) in potential crisis. The Russian Federation has inherited most of the public health resources and equipment of the former Soviet Union but cannot support its network of hospitals and research facilities.

The failure of centralized economies, combined with exhaustive military spending, has caused major economic stagnation over the past decades. Government data confirm that over 71 million former Soviets are destitute, living on an equivalent of U.S. $15 a month or less. Indeed, many of the health problems described above are emerging during the greatest period of economic transition and social dislocation to which a civilian population in nonwartime has been subjected in this century.

Obstacles to reform

The lack of economic stabilization stands as the greatest obstacle to sustainable health care reform in Eurasia and eastern Europe. The most important task facing each nation will be to restructure its industrial base and regenerate the economy. While the economic problems are both complex and broad, and thus can be discussed here only to a limited extent, it is certain that an effective restructuring of the health systems of these nations will not be possible until basic economic issues such as the nature of private ownership, interconvertibility of currencies, inflation, and other hurdles to market-based economies are overcome. Any general strategic intervention in the economic sector needs to consider health care issues, which, if unattended, will deteriorate and may undermine overall economic recovery. It will be more cost-effective to address certain issues immediately, rather than allow crises to emerge that later might require massive international humanitarian aid packages.

The health services sector needs large sums of money to overcome the consequences of previous government policies. Decentralization of manufacturing will be essential prior to the development of manufacturing capabilities for health care supplies and technology. The most immediate requirements are for new equipment and drugs, means to halt deterioration of the health infrastructure, and funds to compensate for low wages in the health sector. Foreign business interests that will be vital in supporting the health sectors of the newly emerged Eurasian states must be confident both in their ability to repatriate profits and in the long-term political stability of the region.

Seventy years of communism and the sociocultural and political climate have made it doctrinally difficult to endorse the idea of free enterprise in health services.

Fear of the repercussions of privatization is strong among the public, physicians, and medical administrators. Concerns have been expressed that reform may be derailed by the hardships people will have to endure during this transformation and that regression to authoritarian government could be imminent. To a large extent, health care reform must await economic recovery; in the process, however, there is the risk that deteriorating health conditions and lack of access to care will exacerbate human misery and add to political destabilization.

Searching for solutions

What measures *can* be taken in the near term to facilitate improvements in health services and health status and thus possibly ease the social transition? As Eurasian and eastern European nations recast themselves politically, economically, and socially, a process of rigorous critical self-examination is occurring. Eurasians are looking to Western concepts and institutions such as democracy, government accountability, and free-market economics as potential models.

As an economic and military superpower, the United States is understandably the object of much Eurasian reform interest. The U.S., however, continues to struggle with its own "health crisis"; 37 million citizens lack any health insurance, and one-fourth of the population is underinsured. The U.S. ranks 20th internationally in infant mortality and 9th in life expectancy at birth. These figures are shocking, especially in light of the size of the nation's health expenditures, which amount to 13% of GDP.

Eurasian and eastern European health planners are faced with strategic choices in restructuring health care, and few desirable or applicable models offer guidance. Eurasians need to resist the temptation of emulating and duplicating the U.S. health care experience. In assessing options for reform, it may be ill-advised for Eurasians and eastern Europeans to discard all values that have been associated (at least rhetorically) with socialism. Abandoning the objective of universal access to health care in the movement to a market economy could be regressive. As a command economy is decentralized and privatized, it may be unwise to diminish the contributions of modern governments to health care infrastructure, medical research, and disease monitoring and prevention.

Opportunities for reform. Eurasian and eastern European populations have high rates of literacy and educational attainment, and concepts of disease causation, prevention, and public health are largely derived from modern medicine. There is less polarization with respect to sex and less repression of women than in many less developed nations. Because international health interventions frequently rely upon the development of women's knowledge and skills to promote health and prevent disease, the women of eastern Europe and several Eurasian nations represent ideal candidates for targeting effective assistance. Pediatric nutrition or immunization programs, for example, can benefit from women's higher status and educational levels. Shifting from the delivery of services centered in hospitals and clinics to prevention of disease in the community is another measure that will be critical. Further, major shifts in health-related behaviors are needed. For example, cigarette smoking, which is particularly widespread, must be reduced. Lung cancer rates among young men in eastern Europe are approaching the highest levels ever recorded and will be reflected in declining life expectancy.

Because the public associates free health care with substandard care, a co-payment system of insurance is likely in the development of a new health infrastructure. Russia, for example, has proposed employer-based health insurance and decentralized, competitive bidding for hospital and specialty care; as of 1993,

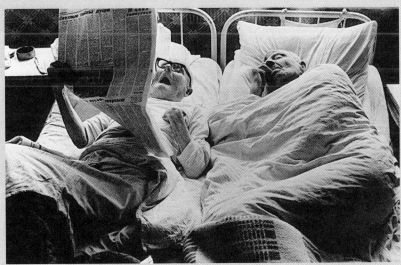

Pozerskis—Rapho

The beds of these aged pensioners have been pushed together in a crowded Russian hospice. Health care reform in Eurasia must await economic recovery. Meanwhile, deteriorating health conditions and lack of access to care could well exacerbate the extent of human misery.

hospitals were to begin charging for services, with payment by private or state-run insurance companies. The problem with employer-paid insurance, however, is that large portions of entire industries are losing money, and wages are far too low for employees to be required to pay. One in seven companies may go bankrupt, and new ones that are key to economic recovery are the least able to afford health insurance. It remains unclear how a safety net can be created for the millions expected to become unemployed by the time the new system is fully operational and for the millions of others caught in the transitional phase who must pay for insurance themselves.

As already noted, Eurasia needs much greater integration of services, bringing together disparate elements of primary health care into comprehensive service programs. Consolidation of the nearly 24,000 small hospitals (four times the number found in the U.S.) that consume 80% of the health care budget will be essential. Vital to improving public health status will be improved coordination of regional systems and redistribution of health facilities as well as strengthening of health services in rural areas. Efforts to improve management skills of both health care facilities and insurance funds are needed. At the same time, competent evaluations will need to be carried out to assess effectiveness of health care provision. Medical training will need to be restructured, with a much greater focus on primary care. Wage increases for medical personnel will be necessary throughout the region, and the numbers are daunting: Russia alone has about 700,000 physicians, 1.8 million nurses, and 1.3 million other health workers.

Entrepreneurial support. The vehicle of joint business ventures is one option that could provide new opportunities for international public health collaboration between the West and Eurasia/eastern Europe. As Eurasian and eastern European business sectors develop, thousands of multinational corporations will be competing for the new markets. Governments could optimally seek to ensure coordinated social and economic development that balances public and private as well as domestic and international interests. Health ministries could encourage international joint ventures with Western businesses that voluntarily integrate public health programs related to the venture product or service. Thus, as entrepreneurial activities develop, there would be strengthening of public health at a low cost.

One approach might be to use distribution networks for specific consumer products or services for health education and promotion. Even product advertising could include specific health messages. Foreign automotive manufacturers, for example, could collaborate with Eurasian governments in establishing vehicular safety and seat belt or child seat education programs. Food suppliers might conduct nutrition education pro-

grams as part of their product promotions. Because television is available in nearly 90% of Eurasian homes, this could provide an opportunity for extensive health education.

Newly acquired management skills that have proved effective in Eurasian and eastern European businesses might also be applied directly to health. As computer-based information systems in the civilian sector undergo rapid development in a market economy, these could be linked with, and utilized for, product-related health communications.

Very importantly, pacing reform through public-private integration of health responsibilities and activities in the above manner has the potential to reduce public anxiety by demonstrating that private-sector involvement in health care does not mean a loss of social equity or universal access to care. As Eurasian and eastern European societies become more socio-economically stratified in a market economy, government and international business contributions to health can mitigate resentment and decrease risk of a public backlash from citizens who feel disenfranchised from social advancement. Moreover, engaging Western business interests may increase the net health resources available to the region. Public-private health collaboration through joint ventures offers governments the ability to integrate private economic growth with continuing public sector contributions to social welfare, and resource savings may be generated in the long term from the prevention of disease.

What the West can do. Many Eurasian and eastern European health problems can be prevented or rapidly remediated. Improved disease surveillance, reduction of health-jeopardizing behaviors through health education, and environmental improvement would offer substantial gains and help reverse the regional decline in health status. These strategies need not be very costly. For the most part, the Eurasian states fall between the industrialized and less developed nations in terms of socioeconomic level of development and major health indicators. People are in better health than in the Third World, and reorienting and expanding existing public health activities may greatly improve health outcomes through a modest investment of aid targeted at specific components of the health care system.

Huge outlays of Western international aid are not of themselves a solution; moreover, such outlays seem unlikely in light of the pressing economic problems in the West and the persistence of need among traditional aid recipients in the Third World. Western aid can also have the counterproductive outcome of encouraging dependency. Therefore, building capacity within Eurasia and eastern Europe for state-of-the-art professional training of current and future health care providers is much more likely to achieve a broad-based strengthening of the primary care and public health systems—and to do so at a cost the West can afford.

Important educational reforms in the health professions can come about only if there is Western collaboration with Eurasian and eastern European institutions to formulate culturally appropriate primary care and public health curricula. These curricula need to focus on prevention of disease and health promotion and to address both the sociocultural heterogeneity that is found in Eurasia and eastern Europe and the differing levels of baseline health that exist from nation to nation. Considerable differences also occur regionally within larger states such as Russia. For example, most health indicators in Russia deteriorate as one moves from Moscow to Central Asia and the Far East (Siberian male life expectancy, for example, is 48 years, compared with 64 years for male Moscovites). Curricula thus need to be developed with at least three variants—Europeanized, Islamic Central Asian, and Far Eastern. If international expertise assists Eurasian and eastern European primary care and public health training efforts without projecting a Western or any specific national model on these populations, the people of these nations would benefit from improved delivery of public health services by better trained, more highly skilled practitioners. Undoubtedly, an epidemiological impact would be observed in reduced morbidity and mortality.

Beyond philanthropy: interdependence in health

Despite the possibilities just described for Western assistance to help Eurasia emerge from its present health crisis, it may not be entirely clear why such aid would be in donor (Western) self-interest. In other words, what benefits will the West in general (and the United States in particular) derive from offering health assistance to these new states?

U.S.-Eurasian interdependence already exists at many levels and in many sectors in addition to health. The development of new markets for a wide variety of U.S. products to improve global trading opportunities is vital to the U.S. and other economies. Eurasia represents the most sophisticated untapped market for international trade in the world and as such is crucial to the economic future of the West. Without a decent health infrastructure, Eurasia is unlikely to become a major trading partner for Western nations. Health care is one of the largest and most rapidly expanding sectors in many Western economies, and in an increasingly competitive global economy the lessons learned and linkages formed through international health contacts will benefit future trade partnerships. Indeed, international business interests will inevitably benefit from product publicity and positive public image building that results from promoting health.

While decent health care is no panacea for preventing Eurasian political instability, it is obvious that deprivation of food and medicine, so vital to health, would serve only to foment social dissatisfaction and political extremism. Military spending by most Western nations continues to be high, and the waning of the Soviet threat has fueled hopes for conversion of these resources to domestic needs. This may not be possible, however, if Eurasian political dialogue decays and civil unrest becomes widespread, as has occurred in the former Yugoslavia. Assistance to improve the Eurasian health infrastructure is one of the best and least costly strategies for preventing such regional civil deterioration.

In terms of health per se, because Eurasia represents one of the largest populations in the world as yet relatively uninfected by HIV, the threat of the disease's spread must be addressed. Global AIDS control will be even more elusive than it already is if the industrialized nations do not aggressively seize the opportunity to avert an epidemic in this region.

The magnitude of the environmental crisis in Eurasia, which constitutes one-sixth of the planetary landmass, has direct implications for Western nations. There are at least 1,200 radioactive waste sites in Eurasia, and as many as 17,000 containers of solid and liquid nuclear waste have been dumped into ocean waters. The repercussions in Europe of the Chernobyl nuclear catastrophe are still being felt, which clearly argues against viewing such matters as a purely national problem. (Fifteen other Chernobyl-type reactors are still in operation in Eurasia.) Similar situations exist for many other nonradioactive pollutants of global concern; thus, environmental interdependence is intimately related to the health status of all nations.

The large and sophisticated health systems of the West surely have something to offer (albeit lessons learned through failure as well as success) to these newly emerging states. Nonetheless, many will wonder why, after spending trillions of dollars building defenses against the Soviet Union, and with significant economic problems of their own, the industrialized nations should now offer health assistance to their former foes.

Today the most credible strategic threats from Eurasia emanate not from its military force, four million strong, but from political instability, ethnic violence, border violations, and mass migration of refugees. The West should recognize its collective self-interest in trying to manage global health problems—a task that will be virtually impossible *without* capable Eurasian partners. Persistent deterioration in health status will only fuel political and social radicalization. The West is in a position to implement cost-effective strategies to assist the underserved peoples of Eurasia, strengthen and expand programs to control regional and global health problems, and by so doing support the continued evolution of pluralistic, democratic civil societies in this large region of the world.

Genetics

The year 1993 marked the 40th anniversary of the elucidation of the molecular structure of DNA. The commemoration of this momentous discovery prompted many biologists to reflect upon the progress that has been made in the science of genetics. James Watson (corecipient with Francis Crick and Maurice Wilkins of the 1962 Nobel Prize for Physiology or Medicine for their explication of DNA's structure) observed that, by his reckoning, genetics was now in its sixth period. According to Watson, the science has passed through: (1) the Mendelian era, when observing the transmission of physical traits from one generation to another was the key to visualizing genes in action; (2) the DNA era, when the workings of that molecule became apparent; (3) the period of the genetic code, in which scientists learned how the information encoded by DNA is translated into proteins; (4) the era of gene control, in which biologists became aware of the roles of certain DNA sequences that act as "off" and "on" switches in the process of transcribing the genetic information; and (5) the era of recombinant DNA technology, in which genes are copied and harnessed to produce their protein products in quantity.

The present period, which Watson characterized as the era of human genome sequencing, is expected to yield a description and location of each of the approximately 100,000 human genes. The use of tests based on the genes identified to date has brought scientists to the threshold of a seventh period—the era of genetic prediction, in which, Watson foresees, medical geneticists will be able to diagnose a vast number of disorders by identifying the genetic aberration responsible long before the disorders become manifest.

Huntington's gene: long road to discovery

The identification of the Huntington's disease gene in March 1993 was greeted with jubilation and relief. Although the investigators had discovered early in their research that the gene is located near the tip of the short arm of chromosome 4, the gene itself eluded them for almost a decade. Their quest was frustrated by false leads, dead ends, and unexpected setbacks.

Huntington's disease is a progressive neurological disorder that does not manifest itself until the fourth or fifth decade of life. It is characterized by uncontrollable movement and dementia and is ultimately fatal. About 30,000 people in the U.S. are affected, and another 150,000 are at risk of developing the disease.

In the early 1980s a team led by psychologist Nancy Wexler of the Hereditary Disease Foundation, Santa Monica, Calif., and molecular biologist James Gusella of Massachusetts General Hospital, Boston, collected hundreds of blood samples from Venezuelan families in whom Huntington's was widespread. They then extracted samples of DNA from white blood cells. By comparing the DNA of people who had the disease with that of relatives who had escaped it, the investigators were able to identify so-called molecular markers, characteristic sequences of DNA that heralded the disease gene within a given family. The markers became the basis of a prenatal diagnostic test that was about 97% accurate in predicting the likelihood of an individual's developing the disease. Having come this far, Gusella and Wexler felt certain that the gene itself would be found quickly. They were thus unprepared for the many obstacles and disappointments they would encounter over the next nine years.

The effort to identify the Huntington's gene was noteworthy for several reasons other than its duration and difficulty. One is that the search firmly established a new term, *RFLP* (or "riflip"), in the biologist's vernacular. The term is an acronym for restriction-fragment length polymorphism—a distinctive stretch of DNA that differs in length among different individuals. RFLPs have enabled scientists to trace the manifestation of disease through the generations of an affected family

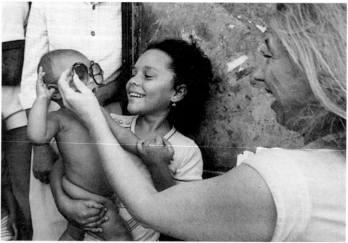

Venezuelan children have some fun with Nancy Wexler, one of the leaders of the decade-long quest for the Huntington's disease gene. Venezuelan villagers were instrumental in the research that led to the identification of the gene in March 1993.

and ultimately to the actual DNA responsible for the defect. In such a quest, geneticists are guided by RFLP markers, which, while they may not be associated with any observable traits, seem to accompany the disease gene as it is passed through the generations. If the gene and the marker remain closely associated, biologists assume that they lie close together on the chromosome. By examining DNA from members of several affected families, researchers can develop a wide assortment of markers, enabling them gradually to close in on the disease-causing gene.

Another remarkable feature of the Huntington's investigation is that it underscored the advantage of collaborative efforts in finding genes. Although the search began as a competition between several teams of investigators, it ended up as a collective effort of the Huntington's Disease Collaborative Research Group, which included 58 scientists from a number of institutions in the U.S. and the U.K.

Finally, the hunt for the Huntington's gene illustrated the importance of scientific tenacity. Although by the mid-1980s the map of chromosome 4 was peppered with markers that seemed to be close to the actual gene, there was no indication which stretch of DNA harbored it. The gene's location near the telomere, or end, of the chromosome also enhanced its ability to escape detection because the researchers were unable to home in on it from two directions.

The point of greatest interest in the newly identified gene is the repetition of a sequence of three of the nucleotides, or bases, that constitute DNA—cytosine, adenine, and guanine (CAG). In those who have the disease, this CAG triplet is repeated not once but many times, in what some authorities have referred to as a "stuttering," or "accordion," effect and others have likened to the action of an office copying machine gone berserk. The number of repetitions present appears to vary proportionately with the intensity of the disease. Thus, when the researchers examined the gene in 173 people who were not at risk for the disease, they found that most had fewer than 24 repetitions of the CAG triplet. In comparison, the number of these trinucleotide repeats in Huntington's patients ranged from 42 to 100. People who have the greatest number of repetitions seem to develop the disease earlier and have more devastating cases. Moreover, the repetitions seem to foster a climate of genetic instability conducive to further mutation, resulting in further increases in the number of repetitions in successive generations.

Although scientists do not yet know the function of the protein for which the gene codes, given the name *huntingtin* by the research collaborators, identification of the gene has provided medical science with a powerful diagnostic tool. By calculating the number of CAG repetitions in people at risk, geneticists can determine not only whether they will develop the disorder but approximately when they will begin to have the first signs of the condition. The same procedure could also potentially detect individuals who have higher-than-normal numbers of repetitions but no evidence of the disease. Although such people are at little risk of developing the illness themselves, their children are likely to have even more CAG repeats and thus an increased risk of Huntington's disease.

"Stuttering" genes

The Huntington's gene is not the first such "stuttering" gene to be associated with hereditary disease. A similar pattern of trinucleotide repeat mutations is shared by three other disorders: myotonic dystrophy, a debilitating neuromuscular disorder; Kennedy disease (also called X-linked spinal and bulbar muscular atrophy), a degenerative neurological disorder; and fragile X syndrome, the most common genetic cause of mental retardation. In all four of these diseases, the mutation is characterized as "dynamic." Unlike static mutations, which are responsible for most previously identified hereditary disorders, dynamic mutations are not likely to be copied intact from parental DNA. Instead, they are apt to be subject to additional mutation and, in most cases, produce escalating numbers of the repeated DNA sequence in each succeeding generation. For example, a team of Baylor University (Waco, Texas) researchers studying myotonic dystrophy reported in April 1993 that among 110 parent-child pairs at risk for the disorder, mothers who had no symptoms and had as few as 50 trinucleotide repeat mutations bore children with more than 700 repetitions. These children had evidence of the condition at birth. (There were also some instances in which fewer repetitions were seen in subsequent generations.)

Scientists speculate that the increase in the number of trinucleotide repetitions is due to the activity of DNA polymerase, the enzyme entrusted with copying DNA sequences during replication. They theorize that the polymerase gets "stuck" on a particular sequence, in much the same way as a needle on a scratchy record becomes trapped in a single groove. At present, geneticists counseling prospective parents at risk for any of these disorders cannot predict the number of trinucleotide repetitions a parent may pass on to a child. They have, however, developed some benchmarks for each disease, enabling them to distinguish a normal number of repetitions from numbers signaling that a person is at risk of having offspring with the disease and numbers likely to represent full-blown disease.

Lorenzo's gene

The identification of the gene for X-linked adrenoleukodystrophy (ALD), the disorder now familiar to many people from the movie *Lorenzo's Oil,* was reported in February 1993, just as the film was finishing a long run in U.S. theaters. However, it was not yet apparent whether the discovery, made by a team of investigators from the U.S., France, and Germany, would lead to a treatment for ALD more effective than the mixture of erucic acid and oleic acid concocted by Augusto and Michaela Odone for their son, Lorenzo.

There are two primary forms of ALD, both of which affect only males and thus have been assumed to be transmitted by a defective gene on the X chromosome. (Since males have one X and one Y chromosome—as opposed to females' two X's—a defective gene on the X chromosome would not have a normal counterpart.) Childhood ALD usually begins between ages 5 and 12 and progresses rapidly, devastating the central nervous system within a few years. The adult form, called adrenomyeloneuropathy, arises between the ages of 15 and 30 and may affect only the adrenal glands and the peripheral nerves. Both versions are known to be a result of failure of the body to break down fatty acids. The accumulation of long chains of fats in cells somehow destroys the myelin sheaths covering the nerves and interferes with adrenal function.

In searching for a genetic aberration that might be responsible for ALD, the international team turned its sights on genes that encode proteins found in peroxisomes, specialized organlike structures in the cell membrane. Peroxisomes are responsible for a variety of metabolic functions, including the oxidation of fatty acids to provide energy. The researchers intended to purify their prime suspect, VLCFA-CoA synthetase—an enzyme that plays a role in breaking down very long-chain fatty acids—and to use the genetic code for the enzyme to devise a synthetic gene capable of encoding it. The synthetic gene, which would bind to its counterpart on the X chromosome, could then be used to find the VLCFA-CoA synthetase gene.

When they were unable to purify the enzyme, the researchers were forced to pursue an alternative strategy. They searched the DNA of families at risk for ALD, looking for markers on the X chromosome in individuals who either were carriers of ALD or had the disease. They then copied several DNA sequences near the markers and tested each one to determine what kind of proteins it encoded. The gene that seemed to fit the bill encoded a protein the investigators named ALDP, which helped to transport molecules into the peroxisome. When they looked at the DNA of individuals with ALD, the research team found that many people had obvious mutations in the ALDP gene. ALDP probably works by carrying the enzyme VLCFA-CoA synthetase into the peroxisome, but more research is necessary to verify the role of the protein and to determine how this information might be used to develop a treatment for ALD.

Other successful searches

In addition to the finding of the genes for Huntington's disease and ALD, the past year was marked by

several reports of success in efforts to identify other disease-causing genes. Researchers at the University of Washington announced that they had found a gene on chromosome 14 that, when defective, causes a rare familial form of Alzheimer's disease. Previous studies had linked inherited forms of the disease to genes on chromosomes 19 and 21. The new finding prompted authorities in the field to speculate that a variety of biological pathways may lead to this dementing illness.

An international team led by Robert H. Brown, Jr., at Massachusetts General Hospital in Boston, Robert Horvitz at the Massachusetts Institute of Technology, and Teepu Siddique at Northwestern University Medical School in Chicago identified a gene on chromosome 21 that they believe is responsible for many cases of amyotrophic lateral sclerosis (ALS), the degenerative neurological disorder also known as Lou Gehrig's disease. The gene directs the synthesis of an enzyme called superoxide dismutase, which destroys highly reactive compounds that apparently damage motor nerves. Two other genes code for different forms of the enzyme, and the same researchers were investigating the possibility that mutations in these genes may cause other forms of the paralyzing disorder.

One particularly remarkable ALS patient is Stephen Hawking, the brilliant English physicist who has survived for nearly three decades with a disease that is usually fatal within five years after symptoms appear. In 1992 Hawking was the subject of a documentary based on his life and his best-selling book about the universe, *A Brief History of Time.*

Other announcements of the past year concerned the discovery of the genetic defect that causes severe combined immunodeficiency (SCID), the congenital disorder that affected the Houston, Texas, youngster—David—who lived most of his 12 years in a sterile "bubble" because his immune system was unable to fight infections; a gene identified by Finnish researchers as either a cause of non-insulin-dependent (type 2) diabetes or a marker for the pathogenic gene that leads to development of the common, adult-onset form of the metabolic disorder; and a mutation responsible for familial hypertrophic cardiomyopathy, a type of heart disease that, if undetected, can cause sudden death in young people, notably athletes.

Cancer genetics

While all forms of cancer involve mutations in genes that regulate cell growth and proliferation, most of these changes occur over the course of a lifetime. A few such mutations are inherited, however, and therefore the gene defect is present at birth. In 1993 investigators came closer to identifying two such genes, one responsible for breast cancer and one believed to predispose those who inherit it to colon and possibly other cancers.

Breast cancer and the BRCA1 gene. Inherited muta-

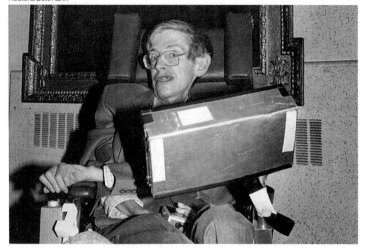

With the aid of an electronic voice synthesizer, Stephen Hawking, the brilliant physicist who suffers from amyotrophic lateral sclerosis (ALS), announces the publication of his book A Brief History of Time *in 1988. Confined to a wheelchair most of his adult life, Hawking has nonetheless lived many years longer than most of those stricken with the degenerative neurological disorder. In 1993 an international team of scientists studying ALS found a gene they believe is responsible for one form of the disorder.*

tions in three genes—p53, a tumor suppressor; ER, the estrogen receptor; and BRCA1, the function of which is yet to be identified—have been associated with breast cancer. Of these, the gene called BRCA1, which has been traced to chromosome 17, seems to be responsible for the disease in families at high risk for the disease and in families in which both breast and ovarian cancers are highly prevalent.

In April 1993 researchers from the University of Michigan and the Dana-Farber Cancer Institute, Boston, reported that they had used molecular markers on chromosome 17 to identify those women in families with high rates of breast cancer, ovarian cancer, or both who have inherited the abnormal form of the BRCA1 gene.

Cancer specialists believe that inherited gene defects are responsible for 5 to 10% of all cases of breast and ovarian cancer and are carried by one woman in 200–400. Women who inherit a defective copy of the BRCA1 gene are estimated to have an 85% chance of developing breast cancer over their lifetime. On the other hand, women in the same family who have not inherited the defect are likely to have only a 10–11% lifetime risk—the same as the general population.

The researchers predicted that once the gene itself had been identified, a test for the defective form could be made available to millions of women. They cautioned, however, that widespread genetic testing for breast cancer could have enormous social, psychological, and economic ramifications.

Colon cancer gene. Over the past few years several genes, including p53 and DCC, have been implicated in the sequence of cellular mutations that leads to the development of colon cancer. In May 1993 a collaborative group of Finnish and U.S. researchers announced the discovery of a gene that may be responsible for a cell's susceptibility to such mutations. Although the gene has not been specifically identified, a trail of markers has led the investigators to chro-

mosome 2. The gene, which may be carried by one in every 200 people, was dubbed "FCC" for "familial colon cancer" by team leaders Albert de la Chapelle of the University of Helsinki, Fin., and Bert Vogelstein of Johns Hopkins University School of Medicine, Baltimore, Md. Its activation appears to trigger a host of mutations on a variety of chromosomes, perhaps by provoking errors in the DNA-copying process that precedes cell division.

Human Genome Project: three years of progress

As the international effort to identify, map, and sequence every human gene progressed, those involved were optimistic that the task would be completed in advance of the 2006 target date. Craig Venter, a former National Institutes of Health (NIH) researcher, who established the Institute for Genomic Research in Germantown, Md., in 1992, has predicted that a nearly complete account of the human genome will be available on computer by mid-1994. Venter's projection was dependent on the use of robotic sequencers, which are currently capable of identifying 500 to 1,000 gene sequences a day. This rate attests to the rapid acceleration of the pace of gene identification since the inception of the project; the number of genes identified during all of 1988, for example, was slightly over 700. Daniel Cohen of the Center for the Study of Human Polymorphism, Paris, made similar predictions, vowing to produce a physical map on which genetic markers are aligned according to the actual number of DNA bases between them.

Predictions of an early conclusion to the project seemed plausible in light of the announcement in October 1992 that two chromosomes—Y and 21— had been completely mapped, the former by David Page and colleagues at the Whitehead Institute, Cambridge, Mass., and the latter by researchers at the Paris center. Both groups produced physical maps on which genetic markers, formerly located only by genetic linkage (their relative distance from one another), were aligned according to the actual number of DNA bases between them. At the same time, scientists in Paris and at the NIH published linkage maps for 23 other chromosomes. Not only is the acceleration of gene mapping expected to bring to a close the era of concerted searches for single genes—like those responsible for Huntington's disease and ALD—but identifying most remaining genes is expected to come as a matter of course, an outcome of the stunning progress of just three years' work.

Folic acid and birth defects

In September 1992 the U.S. Public Health Service (PHS) recommended folic acid supplementation for all women of childbearing age—a low-tech but apparently highly effective approach to preventing birth defects. Folic acid, a water-soluble vitamin involved with vitamin B_{12} in DNA synthesis, seems to affect the occurrence of the group of congenital abnormalities known collectively as neural tube defects (NTDs). Each year about 2,500 babies in the U.S. alone are born with NTDs; the most common are anencephaly—in which the brain does not develop fully—and spina bifida—in which the tissue surrounding the spinal cord fails to completely cover it.

Folic acid had for many years been believed to help prevent recurrence of NTDs and was prescribed during pregnancy for women who had previously borne affected infants. The PHS based its new recommendation on the early results of a Hungarian study indicating that women who take supplemental folic acid from at least one month before conception through the third month of pregnancy significantly reduce the risk of NTDs. A subsequent U.S. study, reported in March 1993, indicated that a 0.4-mg dose—the amount usually included in commercial multivitamin supplements (and twice the recommended daily dietary allowance)—is enough to prevent NTDs. Moreover, unlike the higher folic acid doses that have been recommended in past studies, the 0.4-mg dose will not disguise the effects of vitamin B_{12} deficiency, which, if undetected, can cause neurological damage in women.

Prenatal diagnosis: safety questioned

Meanwhile, several reports raised fears that chorionic villus sampling (CVS), a high-tech approach to prenatal diagnosis of birth defects, might be causing congenital abnormalities rather than helping to identify them. CVS is a technique in which a few placental cells are extracted via a fine hollow needle inserted into the womb. DNA extracted from these cells is subsequently examined for genetic defects. Because CVS can be performed as early as the eighth week of pregnancy, it allows women more time to consider the option of terminating the pregnancy than does amniocentesis, which is commonly performed after the 15th week.

By June 1992 three separate reports, from England, Italy, and the U.S., indicated an unexpectedly high rate of certain birth defects—missing or shortened fingers and toes and malformed jaws or tongues—among babies born to women who had undergone CVS. Other, larger studies had found no such defects, however.

That same month, the NIH and the American College of Obstetricians and Gynecologists convened an international conference to evaluate the safety of the procedure. Several experts speculated that abnormalities like the ones reported might result from the disruption of blood flow to the placenta during CVS. Others believed that the defects resulted from a lack of skill on the part of physicians performing the procedure rather than being an effect of the procedure itself. The groups concluded that the evidence was not strong enough to advise women to avoid CVS. Nonetheless, many experts now believe the procedure is not as safe as it was originally thought to be.

Dad's legacy

While mothers-to-be have long been warned not to smoke, drink alcohol, or engage in other unhealthy behaviors during pregnancy, evidence is beginning to indicate that prospective fathers should also avoid certain risky exposures. At the first multidisciplinary conference of its kind, held at the University of Pittsburgh, Pa., in September 1992, a group of scientists considered mounting evidence that paternal exposure to certain environmental toxins can produce birth defects. The panel agreed that studies had failed to demonstrate an elevated risk of childhood leukemia in the offspring of men occupationally exposed to radiation, but they found reason to suspect that paternal exposure to chemicals such as solvents and pesticides may indeed be responsible for birth defects.

A study by researchers at Temple University, Philadelphia, reported in October 1992, suggested that cocaine can filter into seminal fluid and bind to sperm. Because the substance does not impair sperm function, it is carried into the egg. Although paternal cocaine use has not yet been linked to any specific birth defects, it apparently may have damaging potential.

Many researchers are now calling for additional studies to determine exactly how damaged sperm may produce developmental abnormalities. Most authorities agree that the conventional wisdom—which holds that damaged sperm are harmless because they are rendered incapable of fertilization—needs to be revised. The March of Dimes Birth Defects Foundation agrees. It has launched a "Men Have Babies, Too" campaign to inform dads-to-be of their role in ensuring the health of their offspring.

—*Beverly Merz*

Special Report
Reflections on Solving the DNA Puzzle
by Francis H.C. Crick, Ph.D.

We wish to suggest a structure for the salt of deoxyribose nucleic acid (DNA). This structure has novel features which are of considerable biological interest.
—*Nature*, April 25, 1953

Forty years ago, in April 1953, James D. Watson and I suggested that DNA had the shape of a very long double helix, consisting of two chains twined round one another and fitting neatly together so that the shape of each was the precise complement of the other. A month later we spelled out just how such a structure might be replicated in the cells. These ideas made it highly plausible that genes were made of DNA and that the genetic information was carried by the precise sequence of DNA's four bases, or building blocks (simple compounds known as adenine, guanine, cytosine, and thymine).

Picking a career: the gossip test

How did I, a physicist by training, come to be involved in such a discovery? During World War II, I worked as a scientist for the British Admiralty, spending most of my time designing and testing new circuits for magnetic and acoustic mines. When peace finally came, I was uncertain what to do. I could have stayed on at the Admiralty but felt no urge to spend the rest of my life designing weapons. As there was little else I knew about, I had a rather wide array of choices open to me, an unusual situation for someone already 30 years old. I realized this was a unique opportunity, which might never come again—to start afresh—and I would be wise to select something that interested me deeply. But how to find out one's real interests? I decided to use what I call the gossip test (gossip being talking about something with relish, even if one is not in full possession of the facts). Using this method to analyze my conversations—with myself and others—I narrowed my choices to two broad areas of science: one involving the borderline between the living and the nonliving (today known as molecular biology) and the other the nature of consciousness (how the brain works).

With financial support from the British Medical Research Council (MRC) and with some help from my family, I went to the University of Cambridge, arriving there in September 1947. At first I worked in a tissue culture laboratory and tried to teach myself biology and chemistry in my spare time. A little under two

years later, I transferred to the physics department, the renowned Cavendish Laboratory, where a small group (also financed by the MRC) headed by Max Perutz, under the guidance of Sir Lawrence Bragg, was trying to solve the three-dimensional structure of a protein by diffracting X-rays from certain protein crystals. With a little help, I taught myself X-ray crystallography and resumed the attempt, abandoned because of the war, to get a Ph.D.

By that time I had decided that the most important problem in biology, at this level, was the physics and chemistry of genes—what they were made of, how they were replicated, and how they influenced the cell. I had formed the opinion, not entirely novel, that what a gene did was to carry instructions for producing the amino acid sequence of a protein, but of what genes were made I was less sure. Earlier, scientists had believed that genes were themselves made of protein, but certain experiments hinted that perhaps DNA was

In 1953, when Francis Crick (with pointer) and James Watson were constructing their now-famous double helix model, little did they know the impact their discovery would have—let alone that they would win a Nobel Prize.

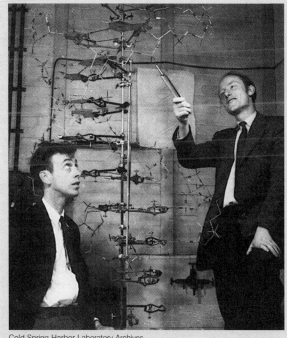

Cold Spring Harbor Laboratory Archives

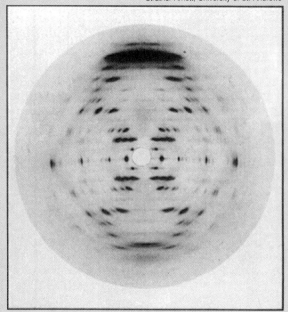

The crosswise pattern of X-rays diffracted from the atoms in a DNA crystal suggest its helical structure. Such X-rays helped but did not provide the answer to the puzzle Crick and Watson were trying to solve in their Cambridge lab four decades ago.

also important. My friend Maurice Wilkins (also trained as a physicist and supported by the MRC) at King's College of the University of London was trying to solve the structure of fibers of DNA. Rosalind Franklin, a trained crystallographer, was working with him on the problem.

A little later, in the fall of 1951, Watson arrived in Cambridge, a young American of 23, already with one year's postdoctoral experience in Copenhagen. He, too, had decided that the physical structure of genes was the key problem in molecular biology and had come to help our colleague John Kendrew. For the better part of two years, Jim and I thought and talked about the problem (while I was also working to produce a Ph.D. thesis on protein structure) and from time to time visited King's College London, where X-ray diffraction experiments were being done.

Confounding configuration

DNA is a polymer, a long molecule made by the joining, head to tail, of four similar but distinct subunits called nucleotides. In the early 1950s the *general* chemical formula for DNA had already been established, though the exact base sequence of any bit of DNA was still quite unknown. An organic chemical can be thought of as made up of a set of round balls (atoms) joined together by stiff pieces of wire (chemical bonds). At that time the distances between each type of atom—the length of each particular chemical bond—and the angle between each pair of adjacent

bonds were known fairly accurately from studies on other compounds similar to DNA but much smaller. This being so, why was the three-dimensional structure a problem? Surely all this available information would give the shape of the molecule. But that was not the case because within molecules there is fairly free rotation about all the *single* chemical bonds, whereas the double and triple bonds, when present, are relatively fixed. Thus, DNA could in theory take many shapes since it had several single bonds in every crystallographic repeat. How could one determine which configuration the molecule, influenced by the weaker and less well-defined bonds between more distant atoms, would actually take?

The obvious way would be to take some sort of picture of it. Visible light was hopeless since its wavelengths are hundreds of times longer than the diameter of the DNA, which makes it far too coarse a probe to resolve the internal details of the structure. The electron microscope was not suitable. There remained X-rays. Their wavelengths are short enough, being about the same length as the typical distance between adjacent atoms, but, unlike light, they are difficult to focus satisfactorily, so instead of a true picture one merely gets a diffraction pattern of the structure. Even to obtain the diffraction, it is necessary to have many molecules together in an ordered array, such as a crystal or a paracrystal, to get a big enough ratio of signal to noise.

What actually diffracts the X-rays is the cloud of electrons surrounding each atom. The X-ray diffraction pattern caught on a series of photographic films (or by Geiger counters) is a three-dimensional "wave analysis" of the 3-D pattern of electron density. Given the position of all the atoms, it is a straightforward but tedious process to calculate the magnitude of all the spots on the X-ray pictures.

Unfortunately, the reverse is not true. If we had *all* the parameters of the diffracted pattern, then, again, a mathematical synthesis would yield the required 3-D electron density; alas, the darkness of each X-ray spot on the film gives only the *amplitude* of each "wave," not its phase. Thus, the picture contains just half the information needed to solve the structure automatically without further assumptions—a maddening restriction.

Small structures can be solved because one can assume that what is diffracting is a set of compact atoms, but DNA is too large a structure for such a method to apply. There is a further snag: the crystalline, or semicrystalline, arrangements of DNA are irregular, so that the information is smudged; the X-ray spots that would correspond to the higher resolutions are missing. Thus, even if the missing phases were provided in some way, one could not hope to resolve individual atoms, only groups of atoms. One way to obtain the phases is to add heavy atoms to the structure in definite places and then compare the

306

resulting diffraction patterns, with and without these reference points. However, this method could not be used on DNA.

Charting new territory

In brief, no method was available to solve the structure in a straightforward way. The information actually available was of two main kinds: first, the chemical formulas plus the parameters for bond lengths and angles, not by themselves enough to define DNA's structure, and second, a limited number of X-ray spots, also insufficient to give the structure without further assumptions. The obvious approach—following the example of Linus Pauling, who had in 1951 discovered the α-helix of proteins—was to see if the *combination* of these two very different sets of data could provide a plausible answer. This meant building an accurate scale model and playing with it until a structure was found that fitted the X-ray data satisfactorily.

Fortunately, some bits of information could be obtained directly from the data. The *positions* of the X-ray spots give unambiguously the size of the repeat unit (known as a unit cell) in space. In favorable cases the pattern shows the *symmetry* of the unit cell. Given this information, it is possible to deduce the size of the asymmetrical unit—the minimum bit of structure that, operated on by all the symmetry elements, will give the entire DNA crystal. From the density of the material, which was not always easy to measure because of the variable water content of DNA fibers, it was then possible to calculate how many atoms there are in the smallest crystallographic repeat.

When the above approach was taken by our colleagues at King's College London in the early 1950s, it was found that the unit cell was always very large and the apparent asymmetrical unit was only a half or a quarter the size. Though researchers could infer that the structure had either two or three chains in it (probably the former), it was far too big to obtain the atomic positions by any orthodox method. But there was a ray of hope. The backbone of the molecule was chemically very regular. Was it possible that, in spite of the variety of base sequences, the backbone formed a regular helix? If so, the true asymmetrical unit might be just one nucleotide (or, as we would say now, just half a nucleotide pair). Could the structure then be solved with this additional assumption?

Gaining ground quickly

The answer turned out to be yes. By paying attention to the strong features of the X-ray data, it was possible to deduce certain general features of the structure—the way the bases were stacked, for example. Moreover, in 1952 several of us had worked out the mathematical theory for the diffraction pattern of a regular helix. The theory predicts that for a helix, no matter what the exact arrangement of the atoms, there will be a large vacant region of the X-ray photograph—the helix's "signature." From this information one can deduce the parameters of the helical screw axis, which carries one nucleotide pair into the next one. The detailed symmetry of one of the unit cells also suggested that the backbones of the two chains, although helically intertwined, ran in opposite directions.

Only one further concept needed to be resolved. How did an irregular base sequence form such a regular structure? Once we realized, in March 1953, that the bases, though differing in size, could be matched up to give base pairs of identical size and shape, the structure of DNA simply fell out. The two strands of the double helix are held together by weak hydrogen bonds between complementary base pairs (adenine always pairing with thymine, cytosine always pairing with guanine). It took only a day or so to build a rough model and a few more days to produce a more refined one. Moreover, the model of DNA explained, in a natural way, the one-to-one base ratios discovered a few years earlier by Erwin Chargaff.

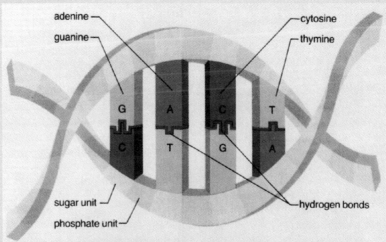

The genetic information is carried by the precise sequence of DNA's four bases: adenine (A), guanine (G), thymine (T), and cytosine (C). The structurally similar compounds cytosine and thymine bond only with structurally similar guanine and adenine, respectively.

adenine
guanine
cytosine
thymine

G A C T
C T G A

sugar unit
phosphate unit
hydrogen bonds

All too easy?

The path to the double helix was a twisted one, involving many detailed technical considerations and quite complicated chains of argument. It is hardly surprising that there were many false starts and trails. In 1952 we built a totally incorrect model because of a misunderstanding about the water content of DNA fibers. For quite some time Franklin thought she had evidence that one form of DNA was *not* helical (she was, of course, wrong). Early in 1953, Pauling produced a three-chain model, which we knew was incorrect and which prompted us to try again. These were all customary vicissitudes of research, particularly of the kind of research done at the frontiers of knowledge.

The accounts have sometimes been distorted by an undue emphasis on the personal factors involved, which has often disguised the real though guarded collaboration of almost all the people concerned. Scientific research is a cooperative venture, even if competition will keep breaking through.

I am often asked what I felt at the time of our discovery. Before we had the vital idea of exactly how to pair the DNA bases, we were constantly baffled since the various bits of data never seemed to fit together properly. After Jim figured out the base pairing, everything suddenly fell into place. During the actual model building, I was mostly in a state of constant enthusiasm (Jim had occasional spasms of doubt). Any enthusiasm, though, had to be tempered by the knowledge that our idea was only a hypothesis and might well be misguided or even wrong. But most of this time I was so busy trying to avoid awkward atomic contacts and measuring the coordinates of

A laboratory gene-tranfer technique now enables the replacement of a crucial enzyme that patients born with an inherited immune-deficiency disorder lack—one of many breakthroughs made possible by the elucidation of DNA's structure.

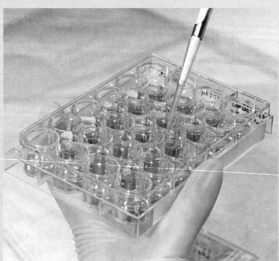

National Institutes of Health, Bethesda, Maryland; photograph, John T. Crawford

the atoms that I hardly noticed how I felt. As we were constructing our model, we had only a rough idea of the experimental data that had been obtained by Franklin and Wilkins at King's College, so shortly thereafter, when we saw the drafts of their papers, we were greatly encouraged to learn how well their data turned out to fit the double-helix pattern.

While we did realize that if we were correct, our "discovery" would be very important for biology, the idea that we might get a prize for it (let alone a Nobel Prize) never entered my mind (until many years later). In addition to my work on solving DNA's structure, I was also spending a good part of my time that summer finishing my Ph.D. thesis (which focused on other work, dealing with proteins and polypeptides). Our papers on the double helix were not part of the body of my thesis. I was also preparing to go to Brooklyn, N.Y., to do postgraduate work for a year.

Eureka!

The structure of DNA is now well established; time has shown that our model was correct, that the DNA molecule really is a right-handed double helix. DNA really is the universal hereditary material, carrying genetic instructions from one generation to the next. (For certain small viruses, it has been discovered that the genetic messages are carried by DNA's close relative RNA, which in some cases may even be single stranded.)

What has happened since the discovery for which Watson, Wilkins, and I received the Nobel Prize for Physiology or Medicine in 1962? More than I or my codiscoverers could ever have fathomed! A virtual explosion of biological knowledge—a revolution in genetics. That a substantial part of these new foundations of knowledge has sprung from the understanding we gained 40 years ago of the structure of DNA is indeed gratifying. What a wonderful flowering of the small seed that grew in our lab at Cambridge, nourished many years ago by the MRC!

When the structure of DNA was first suggested, many people either ignored it or disbelieved it. Then it was said that although it might be correct, it was of little use to anyone. More than a decade ago, the revolution in molecular biology that enabled scientists to cut, splice, and redesign the hereditary material for the first time led some to believe DNA was too dangerous to play with, though these fears proved greatly exaggerated. Then Wall Street decided that, by God, one could make money out of it. (Some might say there could be no better testimony to its usefulness.) And today it is even fashionable: a manufacturer of cosmetics now markets a "DNA" scent, sold in swirly, helix-shaped bottles.

And what am I doing now? I'm following that other path uncovered by my gossip test over three decades ago: I'm trying to find out how the brain works.

Special Report
The Promise of Gene Therapy
by Edward P. Cohen, M.D.

Severe, lifelong, and chronic diseases result from defective genes. They include such common inherited afflictions as cystic fibrosis, muscular dystrophy, and sickle-cell disease. Until recently medical science could offer no hope of a cure for these diseases; only the symptoms could be treated. In the past few years, however, advances in molecular biology and biotechnology have allowed researchers to add normal, nondefective genes to patients' gene-defective cells, an achievement having important implications for the treatment of diseases caused by genetic defects. In fact, there is real optimism that certain hereditary diseases may soon have permanent cures.

Sickle-cell disease: gene therapy candidate

Many targets exist for human gene therapy. A prime candidate is sickle-cell disease (sickle-cell anemia). The disease is caused by a defect in the gene for hemoglobin, the substance inside red blood cells that carries oxygen to all the cells and tissues of the body. The structure of genes determines the structure of the body's various protein molecules, and the defective hemoglobin gene specifies an abnormal molecule of hemoglobin. The defective hemoglobin carries oxygen, as does normal hemoglobin. The problem is that it causes the red blood cells that contain it to take on a sickle, or crescent, shape when the level of oxygen in the blood is low. This can happen, for example, when the person with the disease has a lung infection and experiences difficulty breathing or travels in an aircraft in which the amount of oxygen in the air is low. The sickle-shaped red blood cells are stiff—normal red cells are pliable round disks—and they clog small blood vessels, interfering with blood flow and causing severe pain and damage to the person's muscles, brain, kidneys, and other organs and tissues. Current treatment calls for giving the patient medication to control the pain (some patients become drug addicts from the chronic use of narcotics) and transfusing fresh normal blood when the blood count falls. These temporary measures do not solve the problem, however. The underlying cause, the defective gene for hemoglobin, is still present, and eventually pain and damage will recur.

Where do defective genes for sickle-cell disease and other genetic disorders come from? Like all the genes in the human body, they are inherited from one's parents. The defective genes are present because, from time to time, normal genes undergo accidental mutations, or changes in molecular structure. Mutations in germ cells—sperm cells in the testes and egg cells in the ovaries—are passed on from parents to child. (Mutations in cells elsewhere in the body, called somatic mutations, are not inherited.)

Normally, two identical or nearly identical genes for each kind of protein are inherited, one from the mother and an equivalent one from the father. Each cell of the body contains a copy of the maternal and the paternal genes, which were first brought together in the fertilized egg at conception. In some instances the two inherited genes for a given protein are not the same. A gene pair of this kind is called heterozygous, in contrast to the homozygous condition, in which both genes are essentially identical. Individuals, for example, who are heterozygous for hemoglobin have one normal and one defective gene. Such persons, who are said to have sickle-cell trait, may experience no symptoms of the disease because the expression of the normal gene compensates for that of the defective one. On the other hand, individuals who inherit two defective hemoglobin genes, one from each parent, have sickle-cell disease. Both genes are abnormal, and there is no normal hemoglobin to compensate. Such individuals are homozygous for the sickle-cell gene.

Sometimes defective genes confer a survival advantage, which helps explain why they persist and spread despite their harmful effects. One theory postulates that individuals with sickle-cell trait are more capable of resisting the blood parasite that causes malaria than those with two normal hemoglobin genes. Individuals who most commonly inherit defective genes for hemoglobin live in or derive ancestrally from parts of the world, Africa, for example, in which malaria is endemic.

The first target

Severe combined immunodeficiency (SCID), another example of an inherited disorder, is much rarer than sickle-cell disease and ordinarily is fatal. The immune system of an individual with SCID is severely impaired, and death from common infections often occurs at an early age. Probably the most well-known victim of SCID was David, the Texas youngster known as the

309

"bubble boy," who lived in a sterile environment within a plastic enclosure until shortly before his death at age 12.

One form of SCID results from the inheritance of two defective genes for a key enzyme, adenosine deaminase (ADA). The enzyme destroys a by-product of cell metabolism that would otherwise accumulate in cells of the immune system. Persons who are heterozygous for the defective ADA gene remain well. In persons who are homozygous for the defective gene, the deficiency in ADA results in the buildup of the by-product, which kills immune cells. Without these cells the immune system is severely crippled.

Until recently the only long-term treatment for SCID was a transplant of bone marrow from a healthy individual with normal genes for ADA. In this procedure the patient's marrow is destroyed, usually with high doses of X-rays or toxic drugs. Afterward, normal donor marrow is given to the patient, usually by injection. Cells in the donor marrow called stem cells "colonize" the patient's marrow, where they proliferate and function normally. The cells form red blood cells, phagocytic white blood cells to protect against infection, and lymphocytic white blood cells to restore the immune system, and they carry the gene for normal ADA. In about two-thirds of cases, however, a suitable, matched donor cannot be found. Unless the donor and the patient with SCID are closely matched genetically—close blood relatives have the best chance for a good match—the transferred marrow begins an immune attack against the patient. Improperly matched patients can die from such a reaction, called graft-versus-host disease.

With the advent of gene therapy, persons with SCID now have an alternative to marrow transplant. The gene specifying a nondefective, functioning ADA enzyme can be transferred to the patient's cells, and the patient can enjoy a normal existence. The first such gene transfer was done in 1990 at the National Institutes of Health (NIH), Bethesda, Md. Using the same strategy, medical scientists hope one day soon to devise a comparable treatment for persons with sickle-cell disease.

Techniques for moving genes

How is gene transfer accomplished? There are several approaches, but the most promising of them uses cell-infecting viruses called retroviruses to carry the normal gene into cells having defective genes. Since 1990 retroviral gene transfer has been used to treat SCID and other genetic diseases. Retroviruses are used because the genetic material of the virus integrates into the host cell's genome; that is, it actually joins and becomes part of the DNA of the cell that it infects. AIDS, a result of infection with the human immunodeficiency virus, is the most notorious retrovirus-caused disease.

For the purposes of gene therapy, researchers modify a retrovirus so that once its genes are integrated into those of the host cell, it can no longer replicate and infect other cells. Thus, a retrovirus that has been modified to carry, say, a normal ADA gene will take that gene into the defective cells of patients with SCID. The great advantage of the approach is that the normal gene will function inside the infected cell for the cell's life-span, just like a gene inherited from one's parents. And, when the cell divides, the transferred gene will be copied along with the inherited genes.

How the viruses are modified to carry normal genes but not to cause a widespread infection is based on a knowledge of viral genetics. An unmodified infectious retrovirus carries two identical RNA molecules, the genetic material of the virus. The molecules contain all the components necessary for the life cycle of the virus, including genes specifying its structural protein, a protein for its capsule, and a protein for replicating (copying) viral RNA. During the process of infection the virus particle binds to a receptor molecule on the surface of the cell and is taken inside. Once in the cell, the particle sheds its outer capsule, exposing its RNA. Then, by means of a special viral enzyme, reverse transcriptase, a DNA copy of the viral RNA is made. Both RNA strands are copied into double-stranded DNA copies of the RNA molecule. Afterward, the viral DNA copies are inserted into the large DNA molecules, the genome, of the infected cell. For most retroviruses the insertion point is random. Thus, integration of the viral DNA may occur at any place in any of the various chromosomes of the cell.

In some instances the inserted genes of the unmodified virus do not function immediately and are not expressed as protein. These latent viral genes are duplicated along with other genes when the cell divides. The viral genes remain "silent" for many cell generations until, often for an unknown reason, they become activated in an individual cell. Enzymes that are already present in the infected cell and that are used for normal cell processes are recruited to copy the viral DNA sequences into RNA molecules. The two strands of full-length viral RNA are then packaged into infectious viral particles and shed from the membrane of the infected cell. They then spread and infect other cells, and the process of reverse transcription, integration, and later expression is continued.

For gene therapy a "crippled," replication-defective virus is prepared. The genes required for viral replication and cell-to-cell spread are removed. What is left is a modified virus that can infect only one cell but is still able to produce viral proteins and to integrate its genes into the cell genome.

To take the normal genes into the defective cells, a molecule of genetic material called a plasmid is prepared. The plasmid contains the normal gene to be used for therapy along with "promoters," stretches

310

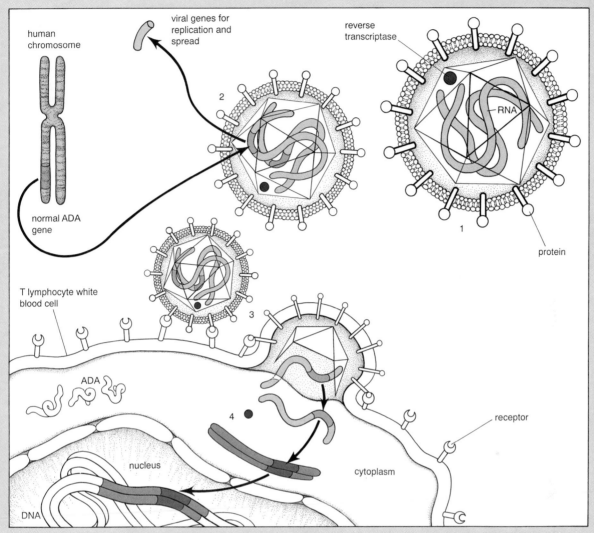

human
chromosome

viral genes for
replication and
spread

reverse
transcriptase

2

RNA

1

protein

normal ADA
gene

T lymphocyte white
blood cell

3

ADA

4

receptor

nucleus

cytoplasm

DNA

Retroviral gene therapy has been used to deliver normal genes for adenosine deaminase (ADA) into the cells of patients with defective ADA genes. A retrovirus possesses its genetic material in the form of RNA; it also contains the enzyme reverse transcriptase and an outer coat studded with protein (1). For gene therapy a normal ADA gene is added to the viral RNA, while genes that enable the virus to reproduce are removed (2). White blood cells from the patient are then exposed to the modified virus, whereupon proteins on the virus' surface attach to receptors on the target cells (3). The virus then delivers its gene package to the cell, whereupon the virus' reverse transcriptase converts the RNA to DNA. The DNA integrates into the cell's nuclear DNA, allowing production of ADA in the cell to begin (4). Cells so treated are then returned to the patient.

of DNA that switch on the transferred gene. Both the plasmid and the replication-defective virus are transferred into a "packaging" cell, a specially prepared cell that allows the replication-deficient viral genes to encapsulate themselves along with the plasmid into viral particles. The modified viral particles, which now carry the therapeutic gene, are then allowed to infect target cells of the patient. The usual procedure is to remove cells from the patient—for example, white blood cells from a child with ADA deficiency—and expose the cells to the modified virus. After infection, the cells are returned to the patient, usually by intravenous injection. Once the therapeutic gene is inside

the cells, it is integrated into the genome. And, as the cell divides, that gene is copied and passed on to the daughter cells. If, for example, the defective virus carrying a gene specifying ADA is used to infect cells from a patient with SCID, each of the infected cells will form the normal enzyme. And, as long as those cells divide, each daughter cell will receive a copy of the normal gene as well.

One problem that had to be solved for retroviral gene transfer to work is that the efficiency of transfer is low—not every cell is infected by the modified virus. To ensure that only infected cells carrying the normal gene are returned to the patient, the plasmid is given a second gene, one that confers resistance to an antibiotic that kills any cell failing to take up and integrate the transferred genes. After the patient's cells are exposed to the virus, they are treated with the antibiotic, which eliminates all but those cells that have accepted and integrated the therapeutic gene.

Safety of retroviral gene therapy

Why is such great care taken to prevent retroviral replication in the patient who is to receive gene therapy? Because the genes of retroviruses integrate into the DNA of the cells that they infect, they act in a fundamentally different way from other viruses and can have serious potential effects.

The viruses that cause common infections, such as chicken pox or the common cold, do not tamper with the genome of the infected cell. Whereas they do cause damage to and may kill the cells they infect, eventually the immune system responds and eliminates the virus. The genes of retroviruses, because they integrate, remain silent and go unrecognized by the immune system. More important, because they integrate randomly, the precise point of insertion into a chromosome can affect nearby normal genes involved in regulating cell division or can alter the extent of a cell's response to external signals. Because such changes in individual cells could allow progressive cell division and uncontrolled growth, an uncontrolled retroviral infection could lead to cancer.

Could a retroviral infection in patients given gene therapy lead to cancer? Whereas this theoretical possibility has not happened, three of eight laboratory rhesus monkeys given bone marrow cells that had been infected with large numbers of replication-competent retroviruses developed lymphoma, a cancer of lymph nodes. Because the chance for cancer exists, only carefully modified retroviruses are used for gene therapy.

Research physicians in the U.S. who wish to use retroviruses to treat genetic disorders are required to pass several stringent reviews by both local and national committees. The NIH's Recombinant DNA Advisory Committee comprises physicians and research scientists as well as ethicists. The Center for Biologics Evaluation and Research at the Food and Drug Administration is staffed by experts with a special knowledge of gene therapy techniques and applications. Both committees require absolute, firm evidence that the virus and the cell line used for packaging do not contain retroviruses capable of replication. The complete structure of the virus has to be determined in each case and shown to be free of genes capable of viral replication and cell-to-cell infection. In addition, proof that the material to be administered to the patient is not contaminated with other infectious agents, such as hepatitis virus, is absolutely necessary. Only then, with careful consideration of the risk to the public and the potential benefit to the patient and in light of the severity of the patient's disease and life expectancy, can gene therapy be considered.

Usually, approval is given to allow treatment of a limited number of severely ill patients. Patients who receive gene therapy have no other remaining options for effective treatment. Consequently, patients with sickle-cell disease, who can be treated with blood transfusions, are not candidates for gene therapy at present. Further experience, to be certain that retroviral gene transfer is without harm, must be gained before it can be widely employed for sickle-cell disease and other relatively less grave genetic disorders.

Early successes

In the carefully selected cases in which gene therapy has been used, results have been dramatic. The first ones, carried out in late 1990 and early 1991, involved two young girls (four and nine years old), both born with ADA deficiency and subject to frequent life-threatening infections. In gene therapy protocols conducted by R. Michael Blaese, Kenneth W. Culver, and W. French Anderson of the NIH, long-lived white cells, lymphocytes, from the patients' blood were removed and infected with a modified retrovirus carrying a normal gene for ADA, control elements, and a gene conferring resistance to an antibiotic (neomycin) that is toxic to uninfected cells. After selection in the laboratory with neomycin, the gene-altered cells were returned by intravenous injection to the patients. Gradually the levels of metabolic by-product fell, and the lymphocyte count began to rise. Now both children lead essentially normal lives and are capable of resisting infection.

Nevertheless, since the cells taken from the girls for retroviral gene transfer were blood cells, production of the enzyme continued only as long as the gene-modified lymphocytes remained alive. Normal blood cells have a finite life-span and a limited proliferative capacity. Thus, for the two girls gene therapy has not been a permanent cure, and reinfection of fresh cells from the patients has been necessary from time to time.

A permanent cure for ADA deficiency would require gene transfer into stem cells, the blood-cell progenitors found in the bone marrow. Stem cells have an indefinite proliferative capacity. However, since they are few in number, the difficulty in isolating them for gene therapy poses a serious practical problem. It also constrains the application of gene therapy to more common genetic diseases, such as sickle-cell disease, for which temporary treatments are available. There is a safety consideration, too, since once infected, the genome of stem cells would remain altered for the patient's life. Thus, until medical scientists gain further knowledge of the risks and disadvantages of the procedure, treatment of nonfatal diseases will be delayed. In 1993, because of the life-endanger-ing severity of SCID, the Recombinant DNA Advisory Committee gave Blaese, Culver, and other researchers approval to use stem cells for gene therapy. In mid-1993 two newborn boys received this type of therapy for what doctors hoped would be a truly permanent cure for their ADA deficiency.

Individuals who are born with a genetic disease known as familial hypercholesterolemia have extraordinarily high levels of cholesterol in their blood, more than three times normal, and they often die from fatal heart attacks at young ages. Familial hypercholesterolemia results from the failure of the body to form receptors on the surfaces of cells that capture low-density lipoprotein (LDL), which is rich in cholesterol. Normally the body transports cholesterol in the bloodstream from one cell to another in lipoprotein vesicles. The vesicles are captured by cell-surface receptors that take the cholesterol out of the blood and into the cell; the process is essential for normal cell function. Patients with familial hypercholesterolemia possess a pair of defective genes for the LDL receptor, and high blood cholesterol levels result. James M. Wilson, now at the University of Pennsylvania, developed a protocol for treating the disease in which a functional LDL receptor gene is transferred into liver cells of the patient. In the procedure a small portion of the liver is surgically excised and infected with a retrovirus containing a normal gene for the receptor. The genetically altered liver cells then are injected into the vein that carries blood to the liver. The cells rejoin the liver, where they form the LDL receptor and begin clearing excess cholesterol from the blood. The early results of patients so treated were promising.

Other viruses as gene carriers

Retroviral gene transfer is not suitable for all genetic disorders. Because of the nature of retroviral infection, the transferred therapeutic gene integrates into the genome of the infected cell only when the cell divides. The cells of most tissues—for example, skin or the tissue lining the airway—consist of nondividing cells or cells that divide only infrequently.

Other strategies are used to introduce genes into nondividing cells. Although they also involve the use of genetically modified viruses that infect, the therapeutic gene is not integrated into the genome of the infected cell. Viruses analogous to those that cause measles or mumps can be used for this purpose. An example is the adenoviruses, a group of viruses that in humans specifically infect cells of the upper respiratory tract and the bronchi, the tubes in the lungs that carry air. Upper respiratory tract infections similar to the common cold are often caused by adenoviruses.

Patients with cystic fibrosis have a defect in the gene for a transmembrane regulator, a large, complex protein that transfers sodium ions between the inside and the outside of the cell. The defect results in thick, sticky sputum that clogs the respiratory tract, and children with the disease suffer repeated, chronic respiratory infections that damage the lungs and eventually lead to bronchitis and emphysema. Death often occurs before age 20. The experimental gene therapy protocol, still in its early stages, involves modifying an adenovirus to carry the gene for the normal transmembrane regulator. The modified virus is then inhaled by the patient, and the normal gene is carried into cells of the trachea and bronchi. Since the transferred gene is not integrated into the genome of the cell and the infected cells do not proliferate, the treatment is not permanently curative and must be repeated.

Genetic modification as cancer treatment

In addition to the treatment of genetic disease, genetic alteration of cells is being used as an experimental approach of great promise in the treatment of patients with cancer. Cancer cells divide frequently as the tu-

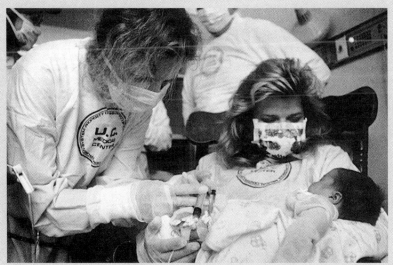

Paul Fusco—Magnum

Zachary Riggins is one of two newborn boys with ADA deficiency who were treated in May 1993 by means of a gene therapy procedure that had the potential to achieve a permanent cure. Immediately after Zachary was born, stem cells were isolated from a sample of blood from his umbilical cord, given a normal gene for ADA, and then injected back into his body. Stem cells, the progenitors of the body's blood cells, can proliferate indefinitely. Doctors hoped that the gene-corrected stem cells would take up permanent residence in their normal location, the bone marrow, and thus ensure Zachary a lifetime supply of ADA.

mor grows and spreads throughout the body. Since retrovirally transferred genes integrate only in actively dividing cells, the transfer of a gene that, once expressed, will help kill the cell represents a new form of treatment selective for cancer cells.

One group of targets for this approach is brain tumors, which are composed of frequently dividing cells in the brain. Normal brain cells do not divide. The therapy uses a replication-defective retrovirus that is modified to carry the gene for thymidine kinase, an enzyme normally present in a common virus, herpes simplex. When the retrovirus is introduced to the tumor site, the gene for thymidine kinase integrates selectively into the genome of a patient's dividing tumor cells, which then secrete the enzyme. Subsequently, the patient so treated is given the antiviral antibiotic ganciclovir, which acts by killing any cell that forms thymidine kinase. Thus, only cells forming thymidine kinase, i.e., brain tumor cells, are destroyed. Unlike the retrovirus used to treat SCID, the modified anticancer retrovirus is administered directly into the tumor with a fine needle.

In related approaches to cancer treatment, defective retroviruses are being used to carry genes for cytokines into tumor cells. Cytokines—interleukin-2 is an example—are soluble hormones of the immune system. They are intercellular messengers, released by one cell and taken up by another. Interleukin-2, for instance, stimulates special functions of certain immune cells as a requirement for the body to develop immunity to common infections. For reasons that are not entirely understood, the formation of cytokines causes malignant cells to be rejected by the body's immune system. The immune system of laboratory mice injected with, for example, cytokine-secreting mouse kidney cancer cells is stimulated to reject the cells, whereas injection with kidney cancer cells that do not secrete cytokines results in tumor growth and eventual death. Secretion of cytokines by cancer cells appears to stimulate the immune system to recognize the malignant cells as foreign. Of special relevance to gene therapy approaches to cancer treatment is the finding that mice whose immune systems were stimulated to reject the cytokine-secreting cancer cells also developed immunity to nonsecreting cancer cells that were present elsewhere in the animals.

Steven A. Rosenberg of the National Cancer Institute recently extended these findings to the treatment of patients with malignant melanoma, a severe form of skin cancer. Rosenberg removed portions of patients' tumors, infected them with a replication-defective retrovirus carrying the gene for interleukin-2, and then returned the gene-altered melanoma cells to the patients as a tumor "vaccine." As in the studies in mice, the altered cells were rejected by the patients' immune systems. Since the cancer patients who were chosen for these early studies had advanced,

widespread disease, the treatment was not curative. A related nongenetic treatment under study, the direct intravenous administration of large quantities of interleukin-2, resulted in inhibition of tumor growth in a significant proportion of patients with melanoma; however, it often caused serious side effects. By contrast, the slow, continuous secretion of interleukin-2 by the genetically modified cells avoided the toxicity of the intravenous administration.

Tae Sung Kim and this author at the University of Illinois at Chicago treated mice with melanoma with mouse cells genetically modified to secrete interleukin-2 and to express unique molecular surface structures associated with melanoma cells. The treated mice survived longer than untreated mice with melanoma. As in most studies involving tumor immunotherapy, the melanomas eventually recurred. Analysis of the melanoma cells from the recurrent tumors indicated that they had developed resistance to the attack of the immune system. Such outcomes suggest that gene therapy for cancer will not eliminate all of a patient's tumor cells. Additional treatments, such as chemotherapy, surgery, and radiation, will likely be required.

Bright prospects

By mid-1993 the Recombinant DNA Advisory Committee had approved more than 30 gene therapy protocols and was considering over a dozen more. In addition to approved protocols for treating patients with malignant melanoma, SCID, cystic fibrosis, hypercholesterolemia, and lung cancer, among others, the committee will consider innovative protocols for ovarian cancer, AIDS, and tumors of the brain. Protocols—for example, for SCID and hemophilia—are also being developed and tested by researchers in countries other than the U.S. Although gene therapy is in its earliest stages, its potential is so great that more and more studies will be undertaken in the hope that the treatments can be extended to large numbers of patients.

Concerns have been voiced that the ability of medical scientists to alter one's genes will challenge the fundamental integrity of human life and that in the future this knowledge will be extended from genetic treatment to genetic "enhancement"; i.e., to provide genes for such traits as intelligence, beauty, height, or athletic prowess. In human beings the complexity and probable number of genes governing traits considered desirable is so great that it appears unlikely that such modifications can be successfully achieved in the foreseeable future. Furthermore, nature will continue to alter genes through random mutations, with occasional adverse results. Nevertheless, it is not too soon for society to begin considering the many social and ethical questions inherent in the application of this rapidly evolving technology.

Health Care Law

By mid-1993 over one million people in the U.S. alone had become infected with the human immunodeficiency virus (HIV), the virus that causes AIDS. More than 160,000 Americans have died of AIDS since 1981. And as the incidence of HIV infection rises, more people are being drawn into legal battles concerning the disease. The most notorious court cases are those in which people with AIDS have been criminally prosecuted and sometimes convicted of attempted murder for spitting on, biting, or spattering infected blood on others.

The majority of legal cases, however, are much less dramatic. They revolve around aspects of everyday life, such as employment, housing, insurance, child custody, and wills. Discrimination is a major issue in virtually all of these areas and has been the focus of many legal cases involving HIV and AIDS.

Among the most serious problems that AIDS patients face are finding doctors and dentists willing to treat them and having the means to pay for any care they do get. Health care professionals who are HIV positive have also faced discrimination—in fact, doctors, dentists, nurses, and others have found themselves without jobs after their HIV status was disclosed. The following examines how selected recent court rulings and legislation have affected health care for people with AIDS.

Limiting insurance benefits

Perhaps above all else, people with HIV require access to medical care—for monitoring of their immune status, prevention and control of opportunistic infections, and treatment of life-threatening complications of their illness. Because many have lost their health insurance coverage, however, access to care is becoming increasingly difficult. In the U.S., getting medical care depends upon having the financial resources—usually in the form of health insurance—to buy necessary services. The cost of health care for people who are infected with HIV but do not have AIDS has been estimated at approximately $10,000 per year. The lifetime cost of treating symptomatic AIDS, according to a 1992 estimate, is about $102,000. Although such costs are commensurate with those of treating other serious or chronic illnesses, such as heart disease, they are clearly higher than most individuals can afford out-of-pocket. Thus, like most chronically ill people, those infected with HIV rely on health insurance to pay for the care they need.

The majority of Americans are covered by health insurance plans provided by their employers (or the employers of their spouses or parents). In recent decades the soaring costs of health care have made it difficult for many employers, especially small businesses, to provide insurance coverage for all medical

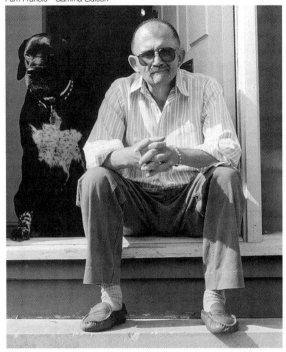

The court ruling in the case of John McGann—a Texas music store employee who filed insurance claims for AIDS-related treatment—established that an employer can limit benefits paid to those with certain medical conditions.

care. Many companies have attempted to control costs by introducing so-called managed-care plans that limit the choice of providers, coordinate care through a single provider, require patient co-payments, and include substantial deductibles. For the most part, however, even these measures have failed to keep health insurance premiums in line with the annual rate of inflation. Inevitably perhaps, some employers have tried to limit—or in some cases eliminate—medical benefits for employees with HIV infection or AIDS. The crux of the legal issue in such cases is whether it is lawful to limit benefits for one disease but not for others.

The McGann case. John McGann, an employee of a Houston, Texas, music store, raised this question in federal court. His employer provided employee health insurance with lifetime medical benefits of up to $1 million per employee. In 1988, however, after McGann filed claims for AIDS treatment, his employer changed its insurance, capping the lifetime medical benefits for AIDS at only $5,000. McGann challenged the new limit, claiming that it violated the 1974 federal Employee Retirement Income Security Act (ERISA). Section 510 of ERISA prohibits discrimination against an employee for exercising any right under an employee benefit plan, including health insurance plans.

In 1991 the U.S. Court of Appeals for the 5th Circuit heard the case in *McGann v. H & H Music Company* and ruled against McGann. The court found that employers have an absolute right to change the terms of employee benefit plans and that the cap on AIDS benefits was not the kind of discrimination that ERISA prohibits. The ruling also stated that section 510 was intended to prevent employers from retaliating against an individual employee; it would, for example, have protected McGann from being fired simply because he had filed costly health insurance claims. But, said the court, the change in plan benefits was not directed against McGann personally, even though no other employees of the store had AIDS. Rather, the change in coverage was intended to save money and applied to all employees. The court also found that employees have no right to insist that a company health plan remain unchanged, as employers must be free to adjust the coverage as needs alter.

The court did not consider that H & H Music was wrong in assuming that it was more expensive to treat AIDS than other diseases. Instead, its ruling underscored the employer's prerogative to choose the benefits it offers—even if the choice is based on misinformation or downright prejudice. In this respect the court may have gone too far. However, its decision can be seen as consistent with earlier U.S. Supreme Court decisions, which held that ERISA does not require employers to provide any health insurance at all, nor does it forbid discrimination in the benefits they choose to offer.

In November 1992 the Supreme Court refused to hear an appeal of the McGann case. Two months later in another case, another federal appeals court upheld a $25,000 cap on health insurance benefits for AIDS, relying on the reasoning in *McGann*. Thus, ERISA is not likely to protect employees with AIDS (or any other disease, for that matter) from losing their employer-provided group health insurance. Although the McGann case happened to concern AIDS, the decision applies to all medical conditions.

Congress could change this situation by amending ERISA to require employers to maintain current levels of insurance coverage, and legislation has been proposed that would do just that. However, because not all employees are covered by health insurance, amending ERISA would not help everyone. The real challenge is ensuring that adequate insurance coverage is available to everyone in need of medical care. Accomplishing this goal will require more fundamental reform of the health care system. However, McGann's experience points to the need to ensure that AIDS is covered to the same degree as other diseases. There is ultimately no financial saving in denying coverage to people with AIDS. This simply forces them to rely on Medicaid or other public programs, thus shifting the cost of their care from employers to government and, finally, to the taxpayers.

Insurance and the Americans with Disabilities Act. Mark Kadinger, a Minnesota electrician, died of AIDS in November 1992. Like McGann, Kadinger faced a cap on his insurance benefits, although he was insured not by his employer but by his labor union. The limit in Kadinger's case—$50,000—was higher than in McGann's but still not high enough to cover his medical bills. Instead of challenging the cap under ERISA, however, his estate sued the union, the International Brotherhood of Electrical Workers, claiming it had violated the 1990 Americans with Disabilities Act (ADA), which was enacted to prohibit discrimination against people with disabilities. Its employment provisions specifically forbid discrimination in many of the conditions of employment, including fringe benefits such as health insurance. People with HIV or AIDS are among those who qualify as disabled under the ADA.

It might seem reasonable that this federal law would prohibit disease-specific caps on benefits that affect employees who qualify as disabled. The ADA, however, contains a specific exemption concerning insurance, under which "ordinary" insurance practices are permitted, and such practices, by definition, may discriminate among different medical conditions or disabilities. In passing the law, however, Congress did not specify which practices were considered "ordinary" and necessary and which might be unjustified.

Regulations and guidelines of the Equal Employment Opportunity Commission (EEOC), the agency that administers and enforces most of the ADA provisions, state that the act permits limits on medical benefits, but these must apply equally to disabled and nondisabled employees. Thus, if Kadinger's union had limited all medical benefits to $50,000 per employee, regardless of medical conditions, it would not have violated the ADA. Like ERISA, the ADA does not require that any health insurance benefits be provided at all, nor does it say that benefits that are offered voluntarily must provide a particular level of coverage.

EEOC guidelines also permit health plans to limit coverage for specific medical procedures, such as numbers of blood transfusions or inpatient days in a hospital. However such rules could be used to selectively limit procedures for certain diseases that are regarded with disfavor. While the ADA prohibits employers from using health insurance limits as a subterfuge for discrimination against disabled employees, in practice it may be difficult to distinguish between limits intended to save money and limits intended to discourage disabled job applicants.

Federal and state antidiscrimination laws, including ERISA and the ADA, are intended to prevent discrimination based on irrational prejudice. Most of the time, reductions in health benefits are motivated by the desire to save money. When such cutbacks affect only AIDS, however, and benefits for conditions that entail similar costs remain unlimited, it is reasonable to suspect that prejudice, not responsible accounting, may be at work.

This concern led the EEOC to issue an interim guidance statement in June 1993 under which insurance limits will be considered discriminatory if they single out a particular disability. Employers then bear the burden of proving that the provision is justified by the risks or costs associated with the disability. An acceptable proof would be to show that the benefit limit is based on legitimate cost information. Capping of benefits could also be justified by the employer's showing that it is necessary to preserve the insurance plan's financial soundness or competitiveness and that other cost-saving alternatives *not* based on disability are not feasible. This new provision may prevent employers from making assumptions about the cost of treating AIDS without checking the facts.

Refusal to treat

Even if people with HIV can pay for their medical care, it is not always easy for them to obtain care. Early in the epidemic, many doctors were reluctant to treat patients with HIV, fearing that they themselves were at risk of becoming infected. Better information about the transmission of the virus helped convince most doctors that they could protect themselves adequately by the wearing of gloves and similar measures, known collectively as universal precautions, when dealing with blood and bodily fluids. Such measures also protect them from exposure to hepatitis B, another blood-borne virus that can be fatal. Although some doctors may grumble about having to use universal precautions, most health care professionals agree that these methods have made the practice of medicine safer all around.

Both the American Medical Association and the American Dental Association have stated that their members have an ethical duty to treat HIV-positive patients. Nonetheless, a minority of doctors, dentists, nurses, and other health care professionals object to treating people with HIV, either because they are especially afraid of becoming infected or because they do not like some groups of people—such as intravenous drug users—who have a disproportionately high incidence of HIV infection. In one such case, Donald Clausen, a Minnesota dentist, refused to continue to treat one of his patients after the patient told Clausen that he was HIV positive. Clausen canceled an appointment to clean the patient's teeth and instead referred him to the University of Minnesota, claiming that he did not know enough about the infection to give patients with HIV proper dental care. Clausen did not check with the patient's doctor or a specialist in HIV infection to see whether such a patient needed to be treated differently from others.

The individual in this case complained to the state's Human Rights Department, which found that the dentist had unlawfully discriminated against his patient on the basis of a disability. The Minnesota Court of Ap-

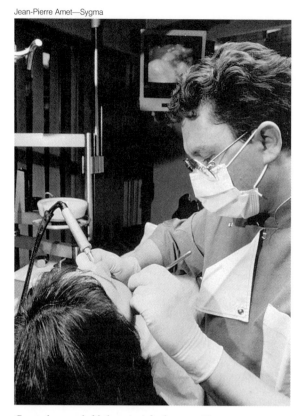

Courts have upheld the principle that practitioners may not refuse treatment to people who are HIV positive, emphasizing that the routine use of universal precautions is the most certain way to prevent transmission of HIV in the health care setting.

peal upheld that decision in October 1992, noting that there is no medical reason for a dentist who uses universal precautions, as Clausen did, to refer a patient with HIV elsewhere. Thus, the dentist's claim that he was unable to treat an HIV-positive patient was found to be a pretext for unlawful discrimination.

The fact that HIV-positive patients have been turned away lends credence to the fears of people with HIV that they will be unable to find caregivers if they reveal that they are infected. Some health care professionals have urged that patients disclose their HIV status and have called for laws that would permit doctors to test patients for HIV without the patients' consent. It is a matter of general legal doctrine, however, that patients have the right to refuse to undergo any kind of testing as part of their right to accept or refuse any treatment or diagnostic procedure. In addition, many states have passed legislation specifically prohibiting HIV tests without the patient's prior written informed consent. Many also prohibit disclosure of test results without the patient's permission.

The reason for such laws is twofold. First, the disclosure of a positive HIV test can have serious repercussions, possibly causing the patient to lose health care, employment, housing, or insurance or to be ostracized by friends and family. Second, it is not always necessary for doctors and nurses to know an individual's HIV status in order to provide care. Of course, the physician who is treating the HIV infection itself needs to know. Often, however, the desire to know is based not on the patient's medical needs but on the doctor's curiosity or personal fears. Furthermore, a patient's test results are not always a reliable indicator of infection. Because there is a window of time between initial HIV infection and the appearance of antibodies detectable by current blood tests, a patient can be infected for weeks to months before testing positive for HIV. For this reason, responsible health professionals use universal precautions with all patients.

Tolerable risks

Fear of AIDS often bears little relation to the actual risk of contracting the disease. For example, many people may believe that going to a doctor or dentist who is HIV positive puts them at significant risk of infection. In actuality, health care professionals are far more likely to be exposed to HIV by their infected patients than the other way around. Moreover, since all the evidence indicates that the risk to health care workers is itself very small, the risk to patients is negligible.

A few years ago, however, when the source of HIV infection of Kimberly Bergalis, a young Florida woman, and four others was traced to the dental practice of David Acer, considerations of statistical risk were forgotten. The publicity surrounding the case of Bergalis, who died of AIDS in December 1991, inspired several legislative proposals and court decisions intended, basically, to achieve the impossible—to protect patients from any risk whatsoever. In July 1991 Sen. Jesse Helms (Rep., N.C.) sponsored a bill to impose a $10,-000 fine and a 10-year prison sentence on HIV-positive doctors who treat patients without disclosing their HIV status. The bill did not pass, but there followed a year of intense public concern over the potential risks posed by HIV-infected health care professionals. Despite an extensive investigation, the precise way that Acer's patients became infected was never discovered. The virus may have been transmitted as a result of poor infection-control practices, although this was never proved. The mystery of how Acer's patients acquired the virus deepened in 1993 when it was revealed that a sixth patient treated by him had been infected; unlike the earlier cases, she had never undergone any invasive dental procedures of the type that might offer an opportunity for transmission of HIV.

Also in the summer of 1991 the Centers for Disease Control and Prevention (CDC), attempting to calm public fears of HIV transmission in the health care setting, called upon all health care workers to ascertain their HIV status; those who were HIV positive, the CDC said, should voluntarily refrain from performing "exposure-prone invasive procedures." The problem

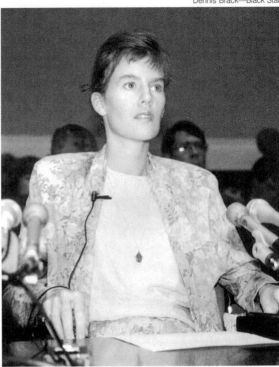

Despite the fears aroused by the case of Kimberly Bergalis, one of six Florida patients who contracted AIDS from an HIV-infected dentist, experts have reassured the public that the risk of practitioner-to-patient transmission is negligible.

was that no one knew for certain which procedures might expose a patient to infection. The CDC, therefore, asked a number of medical professional groups to compile a list of such procedures. The organizations refused on the grounds that (a) the task was impossible, and (b) a list would create a false sense of security. They pointed out that in the more than a decade since AIDS was first identified, only one health care professional—Acer—had been found to have transmitted the virus to patients, and no one knows how it happened. Medical and public health organizations attacked the CDC recommendations, and the agency attempted to revise them, but as of mid-1993 no satisfactory alternative had been approved.

The public's fears about the potential of health care workers to spread AIDS are understandable, but this does not mean that they are justified. Moreover, public anxiety alone has never been a sufficient reason for draconian measures to eliminate a public health risk. Law and social policy must take into account the costs and consequences of such measures. By way of analogy, as many as 40,000 lives could be saved each year if automobiles were banned in the U.S. They are not banned, of course, because the benefits of cars are believed to outweigh the risks. Recommendations that HIV-positive health care professionals be removed from practice are attempts to eliminate the risk of transmitting HIV to patients, but they would do so at the expense of the practitioners' liberty. Not only is complete elimination of risk an unattainable goal, the means of achieving it contravene the laws regarding discrimination against people with disabilities.

The ADA is only the most recent and widely applicable law prohibiting discrimination against disabled people. The federal Rehabilitation Act of 1973 bars discrimination on the basis of handicap in programs and activities that receive federal funding. Most states have similar laws to protect their residents. These laws embody a social policy that the perceived risks posed by a disability should be tolerated in order to permit disabled people to participate in society to the same extent as others. In particular, the disabled may not be denied employment simply because they might pose some risk to others.

When "risk" is "significant"

Under the ADA (and the Rehabilitation Act), employers may not discriminate against a disabled person unless that person is not "otherwise qualified" to perform the job. An infectious disease is a disability protected under the federal laws, and the only thing that would prevent an infected individual from being "otherwise qualified" would be if there was a "significant risk" of that individual's transmitting the disease to others in the workplace.

A "significant risk" is more than a risk. In a 1987 decision the Supreme Court found that the determination of a significant risk must be based on reasonable medical judgments about how the disease is transmitted, the duration of the risk, the severity of the potential harm if the disease is transmitted, and the probability of transmission. Thus, the potential for serious harm is not significant if there is a low probability that it will actually occur. For purposes of antidiscrimination law, therefore, the risk that a doctor, dentist, or other health care practitioner will transmit HIV to a patient is not significant. This means that, by itself, being infected with HIV is not a sufficient basis for discrimination against health care workers.

When faced with actual cases in which hospitals have fired HIV-positive doctors or withdrawn their privileges to practice, however, some courts have ignored these established principles of antidiscrimination law. For example, in 1987 William Behringer, an otolaryngologist and plastic surgeon, was diagnosed with AIDS at the Princeton, N.J., hospital where he practiced. His co-workers learned of the diagnosis almost immediately through hospital gossip; this, in effect, violated his privacy as a patient. The hospital's board of trustees then adopted a policy that effectively barred Behringer from performing surgery. Behringer claimed that the policy violated New Jersey's antidiscrimination statute. The Superior Court of New Jersey acknowledged that to bar him from practice

the hospital was required to prove that if Behringer performed surgery—using appropriate precautions— a "reasonable probability of substantial harm" would be created. Then, however, the court proceeded to ignore this probability test. Finding that "a risk of transmission, however small, does exist," the court upheld the hospital's action, apparently because, in its eyes, the possibility of serious harm (*i.e.*, death from AIDS) outweighed the law's requirement that there be a significant risk of that harm's occurring. The court did not consider that a patient who transfers from the care of an HIV-positive doctor to that of an HIV-negative doctor is exposed to different, but not necessarily lower, risks.

In another case a Louisiana hospital fired a licensed practical nurse for refusing to disclose the results of his HIV test. The hospital said that the nurse was "known to be a homosexual" and claimed that it needed to know whether he was HIV positive in order to comply with infection-control guidelines. This was not true since the hospital could simply have treated the nurse as if he were infected and required him to use universal precautions. There is little doubt that the nurse was fired because he was suspected of being HIV positive, a violation of the antidiscrimination law. However, the U.S. Court of Appeals for the 5th Circuit accepted the hospital's pretext. Although it correctly stated that the hospital could not fire the nurse unless he posed a significant risk of harm to others, and it acknowledged that the risk of transmission was extremely low, the court nonetheless upheld the firing because the potential harm—should it ever occur— would be great. In so doing, the court conflated a risk of harm with harm itself. Moreover, since the nurse did not perform any invasive procedures and used universal precautions, the risk was negligible.

Such cases illustrate how judges who ostensibly understand antidiscrimination law and can apply it correctly in cases involving most disabilities may lose their objectivity when it comes to AIDS. There are indications, however, that such cases may become a thing of the past as people begin to appreciate that an individual with HIV is not inherently dangerous. Rather, any risks to others arise from things the individual does or does not do.

A recent case in New York illustrates the dawning of this new appreciation. When a qualified pharmacist applied for a job at the central pharmacy of the Westchester County Medical Center, a preemployment medical examination revealed that he was HIV positive. The hospital then refused him the job, and the pharmacist complained to the federal Office of Civil Rights. That office found that the hospital had violated the Rehabilitation Act by refusing to hire a qualified employee who posed no significant risk to patients. Finally, after several years of dispute, the man was allowed to begin work at the medical center.

The goal: justice for all

People who are infected with HIV face many forms of discrimination. In the area of health care, laws that protect most people against discrimination do not yet adequately protect people with HIV. In part this is because the law does not prohibit discrimination that results from efforts to save money. ERISA, for example, allows health plans to provide differential benefits as long as they are used to control costs and not to retaliate personally against an individual employee. The ADA permits the coverage offered to disabled people to be different from that offered to others if the difference is justified by cost.

Laws that bar discrimination based on personal prejudice should protect those who are HIV positive from being refused employment or medical care. However, a few courts appear to have allowed fear of AIDS and misinformation about how it is transmitted to influence their decisions. This not only weakens confidence in the law, it undermines the social goal of preventing discrimination in all its forms. Moreover, if judges misapply the law in cases involving AIDS, they may also do so in cases involving heart disease, cancer, or traumatic injuries.

By themselves, laws cannot root out prejudice or make people good. They can only set the rules for social behavior and punish those who break them. As the public becomes more familiar with the facts regarding AIDS, misunderstandings that create prejudice should diminish and with them the need for legal action to ensure fair treatment of people living with HIV.

—Wendy K. Mariner, J.D., LL.M., M.P.H.

Health Policy

Not terribly long ago most Americans would have considered it unthinkable that anything approaching a health care crisis could occur in their country. Major U.S. cities and small towns alike boasted shiny new hospitals; technology and research seemed destined to find a cure for almost every imaginable disease; modern medicine and pharmaceutical wonder drugs had won the battles against smallpox, polio, and other devastating infectious diseases that had once threatened entire populations. Even many diseases associated with poverty, such as tuberculosis and some sexually transmitted diseases, appeared to be on the decline (although poverty, unfortunately, was not).

Continuing U.S. health care crisis

Today, however, the numbers are familiar to even the most casual student of contemporary issues: health care expenditures have skyrocketed to over 12% of gross national product (GNP). Employers especially have borne the brunt of this inflation; in 1988 alone, health insurance premiums for U.S. businesses rose by 18.6%. Small businesses and large corporations alike are threatening to eliminate health benefits for employees to cut their costs, and individuals are desperately trying to hold on to some form of health insurance by accepting larger deductibles (the amount of money the patient pays out of pocket before the insurance plan becomes activated) and co-payments (the portion of the cost the patient must shoulder after the insurance policy has paid its share).

U.S. health care expenditures increased by approximately $580 billion between 1960 and 1990, when they totaled $30 billion and $610 billion, respectively. Yet vast numbers of American now have no insurance, and thus their access to care is sharply limited. Although estimates vary, it is generally accepted among policy analysts that between 35 million and 40 million Americans either have no health insurance or are inadequately insured.

Meantime, AIDS, a resurgence of tuberculosis, violence in U.S. cities, drug abuse, and other "social pathologies" associated with poverty and despair have placed added burdens on the nation's health system. The groups who tend to be most affected by these conditions include minorities, the homeless, women, children, and the elderly—those least likely to be covered by insurance. In addition, the overall aging of the population portends a further increase in the need for long-term care. Nevertheless, medical insurance is being cut back for many retirees.

The present policy debate

When presidential candidate Bill Clinton promised a comprehensive national public health policy, many policy analysts rejoiced. For years there has been a movement among some health professionals and policy experts to steer U.S. health care closer to something approximating a European or Canadian system. According to these views, health care needs cannot be successfully addressed by a system whose primary goal is profit. In other words, health is not produced and sold by the item, it cannot be priced according to pure market determinations, and huge profits cannot be reaped from the provision of health care to poor people. Like education, police and fire protection, and national security, health is a "public good" rather than a commodity, and it should not be available only to those with the money to pay for it.

There continues, however, to be a well-entrenched resistance to increased governmental involvement in health care. Advocates of the current U.S. approach point out that nationalized systems can be encumbered by long waits, stifling bureaucracies, and questionable quality. They point to the crown jewels of U.S. health care—the world's finest surgeons, the most sophisticated hospitals with the best-trained specialists and state-of-the-art technology, and a seemingly endless supply of miracle drugs and technological interventions for acute conditions—as evidence that the

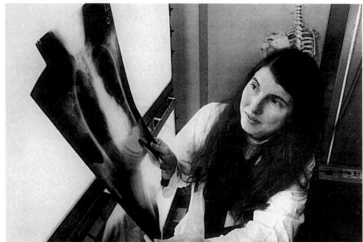

Physician and health policy analyst Steffie Woolhandler of Harvard Medical School is among those who believe that privatization of health care in the U.S. would be too costly. As a cofounder of the group Physicians for a National Health Program, she supports a publicly funded insurance program that would largely circumvent the private insurance industry as it now exists.

health care industry can "do well by doing good." In this view the marketplace is the most efficient distributor of goods and therefore should also be the setter of prices. It is also suggested that the people in the United States are loath to pay more taxes for new government programs and that the imposition of a new government bureaucracy to administer or provide health care would significantly lower quality of care.

Underneath both these arguments lie many unanswered questions. It is true that the Pentagon and the U.S. Postal Service, as two examples, have shown that governmental bureaucracies can be inefficient and inflationary. However, as policy analysts David Himmelstein and Steffie Woolhandler of Harvard Medical School, cofounders of the group Physicians for a National Health Program (discussed below), have pointed out, privatization has its costs as well. Himmelstein and Woolhandler estimated in 1986 that administrative costs alone—insurance program administration and overhead, hospital and nursing home administration, and physicians' overhead—accounted for $77.7 billion of national health care expenditures in 1983. The exact numbers have been disputed, but few argue that maintaining a commercial operation on the scale of a large U.S. hospital or maintaining a working industry on the scope of the U.S. insurance industry is extremely costly.

The assumption that most Americans distrust federal participation in health care has also been challenged. In 1984 Vicente Navarro, professor of health policy at Johns Hopkins University, Baltimore, Md., analyzed the results of published nationwide polls conducted between 1976 and 1983—before the current health policy debates and during a time when it appeared as if health maintenance organizations (HMOs) might yet succeed at their appointed mission of cutting costs. He found that the majority of Americans even then supported federal government health expenditures for the poor, elderly, and handicapped

and also that most Americans felt that deficit reduction should be attained through cutting military spending and increasing corporate taxes—instead of cutting social services including preventive health programs and medical care. Navarro interpreted these results as indicating that "the popular mandate is for national health policies that include . . . expansion of government health expenditures for the aged, handicapped, and the poor."

However, as noted above, American health care is world renowned for its technical splendor, the expertise of its personnel, and its ability to intervene successfully in serious and life-threatening health conditions. The ability of a national public-sector system to satisfy Americans, immersed in a culture of individual choice and consumerism, is untested. The historical role of the American public hospital as "provider of last resort" for the poor and uninsured may make the idea of using a public system distasteful to many class- and image-conscious American consumers.

Furthermore, existing public systems in other countries are far from perfect. Tales of bureaucratic bungling and insufferably long waiting periods for routine care and surgery have soured some American observers on the very idea of a public system. Recently, some British policy makers have suggested that their National Health Service (begun in 1948 and offering every citizen access to care without payment at the time of need) now needs to be streamlined by limitations on or even denial of care to smokers and others whose lifestyle choices may have impinged upon their condition. Such draconian solutions are anathema to most Americans and may have served to heighten their distrust of public-sector medicine.

Probably the most important barrier to the success of a national health care system in the U.S., however, is political. The country's history of private-sector emphasis in health policy is partly due to its cultural bias toward individualism and independence—and away from governmental intervention in private affairs. This philosophy has been supported and nurtured historically by private-sector health care interests.

Today more than 200 powerful medical-industry political action committees (PACs)—including the American Medical Association, the American Hospital Association, the insurance industry, and representatives of the pharmaceutical industry—exist solely to influence U.S. health care policy; these PACs contributed more than $60 million to candidates running for political office between 1980 and the first six months of 1991.

Public good, private profit

The structure of U.S. health care has for years been largely defined by private-sector initiative. A look at early U.S. health care policy is instructive. The Flexner report of 1910, financed and conducted largely under the auspices of the Carnegie Foundation, played a major role in defining U.S. medical education and eliminating alternative practitioners such as homeopaths and naturopaths from the mainstream of American medicine. Some years later fee-for-service payment, where care is paid for "after the fact" on a procedure-by-procedure basis, was firmly institutionalized by the introduction in the 1930s of Blue Cross/Blue Shield insurance. Fee-for-service has historically been seen as a boon to hospitals and physicians, who could reap extra profit through performing additional procedures and prescribing additional medications, all of which would be reimbursed by insurers. The patient, meanwhile, was largely insulated from the actual cost of this care. For these reasons fee-for-service health care financing is also considered inflationary.

The implementation of the entitlement programs Medicaid and Medicare in the mid-1960s not only provided the poor and the elderly with necessary care, it further entrenched the fee-for-service model. According to some policy analysts, that model not only benefits private-sector providers and insurers but also emphasizes individual patients' existing problems (rather than an ecological or social model of disease prevention). In this view it might work to the detriment of some patients, whose health problems may be due to social or environmental factors.

Recent history: vision and compromise

Most of the major health care policy initiatives of the past 25 years have continued to be the result of compromise between the ideal of comprehensive national health care and the political realities of operating in the context of the above historical private-sector orientation of the U.S. public policy debate. In the 1970s a plethora of proposals from various sources and constituencies for a national health care policy began to appear on the floor of Congress. Only one, the Kennedy-Griffith proposal, would have excluded the private insurance industry from participation in a

national system. An alternative version, the Kennedy-Mills proposal, was eventually introduced as a compromise because, as was explained in a *New York Times* editorial (April 7, 1974):

To retain the insurance companies' role was based on recognition of that industry's power to kill any legislation it considers unacceptable. The Bill's sponsors thus had to choose between appeasing the insurance industry and obtaining no national health insurance at all.

Fee-for-service remained virtually unchallenged until the implementation of the HMO model—more broadly known as managed care—under the Reagan administration. HMOs are based on prospective payment (instead of the "retroactive reimbursement" model of fee-for-service). Because a specific amount of money is allocated for specific illnesses and procedures, there is little incentive for providers to pad their bills by performing unnecessary procedures or for patients to seek superfluous or unnecessary care without concern for cost.

HMOs represented yet another example of the compromise between advocates of a coordinated national health policy and advocates for the private sector. They provided a means for individuals who were members of employee groups to save money on their care and at the same time for businesses ostensibly to reduce overall health spending. HMOs were implemented largely in response to activism by advocates representing the private sector who had become alarmed at the increasing cost of employee health insurance. HMOs were not envisioned as a means of meeting the needs of the uninsured. They were designed primarily to ease the cost burden on business and to finance the care of already-ensured employees in a more efficient manner. In 1981, according to San Francisco policy analyst Thomas Bodenheimer, managed care plans represented 4% of employer-sponsored health insurance; by 1987 they represented 60%. Yet health care costs have continued to soar despite business' overwhelming move to HMOs.

Rather than shape public policy, the U.S. government often imitates private-sector behavior. In 1983 in response to a growing conservative and middle-class outcry over the cost of providing human services to the poor (the so-called tax revolt), the federal government initiated the prospective payment system (PPS) under Medicare. Hospitals bill the federal government for the Medicare cases they have seen over a particular time period, and they are paid according to the diagnosis-related-group (DRG) categories into which their patients' medical conditions have fallen during that period. DRGs are used to delineate specifically the maximum allowable payment for each medical condition; their rates are determined by the Prospective Payment Assessment Commission (ProPAC) and can be modified or altered according to changes in cost. Patients, under the PPS plan, are not required to select from a predesignated group of providers, as they usually are under private-sector prospective payment plans. However, because increasing numbers of physicians are reluctant to accept publicly insured patients, people on Medicaid and Medicare have a more limited pool of providers to choose from than their privately insured counterparts.

Managed competition: the latest compromise

Despite the recommendations of some policy analysts that the U.S. adopt a comprehensive, public-sector, single-payer health care system, history suggests that further compromises between compassion and pragmatism are likely. Although by late summer 1993 President Clinton had not yet announced the details of his health care proposal, on the basis of the work of the President's Task Force on National Health Care Reform, headed by Hillary Rodham Clinton, indications were that it would be based on the "managed competition" model that has long been advocated by the Stanford University economist Alain Enthoven. In essence, this model proposes to limit unfettered market activity among providers without challenging the basic private-sector structure of the U.S. health care system. Like previous models, it represents a compromise between the idealistic vision of universal access and a pragmatic reluctance to challenge long-established private-sector orientation.

Under managed competition the country would be divided into designated geographic areas; within each of these areas, a collective purchasing agency called a Health Insurance Purchasing Cooperative (HIPC) would be created. The HIPC would negotiate contracts between private health plans and large groups of prospective members. Managed competition assumes that most of these competing health care plans would be managed care plans—prepaid, largely employment-based, HMO-type membership plans—administered and operated either by large insurance companies or by already existing medical facilities. For each geographic area there would be a minimum of three competing insurers.

All plans would be required to provide a basic package of benefits; this package would be drawn up by a national authority, much as ProPAC currently designates DRGs. Consumers could enroll in more expensive plans that offered more comprehensive services, but they would have to pay out of pocket for the extra premiums.

People without employment-based coverage would enroll in a plan subsidized through a public insurer. The poorest individuals (below the poverty line) would receive additional subsidies and would be able to choose any plan with a premium at or below the national average; the premium would be paid by public funds. Unemployed individuals at or up to 50% over the poverty line could also enroll in the plan, which

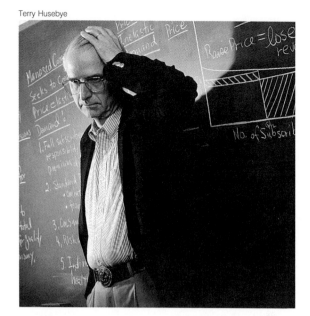

Economist Alain Enthoven, whose ideas have influenced reform of health systems in Europe, is the originator of the "managed competition" health care policy model—a compromised version of which is a key contender for adoption in the United States.

would have sliding scale, with public funding paying the balance of their premiums.

The basic philosophy behind the managed competition model is that competition among health plans will provide incentives to improve both cost effectiveness and quality of care. Consumers will have a choice between cost and comprehensiveness; the appropriate balance between bare-bones coverage and more expensive, more comprehensive coverage will be determined by the market. The poor, in theory, will be covered adequately by the publicly subsidized health plans.

Opponents of this model say that in many parts of the country—the sparsely populated rural Southwest, for example—there are insufficient numbers of residents to support three large-scale, competing health organizations; thus, one or two insurers could end up monopolizing coverage for an entire area. Some also question whether relegating the poor to an alternative, publicly subsidized insurer would raise the specter of two-tiered care—*i.e.*, a bare-bones plan for the poor, a more comprehensive and better-funded plan for everyone else. Clearly, the tension between policy makers' proposals and the political agenda of health care industry representatives is far from resolved and will continue to inform the national health care debate for some time. Although on Feb. 17, 1993, President Clinton had announced that health care legislation was top priority "this year—not next year, not five years from now," passage of a comprehensive health care bill before 1994 seemed unlikely.

323

Meanwhile, however, on the state level the issues have progressed beyond debate. States have been busy initiating their own strategies to cut costs and improve access while at the same time attempting to mollify both advocates of affordable care as a right for all and representatives of private-sector concerns. How well these state-level initiatives succeed may well determine the direction that national health care policy in the United States will ultimately take.

States lead the way

State governments, like the federal government, face powerful political challenges in implementing public health care policy. Lobbyists representing patients, physicians, the hospital industry, the insurance industry, and other players pressure legislators to modify initial proposals so all vested interests may be represented. Thus, state policy represents compromises similar to those seen in national initiatives.

Hawaii. The pioneer state in implementing an active policy to address health care issues was Hawaii. Since the mid-1970s Hawaii's state law has required all employers to provide comprehensive insurance to their workers; workers may be asked to pay up to 50% of the premium or 1.5% of their wages, whichever is lower. Hawaii's state health insurance program is managed under contract by two private insurers: the Hawaii Medical Services Association (HMSA), a Blue Cross affiliate, and Kaiser Permanente, the state's largest HMO. The majority of Hawaiians are insured by HMSA.

Hawaii has addressed an issue crucial to state-level health policy: the problems small businesses have in paying for health insurance premiums. All Hawaiian businesses of 100 or fewer employees pay a standard rate; their employees are members of a "risk pool," and they can choose either HMSA or Kaiser Permanente as their insurer. Since the late 1980s other states have followed Hawaii's lead in implementing health care "reforms" (the term usually used by state-level policy makers for local policy initiatives).

Massachusetts. In 1988 Massachusetts approved a universal health care law. In that state approximately 100,000 formerly uninsured residents now qualify for, and receive, basic health insurance. Financing is primarily drawn from a statewide pool into which all employers must contribute. The Massachusetts model differs from the standard "pay-or-play" model in that employers are not required to provide insurance; they only must contribute to the statewide pool. Although the Massachusetts plan was hailed during its inception as a landmark attempt to provide universal health coverage, opposition from small businesses has combined with a statewide economic recession to slow implementation. The plan's future is now in question.

Florida. Florida has used the pay-or-play concept as a kind of carrot-and-stick approach toward employers.

A voluntary plan whereby employers will meet targets for expanded employee coverage or face a mandate to do so has been put in place and will be fully operational by 1995. The state will attempt to lower costs and encourage participation by putting together a pooled purchasing arrangement as well as expanding its Florida Health Access Corporation, which currently provides HMO coverage to approximately 10,000 enrollees in 2,300 small businesses. Because the Florida model is strongly employer based, unemployed people will not receive much relief in terms of health insurance affordability.

Colorado. In Colorado, pay or play has been refined to "pay—or else." Under a proposed bill the state would require that employers pay a flat amount for every full-time employee—with a cap, probably of no more than 7% of each employee's salary—into a fund toward the cost of employee health insurance.

Colorado also proposes having employees foot a portion of their health care insurance bill through premium contributions—amounting to 2% of their gross income or about $50 per month, whichever is less. Actual health insurance coverage would be provided by a limited number of private insurers; individuals and families could enroll in any plan, and the state would then contribute a fixed amount per individual. This is a variation on the managed competition model.

Cost control, of course, is a central feature of the Colorado model as it is in every other state proposal. Colorado will provide incentives for managed care instead of fee-for-service, and it will mandate a basic-benefits package that will stress preventive care. Competition among insurers would take place on the basis of benefits or services offered, instead of price.

Oregon. Some state initiatives have attempted to aggressively cut costs through creative interference in the unfettered free-market process. Most of these strategies have involved defining a basic-benefits package that will be available to all citizens; in this view, unlimited access to unlimited care would be inflationary and would not serve either the financial or the health needs of a state.

Oregon has implemented a law that, like Massachusetts' law, will include a mandate for employers to contribute to a statewide pool. It also, however, includes a highly controversial rationing component; health conditions are divided into three categories on the basis of their "worthiness" for coverage—"essential," "very important" (to be funded to the extent possible), and "valuable" (to certain individuals but less likely to be cost-effective or produce long-term gain). The last category includes certain conditions that lead to long-term disability such as severe brain injury; it also includes extremely premature infants, who require highly costly neonatal intensive care but often do not survive or have lifelong disabilities even with that care, and cancer and AIDS in their advanced (and

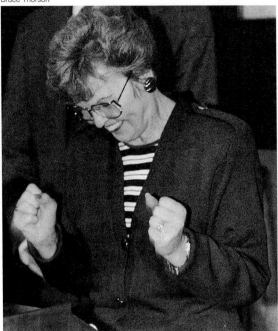

Bruce Thorson

Oregon's recently implemented health care initiative, supported by Gov. Barbara Roberts, includes a controversial rationing component, which ranks health conditions on the basis of their "worthiness" for coverage.

likely terminal) stages. Such prioritizing has been vilified by advocates of the disabled, who maintain that it perpetuates stereotypes about people with disabilities and assumes that their quality of life is somehow less important than that of people without such problems.

Minnesota. The basic-benefits issue has been approached somewhat differently in the state of Minnesota. There, all citizens who do not qualify for Medicare or Medicaid may purchase insurance with the aid of a state subsidy that is based on income. The subsidy is funded through an increase in the cigarette tax; a 2% surcharge on all hospital, physicians', and dental bills; and a 1% tax on all HMO and nonprofit insurer's bills. Private insurers provide the coverage, assisted by the state subsidies; currently the total monthly premium for the state's insurance scheme, MinnesotaCare (formerly HealthRight), is $432. A family of three earning $10,000 annually will pay $12.53 per month, whereas a family earning $30,000 annually will pay the full $432 premium.

The Minnesota law divides services into three groups: (1) "basic services" (for which there should be unlimited access to all), (2) "desirable services" (for which financial barriers to access should be reduced), and (3) "optional services" (to which the government is not required to reduce barriers). "Limitation of disability" is a criterion, along with promotion of public health and reduction of suffering, for basic care. Thus, although the private insurance industry remains the

financier of Minnesota's plan, insurance must be available to the sick and disabled—not just the healthy, young population traditionally sought by insurers.

Vermont. In Vermont, the only state with a physician-governor, an aggressive and comprehensive health care reform bill, to take effect by 1995, has been enacted. Democrat Howard Dean, now in his second term of office in a traditionally conservative state where distrust of government runs high, has stated that his objective is "to make health insurance work for everybody." A new Vermont Health Care Authority has been authorized to design several alternative models for legislative consideration including a single-payer and a multiple-payer plan. The aim is universal access with centralized planning and global budgeting.

The state will provide a uniform set of minimum benefits for all Vermont residents, create cost-containment incentives, and establish a purchasing pool for all state and municipal employees who choose to participate. A particularly unique element of Vermont's proposal is a set of incentives to increase the physician supply in the state's impoverished rural regions, which have few or no doctors.

For the present, Governor Dean believes that state approaches to health policy reform are the only ones that will work. In particular he points to the Medicare system as "a wonderful ad for why the feds should never be allowed to run a national health care system."

New York. New York, long a stronghold of aggressive public involvement in health care and other human services, has designed one of the most comprehensive of any state approaches. Called the Universal New York Health Care Plan (UNY*Care), it would be based upon a set of guaranteed benefits for all state residents, with some additional benefits for the poor.

New York has also included a variation on pay or play in its proposed system. Employers who do not provide health care would pay a tax to subsidize premiums and self-pay expenses by low-income people. Catastrophic-illness benefits would be available to all New Yorkers for inpatient care above $25,000 and major medical coverage above $25,000. Individuals who are self-employed as well as the unemployed would be able to purchase basic health insurance coverage through UNY*Care; those whose incomes were below 200% of the poverty level would receive additional state subsidies.

UNY*Care would be among the most centrally controlled of any proposed state plan. The state would establish a public authority to administrate insurance; in effect, this authority would act as a single payer. It would set rates statewide and establish a set of guidelines for provider payment that all insurers would adhere to. The UNY*Care system would be financed through money raised from employers' purchasing insurance, taxes on those employers who did not provide insurance, and general revenues.

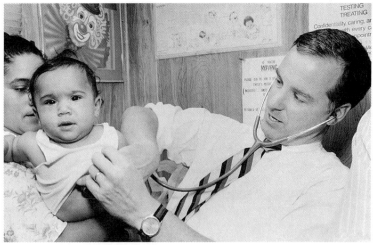

Vermont pediatrician and governor Howard Dean has made universal health insurance that "work[s] for everybody" a banner issue in his state. A unique feature of Vermont's health plan, which will take effect in 1995, is the provision of incentives to increase the supply of physicians who serve the state's impoverished rural regions. Dean has said that his state's approach to health care reform offers a model for the nation.

An even more sweeping plan has been put forward for the state of New York by Assemblyman Richard Gottfried. The Gottfried model would be a single-payer system similar to Canada's; it would be tax financed and cover an expanded range of services for all New York residents. Another proposal, that of the New York Hospital Association, would extend employer-based coverage to all employees and dependents, with subsidies for low-income individuals not eligible for Medicaid. Rates would be set by an independent commission, but insuring would be done through the private sector.

Washington. Several states have proposed a kind of "cookbook" approach to health care reform; these approaches combine elements of several different payment and health care delivery models. Washington has long been a health care innovator; Seattle has one of the country's most effective networks of community-based clinics, known both for its success and for the unusual autonomy individual providers enjoy. Several proposals are currently being debated in Washington.

The state's Health Care Reform Act of 1992 was defeated in the legislature, but elements of that proposal remain dominant in Washington's health care reform debate. Three mechanisms of coverage would exist under this model: a pay-or-play requirement for employers; insurance reform that would guarantee all employers access to community-rated policies for their workers (including guaranteed availability and renewability); and a Basic Health Care Plan that would offer subsidized insurance for individuals with incomes below 200% of the poverty level. The plan would be financed by additional taxes on alcohol and tobacco products as well as a tax on all insurance premiums sold in the state. Cost control would focus on provision of a uniform benefit plan that all insurers would be required to offer. As in some other states, insurers could compete in terms of the benefits packages they

offered but not in terms of how much they would charge for the basic-benefits package, and there would be a cap on allowable annual increases in the cost of this package.

California. California is also currently considering a set of proposals that would fuse elements of diverse models. California's insurance commissioner, John Garamendi, has proposed a system with some similarities to the managed care model first proposed by Enthoven. The Garamendi proposal places the burden of cost control squarely on the shoulders of insurers. Regional purchasing corporations would collect premiums, certify participating health care plans, and then purchase individual health insurance from private insurers. For each enrollee the insurer would be given a flat fee (adjusted for that enrollee's age and gender). Individuals could choose among plans, but a basic package (delivered on a managed care basis) would be available to all. More comprehensive plans could be purchased by an individual willing to pay extra for the extra benefits.

Competition: boon or bane?

Although, as mentioned above, the philosophy of free-market competition continues to drive most federal and state health care policy, there is evidence that, in fact, competition may not be the sole answer to either cost or quality issues. Hawaii's system, dominated by two insurers instead of a multitude of smaller, competitive entities, has managed both to cut costs and to maintain a high quality of care. In Rochester, N.Y., a local initiative has approximated a private-sector version of the "single-payer" model, which advocates of a national health care system have been suggesting for years.

Rochester is a company town whose political and economic processes are dominated by Eastman Kodak and Xerox. The city's health care strategy is based upon the concept of "community rating": each citizen pays exactly the same premium for health insurance as Kodak or Xerox pays for an employee. Any citizen of Rochester or its principal suburbs is eligible to purchase insurance. Individuals who are at higher risk do not have to pay higher premiums; this makes insurance affordable to many. The self-employed, those who work in hazardous jobs, or those who are otherwise in high-risk categories—as well as people with preexisting conditions—are thus eligible for insurance. The risk is spread across the entire population and is thereby lessened for any individual. Only 6% of Rochester's citizenry lacks coverage, as opposed to the nationwide average of 14%.

Blue Cross has found that the high volume of patients that Rochester's system attracts offsets the presence of high-risk people. It can offer lower premiums—an average of $2,378 per household in 1991, as opposed to the New York state average of $4,361 and the national average of $3,684. The insurance company's overall expenditures have been reduced also because there are fewer uninsured people receiving free care in Rochester; formerly, doctors providing free care compensated for their losses by charging their Blue Cross patients more and passing the costs on to the company.

Another important element of Rochester's success in containing health care costs has been a state law that limits hospital capital expenditures. Duplication of facilities is reduced, further lowering waste and hospital charges. The hospitals have agreed which institutions should perform specialized services, such as organ transplantation and open-heart surgery, and they no longer compete for the technology and personnel to attract these patients.

Advocates of a public health care system decry the corporate dominance in the Rochester model; there is no institutionalized mechanism for providing coverage to the very poor—Medicare and Medicaid must still bear that burden—and some observers have suggested that hospitals in certain communities have insufficient beds and facilities for treating their patients. One hospital administrator called this a "subtle form of rationing." Rochester, however, presents an interesting challenge to the philosophy of competition as a cost-cutting device. Cooperation seems to have made the city's hospitals more efficient without lowering the quality of care. In fact, the system of allocating specialized services to those institutions most qualified to perform them may eventually lead to better care and a greater number of positive outcomes.

Advocacy groups enter the fray

Not only legislatures have been wrestling with the health care policy issue. Some groups traditionally considered opposed to any governmental intervention in health care delivery, such as physicians and insurers, have added their voices to the debate.

The group Physicians for a National Health Program may not represent the mainstream opinion among American doctors, but its proposal for a comprehensive national health system has received wide public attention. This group proposes a publicly funded insurance program that would largely circumvent the current private insurance industry. Under its model, hospitals and nursing homes would be provided an annual budget to cover all operating expenses. Patient costs would be paid through either a fee-for-service system, with fees determined by state boards; an annual global budget, paid directly to institutions such as hospitals, clinics, and physicians' group practices to cover costs of care; or a prepayment system similar to current HMOs. All physicians working for such institutions or groups would be salaried.

A similar comprehensive proposal has been put forth by Nurses for National Health Care. Unlike Physicians for a National Health Program, the nurses' group has turned to an existing bill that was being considered in both houses of Congress in 1993. This bill, the American health security bill, proposes a single-payer system financed through a combination of payroll taxes, premiums adjusted with higher rates for those with higher incomes, and an increased income tax for individuals in high-income groups. Nurses for National Health Care favors this model especially because it

A Xerox Corp. employee pays a high monthly premium in order to be able to have her daughter treated by a private practitioner rather than a physician who practices with one of the company-supported health maintenance organizations.

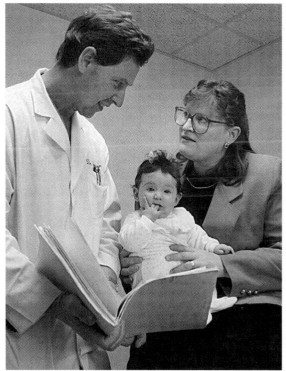

Stephan Castagneto—The New York Times

advocates a strong role for states in administering the program and acknowledges that different regions of the country have different needs, which can best be met by local initiatives. The bill also emphasizes preventive care, and it includes mid-level practitioners such as nurses as providers. Controls on state administrative expenses and prescription drug prices are included in the bill.

Probably closer to conventional mainstream opinion among caregivers is the proposal put forth by the American College of Physicians, the nation's largest medical specialty group, representing internists. This plan recommends universal insurance delivered with a mixture of public and private financing. Employers could either insure their own employees or pay a tax so their workers could participate in a publicly sponsored insurance plan, which would eventually replace currently existing state and federal entitlement programs for specific groups. Funding would derive from the payroll taxes, increased taxes on alcohol and cigarettes, and income-based premiums. General tax revenues would also fund a portion of this plan.

Competition among private insurers is a cornerstone of the American College of Physicians' model; all insurers would offer similar coverage, but they would compete on the basis of prices offered to employers. Individuals unable to participate in such a national system—because of their geographic location, extreme poverty, or other reasons—would be served by an expanded public health system that would include community-based health care centers, local health departments, and the National Health Service Corps, which sends physicians to federally designated medically underserved areas.

Critics of this plan look with disfavor upon the continued strength of the insurance industry as well as the potentially "two-tiered" division of care between those who participate and those who are served by the public sector. It does, however, incorporate many of the elements of more wide-ranging proposals— public financing, state-level administration, and mandated employer participation.

Perhaps the most surprising entrant into the debate on national health policy has been the insurance industry. In 1992 the Health Insurance Association of America (HIAA) went public with a proposal that includes universal coverage with a guaranteed package of basic benefits. HIAA has also suggested incentives for providers to eliminate unnecessary testing and other costly procedures. Employees would not be taxed on their premiums, but they would pay taxes on any additional amount of coverage over the basic package that was purchased by their employers.

Cost cutting is a major agenda item for the health insurance industry. The proposed bill would prohibit provider "cost shifting"—the practice of charging insured patients more in order to make up for money lost treating uninsured patients or patients insured by Medicare or Medicaid.

Hospital associations have criticized HIAA's bill for these restrictions and for its stringent limitations on how much money can be paid. Advocates of an overhaul in the basic finance structure of American health care tend to believe that at the very least, insurers should be prohibited from charging higher premiums to sick and high-risk people. The HIAA proposal prohibits exclusion of people with preexisting conditions, but it places little restriction on how much their premiums may be.

Many voices, difficult choices

The debate on national health policy, as outlined here, is far more than a trading frenzy in the free market of ideas. It represents a complex and constantly shifting array of political and economic self-interests among some of the country's most powerful groups. Although some consumer groups, *e.g.,* the American Association of Retired Persons, have come forth with proposals for national health reform, most public attention has focused on the plans coming from the nation's capital and from such organized bodies as the American College of Physicians.

To choose among these vested interests will not be easy, especially in an age where public opinion of government is at an all-time low. Compromises such as managed care, although they appear initially to be attractive, may be insufficient to quell the tide of opinion demanding more fundamental changes in the system.

It may be instructive that few of the proposals being most widely discussed today resemble managed competition in the way it was originally proposed by Enthoven and as it has been suggested by the Clinton administration. Some policy analysts have suggested that managed competition, with its emphasis on free-market solutions combined with the limitation it places on entry into the market, will please no one. Those who propose a system-wide overhaul on the scope of that suggested by Physicians for a National Health Program hope that if this happens, it will force the country to consider a more comprehensive overhaul of the system.

On the other hand, recent history shows that failure of governmental programs often leads to political timidity. It is widely perceived that the social programs of the 1960s did not work, and so today it is politically risky to suggest even moderate public spending to address social concerns. If Clinton's plan, once put forth, does not succeed, the result may be the opposite of what the activists have in mind: disillusionment with governmental intervention in public health and a return to market-based attempts to solve the national health care crisis.

—David Whiteis, Ph.D.

Special Report
Public Health in the U.S.—
Not Making the Grade

by Joyce C. Lashof, M.D.

• In the state of Alabama 19% of the population has no health insurance; 20% of drinking water is unsafe; the tax on cigarettes is 17 cents per pack; 24% of the population is obese; and $58.42 is spent per person on sanitation and sewerage.

• In Wyoming 12.5% of the population is without access to primary health care; there is no measurable pollution; 85.9% of the population has a high school degree; 59.6% of car passengers over age 18 do not wear seat belts; and there is one public health worker per 14.7 residents.

• In Missouri Medicaid spending is $115.11 per capita; there are 10.5 cases of occupational injury per 100 full-time workers; the childhood poverty rate is 18%; 15.5% of adults report binge drinking—consuming five or more drinks on one or more recent occasions; and the state government spends $74.35 per person on community health programs.

That was how three U.S. states (selected arbitrarily from the beginning, middle, and end of the alphabet) fared on *America's Public Health Report Card,* issued one week after the November 1992 national election. The *Report Card,* a 65-page document, was a first of its kind. It rated each of the 50 states and the District of Columbia on their public health performance in a way that no previous assessment of the country's health had.

Why a "report card" on health?

Health care reform figured prominently not only in the presidential election but in many state races as well. Finding solutions to the current dilemma of increasing health care costs and decreasing numbers of people with adequate health insurance is now a top priority of the administration of Pres. Bill Clinton. In issuing the *Report Card,* the American Public Health Association (APHA) sought to focus the nation's attention on critical issues that need to be addressed as the country pursues the debate on health care reform in earnest.

The APHA was founded in 1872 and is the largest organization of public health professionals in the world, with more than 50,000 members from 77 public health occupations. In keeping with its mission to improve the health of the American people, the association provides leadership in the formulation of health policy—policy that focuses on the important interrelationship of health and quality of life.

The need for health care reform in the United States is easily seen when its health statistics are compared with those of the rest of the industrialized world. In fact, the U.S. is doing worse than many less developed countries, now ranking 20th in infant mortality, worse than Hong Kong, Singapore, and almost every country in western Europe; 28th in the incidence of low-birth-weight babies, behind Jordan, Ireland, and Costa Rica; and 9th in life expectancy. Yet the U.S. spends over $800 billion a year on health care—more than any other nation.

While such numbers are revealing, there is a need to look *behind* them to understand *why* the country ranks so poorly. That there is a marked disparity in health status related to socioeconomic status and racial and ethnic background has long been recognized. Death rates among low-income populations are twice the rates among those with the highest income. Thirteen percent of black infants are born at low birth weight, compared with 6% of white infants. The risk of heart disease is more than 25% higher for low-income people than for the overall population. The incidence of cancer increases as income decreases, and survival rates are lower for low-income cancer patients. But much of the current public debate and many of the specific issues for which various solutions are being proposed relate to how to pay for medical care and not how to ensure a healthy population.

Access to medical care is essential, but a great deal of disease is preventable or postponable. The nation now devotes a significant portion of the medical care dollar to high-technology specialty care for illnesses that should have been prevented or treated at a much earlier stage. The determination of what measures beyond the provision of medical care will be needed to improve the country's dismal health statistics necessitates scrutiny of *all* of the conditions that influence a person's health.

Poorer health status of blacks, Hispanics, and Native Americans has been widely documented. Why do these groups bear the brunt of poor health and have such excess mortality? Much of the health differential can be attributed to economic status, but there are many other, often overlooked, factors that directly affect health. It was thus a broad array of health determinants—factors pertaining to income, occupation, education, environment, community living conditions, lifestyle, and access to preventive health services—that the *Report Card* evaluated.

Measures of health

To assess how well or poorly a state was doing in providing conditions conducive to health, the APHA chose not to use the usual measures of health status—*i.e.*, infant mortality, life expectancy, and disease-specific mortality. Rather, data in five areas that the association considered essential to building a healthy society were selected: (1) medical care access, (2) healthy environment, (3) healthy neighborhoods, (4) healthy behaviors, and (5) community health service. Within each of these broad categories, specific indexes were chosen (25 in all).

The APHA was not in a position to develop new data but depended on the availability of existing, comparable data from many sources for as many states as possible; unfortunately, in some cases data were not available. The investigators were limited by time and resources, having approximately six months to gather the data and prepare the report. The goal was to have the *Report Card* completed in time to be of value to a new administration and the American public as the nation turned its attention to the domestic agenda.

How the states fared

How well did the states do? What did the *Report Card* reveal about the country's overall public health performance? The following summarizes—in a necessarily abbreviated fashion—the findings on a category-by-category basis.

Medical care access. To determine access to medical care, data on the percentage of uninsured, the number of primary care physicians per capita, the adequacy of prenatal care, the percentage of the population without access to care, the ratio of people receiving Medicaid (the federally administered, state-financed system that pays for care for economically disadvantaged people who meet state-determined eligibility criteria) to the number of poor people, and Medicaid spending per capita were considered. Although these data were drawn from a number of sources, they were available for all states.

There was great variation between the states, and even within states there was often variability in rankings on each of the specific indexes. For example, 26% of the population of New Mexico was found to be uninsured, and only 38% of its poor people received Medicaid, whereas only 8% of the population of Rhode Island lacked health insurance, and virtually all of its poor received medical assistance from the government. In the District of Columbia 19% of the population was uninsured, but 96% of its poor received Medicaid. Overall, the Northeast fared best for this category, and the South and Southwest fared worse. Generally, how well a state ranked was a reflection of that state's general economic condition. The range of scores for the particular indexes is shown in the table.

Healthy environment. A healthy environment was considered one in which citizens are protected from environmentally caused illness and injury (including occupational injuries and diseases) and environmentally induced ("man-made") cancers. When the environment in which people live is conducive to health, there is a reduced need for expensive treatments and hospital stays and thus a reduction in overall cost of medical care. To evaluate how well a state was doing in providing a healthy environment, the APHA used the following four indexes: the Environmental Protection Agency's Pollution Standard Index, which measures the presence of such pollutants as ozone, carbon monoxide, sulfur dioxide, and fine particulate matter; the percentage of a state's population drinking water from a community source that was in violation of the Safe Drinking Water Acts of 1974 and 1986; the percentage of the population that had a fluoridated drinking water supply (important for dental health); and the number of recorded cases of occupational injury and illness per 100 full-time workers—a statistic obtained from the Bureau of Labor Statistics.

Again, there was often great variability in how the individual states ranked on each of these indexes (*see* table), rural states in general having a low pollution index but a significant percentage of their citizens using unsafe drinking water. Nationwide, the greatest variability was seen in the percentage of the population receiving fluoridated water; in 40% of the states greater than 75% of the population used water that was fluoridated, but the overall range was from 100% in Illinois and the District of Columbia to 2.2% in Nevada. Work-related injury as an index showed the least variability; however, data were unavailable for one-fifth of the states.

Healthy neighborhoods. In trying to determine whether people lived in healthy neighborhoods, the APHA considered a broad range of very disparate factors but ones that have been shown to have significant influence on health. Thus, indexes of poverty such as childhood poverty rate, unemployment rate, and average public assistance payment per family were included. Educational achievement and health status are highly correlated; therefore, the percentage of a population that had finished high school (graduation rate) and education spending per capita were assessed. Another crucial index, the amount of tax a state charges per pack of cigarettes, was chosen because there is now convincing evidence that smoking rates decrease as the tax increases. A high tax on cigarettes especially influences the number of young people who start to smoke. Two other important figures were also considered in assessing neighborhood health: motor-vehicle deaths and violent crime—both of which reflect community living conditions, including the prevalence of alcohol and drug abuse within a community.

Because so many indexes were considered for this category (eight), there was considerable variability both between and within states. Overall, rural states in the North and Midwest fared best; poorer southern states and the larger industrial states with significant problems in their urban centers fared least well.

Healthy behaviors. Individual behavior, although highly influenced by many factors, several of which have already been discussed, profoundly affects health. In fact, it is now generally acknowledged that lifestyle may be the single most important determinant of health. In the U.S. 400,000 deaths a year are attributed to tobacco, and 100,000 are alcohol related. Obesity has been linked to increased risk for diabetes, hypertension (high blood pressure), stroke, coronary heart disease, several types of cancer, and gallbladder disease. Use of seat belts can markedly reduce deaths due to motor vehicle accidents.

The Centers for Disease Control and Prevention, in Atlanta, Ga., in cooperation with state health departments, periodically carries out telephone surveys to determine the frequency of particular behaviors that increase risk of illness and injury. The 1990 Behavioral Risk Factor Survey provided data on nonuse of seat belts, obesity, and binge drinking for all but six states. Data on smoking rates were obtained for all states from studies carried out by the National Heart, Lung, and Blood Institute. As the table shows, the greatest variability was found in nonuse of seat belts. The low of 4.9% was in Hawaii, and the high of 59.6% was in North Dakota. Most states had smoking rates between 22 and 29%, with the lowest rate (15.3%) in Utah and the highest (31.8%) in the District of Columbia. The binge-drinking rates were generally between 10 and 20%, but the District of Columbia had a surprising low rate (5.5%), while Wisconsin had the highest recorded rate (26.8%). Data were unavailable on binge drinking in Alaska, Arkansas, Kansas, Nevada, New Jersey, and Wyoming—all of which were given the lowest score on this index (for the purpose of determining quartile rankings—discussed below). The least variability was seen in the obesity rate, which was generally about 20%.

Community health service. Community health services designed to prevent illness and injury through health education, provision of preventive services such as immunizations and screening for cancer, development of policies that promote health, and regulatory action can go a long way toward improving many of the adverse health indexes already discussed. The *Report Card* attempted to assess how well the states individually—and the country as a whole—were doing in supporting such public health efforts. Three indexes were used: state governments' spending on community programs—primarily preventive services and

Public health in the states		
	best	worst
medical care access		
population uninsured	8%	26%
primary care physicians per 10,000 population	10.9	4.3
adequate prenatal care	85.2%	57.4%
population without access to primary care	0.3%	17.2%
ratio of Medicaid recipients to poor people	5.64	0.34
Medicaid spending per capita	$483.68	$48.55
healthy environment		
Pollution Standard Index	0	224
unsafe drinking water	1%	53%
fluoridated water	100%	2.2%
work-related injury cases	6.4	14.3
healthy neighborhoods		
average public assistance payment per family	$620	$114
cigarette tax per pack	$0.45	$0.03
motor vehicle deaths per 100,000 miles	1.3	3.6
violent crimes per 100,000 people	63	2,142
education spending per capita	$2,320.82	$708.30
childhood poverty rate	5.8%	34.6%
graduation rate	89.3%	55.3%
unemployment rate	3.5%	11.4%
healthy behaviors		
seat belt nonuse	4.9%	59.6%
obesity rate	16.3%	27.4%
smoking rate	15.3%	31.8%
binge-drinking rate	5.5%	26.8%
community health service		
government health spending per capita	$188.36	$26.61
sanitation and sewerage spending per capita	$223.58	$34.89
public health workers per 10,000 population	44.4	5.6

Source: *America's Public Health Report Card*, a project of the American Public Health Association, November 1992

primary care services to the poor (excluding hospital care); spending on sanitation and sewerage; and number of public health workers per 10,000 people.

Unfortunately, the data in this important area were limited and could not be directly correlated to the particular problems of particular communities. What was most striking was how little the states and federal government are spending on community health services. It is generally estimated that of the total dollars the nation as a whole spends on health care, less than 3% is spent on prevention.

The nation flunks

The data presented in the *Report Card* demonstrate quite clearly that no state is doing very well in promoting and protecting the health of its citizens. The report used a quartile overall ranking system. The APHA developed the quartile rankings by measuring each state's performance in each of the 25 subcategories.

The states were then grouped in four quartiles for each of the five basic categories—the first containing the top 12 states, the second containing the next 13, the third containing the next 13, and the fourth, the bottom quartile, containing the 13 lowest-ranking states. Only six states ranked in the first quartile for more than two categories: Hawaii, Maryland, New York, Vermont, Virginia, and Washington. At the bottom were those ranked in the fourth quartile for three or more categories: Alabama, Arkansas, the District of Columbia, Kentucky, Mississippi, Nevada, Pennsylvania, and West Virginia.

Only if every state did as well as the best state for each of the health indexes could the nation be said to be doing well. Moreover, given the country's poor performance when compared with the rest of the industrialized world, even the states that fared best cannot be complacent. Clearly, the status quo is not acceptable.

Seeking remedies

Focus on domestic issues now affords the opportunity for the U.S. to improve its low marks on health. Reforms in many areas that are undertaken with their effects on health in mind could help to eliminate many of the marked disparities in health status that exist between population groups. This is well illustrated by the following three examples:

● Seven percent of all babies and 13% of black infants born in 1990 were at low birth weight. Low-birth-weight infants require expensive neonatal care, and even with that care they often survive only with lifelong disabilities. Family planning, good nutrition, decent housing, and comprehensive prenatal care that offers social support, counseling, and treatment for drug abuse when needed would all markedly reduce the frequency of high-risk babies born at low birth weight.

● The use of tobacco—a substance whose production and advertisement are supported by taxpayers through federal government subsidies and tax deductions—is the leading known cause of cancer deaths in the United States. A recent American Cancer Society study documented that these death rates are increasing, especially among women; it is predicted that the percentage of smoking-induced deaths in women will reach 37% by 1995 (from 25% in 1985). The use of tobacco could be cut, thus reducing the high rates of illness and death due to cancer, cardiovascular disease, and lung disease. Such reductions would be achieved by raising cigarette taxes, eliminating tobacco subsidies and tax write-offs for advertising, and providing help to farmers in developing alternative crops.

● Injuries, intentional and unintentional, are the number one cause of death among both sexes between the ages of one and 44. Many of these deaths would be reduced through increased taxes on alcohol; en-forcement of speed limit, drunk-driving, seat-belt, and child-safety-seat laws; gun control; and, perhaps most important, treatment of the epidemic of violence in the inner cities as a major *public-health* problem—not simply as a law-enforcement issue.

The Clinton administration is committed to reforming the health care system and ensuring access to care for all citizens while also controlling the rate of increase in medical care expenditures. It is likely that some form of health insurance will be enacted by Congress in 1994. But before a comprehensive health care bill can be passed, agreement will have to be reached in a number of areas. At present, consensus is lacking. Surveys indicate that approximately one-third of the American people favor a single-payer, Canadian-style plan; another third favor mandating that employers provide health insurance for employees with the government providing insurance for the unemployed and employees of small businesses; while another third support a "voucher plan" that allows people to buy insurance in an open, competitive market. In view of the strong vested interests of physicians, hospitals, insurance companies, business, and labor, reaching a consensus may take longer than the administration originally envisioned.

The APHA believes that health care is a social right and has long supported the adoption of a universal comprehensive national health program. In 1977 the association endorsed the proposition that "all citizens are entitled to comprehensive health services: these include preventive, educational, diagnostic, therapeutic, health maintenance, and rehabilitative services for all illness categories and health problems associated with living and working conditions." In 1989 the APHA adopted a set of principles that it believed should be incorporated into any national health program—calling for universal coverage, comprehensive benefits, financing based on ability to pay, public accountability, inclusion of disease-prevention and health-promotion programs, and attention to meeting the needs of all populations, including those faced with geographic, physical, cultural, language, and other nonfinancial barriers to care. The APHA believes that these principles could best be met by a single-payer system.

As the debate over the best means of ensuring financial access to medical care is waged, it is important not to lose sight of the basic underlying determinants of health that are so essential to the well-being of all citizens. The APHA is therefore urging citizens and governments alike to use *America's Public Health Report Card* to examine within their own states the particular conditions that most need attention. Ultimately in confronting its health crisis, which affects *all* segments of American society, the nation will have to address the societal inequities that directly or indirectly contribute to health status. Commitment to the common good should be a guiding principle.

Hypertension

The heart is the center of the body's circulatory system, which supplies the tissues and organs with blood, thereby delivering vital nutrients and removing the products of metabolism. The pumping action of the heart causes a pulsatile flow of blood through a series of tubes (arteries) that have a remarkable ability to dilate or contract. The arteries, which carry blood from the heart to the tissues, branch off into vessels of progressively smaller diameter as they distance themselves from the heart, ultimately dividing into millions of tiny arterioles invisible to the naked eye. The greatest resistance to blood flow occurs at this arteriolar level, where pulsatile high-pressure flow is converted to the continuous low-pressure flow necessary for the exchange of material between capillaries (the tiniest blood vessels in the body) and cells. The blood is then returned to the heart through the veins.

Each heartbeat changes the pressure within the arteries. The maximum pressure, reached during the heart's contraction (systole), is systolic blood pressure. The minimum pressure, occurring when the heart relaxes (diastole), is diastolic blood pressure. The difference between the two is called the pulse pressure. Both systolic and diastolic pressures are measured in millimeters of mercury (mm Hg).

The two major factors influencing blood pressure are cardiac output (the amount of blood propelled from the heart as it contracts) and peripheral resistance (the resistance to blood flow exerted primarily by the arterioles). These two factors may change quickly and thus are responsible for moment-to-moment changes in blood pressure. Other intrinsic factors that affect blood pressure but do not usually change rapidly are total blood volume, viscosity of the blood, and elasticity of the arterial walls.

Many factors and conditions regulate cardiac output, peripheral resistance, and blood volume. For example, baroreceptors (pressure sensors located in such vital body areas as the aorta, kidneys, and brain arteries) control nerve impulses flowing to vasomotor centers in the brain that, in turn, send signals via the autonomic nerves to slow or speed the heart rate or to constrict or dilate the arterioles. This feedback system enables the body to make rapid adjustments in blood pressure in response to changes in activity. The adrenal glands and the kidneys produce a variety of hormones that cause increased or decreased excretion of sodium and water, thus regulating blood volume; such hormones may also influence the smooth muscle in the arteriolar wall, thereby changing the resistance to blood flow. Thus, blood pressure is a complex phenomenon regulated by a variety of physiological mechanisms, all of which must work in harmony to meet the variety of urgent adjustments required for the body to function normally.

If any one of these systems or regulatory mechanisms goes awry, blood pressure may increase or decrease inappropriately. Persistently high blood pressure is the hallmark of the chronic disease hypertension. Hypertension usually produces no symptoms and may go undetected for years until its damaging effects appear as heart attack, stroke, kidney disease, hemorrhages in the eyes, or heart failure.

Causes of hypertension

Sometimes kidney disease or impaired circulation to one or both kidneys due to a narrowing of the kidney artery is the culprit; more rarely congenital narrowing (coarctation) of the aorta or an adrenal gland tumor is implicated. However, such a specific cause of hypertension can be identified in fewer than 10% of patients. When no cause can be found, hypertension is called "essential," or primary. The mechanisms responsible for primary blood pressure elevations are varied. The usual mechanism is an increase in peripheral resistance, but among young adults and adolescents increased output of blood from the heart may in some cases be the source of the blood pressure rise. Levels of various hormones produced and secreted by the adrenal glands are elevated in some cases but not in others. Renin, an enzyme released by the kidney, may be present in high, normal, or low amounts.

The fact that hypertension seems to run in families suggests that heredity may be an essential factor in its development, but factors such as obesity, stress, high sodium intake, excessive alcohol consumption, and sedentary lifestyle clearly play an important role in the process among genetically susceptible individuals. Much research is now being conducted to uncover the gene or genes responsible for hypertension and to improve understanding of how lifestyle factors interact with an inherited propensity to develop hypertension. This research ultimately may lead to new approaches that will enable scientists to prevent, or even cure, hypertension. Fortunately, effective treatment of hypertension is possible even in the absence of knowledge about its underlying cause.

Hypertension as a risk factor

More than half a century ago the value of measuring blood pressure was appreciated by the Society of Actuaries. Actuarial data reported in the 1920s systematically documented that high blood pressure levels increased the risk of future complications, thus shortening life. The gradients of risk for sequelae of high blood pressure, such as heart attack or stroke, are continuous and without any apparent thresholds. Table 1 depicts the increased chance of death for men and women as systolic blood pressure rises (based on actuarial data).

In 1947 the Framingham Study began collecting longitudinal health information on the citizens of Fra-

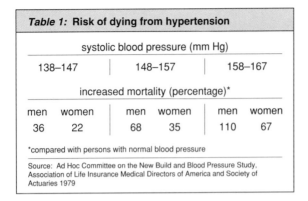

Table 1: Risk of dying from hypertension		
systolic blood pressure (mm Hg)		
138–147	148–157	158–167
increased mortality (percentage)*		
men women	men women	men women
36 22	68 35	110 67

*compared with persons with normal blood pressure

Source: Ad Hoc Committee on the New Build and Blood Pressure Study, Association of Life Insurance Medical Directors of America and Society of Actuaries 1979

mingham, Mass., to improve understanding of risk factors for cardiovascular disease. To measure the risk of cardiovascular morbidity (illness) associated with hypertension, persons free of coronary heart disease were initially classified into two groups according to whether they had hypertension. Both groups have been followed since that time to determine who experiences cardiovascular events. The relative risk of cardiovascular morbidity and mortality (death) associated with hypertension has been calculated at various intervals. For example, the relative risk of having a stroke associated with increasing diastolic blood pressure levels in men and women aged 45–74 years who had no other major cardiovascular risk factors was found to be approximately five times as great among those with diastolic blood pressures above 110 mm Hg as among those with pressures under 80 mm Hg. Framingham data also have shown that even though hypertensive women are less susceptible to cardiovascular disease than hypertensive men, women are by no means immune to the devastating effects of high blood pressure, and the risks rise with increases in blood pressure. In both men and women risk is highest for persons in the older age groups.

In addition, the Framingham Study found that when risk factors other than hypertension (*e.g.,* cigarette smoking, high blood cholesterol, diabetes) are also present, the risk for coronary heart disease increases dramatically. Unfortunately, there is a tendency for more than one risk factor to be found in an individual. A serious U.S. public health concern is that about 25% of all hypertensives are regular smokers; smoking, even in the absence of other risk factors, accelerates the risk for cardiovascular disease. Deaths from hypertension are more common among smokers, and smokers have a fivefold greater incidence of malignant hypertension (a severe form of hypertension that has a poor prognosis) than do nonsmoking hypertensives.

How common is high blood pressure?

Today nearly 50 million Americans (25% of the adult population) have blood pressures of 140/90 mm Hg or more or take antihypertensive medications. This is

14% fewer than the number reported to have high blood pressure a decade ago. It is not clear whether this decline in prevalence represents a real decrease in the number of persons affected, merely some inconsistency in the way this information was collected, or both.

The prevalence of hypertension not only increases with age but is greater for blacks than for whites, and in both races it is more common in less educated groups. Hypertension is particularly prevalent and damaging among persons in lower socioeconomic status groups. During young adulthood and early middle age, more men than women have hypertension, but the reverse is true at older ages. In the southeastern U.S. the black population has a greater prevalence of hypertension and a much higher rate of stroke deaths than do black populations living elsewhere in the country; the exact cause for the higher mortality is unknown, but black women residing in the Southeast are more likely to be obese, and black men in that region are likely to have more severe hypertension—factors that may contribute to their higher mortality.

"Mild" hypertension can kill: new classification

Traditionally hypertension in adults was classified into three categories according to diastolic blood pressure levels: mild (90–104 mm Hg), moderate (105–114 mm Hg), and severe (greater than 114 mm Hg). That changed in 1992 when the Fifth Report of the Joint National Committee on Detection, Evaluation, and Treatment of High Blood Pressure suggested that this classification was misleading because it failed to convey the impact of mild high blood pressure on the risk of cardiovascular disease. Even though a plethora of actuarial and epidemiological evidence exists implicating mild hypertension as an important cardiovascular risk factor, many people equated the term *mild* with "inconsequential" and, therefore, were not motivated to address this important risk factor. Further, the older classification did not permit categorization of isolated systolic hypertension (high systolic blood pressure in the presence of normal diastolic blood pressure), which also increases the risk of nonfatal and fatal cardiovascular events.

Therefore, a new classification was developed describing hypertension in four stages (*see* Table 2). Stage-one hypertension is the most common form of the disease in the adult population, comprising about 70% of all hypertensive individuals. It is responsible for the largest portion of the excess morbidity, disability, and mortality attributed to hypertension. Thus, from a public health standpoint stage-one hypertension is actually a more significant problem than the more severe stage-two, stage-three, or stage-four hypertension. Even though these later stages are associated with greater relative risk of morbidity and mortality for the individual, smaller numbers of individuals are at risk.

Because data are relatively lacking for children and adolescents, percentile levels are used to classify and diagnose high blood pressure in younger people. Blood pressure normally increases from birth to age 18. Children with blood pressures in the 95–99th percentiles are considered to have significant hypertension; pressures above the 99th percentile are designated as severe hypertension.

Lowering high blood pressure: many benefits

Although the risks associated with high blood pressure were well established in the early part of the 20th century, the extent to which lowering blood pressure could reduce risk was unknown for some time thereafter. The lifesaving benefit of treating the most severe forms of hypertension was established in the 1950s shortly after antihypertensive drug therapy became available. Since 1965 a number of clinical trials have shown the overwhelming benefits of treating various forms of hypertension with medications. Protection has been demonstrated against stroke, coronary events including heart attacks, congestive heart failure, death from all causes, and progression to more severe hypertension. Of particular interest have been studies of blood pressure lowering in persons with mild (stage-one) hypertension—most notably, the Hypertension Detection and Follow-up Program. Study results, reported in 1979, showed that after five years a systematic "stepped-care" group who took diuretic (water pill) medication experienced a 20% reduction in mortality, predominantly from cardiovascular diseases, compared with a "referred-care" group who were in the care of their community physicians and received usual care.

Hypertension in older persons is a topic of considerable interest because the disease is so prevalent in this group, and they represent the fastest-growing segment of the population. Sixty percent of non-Hispanic whites, 71% of non-Hispanic blacks, and 61% of Mexican Americans aged 60 years or older have hypertension. In addition, the prevalence of isolated systolic hypertension also increases after the age of 60. The benefit of lowering high blood pressure in older persons has been demonstrated in at least seven large clinical trials. One recent study, the Systolic Hypertension in the Elderly Program, enrolled nearly 5,000 persons aged 60 to 90 years with average systolic blood pressure of 170 mm Hg and diastolic pressure of 77 mm Hg. After 4.5 years a group receiving drug treatment had 36% fewer strokes and 27% fewer heart attacks than a group taking placebos. The benefit was observed among all age, race, gender, and blood pressure subgroups.

Optimizing drug treatment: new standards

Physicians now have a very large variety of antihypertensive medications to help lower blood pressure. Blood pressure medications are divided into several classes according to their modes of action. These include *diuretics,* which enhance urinary excretion of salt and water; *beta blockers,* which slow the heart rate and decrease its output; *calcium antagonists,* which dilate arteries and arterioles by preventing calcium buildup; *angiotensin-converting enzyme (ACE) inhibitors,* which dilate arteries by preventing formation of angiotensin II, a potent constrictor; *alpha-adrenergic blockers, alpha-beta blockers,* and *centrally* and *peripherally acting inhibitors,* all of which dilate arteries by decreasing sympathetic nervous system activity and/or reduce heart rate and output; *rauwolfia,* which dilates arteries and slows heart rate; and *direct vasodilators,* which act directly on the muscle of blood vessel walls.

Because hypertension may be caused by different mechanisms, and drugs may have different side effects, ranging from impaired sexual function in men to fainting, dizziness, headache, fatigue, insomnia, and constipation, selecting the appropriate drug or drugs for a particular patient represents a challenge for both doctor and hypertensive individual. Other factors that may influence selection of medication include the presence of other risk factors or diseases (*e.g.,* a previous heart attack or kidney disease), demographic characteristics (*e.g.,* race and age, concomitant therapy, previous experience with medications), and economic considerations. In some cases drugs from more than one class are prescribed so that the patient has the benefit of several modes of action to lower blood pressure. In these situations less than a full dose of medication is given, thereby minimizing or eliminating side effects and increasing compliance with therapy.

Although almost any class of antihypertensive medication may be given as first-line therapy, the recent report issued by the Joint National Committee indicated that diuretics and beta blockers are preferred because controlled clinical trials have proved that they reduce cardiovascular morbidity and mortality.

Table 2: New blood pressure classifications*

	systolic (mm Hg)	diastolic (mm Hg)
normal	< 130	< 85
high normal	130–139	85–89
hypertension†		
stage 1 (mild)	140–159	90–99
stage 2 (moderate)	160–179	100–109
stage 3 (severe)	180–209	110–119
stage 4 (very severe)	≥ 210	≥ 120

*for adults aged 18 and over not taking antihypertensive drugs or acutely ill
†based on average of two or more readings at two separate visits after initial screening (discontinued terms are in parentheses)

Source: Fifth Report of the Joint National Committee on Detection, Evaluation, and Treatment of High Blood Pressure, November 1992

The other classes of drugs can be equally effective in lowering blood pressure but have not been tested with respect to their long-term effects on illness and death rates. This recommendation reverses what had been a growing trend away from these two drug classes. In the past there was theoretical concern that the use of diuretics sometimes caused metabolic changes, such as rises in blood cholesterol and blood sugar levels, thus negating their benefit in protecting against coronary disease. But these effects appear to be dose related. In earlier studies higher doses of diuretic agents were used than are now customarily prescribed. At lower doses metabolic changes appear to be less of a problem. In long-term studies using diuretics, blood cholesterol concentrations eventually decreased to below the levels observed when patients first entered the studies. Studies are now under way to test the long-term benefits and risks of new classes of antihypertensive medications.

A monumental public health campaign

A National High Blood Pressure Education Program, mounted in 1972 at the direction of Elliot Richardson, then secretary of health, education, and welfare, represents one of the most successful public health campaigns of this century. At that time the results of the clinical trials demonstrating the benefit of lowering high blood pressure apparently were being ignored by the medical community, and many hypertensives were unaware of their condition because it did not produce symptoms. The National Heart and Lung Institute (now the National Heart, Lung, and Blood Institute) initiated a monumental national effort to improve detection and control of this "silent killer" and to develop an education program for health care providers and the public.

Over the next two decades a coalition of 15 federal agencies, approximately 150 national and professional organizations, all 50 state health departments, some 2,000 community agencies, and a variety of other facilitating groups launched comprehensive health-education campaigns that included public service announcements on television and radio and posters at various public transport sites (airports, railway stations, bus stops). The messages encouraged people to have their blood pressure measured. Such screenings were done in shopping malls and at numerous community and civic events. Articles about high blood pressure were published in popular magazines and in newspapers; television shows featured well-known actors and professional athletes such as Ed Asner and Arthur Ashe describing how they managed their high blood pressure. In some communities sixth-grade children were taught how to measure their own blood pressure with reliable measurement devices; they then took blood pressure readings of family members and friends. Churches also were enlisted in the crusade;

the benefits of controlling hypertension were extolled from the pulpit, and church choirs sang the "Hypertension Song." In addition to educating the public on a grand scale, the national program also issued consensus documents for practicing clinicians that brought together the latest data and research findings relevant to medical practice.

The remarkable accomplishments of the national education program have been measured in several ways. The proportion of hypertensives aware of their condition increased from 51% in 1971 to 84% in 1991. The proportion of patients being treated with antihypertensive medication more than doubled, and the proportion with controlled hypertension (defined as blood pressure less than 160/95 mm Hg) increased from 16 to 55%. In addition, visits to physicians for hypertension increased 10-fold, while visits to physicians for all causes remained relatively stable. More important, since the establishment of the National High Blood Pressure Education Program, deaths from strokes have declined 57% and deaths from coronary heart disease 50%. While the precise impact of the national public health effort is difficult to calculate, it is reasonable to speculate that improved detection and control of hypertension *have* contributed significantly.

Prevention: the new battleground

Although treating hypertension has been shown, beyond doubt, to reduce morbidity and mortality, this strategy is insufficient by itself. Even persons with

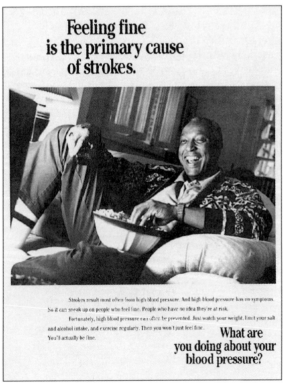

National High Blood Pressure Education Program

well-controlled hypertension have an increased risk of cardiovascular and renal complications compared with persons with normal blood pressure. Cardiovascular complications, in particular, can occur prior to the onset or discovery of established hypertension. The risk relationship between blood pressure and complications is continuous and progressive, even within the *normal* blood pressure ranges. For example, the relative risk of coronary heart disease rises progressively and sizably at every level of systolic blood pressure, from 100–129 mm Hg upward. One very large clinical study estimated that 49% of the coronary heart disease deaths that occurred in more than 360,000 men aged 35 to 57 years were attributable to systolic blood pressure above the optimal level. Significantly, about one-fifth of these deaths were in those with systolic blood pressures of 130–139 mm Hg, which is considered "high-normal" blood pressure. A number of long-term studies have documented a similar increased risk for women. The relationship of "mildly" elevated blood pressure to mortality risk reinforces the importance of preventing hypertension—which is now the primary goal of the National High Blood Pressure Education Program.

Hypertension prevention can be accomplished by two complementary strategies. In the first approach, the objective is to achieve a downward shift in the blood pressure distribution of the entire population. Even a small shift has the potential to produce a sizable reduction in the number of individuals with hypertension and consequently a large decrease in cardiovascular risk. It has been estimated that an average systolic blood pressure reduction of 2 mm Hg within a very large population (not in a single patient) might reduce annual mortality from stroke by 6%, from coronary heart disease by 4%, and from all causes by 3%.

The second disease-prevention approach is a targeted strategy to lower blood pressure among the people who are most likely to develop hypertension. Targeted groups may include persons whose blood pressures are in the high-normal range, those with a family history of hypertension, those of African-American descent, the obese, those who consume large amounts of salt or alcohol, and the physically inactive.

The National High Blood Pressure Education Program recently reviewed 11 potential interventions; of them, four (weight loss; reduced sodium intake to no more than six grams, or approximately one teaspoon, of salt per day; reduced alcohol consumption; and exercise) have been shown to be efficacious. The other seven, which have only limited or unproven efficacy, include stress management, macronutrient alteration (changes in fat, fatty acid, carbohydrate, and protein intake), and dietary supplementation with fiber, potassium, fish oil, calcium, or magnesium.

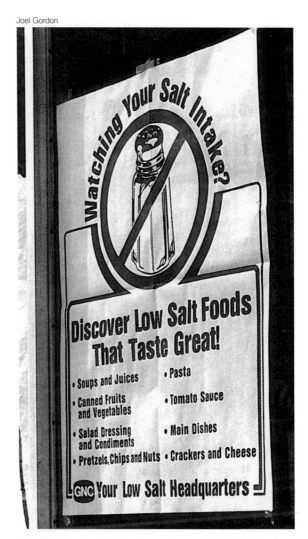

Joel Gordon

Specific strategies that have been shown to be effective in the prevention of hypertension are: weight loss, exercise, reduced alcohol consumption, and consumption of no more than six grams of sodium (one teaspoon of salt) per day.

Because public education has been the foundation of the successful efforts to detect, evaluate, and treat high blood pressure, this approach will also be used in a major prevention campaign. Mass media will be enlisted to convey the importance of consuming less sodium and reducing alcohol consumption. The food industry will be enlisted to promote low-sodium and low-calorie foods in marketing strategies. Restaurants and fast-food establishments are seen as important settings for reducing the caloric content and the sodium, fat, and cholesterol in the foods consumed by the public. Active lifestyles and regular exercise will be encouraged in the population at large and physical education taught in schools.

There is no doubt that substantial gains have been made in reducing the cardiovascular sequelae of hypertension. A variety of scientific disciplines

337

and approaches—including epidemiology, actuarial sciences, clinical trials, basic research, pharmacology, behavioral sciences, and health education—have contributed to unprecedented and vastly favorable changes and represent what can be accomplished when a variety of forces join together to address an important public health problem. Because hypertension *still* burdens society more than any other single health problem, the new strategies aimed at preventing it are all the more important and may provide the key to eliminating its devastating effects.

—Edward J. Roccella, Ph.D., M.P.H.,
Ray W. Gifford, Jr., M.D.,
and Claude Lenfant, M.D.

Infectious Disease

Infectious disease epidemics and pandemics have occurred throughout human history. Progress in medical science has made us less vulnerable to their devastation now than at any point in the past. Nevertheless, the nation's current experience with the human immunodeficiency virus (HIV) and acquired immunodeficiency syndrome (AIDS) is a sobering reminder that serious microbial threats to health remain and that we are not always well equipped to respond to them.

—Emerging Infections: Microbial Threats to Health
in the United States, U.S. Institute of Medicine, 1992

In May and June 1993 at least 16 people on or near the Navajo Reservation in New Mexico and Arizona died of a mysterious flulike illness. On the basis of preliminary evidence, scientists at the U.S. Centers for Disease Control and Prevention (CDC) tentatively identified the culprit as a virus belonging to the group called hantaviruses, similar to one that causes a lethal fever in Southeast Asia. The main host for the virus is a species of rat found in Asia, which may have made its way to the United States as a stowaway on a merchant ship.

Old threats, new urgency

On the scale of potential threats to the public health, an outbreak of hantavirus in the Southwest pales in comparison with the global AIDS pandemic now in its second decade. The outbreak among the Navajo, however, is only one of many "emerging" infections that disease surveillance experts at the CDC and elsewhere are anxiously monitoring. Moreover, its incidence served to dramatically underscore the urgency of a report issued a few months earlier by a committee of the U.S. Institute of Medicine (IOM). The report, *Emerging Infections: Microbial Threats to Health in the United States,* published in October 1992, amounts to a "wake-up call" to a medical community that has grown complacent about the devastating potential of infectious diseases. The authors were 19 recognized infectious disease specialists from across the U.S.

Emerging Infections notes that despite recent medical advances, diseases such as malaria and tuberculosis (TB)—once considered vanquished in the Western world—are striking more and more people each year. A host of other illnesses, such as Lyme disease and AIDS, are more recent entries in the medical annals. Added to this roster are disorders whose causes, once shrouded in mystery, now appear to be microbial. One such ailment is peptic ulcer, most likely caused by the bacterium *Helicobacter pylori.* Another is cervical cancer, which is now linked to particularly malignant strains of the human papillomavirus. Scientists are also seeking infectious agents that might contribute to a host of other common afflictions, including atherosclerosis and rheumatoid arthritis.

Glancing through the medical history books, one gets a sense of the magnitude of the threat posed by emerging new maladies and reemerging nemeses. Influenza, for example, usually a relatively innocuous illness that results only in a few missed days of work

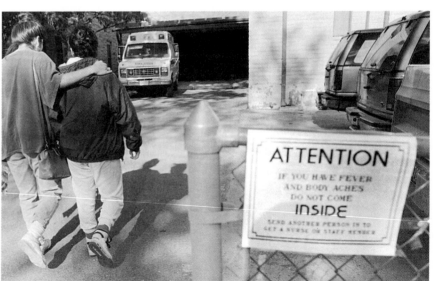

A sign outside the Fort Defiance Indian Hospital in Window Rock, Ariz., in June 1993 reads: "Attention: If you have fever and body aches do not come inside. Send another person in to get a nurse or staff member." The message was intended to keep those with flulike symptoms—who could have been infected with a mystery ailment that had already caused several deaths—away from the building lobby. The outbreak gave a new immediacy to warnings about the threat of emerging diseases.

AP/Wide World

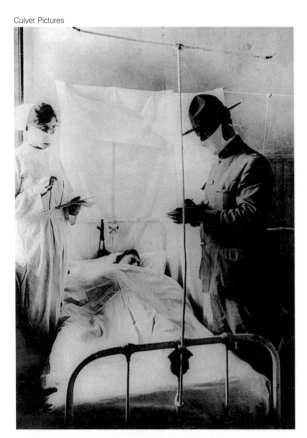

A soldier stricken with influenza in the great pandemic of 1918 is cared for in a New York state military hospital. This outbreak was one of the most devastating in history, causing an estimated 20 million deaths worldwide.

or school, from time to time becomes a major killer. The 1918 influenza pandemic was responsible for the death of more than 20 million people worldwide, including 500,000 in the U.S. The IOM report characterizes that pandemic as "one of the single most devastating outbreaks of infectious disease in human history." While the existence of influenza vaccines makes it unlikely that flu will ever again take such a toll on humanity, the influenza virus remains potentially dangerous. Flu outbreaks in 1957 and 1968 killed a total of 90,000 Americans and cost some $3.4 billion in medical care.

Accounting for "new" infections

Biomedical scientists point to many factors behind the recent emergence of infectious diseases. One is simply the existence of better disease surveillance; respiratory infections due to chlamydia, for example, are reported more frequently these days because they are better recognized. Another, less common factor is the sudden development of genetically altered forms of microbes, exemplified by the periodic appearance of new influenza strains.

More often, however, the emergence of diseases is brought on by the explosive growth of the human population. Many infectious microbes are likely to have existed in nature for years—either in isolated human populations or in animals—and have begun to emerge only with demographic shifts. For example, the spread of Argentine hemorrhagic fever to humans began only after local agricultural practices brought people and the rats that carry the disease into the same environment. Many of the world's most virulent diseases are zoonotic—transmitted from animal to human. Some authorities theorize that AIDS may be one of these.

The magnitude of the zoonotic threat is well illustrated by the frightening case of the Reston virus. In 1990 research monkeys imported by Hazleton Research Products, Reston, Va., were found to harbor a virus that killed nearly every infected monkey. Scientists from the U.S. Army Research Institute of Infectious Diseases discovered that the virus was a close cousin of the Ebola virus, which causes a deadly hemorrhagic fever. In 1976 this agent caused a devastating outbreak of human disease in Zaire and The Sudan that killed 75% of those infected. Compounding the potentially calamitous situation in Reston was the fact that blood tests for antibodies to the virus indicated that it had infected several veterinarians and technicians who worked with or near the monkeys. After several agonizing days, the army researchers determined to their great relief that the Reston virus was not causing any illness in the infected humans.

Many infectious organisms are capitalizing on today's increasingly global economy. One microbe that appears to have widened its horizons thanks to international commerce is the hantavirus mentioned above. Another insidious stowaway is the virus that causes Lassa fever, a disease endemic to West Africa. The IOM report recounts one chilling case history. In 1989, in the midst of the winter influenza season, a man went to a Chicago health clinic complaining of flulike symptoms. As the days passed, the patient became progressively sicker, however, and the illness no longer resembled flu. Finally an astute physician reviewed the man's history and made a correct diagnosis. Shortly before appearing at the clinic, the man had traveled to Nigeria to attend the funerals of his parents, who had died within 10 days of each other of an unknown febrile illness. The Chicago physician guessed that the patient's parents had died of Lassa fever and that the disease was transmitted to him though contact with their bodies before burial. The physician's guess proved correct, but it was too late to save the man's life.

Also appearing to have emerged from the changing interaction of people and the environment is the infectious arthritis-like ailment known as Lyme disease. In the past decade Lyme disease has grown from an obscure malady reported in a few counties in Connecticut to a disease that can strike nearly anyone in the U.S. who ventures into heavily wooded terrain. In 1991 the CDC recorded 9,344 cases of this tick-borne illness, and the true figure, health officials believe, is probably much higher. The industrial revolution indirectly paved the way for Lyme disease by returning agricultural lands in the northeastern U.S. to forestry. Reforested areas became both a home to deer and a site for suburban housing developments. According to the IOM report, "The resulting proximity of people, mice, deer, and ticks has created nearly perfect conditions for the transmission of the Lyme disease spirochete to human hosts."

Rift Valley fever is another disease that appears to be a beneficiary of human-induced environmental change. Transmitted by a mosquito, the virus that causes Rift Valley fever was known for years in Africa as a cause of sickness in domesticated animals and, in rare cases, humans. In 1977, however, the virus infected 200,000 Egyptians, killing 600. Public health experts now blame the outbreak on the Aswan Dam, the construction of which flooded many hectares of land along the banks of the Nile River. The flooding, in turn, led to ideal breeding conditions for the mosquitoes that carry the illness.

Paying the price for complacency

Despite its many advances, modern medicine has unwittingly contributed to the emergence of infectious diseases. The development of antibiotic drugs is a case in point. As recently as 50 years ago, physicians were all but impotent in the face of bacterial infections. This situation changed during World War II, however, when penicillin, a substance derived from mold, came into widespread use. Penicillin heralded the advent of an entirely new class of drugs, the antibiotics, capable of curing almost any bacterial disease. But the

very success of these so-called wonder drugs, as the IOM report notes, fostered a "mood of complacency" in the medical community. Perhaps no other disease illustrates this point as well as pulmonary TB, a bacterial infection that destroys lung tissue. Drugs effective against TB have been available since the 1950s, when the incidence of the disease began to decline in developed countries. Nevertheless, TB continued to be a major killer in the less developed world.

In the mid-1980s, however, countries with a low incidence of TB began to experience a resurgence. In the U.S., for example, the number of cases jumped from 22,201 in 1985 to 26,283 in 1991. Behind TB's comeback, according to health officials, are a number of social factors, including an increase in homelessness, poverty, and drug abuse. Another factor is the rise of drug-resistant TB organisms. In patients unwilling or unable to comply with the prolonged treatment regimen—lasting six months or more—these drug-resistant strains flourish. But probably the most important factor in the reemergence of TB is the AIDS pandemic. People infected with HIV are about 500 times as likely to develop TB as are uninfected individuals. Moreover, in AIDS patients and others with weakened immune systems, TB becomes entrenched and extremely difficult to treat.

During the 1960s and '70s, when TB was on the decline in Western countries, the development of new TB drugs was a low priority, and few such agents were introduced. At the same time, TB organisms were evolving into tough new, drug-resistant strains. Thus, the medical community now finds itself ill-equipped to grapple with emerging multidrug-resistant forms of TB, and this is a problem the IOM report characterizes as a "major threat" to health in the U.S.

The resistance of microbes to drugs, as exemplified by TB, is playing a growing role in the emergence of

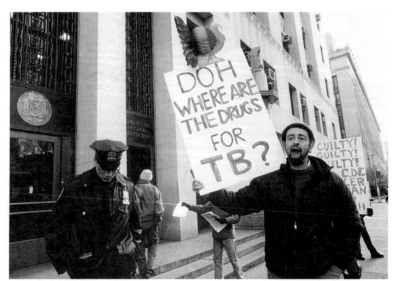

Outside the offices of the New York City Department of Health, demonstrators from ACT UP (the AIDS Coalition to Unleash Power) protest the failure of public health authorities to deal effectively with the resurgence of TB, a disease that is especially difficult to combat in people whose immune systems are weakened by HIV. Widespread complacency engendered by the decline of TB in the West in recent decades has left medical science unprepared for the drug-resistant TB strains that are now emerging.

Meryl Levin—Impact Visuals

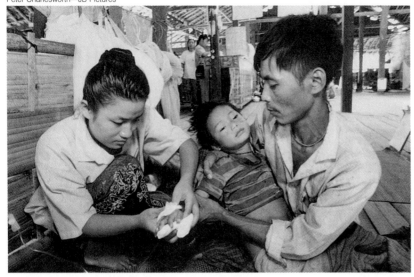

A young malaria victim receives treatment at a hospital in Thailand. Despite intensive eradication efforts, malaria still claims over one million lives annually in tropical regions of the world. The failure of the campaign against the disease is due in large part to the parasite's ability to develop strains that are resistant to drugs.

infections. Resistance springs from the fact that in all living things, no two mature organisms are genetically identical. In the case of disease-causing organisms, some individuals in a population may not possess the genes that account for the species' vulnerability to a particular drug. These genetic mutants, capable of resisting the effects of one or even many drugs, are the most likely to survive. They also have a better chance of reproducing, thus increasing the drug-resistant population.

Another disease that is becoming especially refractory to existing treatments is malaria, which worldwide kills about one million people—mostly children—every year. While malaria remains a huge threat to people in less developed countries, its significance has declined substantially in the U.S., from some 500,000 cases a year in the early 1900s to about 1,200 cases a year in the 1990s, most of them in newly arrived immigrants and travelers returning from endemic regions. As recently as 1988, however, an outbreak affecting 30 people occurred in California. Many varieties of the mosquito-borne protozoan that causes malaria are now resistant to drugs once used against them. The rise of drug-resistant strains, coupled with the periodic resurgence of the disease, prompted the IOM report to warn against the possibility of future malaria epidemics in nonendemic areas.

Ironically, the success of vaccines against many infectious illnesses has also contributed to the reemergence of certain diseases. The proliferation of vaccines against such once-dreaded killers as diphtheria, measles, and polio began at about the same time as antibiotics began to be widely used. Perhaps the crowning achievement of vaccine technology so far has been the eradication of smallpox, a disease that killed about 400,000 people a year in Europe during the 17th and 18th centuries. In 1967, shortly after the development of an improved vaccine against smallpox, the World Health Organization (WHO) began an intensive effort to eradicate the disease, which at that time continued to flourish in 44 countries; four years later only 16 countries reported cases of smallpox. By 1977 the last known smallpox case in the world had been diagnosed in Somalia. Two years later WHO declared the world rid of this ancient scourge.

Given the resounding success of the international campaign against smallpox, why, one might ask, are any vaccine-preventable diseases still posing a major public health problem? It is instructive to look at the example of measles. After an effective vaccine for measles came into use in the United States in 1963, the number of cases dropped from a few hundred thousand per year in the early 1960s to fewer than 2,000 in the early 1980s. This trend began to reverse itself in 1989, however, and during the major 1989–90 measles epidemic, there were a total of 55,000 recorded cases. The reemergence of measles, unlike that of TB, could not be blamed on a lack of effective drugs or the rise of a predisposing illness such as AIDS. Rather, epidemiologists attributed the measles surge to the fact that many children simply were not getting immunized against this common and easily preventable infection.

Finally, modern medical practices sometimes inadvertently lead to the spread of infectious disease. About 5% of people who are hospitalized contract infections that they did not have when admitted. These nosocomial, or hospital-acquired, infections account for about 20,000 U.S. deaths a year and represent billions of dollars in health care costs.

Enhanced surveillance: a critical need

The final chapter of *Emerging Infections,* entitled "Addressing the Threats," deals with the pressing question of how to combat emerging infections. Since prompt recognition of an outbreak is crucial to disease control, public health experts agree that surveillance is an important priority. Most surveillance consists of the gathering of data ("passive" surveillance). The CDC's National Notifiable Diseases Surveillance System, established in 1961, relies on physicians and hospitals around the U.S. to voluntarily report cases of 53 "notifiable" infectious diseases. State health agencies must report all cases of those diseases requiring quarantine: cholera, diphtheria, plague, smallpox, infectious tuberculosis, viral hemorrhagic fevers, and yellow fever. In addition, the CDC has established the National Nosocomial Infections Surveillance System, which collects data from a network of 120 hospitals. The IOM report recommends that the network be enlarged and expanded in scope to include data on antiviral drug resistance and rates of illness and death due to nosocomial infections.

The authors of the report believe that disease surveillance in the U.S. is seriously in need of improvement. They point out that an outbreak of any disease not on the CDC's list could go undetected until well after it had begun to threaten human health. The report cites the CDC's action plan for tuberculosis as an example of how the system functions at its best. In December 1991 the agency brought together a task force to advise it on how to tackle the growing problem of drug-resistant TB. These experts devised a plan consisting of several specific objectives—intensification of epidemiological studies and surveillance, expansion of basic research on the mycobacterium that causes TB, and improvements in patient management. The IOM report suggests that an expert panel like the one assembled to advise on TB could give the

CDC broader recommendations on improving overall disease surveillance.

Even more troubling than the deficiencies in the U.S. surveillance system is the state of international disease surveillance. For years the U.S. government, primarily through the National Institutes of Health (NIH) and the Department of Defense (DOD), has supported overseas laboratories for detecting infectious diseases around the globe. In the past two decades, however, many of these labs have closed or shifted away from surveillance work, leaving a critical gap in the network. Laboratories staffed by DOD personnel—such as the U.S. Army Medical Research Unit in Kuala Lumpur, Malaysia, which conducted groundbreaking work on the mite that causes one form of typhus—are closing as well.

Nonetheless, many important facilities continue to perform the vital function of disease surveillance. The NIH directs an international group of laboratories that conduct research on tropical diseases, and the CDC participates in WHO's global influenza surveillance network, which alerts vaccine manufacturers to changes in the prevailing influenza strains. These efforts, however, fall short of an effective global surveillance system. At a minimum, the IOM report states, any global network must have the following characteristics:

• a mechanism for detecting clusters of new or unusual diseases
• laboratories capable of identifying and characterizing infectious agents
• a database to record reported cases and to disseminate information
• a mechanism to provide feedback to reporting agencies and individuals for the purpose of mobilizing effective intervention in the event of a disease outbreak

Effective intervention

Surveillance of emerging infectious diseases becomes an academic pursuit if health organizations are unable to mount a successful campaign against the threat. As in any combat situation, it is the "soldiers in the trenches" who provide the first line of defense. In the case of the CDC, this function is fulfilled by the Epidemic Intelligence Service, which trains health professionals to conduct epidemiological research in the field. This 40-year-old program has helped the CDC solve many mysterious outbreaks—including epidemics of Hong Kong influenza, Legionnaires' disease, and toxic shock syndrome. The IOM report recommends that the CDC expand the service, both at home and abroad, and suggests that Congress consider legislation to fund a program to increase the number of trainees in public health, epidemiology, infectious disease research, and medical entomology (the study of insects that transmit disease).

As noted above, another line of defense is provided by the overseas infectious disease laboratories

Despite the existence of sophisticated facilities for studying infectious agents, many authorities caution that the surveillance system must be improved if emerging diseases are to be discovered in time to prevent potentially lethal outbreaks.

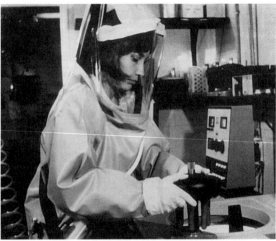

The New York Times

of the DOD. Once there were 20 such labs; now there are only seven, located in Brazil, Egypt, Indonesia, Kenya, Korea, Peru, and Thailand. These laboratories, which have tended to focus on diseases that afflict the military, have gained international renown for both basic research on infectious organisms and applied research (*i.e.,* testing of new drugs and vaccines). The IOM report recommends that the U.S. continue funding these labs and take action to prevent any more of these facilities from closing.

Probably the most cost-effective way of combating emerging infectious diseases is to prevent them in the first place. An effective vaccine saves considerably more in health care dollars than it costs to produce. For example, the recently developed vaccine against the bacterium *Haemophilus influenzae* type B—the most common cause of meningitis in infants—has already dramatically reduced the incidence of this infection in the U.S. On the basis of an effectiveness rate of 72%, vaccinating U.S. infants would save $465 million in treatment expenses. Production and distribution costs for the vaccine would amount to $106 million, netting a saving of $359 million.

The vaccine business can be a risky one for drug manufacturers, however. Because public health authorities sometimes can only speculate on which vaccines—and what quantities of them—might be needed in the future, manufacturers often cannot justify producing a particular vaccine; the costs, including liability for injuries or deaths resulting from vaccine administration, may outweigh potential profits. In fact, since 1985 concern about liability has driven half of all U.S vaccine manufacturers out of the market. This situation puts the U.S. at a disadvantage not only in responding to emerging new diseases but also in combating recurrences of diseases for which effective immunization exists.

The following "worst-case" scenario, imagined by the authors of *Emerging Infections,* persuasively illustrates their point about lack of preparedness:

Consider the city of New Orleans, with a population of about 500,000 people. Early in this century, in cities along the lower Mississippi River, deaths from yellow fever were as high as 50 percent of those infected. We know that the insect vector for yellow fever, the mosquito *Aedes aegypti,* is still in the area in abundance, as is a newly introduced potential vector, *Ae. albopictus.* . . . Were yellow fever to break out in New Orleans and a determination be made to vaccinate the city's population, the existing North American vaccine supply would be exhausted within several days. . . . We could project with some confidence that 100,000 people would become ill with yellow fever and that 10,000 would likely die within a 90-day period. In addition to the loss of life, monetary costs to the health care system and to the New Orleans economy can be predicted to be in the tens of millions of dollars.

To remedy the inadequacy of current vaccine stock as well as provide for increased vaccine research and development, the IOM report recommends that the U.S. stockpile selected vaccines and develop a "surge" ca-

pacity for vaccine development and production. The report envisions two possible means of accomplishing this objective. One would be for the government to support vaccine manufacturers by providing purchase guarantees, analogous to farm commodity loans, to companies willing to maintain vaccine stocks. Another method would be to build federal facilities for vaccine research, development, and production.

Still another way to nip emerging microbial infections in the bud would be to control the vectors, or sources, of these microbes. According to the IOM report, the U.S. and other developed countries "have been able to free themselves to a remarkable degree from the burden of vector-borne diseases." An example of one successful effort is California's mosquito-control program, which, on a relatively modest budget ($48.9 million in 1991 for an area covering 20 million people), provides surveillance and intervention against mosquito-borne encephalitis, plague, and malaria. However, pesticide laws are hampering the ability of federal, state, and local agencies to intervene against disease vectors. The Environmental Protection Agency (EPA), responding to concerns over the health effects of pesticides, has developed strict standards for registering these products. Many companies have declined to follow the standards, opting instead to discontinue selling certain pesticides on U.S. markets. To remedy this situation, *Emerging Infections* recommends that the EPA develop alternative procedures for licensing—and stockpiling—pesticides necessary to curtail disease vectors.

Finally, if prevention fails, public health organizations will have to turn to antimicrobial drugs. As discussed above, the major problem with current drugs on the market is that infectious organisms increasingly are becoming resistant to available therapies. To help stem the tide of drug resistance, the report recommends that the U.S. government better educate health care personnel, veterinarians, and agriculturalists about the importance of using antimicrobials sparingly and "rationally."

The need for vigilance

Perhaps there will never be another Black Death, the pandemic of bubonic plague during the Middle Ages that killed some 25 million people—at least a fourth of the population of western Europe—in four years. Even today, however, cases of bubonic plague pop up in all parts of the world. The lesson of history serves as a reminder of the awful power of this disease and the need to remain watchful. Vigilance, in fact, is the key to prevention and control of any disease outbreak—from the current AIDS pandemic to future, unknown killers. This is the overriding message of the IOM report, one its authors hope the public health community will take to heart.

—Richard Stone

Special Report
John Snow Gets His Monument: London's Tribute to a Medical Pioneer

by Stephen Lock, M.D.

In July 1992 in the heart of London, an unusual memorial was unveiled to John Snow, one of medicine's most original thinkers, who is best remembered as the "father of 'shoe leather' epidemiology." Just opposite the John Snow public house now stands a single-handled pump—commemorating this medical pioneer's role in stopping one of the worst outbreaks of cholera ever experienced by Britain, during the epidemic years of 1854–55.

Revered by modern epidemiologists, Snow is less well known by other physicians and even less so by laypeople. Moreover, as so often happens, the choice of the pump as a tribute is based on a legend that, however picturesque, misrepresents and even diminishes Snow's signal contribution.

Who was Snow?

Who exactly was this 19th-century physician, and why should his work still be the subject of discussion and—indeed—debate almost 140 years after he came briefly onto center stage? And is it possible now to distinguish between the myths about Snow and his real contributions?

Snow was born in York in 1813. He studied medicine by apprenticeship and started his medical career in 1838 as a family physician in Frith Street, in London's raffish and poverty-stricken Soho district. Although by 1854 he had moved his home and practice a few hundred meters away to the more fashionable Sackville Street, just off Piccadilly, he still attended patients in his original neighborhood, and it was this part of London that suffered in particular during England's third major outbreak of cholera. In a small locale with a diameter of only about 230 m (250 yd), in the 10 days from Aug. 31 to Sept. 9, 1854, over 500 people died. This figure undoubtedly would have been much higher if three-quarters of the area's population had not already fled.

Legend has it that Snow, whose interest in cholera dated back as far as 1848, recognized that the disease originated from a pump on Broad (now Broadwick) Street, which supplied water to the neighborhood. According to this version of the story, he boldly immobilized the source of the disease in a single dramatic gesture; he removed the handle of the pump, whereupon the epidemic stopped. In truth, five years had passed since Snow had first suggested that cholera

was principally spread by water, proposing this theory in a 31-page pamphlet published in 1849. What he really did in 1854 was suggest to the local Board of Guardians that the pump handle be removed—and the water supply thus curtailed—and, rather reluctantly, the authorities followed his advice. By then, however, the epidemic had already begun to subside; thus, while there conceivably could have been a second wave of cases, the removal of the pump handle came too late to have any major effect.

For Snow, the episode of the pump served mainly to graphically demonstrate his original hypothesis. His subsequent additional painstaking research, published in 1855 in his book *On the Mode of Communication of Cholera,* was initially attacked or ignored and then belatedly and grudgingly accepted. Finally, he was praised for his perspicacity. By then, however, Snow was dead, having succumbed to a stroke in 1858 at the age of 45.

Spread of a dread disease

Cholera is a disease of the digestive system. Once ingested, the causative organism, the bacterium *Vibrio cholerae,* settles in the intestines. There it multiplies and, after an incubation period of a few hours to four days, produces the characteristic symptoms: vomiting and the purging of enormous quantities of watery diarrhea. The latter contains shreds of the lining of the intestines—so-called rice-water stools. As the result of losing such great quantities of water and salts, patients become shrunken and shriveled from dehydration. They develop painful cramps in the limbs and chest, and many succumb a few hours to days afterward from shock. Among those affected by the classic form of the disease, the death rate is 40–60%.

Nowadays the picture is often different. In the majority of industrialized countries, the water supply is safe. Sensible travelers to cholera-endemic areas not only avoid drinking suspect tap water but also refrain from eating shellfish and uncooked fruit and vegetables, as contaminated foods, too, are a potential mode of transmission. Moreover, in healthy, well-nourished adults the bacterium often fails to get a foothold since it may be killed by stomach acids during the normal process of digestion. Even if infection does result, it may give rise to nothing more than looseness of the bowels. A moderately effective vaccine is available for

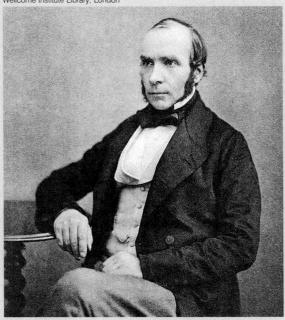

The English physician John Snow's pioneering investigation into the source of an 1854 cholera outbreak in London earned him the title "father of 'shoe leather' epidemiology" and a reputation as one of medicine's most original thinkers.

travelers, and for those who still develop the full-blown disease, there is readily administered, inexpensive, and effective treatment, which centers on replacing the enormous losses of fluid and salts with oral or intravenous infusions. Sometimes antibiotics such as tetracycline are used, in conjunction with rehydration therapy, to kill the bacterium.

In Snow's day, however, nobody recognized the cause of cholera, let alone had the modern resources to treat the disease. If anything, the treatments relied upon at that time did more to hasten the patient's end than to delay or prevent it. There were many and varied measures, ranging from the most common treatments—bleeding of the patient (through the use of leeches) and inducing vomiting with powerful purgatives—to blistering the skin with nitric acid, administering electric shocks, and "bathing" the patient in hot air by means of a device that fit under the bedclothes (the rationale being to warm the cholera victim's characteristically cold skin). It is therefore not surprising that a candid German physician declared in 1833, "We know of absolutely no other disease in which the utter powerlessness of the healing art is manifested as cholera."

One great difficulty in the 1800s was terminology. For centuries all sorts of diseases characterized by looseness of the bowels had been referred to by physicians as cholera. But there is no certainty that any cases of so-called Asiatic cholera—or true cholera—the scourge of the 18th century, actually existed be-

fore the 1780s, when there was a small outbreak on the British warship *Seahorse,* lying off the coast of Madras, India.

The year 1817 was critical in the history of Asiatic cholera. In Jessore, India, in the Ganges Delta, there was a major outbreak that spread throughout that country and eventually to the Far East and the Middle East in the first cholera pandemic of global importance. Then during a second pandemic beginning in 1829, cholera spread to Europe and the Americas. During the latter pandemic, the disease traveled slowly overland from India, arriving in Moscow and St. Petersburg in 1830 and thence spreading to Poland, Prussia, and Austria.

The first place to be affected in Britain was Sunderland, a major port in Durham county in the north of England, the disease having been carried by ship from Hamburg, Germany. The first officially confirmed case was that of William Sproat, a boatman, who developed cholera on Sunday, Oct. 23, 1831, dying at noon on the following Wednesday. In fact, there had almost certainly been sporadic cases in the town since August, and the true initial case was probably that of Robert Henry, a river pilot, who, having guided a ship from the Baltic into the Wear River in early August and out again on August 12, was dead on August 14 after a cholera-like illness.

Over the next 18 months, cholera spread to major towns elsewhere in Britain—and from London to Paris in 1832. In 1831–32 at least 51,000 Britons died, and during the remainder of the century, the country experienced three further major outbreaks: 1848–49 (62,000 deaths), 1854–55 (31,000 deaths), and 1866 (14,600 deaths). As striking as these figures may appear, they need to be placed in historical perspective. In 19th-century Britain about equal numbers of people died from typhus and far more from smallpox and tuberculosis. And, although cholera was often compared to the plague, its relative impact was minuscule. In London, for instance, 0.62% of the population died from cholera in 1849, whereas 15–25% of the entire population succumbed to the "Black Death" in the 14th century.

The most arresting aspect of cholera was its dramatic nature—the speed with which apparently perfectly healthy people were suddenly taken ill with an appalling malady and then died. Not surprisingly, given the universal ignorance about the cause of the disease, some saw it as an instrument of divine wrath. Clergyman fulminated from the pulpit that cholera was sent by God to punish intemperance and loose living. To be sure, most cases did occur among the poor, and early on, a connection between filth and disease was recognized—leading to halfhearted attempts to remove "nuisances" (heaps of manure and the like) and to disinfect the walls of houses inside and out by painting them with chloride of lime.

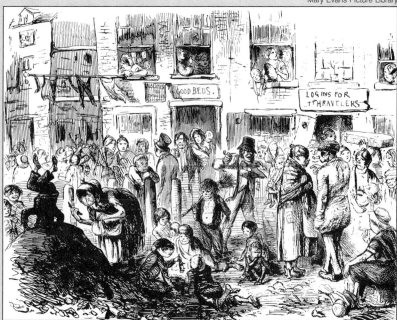

In 1852 Snow had already articulated his theory about how cholera was spread when this cartoon, "A Court for King Cholera," graphically depicting the unsanitary conditions that prevailed in some London neighborhoods, appeared in the periodical Punch. *The famous episode of the pump, however, had not yet occurred.*

"Contagionism" versus "miasmatism"

Medical theories about the spread of cholera fell into two camps. The "contagionists" believed that transmission was through contact between the sick and the well or contact by a healthy person with articles that infected people had touched. The "miasmatists" thought that some infectious agent arose into the air from stagnant pools and heaps of rotting refuse. Such arguments typified the confusion and general ignorance of the times; although in 1840 the great German pathologist Jacob Henle had advanced a version of the germ theory of infection, his ideas were not widely accepted. Nine years later a physician from Bristol, England, William Budd, was to espouse such a hypothesis as a cause for cholera—also anticipating Snow's discoveries by claiming that water was involved. Not only that; Budd also stated that he had found an infective particle, what he called "cholera fungus," in the stools of cholera patients. Budd's concepts received a setback, however, when it was shown that this purported organism, which could be seen under the microscope, was merely one of the normal lining cells of the intestine.

Snow's interest in cholera also dates from this time. He too developed a theory, publishing it in 1849 in the aforementioned pamphlet and also in an article in the *London Medical Gazette*. There were five main points to his theory (which was based on studies not only in London but in other towns, such as Bath and Hull): (1) cholera must be spread by some sort of poison; (2) this poison acts directly on the intestines; (3) the poison must be introduced through the mouth and not by inhalation; (4) all the signs and symptoms of cholera arise as a result of the tremendous loss

of fluid from the intestines; and (5) drinking water, contaminated by water from dunghills and "privies," is almost certainly the cause. Snow's theory, it must be emphasized, was published five years *before* the famous outbreak of cholera in which its validity was proved.

Snow actually anticipated many of the exceptions that might be taken to his reasoning. Birmingham was one notable city that surprisingly had escaped the epidemic. "If effluvia from sewers caused the prevalence of cholera, Birmingham ought not to have escaped," Snow stated, "[but] the water is rendered too impure for any one to think of drinking it. The inhabitants are supplied with water from springs and wells, from the river Taine [now Tain], which is quite uncontaminated by the sewers. In Birmingham, consequently, there is no opportunity for the communication of cholera through the water." Finally, he proposed some remedies, including isolating cholera patients and boiling their soiled linen. He also recommended paying scrupulous attention to cleanliness and avoiding the use of water that had been contaminated with the contents of sewers.

It seems likely that, though Snow's theory was well received by the medical press, it got no further for three main reasons. First, Budd's similar theory had been discredited. Second, most of the medical establishment—including the prominent epidemiologist and statistician William Farr—had always been miasmatists. And, third, by 1849 the epidemic had ceased.

An elegant and persuasive demonstration

"Chance favors the prepared mind," said Louis Pasteur in discussing breakthroughs in scientific research. By the time the 1854 cholera epidemic occurred, Snow's mind certainly was prepared. He could now put his theories to the practical test. When he investigated the Soho outbreak, his suspicions fell straightaway on the Broad Street pump. Upon obtaining the names of the dead in that neighborhood from the General Register Office, he found that nearly all 89 of them had lived near the pump and that no fewer than 69 had been known to use it. It was at this stage that Snow approached the local Board of Guardians, which ordered that the pump handle be removed; the following day it was. Yet an official inquiry soon afterward did not support Snow's views. "The suddenness of the outbreak, its immediate climax and short duration, all point to some atmospheric or other widely diffused agent still to be discovered," wrote the president of London's General Board of Health, adding that there were no grounds for assuming that the disease was transmitted from one infected person to another or by contaminated water.

By then, however, Snow was determined to pursue his study. In support of his incrimination of the pump, he found a local factory where the only water supply was from the public pump; 18 of 200 workmen employed in the establishment had died of cholera. Conversely, in a local brewery, where the workers drank only the beer they produced, there were no deaths. A widow who had moved from Broad Street to Hampstead, then a village on the outskirts of central London, had liked the city water so much that she had a large bottle sent to her new home daily. Snow found that both she and her niece, who had also drunk

Snow's log of cholera cases in the Broad Street area, 1854 epidemic		
date		number of fatal cases per day
August 26		1
27		1
28		1
29		1
30		8
31		56
September 1		143
2		116
3		54
4		46
5		36
6		20
7		28
8	(pump handle removed)	12
9		11
10		5
11		5
12		1
13		3
14–30		18

the Broad Street water, had died of cholera, though Hampstead was otherwise totally free of the disease.

Perhaps the most cogent argument in favor of Snow's theory of how cholera was transmitted came from his 1854 study of the London water supply. Here was one of those natural experiments in which all scientists delight but are rarely lucky enough to encounter in practice. London had always been supplied by several different water companies, and in the case of Soho there were two rival concerns—the Southwark and Vauxhall Co. and the Lambeth Co.—which competed even in supplying houses on the same street. Until 1852 both companies had taken unfiltered water from polluted parts of the Thames; Sir John Simon, one of the key figures in 19th-century English health reform, was to describe the Southwark and Vauxhall water as "the filthiest stuff ever drunk by a civilised community." Then the Lambeth Co. moved its intake to an upper—and pure—part of the Thames; meanwhile, its rival continued to extract its water at London Bridge, in an industrial area on the south bank of the Thames.

Snow compared the death rates from cholera in houses supplied by the two companies. When the inhabitants were uncertain which company provided their water, he was able to recognize the Southwark product because it contained 40 times as much salt as the Lambeth water. The results were clear; deaths

The filth of the London water supply was legendary in Snow's time. A Punch *cartoon from 1850 entitled "The Wonders of a London Water Drop" was accompanied by an editorial that referred to the city's water as "liquid dirt."*

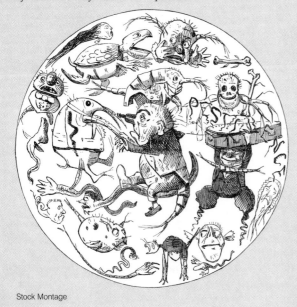

Stock Montage

were eight or nine times as frequent in those houses supplied by the Southwark and Vauxhall Co. Subsequently, Snow confirmed this differential, as did an independent inquiry conducted by the General Board of Health.

In his important 1855 treatise on cholera transmission, Snow expanded upon his earlier theory. The infecting agent in cholera, he believed, was a living cell. He further proposed that this cell multiplied in the patient's body during a delay that accounted for the incubation period of the disease. Finally, Snow held that direct contact between a sick person and one who became a victim was not necessary since contaminated material such as bedclothes could transmit the agent. Snow's account was persuasively presented, addressing the arguments against his hypothesis as well as those supporting it. He applied his theory to the explanation of past epidemics, both at home and abroad, and expressed the hope that the new knowledge could be applied to the prevention of other diseases such as typhoid fever.

Henry Whitehead, who was the curate at the church in the Broad Street neighborhood, was to do equally painstaking research by recording cases in each house. Although at the outset he was strongly skeptical of Snow's proposals, his studies convinced him of their truth. In particular, Whitehead discovered the first, or index, case in the Broad Street outbreak—a baby with diarrhea whose mother had washed its diapers and then emptied the wash water into a cesspit, which was leaking into the well supplying the pump. In retrospect, it was clear that the infant had had cholera and, indeed, the father, a local policeman, subsequently also died of the disease.

Snow's legacy: sound science, clean water

Why were doctors and others so skeptical of John Snow? As so often in Britain, part of the explanation lies in the country's deeply ingrained class system. Although in 1853 Snow, one of the first professional anesthetists, had administered chloroform to Queen Victoria during the delivery of her eighth child (the queen pronounced herself delighted "beyond measure" with the relief she experienced), he was not a member of the medical establishment. The son of a pharmacist, he had come up the hard way, qualifying through apprenticeship and not through being a member of one of the prestigious royal colleges (physicians' associations). He was diffident, was a bachelor, a teetotaler, and a vegetarian, and spoke in a husky, unattractive voice.

Nevertheless, Snow was a genius; not only did he evolve an elegant and consistent theory on the mechanism and processes of cholera, he also showed how the disease could be prevented. While there was to be one further outbreak of cholera in Britain (in 1866), the disease ceased to arouse the dread it had

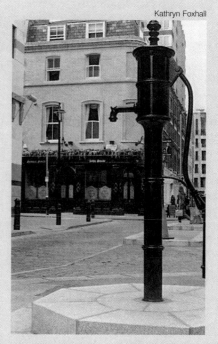

Kathryn Foxhall

A replica of a 19th-century water pump, standing just a few meters from the site of the original Broad Street pump, was unveiled as a monument to London's great epidemiologist in July 1992. Just opposite is the John Snow public house.

previously—although it continued to be greatly feared in other countries, forming, for example, a symbolic backdrop to Thomas Mann's story *Death in Venice*, set just before World War I.

It was left to others to find the actual *V. cholerae* organism—Filippo Pacini, an Italian microbiologist, being the first to see it under the microscope and Robert Koch, in 1883, the first to grow it in the laboratory. Snow's work was a spur not only to the modern discipline of epidemiology but also to the establishment in London and other great cities of a safe water supply and proper sewage disposal, developments that are today taken for granted.

Snow's monument, a replica of a mid-19th-century water pump, was unveiled in a modest ceremony on July 20, 1992. It is situated only a few meters from where the original stood and opposite the corner pub renamed for him in the 1950s. The latter establishment, with its traditional black floor, ochre ceiling, red walls, and snug furnishings, offers a congenial setting for patrons who wish to drink a pint while studying the maps, cartoons, and portraits that decorate the walls, all commemorating the events of nearly a century and a half ago. Visitors can even buy a souvenir of their visit to the historic site—a sweatshirt with Snow's portrait on the front and a chronology of his investigation on the back. Would this dour genius have approved of such commercialism? This author has his doubts. Still, having one's face on a sweatshirt is certainly better than being altogether forgotten.

348

Medical Ethics

Medical ethics in recent months saw continuing developments in the control over death and dying, particularly in the United States and The Netherlands. When a new U.S. president was sworn into office in January 1993, he quickly reversed the stand of previous administrations on several bioethical issues and promised radical reform in health policy. Also, several old bioethical issues—*e.g.*, experimental gene therapy and truth telling to patients—were reintroduced with new twists, and a new debate arose over organ donation by parents.

Control over death and dying

On March 7, 1993, 23-year-old Christine Busalacchi died at Barnes Hospital in St. Louis, Mo. She had been in a persistent vegetative state (PVS) for nearly a quarter of her life, since a car accident at age 17. PVS results from severe damage to the higher brain that renders the person incapable of thought, speech, or voluntary movement of any kind. Busalacchi's brain stem, the section that controls the body's basic physiological functions, survived the accident. With intensive nursing care and artificial feeding, such patients can survive for years, or even decades, even though they have no capacity to experience or interact with their environment.

For over two years Christine's father, Peter Busalacchi, had fought to be allowed to remove the feeding tubes that kept her alive. State officials in Missouri had resisted his efforts to disconnect the feeding tubes and to move her to another state more sympathetic to his intentions. Missouri's new attorney general, who had promised during his 1992 election campaign to end the state's involvement in the case, quickly did so by requesting that the state Supreme Court dismiss the case. The state's lower courts had already given their approval to Peter Busalacchi's plan.

A decade ago the removal of feeding tubes from patients with PVS was extremely controversial and had to be done secretively. Today it is a widely—though not universally—accepted practice. With the collapse of government opposition to the Busalacchi case, it now appears that one troubled issue in death and dying might be resolved, at least for the time being.

The same cannot be said for the activities of Michigan physician Jack Kevorkian. As of early August 1993, Kevorkian had assisted in or been present at 17 suicides. On January 20 he assisted a man for the first time, the previous nine suicides having been women. Although his activities were no longer front-page stories in most newspapers, they continued to be reported and to evoke intense public response.

One issue that lies at the heart of voluntary suicide is whether it is in all cases genuinely voluntary. A document found in the trash of a Kevorkian associate by

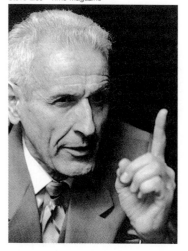

The activities of physician Jack Kevorkian, who continued to help persons with presumably fatal illnesses take their own lives, led the Michigan legislature to pass a law in 1993 making assisting in suicide a felony.

Lynn Mills, a pro-life activist, suggested the possibility that one of the people he had assisted may have changed his mind during the procedure. Hugh Gale, aged 70, suffered from heart disease and emphysema, and Kevorkian provided a mask that delivered carbon monoxide to him. A first attempt ended when Gale reportedly became agitated and said, "Take it off!" The controversy is over what happened during the second, fatal "assist." The recovered document had a section "whited out" that seemed to indicate Gale had once again requested that the mask be removed. Kevorkian's lawyer insisted that the section whited out was erroneous and that Gale had made no protest on the second attempt. With no witnesses willing to testify against Kevorkian and only the ambiguous document as evidence, it was unlikely that prosecutors would press charges.

The Michigan legislature responded to that Kevorkian controversy with a bill that made assisting in a suicide a felony. On Feb. 25, 1993, both houses of the legislature voted overwhelmingly in favor of the new law, which was signed by the governor. The law was designed to be temporary; assisting in suicide would be illegal in Michigan until a special commission appointed to deal with the problem made its recommendations. (On May 16 Kevorkian was at the side of another man who committed suicide but admitted only to being present. However, he did acknowledge his assistance in a suicide on August 4.) The law explicitly permits removing life support in accordance with a patient's wishes, as well as administering drugs to relieve pain even if doing so results in death.

Meanwhile, in the November 1992 elections, California voters rejected a referendum that would have authorized physicians to assist certain patients (*e.g.*, those diagnosed as having less than six months to live) in dying. A similar measure ("Initiative 119") had failed in the state of Washington a year earlier. In Seattle, Wash., however, a new group calling itself

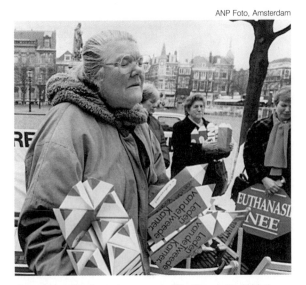

Opponents of euthanasia protest in The Hague. In 1993 the Dutch Parliament approved physician-assisted suicide and euthanasia under certain conditions and thus made legal a long-established practice in The Netherlands.

Compassion in Dying announced that it would provide volunteer health professionals to terminally ill persons who wanted to commit suicide. The volunteers would not provide drugs or other means for the person to take his or her life but would offer advice, counseling, and support.

Such developments, particularly Michigan's hurried effort to deal with a renegade physician, contrast sharply with The Netherlands' unfolding policy on physician-assisted suicide and euthanasia. For many years quite a number of Dutch physicians have openly admitted assisting in suicides and performing active euthanasia. A policy gradually evolved under which physicians who observed certain rules were not prosecuted, despite being in violation of laws against such actions. On Feb. 9, 1993, the lower house of the Dutch Parliament voted 91 to 45 in favor of codifying this unofficial policy into law.

Under the new Dutch law, assisting in suicide and euthanasia remain illegal, but they are permitted for physicians who observe six conditions. First, the request for assistance or euthanasia must be the patient's and must be completely voluntary. Second, the patient must have the information and understanding to make a reasonable decision and to consider the alternatives. (These first two requirements are a part of valid informed consent to any medical intervention.) Third, the patient's decision must be certain—a "lasting longing for death"—not impulsive or the manifestation of a temporary depression. Fourth, a patient must be suffering from what he or she perceives as unbearable and unrelievable pain. Fifth, an independent physician must be consulted about the appropriateness of the requested action. Sixth, the death must be reported, with the physician certifying that the rules have been followed.

Support for physician assistance in dying is strong in The Netherlands. A poll of Dutch popular opinion early in 1993 found that 78% of respondents supported the right of the terminally ill to ask for euthanasia, while 71% agreed that physicians who followed the rules should not have to defend their actions in court. Physicians also appear to have become more willing to admit their involvement in euthanasia. In 1990 only 440 cases were reported (out of an estimated total of 2,300 deaths by euthanasia), whereas in 1992, 1,318 such cases were reported by physicians.

Not everyone is happy with the new law. Protests included one from the Vatican, which compared Dutch euthanasia practices to Hitler's murder of Jews, the mentally ill, and the handicapped. (Dutch Prime Minister Ruud Lubbers, a Roman Catholic, was sufficiently upset at this response that he ordered his Foreign Ministry to file a formal objection to the Vatican statement.) The government estimates that 11% of Dutch physicians oppose euthanasia and assisted suicide and presumably would not take advantage of the legal change. The Royal Dutch Medical Association supports the law.

As in the U.S., the issue of voluntariness persists. Both the old informal and the new formal Dutch rules emphasize that euthanasia must be voluntary. A study by the Dutch government revealed that about 1,000 patients' lives were ended without a recent explicit request of euthanasia. Most of these patients were near death, however, and were not fully conscious. A majority of them had spoken earlier with their physicians about euthanasia, but many had not, and six of the cases involved infants, who could not have consented to euthanasia in any case.

In the U.S., once the right of conscious, competent patients to refuse life-prolonging treatments had been affirmed, voices were soon heard arguing that the right should not be denied to people who cannot at the moment, or perhaps never could, speak for themselves. This position—the right of noncompetent persons to refuse life-prolonging medical treatment—is now widely recognized, although deciding whether the right is properly asserted in a particular case is often difficult. Once euthanasia for the competent has been made legitimate in the U.S., as it has been in The Netherlands, debates over euthanasia for the noncompetent will undoubtedly emerge.

Bioethics under the new U.S. administration

Within two days of his inauguration, U.S. Pres. Bill Clinton acted on a politically important set of bioethical issues when he undid five policies of previous administrations—all touching on abortion. For 12 years the executive branch of the U.S. government had been in the hands of administrations elected with the support of right-to-life groups, whereas Clinton was supported by proponents of the right to choose. He announced the changes on the 20th anniversary of the U.S. Supreme Court decision in *Roe* v. *Wade,* the first such decision to support a woman's right to abortion. On Jan. 22, 1993, the new president threw out a 1988 rule prohibiting any mention of abortion in federally funded family-planning clinics; overturned a 1988 ban against the use of fetal tissue from elective abortions in transplantation research; reversed a 1988 directive that prohibited abortions in U.S. military facilities overseas, even when the woman was willing to pay for the procedure; instructed the Food and Drug Administration to reconsider its policy on the French abortion pill, RU-486, a policy that amounted to a ban on importation; and altered a policy banning U.S. aid to international organizations that performed or promoted abortion as part of family planning.

Right-to-life groups, which could no longer count on sympathy from the government, might now be forced to adopt other tactics, including grass-roots organizing. That the abortion fight can take on tragic dimensions was shown on March 10, 1993, when an abortion clinic physician in Pensacola, Fla., was shot and killed by an antiabortion activist.

As controversial as abortion is, it pales in importance beside another initiative by the new president. Clinton appointed his wife, Hillary Rodham Clinton, to head a task force of some 500 experts whose goal was nothing less than a redesign of the U.S. health care system. Although the quality of health care in the U.S. is generally regarded as very good, an estimated 37 million Americans have no insurance. In addition, the cost of health care continues to soar—growing much faster than overall inflation. American employers increasingly see health care costs as a major impediment to their international competitiveness, and health care consumes an ever growing portion of the gross domestic product.

Bioethicists have debated how a fair health care system should be designed. Though complete agreement has been elusive, most ethicists have concluded that justice would require a system providing health care to all who need it and not only to those fortunate enough to have private or public health insurance. Because economic resources are finite, in a fair system people would get all or most of what they genuinely need and what is likely to provide substantial benefit to them. Services that are only marginally beneficial, or extremely costly, or do not minister to genuine health needs (such as certain cosmetic surgeries) need not be available in a fair system.

It is not clear that the U.S. health reform ultimately agreed to will deal adequately with the issues of access and of rationing. Universal access to health care was one of the central purposes of the reform as initially proposed. That will presumably remain a goal, but economic and political factors could substantially delay its achievement. Further, spokespersons for the plan have been slow to admit the need for rationing.

Care for mental disorders poses another difficult choice for health reformers. Some advocate concentrating on a handful of the most severe disorders that can be treated with drugs. Others stress the value of psychotherapy for a much wider range of mental and behavioral disorders and emotional problems.

Balancing compassion and caution

Research on human gene therapy has been the most closely monitored and rigorously controlled form of human experimentation in history. The prospect of inserting novel or rearranged genes into humans has inspired fears of grotesque harm to the subjects of such experiments, subtle defects passed on to future

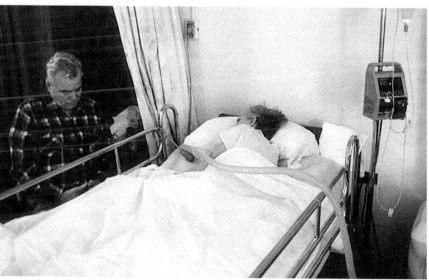

Ruby Washington—The New York Times

Prevented by law from acting as her surrogate in questions of treatment, a man sits at the bedside of his comatose wife. Increasing numbers of jurisdictions are, however, allowing a family member or even a friend to refuse life-prolonging treatment for a noncompetent patient.

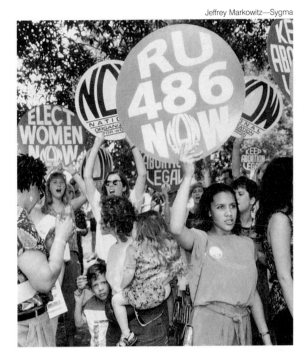

Demonstrators in Washington, D.C., call for an end to the ban on importing RU-486, the French abortion pill. In January, U.S. Pres. Bill Clinton ordered changes in a number of policies on abortion, including a review of RU-486.

generations, and naive or malicious manipulations of body and mind. In the U.S. the fearsome novelty of gene therapy has thus resulted in careful and elaborate screening of all such proposed research with humans. The group that reviews such cases at the National Institutes of Health (NIH) is known as the Recombinant DNA Advisory Committee (RAC). Until the case of Clemma Hewitt, all proposals for human gene therapy had to be approved by the RAC.

Hewitt suffered from a lethal brain tumor that had resisted all established treatments. An entrepreneur-scientist, Ivor Royston, proposed to treat her with an experimental gene therapy protocol—one that had been explicitly rejected by the RAC a year before. Through her husband and sister-in-law, Hewitt had political connections powerful enough to persuade Bernadine Healy, then head of the NIH, to overrule the previous refusal. On Dec. 28, 1992, Healy gave Royston permission to use his experimental method.

Opponents of gene therapy united with the RAC to express their disapproval of Healy's action. The conflict was between scientific and ethical caution on the one hand and compassion for a desperate and dying patient on the other. The rationale in favor of permitting such "compassionate use" exemptions to the usual review process was articulated by Royston at an emergency meeting of the RAC on Jan. 14, 1993: "The best therapy is experimental therapy, because there is no other therapy." In truth, the experiment

on Hewitt was as likely to do her harm or make no difference as it was to help her. Royston's defense of experimental therapies left out any method for distinguishing between those therapies that have a genuine chance of being useful and those with little chance, a distinction review groups like the RAC are intended to make. The mix of desperate patients and enthusiastic scientists is volatile and can lead to regrettable actions. Scientific and ethical review is intended to control such volatility.

In light of public concern over the potential harms and abuses the therapy proposed for Hewitt might bring, the scientific community's stand on experimental therapies was more conservative than it had been about other gene therapy. Opening the door to exemptions based on compassionate use could have the effect of allowing 11th-hour circumvention of the careful review process of the RAC. In its emergency meeting, however, the usually unanimous RAC split in voting for a complicated procedure that for dying patients would permit certain exemptions from its normal review process.

Ethics of truth telling

When Emperor Hirohito of Japan was near death in late 1988, citizens of the U.S. knew that he had cancer. In Japan, however, mentioning cancer is still largely taboo, and it is said that Japanese physicians frequently do not tell their patients they have the disease. Twenty years ago in the U.S., the practice was not much different. The great majority of physicians were reluctant to give such news to patients on the grounds that they would give up hope or become depressed or because they did not really want to know.

Today the overwhelming majority of American physicians say that patients should be told the truth about their condition, no matter how unpleasant. It is widely believed that most patients suspect the truth anyway, that withholding bad news merely contributes to a charade in which patients pretend not to know what their doctors are trying to prevent them from knowing. This realization, coupled with the emphasis on patients' retaining their autonomy as living human beings, which requires them to be informed, underlies the current sentiment in favor of candor.

Antonella Surbone, an Italian physician who has treated cancer patients in both the U.S. and Italy, sparked a debate when she wrote an editorial, published in the *Journal of the American Medical Association,* suggesting that the U.S. practice of truth telling might not be wholly suitable for Italian doctors and patients. A 1986 opinion poll showed the Italian public to be equally divided on whether they wanted the truth from their physicians. Italians for the most part also refuse to see patients as isolated individuals, insisting that when someone is ill it is a problem for the entire family. "The Italian physician remains a powerful, distant figure exercising unilateral decisions on the basis of knowledge that is assumed incommunicable," Surbone wrote.

Although Surbone does not condone the secretiveness historically practiced by her colleagues in Italy, she worries that thoughtlessly importing American practices into Italian medicine may be motivated more by attempts to avoid malpractice than by concern for the patient and that it may thus do more harm than good. Surbone suggests that physicians try always to tell the truth, listen attentively to their patients' subtle requests for information, yet remain sensitive to family concerns.

"Gifts of life" from parent to child

For all of her 21 years, Stacy Sewell's lungs had been attacked by cystic fibrosis, an inherited metabolic disease in which mucus clogs the respiratory tract. In an attempt to save Stacy's life, her father, James, and mother, Barbara, each donated one of the lobes of their lungs to their daughter. The dramatic nature of their gift reignited a debate over whether parents should be permitted to donate organs or parts of organs to their children. When one critic asserted that such donations are coercive, Stacy's parents bristled. Barbara accused critics of being unable to understand how it feels "to be able to take a child you gave birth to 21 years ago . . . and to basically have her be reborn." James said, "We tried to save our daughter. That's all we tried to do." The surgeon who performed the operation emphasized that there was little risk to the parents' health in donating their lung lobes.

In the past several years other parents have donated parts of their livers and lungs to their gravely ill children. In addition, kidney donations between close relations—including but not limited to parents and children—have been quite common for two decades. Kidney donations, because they have a much longer history and occur more frequently, have been studied extensively. One striking finding is that relatives who are potential donors typically make their minds up almost immediately, without prolonged deliberation. To most such donors it seems obvious that family responsibilities—the possibility of saving the life of a close relation—easily outweigh the pain and risk they would experience.

Because the techniques involved are still novel, parents who donate portions of their livers or lungs to their children provoke interest, controversy, and admiration. The public statements of parents such as the Sewells uniformly indicate that they reject any notion that their actions are heroic. Rather, the parents convey a sense of gratitude that they are able to help save their children's lives. It may be that American families exhibit some of the same closeness and moral interrelatedness attributed to the Italian families discussed by Surbone. Moreover, it may be that

"radical individual autonomy" is not an appropriate description of American family life. It can be expected that ideas about individual autonomy with bioethical implications will be both raised and challenged further in the years ahead.

—Thomas H. Murray, Ph.D.

Men's Health

Developments in urology continue to be at the center of issues in men's health. New treatments for both benign and malignant disorders of the prostate are now being tried, and there are basic advances being made in the study of impotence. Although most publicity surrounding the safety of silicone prostheses has involved breast implants, similar questions are being raised regarding penile and testicular implants.

Enlargement of the prostate

As men age, the prostate, the gland just below the bladder that helps produce the fluid that bathes sperm at the time of ejaculation, often increases in size. Such enlargement is known as benign prostatic hyperplasia (BPH). If the enlargement encroaches upon the urinary tube (the urethra), which carries urine from the bladder to the penile opening, obstruction occurs. Symptoms include poor urinary flow, difficulty in starting the flow, frequent urination during both the day and night, and the feeling of an urgent need to urinate.

Until recently over 350,000 men in the U.S. alone were undergoing transurethral prostatectomy (TURP) each year to relieve these symptoms. In this procedure, perhaps the most common surgery in urology, the obstructing tissue is removed under anesthesia with an electrified blade placed in the urethra. The blade "cores" out the prostate, creating a channel that will be adequate for the passing of urine. Complications can include sexual dysfunction and scarring of the urinary passage, which may cause recurrent blockage. In some cases the operation fails to relieve the symptoms.

Many newer surgical procedures are in the early phases of testing. These therapies include heat treatments to shrink the prostate, laser incisions to spring open the obstructing tissue or cause it to fall off, balloon dilatation similar to treatments used to open up blocked blood vessels in the heart and legs, and placement of metal springs to prop open the urinary passage. While the benefits of balloon dilatation appear to be marginal at best and the placement of metal springs has only limited applicability, the other therapies may well come to have an important place in treatment. Each carries with it the possibility of decreasing the three-day hospitalization period required by TURP, as well as avoiding the complications of that procedure. At this point, however, none of these procedures has demonstrated as good a result as TURP,

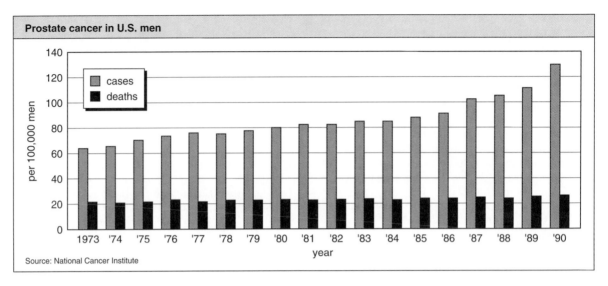

Prostate cancer in U.S. men

per 100,000 men

- cases
- deaths

1973 '74 '75 '76 '77 '78 '79 '80 '81 '82 '83 '84 '85 '86 '87 '88 '89 '90

year

Source: National Cancer Institute

which is still considered the "gold standard" against which newer therapies must be measured.

As more is learned about BPH, it is becoming apparent that some patients who were treated with surgery in the past did not benefit since, despite enlargement of the prostate, the urine stream was not obstructed. Newer studies also suggest that the symptoms caused by obstruction of the urine flow are not always progressive; some patients improve without treatment, and others do not experience any increase in symptoms over many years. For some patients surgical treatment thus can safely be postponed indefinitely. In addition to surgical treatment, medical forms of therapy for benign prostatic enlargement have been developed. A portion of the prostate tissue is composed of smooth muscle, and another portion is composed of glands. Each of these two types of tissue can now be treated with drugs to decrease obstructive symptoms. The muscle tissue can be relaxed with drugs such as terazosin (Hytrin), a common medication used for the treatment of high blood pressure. By relaxing the muscle tone of the prostate, the drug decreases obstruction to the flow of urine, and many patients experience improvement.

Finasteride (Proscar), which was approved for use in the United States in June 1992, acts on the glandular component of the prostate. The drug works by inhibiting production of 5-alpha reductase, the enzyme that converts the male hormone testosterone to dihydrotestosterone (DHT), which is necessary for prostatic growth. Finasteride thus actually reduces the size of the prostate.

The results of treatment with finasteride have been modest, with a 20% reduction in prostate volume on average after several months of therapy. In a study of 1,600 men who took finasteride daily, over 50% reported improved urine flow and 71% had fewer symptoms of urinary distress. Although these results may sound impressive, they are less so when compared with the results of the control group, which was given a placebo. The control group reported a 51–60% improvement, indicating that there was a strong placebo effect in those who received finasteride and suggesting that the symptoms of prostatic obstruction can vary widely in a person over time.

Both terazosin and finasteride appear to be safe and provide a nonsurgical treatment for patients with BPH. Only the informed patient, however, can make an appropriate decision between the options of watchful waiting, medical therapy, and surgery.

Cancer of the prostate

As the second most common cause of cancer-related deaths in men in the United States—after lung cancer—prostate cancer continues to dominate much work in urology. Large-scale efforts to screen for prostate cancer at an early stage are under way, but they are complicated by the unusual patterns of development and epidemiology of the disease. Microscopic evidence of prostate cancer can be found at autopsy in at least 15% of men in their fifties, but this figure increases to 70% of men in their eighties. However, 9 of 10 such cancers remain clinically unimportant (*i.e.,* they do not result in illness) for decades. Such a prevalence of "latent," or "incidental," tumors appears to be unique to the prostate gland and makes the issue of screening extremely complex. Ideally, the physician would like to be able to identify clinically important tumors early and distinguish them from incidental ones. Screening is further complicated by the fact that although the incidence of latent carcinoma at autopsy is similar in different ethnic groups, clinically significant disease is not. Clinically important tumors are, for example, 100 times more common in African-Americans than in native Chinese men (living in Shanghai), with white men in the U.S. falling in between.

Vasectomy and malignancy. Two recent studies, one retrospective and one prospective, have found an association between vasectomy and prostate cancer. The combined studies looked at over 25,000 men with vasectomies and 52,000 men without and showed more than a 50% increased risk of developing prostate cancer 20 years after vasectomy. The studies are considered controversial. No higher death rate was noted in the vasectomy group. A recent survey reported at the 1993 meeting of the American Urological Association found no increase in prostate cancer rates in 8,000 recently screened men who had undergone vasectomy. Nevertheless, the association recommends that men who had a vasectomy more than 20 years ago or who were more than 40 years of age at the time of the sterilization procedure have an annual digital rectal examination and a test to evaluate serum prostate specific antigen level. This is the same recommendation made by the association for all men aged 50 to 70. Although no form of birth control (except abstinence) is free of potential complications, this additional risk of vasectomy must be weighed by men before they undergo the procedure.

Cryosurgery. There have been two standard treatments for localized, and thus potentially curable, prostate cancer. These are radical prostatectomy, a surgical procedure in which the entire prostate and the seminal vesicles are removed, and radiation therapy, given either externally or through radioactive seeds implanted directly into the gland. A new therapy, cryosurgery, in which the cancer is frozen to destroy the malignant cells, is now under investigation.

Cryosurgery has been used for skin and early cervical cancers for many years. However, new technologies were required before it could be used on tumors deep within the body. One requirement was advanced ultrasound to provide guidance for the cryoprobe; another was a probe capable of keeping nitrogen in a liquid state and thus cold enough to freeze tissue. Gary Onik, an interventional radiologist at Allegheny General Hospital in Pittsburgh, Pa., joined with Boris Rubinsky, a biomedical engineer at the University of California at Berkeley, to develop a cryoprobe that could deliver the nitrogen at the temperatures needed.

The combination of these two technologies now allows doctors to completely freeze the prostate by placing liquid nitrogen probes through the skin under the scrotum directly into the gland and to monitor the freezing process with an ultrasound probe placed in the rectum. Because the prostate is so close to the rectum and bladder, the surgeon must take care not to freeze more tissue than necessary. The ultrasound image allows the surgeon to monitor the area of tissue that is being frozen, and a warming catheter is placed in the penis to protect the urethra. Unlike surgery or radiation therapy, the procedure can be repeated if later biopsies show that cancer cells remain. Cryosurgery

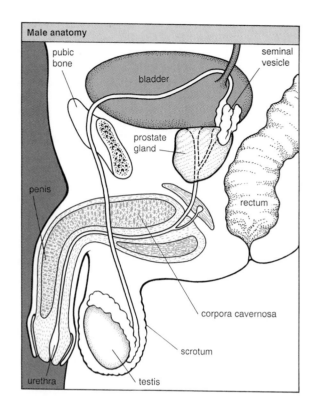

Male anatomy

is a minimally invasive procedure that requires a two-day hospital stay. While there are as yet no long-term data, cryosurgery may ultimately prove to be an effective and low-cost alternative to current therapies. At the present, however, radical prostatectomy remains the most effective treatment.

Impotence

Basic studies of the role of the powerful biological chemical nitric oxide in the vascular system, as a transmitter between nerves, and in the brain are ongoing throughout the world. Advances in the study of male impotence have resulted from this research.

Jacob Rajfer, a professor of urology at the University of California at Los Angeles, performed studies that found that impotence can result when a chain of events dependent on nitric oxide goes awry. Nitric oxide causes the smooth muscle of the penis to relax, allowing the blood to flow in and thus establish an erection. This is the final step in the sequence of events responsible for erection. Taking tissue from 21 men undergoing penile-implant surgery, Rajfer treated the muscles with chemicals to make them contract (the normal state in a flaccid penis) and then exposed them to nitric oxide. This sequence caused rapid and total relaxation of the smooth muscle.

Further studies are needed to determine whether impotence results from nitric oxide's being produced or secreted abnormally or from some other effects of nitric oxide on the ability to produce an erection.

Ultimately, methods of raising nitric oxide levels may come to have a place in treating impotence.

Implants under scrutiny

The first attempts at restoring potency by means of surgical implantation were made in 1936. Initially the procedure involved the grafting of rib cartilage into the penis to stiffen it. The cosmetic results were poor, however, and the rib tended to deform and resorb after a year or so. The first synthetic material implanted into the penis was acrylic, a quite hard and inflexible plastic commonly used in the construction of dentures. The implant was generally placed underneath the skin but above the corpora cavernosa, or erectile tissue, the two cylindrical bodies that become expanded during erection. G. Behri of Cairo was the first surgeon to place polyethylene rods directly into the two erectile bodies so as to provide rigidity for vaginal penetration. While his surgical technique has survived to the present day, the material he used was too rigid to be satisfactory.

The first use of a silicone elastomer prosthesis was reported in 1964 by Harvey Lash, at the Palo Alto (Calif.) Medical Clinic. More recent penile implants were the Small-Carrion silicone semirigid prosthesis and the inflatable silicone implant designed by Brantly Scott at Baylor College of Medicine, Houston, Texas, in the mid-1970s. The latter was the by-product of an artificial urinary sphincter that Scott had developed for the treatment of incontinence. Many new models of implants have since appeared, and up to 300,000 men in the U.S. alone have received either rod-type or inflatable prostheses.

In April 1992, because of unresolved safety questions, the U.S. Food and Drug Administration (FDA) sharply curtailed the use of silicon-gel breast implants. There was some evidence that the silicone gel can leak from an implant and migrate into the body, causing inflammation or, in some women who have received the implants, a strong immune-system reaction similar to an autoimmune disease. Saline-filled breast implants—silicone sacks filled with salt water—remain available. These types of implants are also used in urology and are now under similar scrutiny.

Testicular implants have long been offered to patients who were born with only one testicle or lost testicles as a result of torsion—a twisting of the testicle on its cord—or infection. Approximately 30,000 have been implanted in the United States thus far. The implants, which are purely cosmetic, are constituted of either a silicone gel similar to breast implants or a silicone elastomer, which has more cohesive properties than gel. No studies have been conducted, however, to show that silicone elastomer implants do not leak or even that they are indeed more cohesive than gel.

Silicone-gel testicular prostheses have been voluntarily withdrawn from the market by manufacturers and are no longer available in the U.S. Although the silicone elastomer testicular prosthesis is currently on the market, the potential risk must be weighed against the potential psychological benefit. The American Urological Association notes that if a silicone gel-filled prosthesis is already in place, in the absence of apparent rupture or local complications, the risk of removal may be greater than that of allowing it to remain in place. FDA requirements for additional studies may turn out to be so costly that some companies will reevaluate pursuing the agency's approval, considering the small market for testicular implants.

Early in 1993 the FDA notified makers of saline-filled breast implants that they too must prove the safety of the devices or face having them removed from the market. This position has an impact on urology, as the majority of inflatable penile implants are analogous to saline-filled breast implants. Manufacturers point out, however, that the silicone used in saline-filled implants is harder than that used in silicone-gel-filled implants and is unlikely to migrate if it breaks. Also, far less silicone is used in saline implants.

The current controversy over silicone is based on the overall reaction of the body to the material. For 30 years it was assumed that silicone is inert, compatible with living tissue, and not dangerous to the body's cells. As a class of materials, silicone polymers have thus been considered nontoxic in both animal and human tissue studies. Millions of patients have had silicone implants not only to correct urologic problems and for breast reconstruction but also for reconstruction of elbows, shoulders, temporomandibular joints, and middle ears. The material is also used in wires, silk sutures (which are coated with silicone), and catheters. Many researchers, however, say that the long-term compatibility of silicone with living tissue has never been thoroughly established scientifically. Only recently has the FDA begun to require the manufacturers of silicone breast, penile, and testicular implants to submit data from rigorous trials.

The body appears to tolerate silicone well, forming a natural barrier of fibrous scar tissue around it. The controversy arises from the microscopic examinations of tissue around implants. Silicone implants do sometimes shed microparticles of silicone into the surrounding tissue, which elicit an immune reaction from the body. Generally this is not clinically significant. Despite the tremendous number of silicone-containing penile prostheses that have been implanted in the past two decades, no studies have shown autoimmune problems to be among the complications reported. At this point it can be said that there seems to be little short-term or intermediate-term deleterious effect from this phenomenon. Assessment over a period of 20 years or more, however, will be needed to determine the long-term risks.

—*Philip M. Hanno, M.D.*

Special Report
Health for All:
A Dream Realized in Cuba

C. William Keck, M.D., M.P.H.

Cuba is perhaps best known as one of the last bastions of Soviet-style socialism. In U.S. newspapers, reports about Cuba tend to focus on the negative: the desperation of escaping political refugees; rumors of internal political unrest; speculation about the uncertain future of Cuba after Fidel Castro; and the fervent longings of Cuban expatriates to return to homes they fear they will never see again.

Meanwhile, the story of one of Cuba's most remarkable achievements—its extraordinary health care system—goes largely untold. Nonetheless, it is a story worth telling—a tale of the determination, innovation, and flexibility that have resulted in dramatic improvements in the health status of the Cuban people. Only 30 years ago Cuba ranked among the worst in the world in health care; in 1990 the UN ranked Cuba's health system 31st among those of 191 countries. In recognition of this accomplishment, the American Public Health Association for two consecutive years (1992 and '93) elected Julio Teja Pérez, a physician and the country's minister of public health, to the honorary position of its vice president for Latin America.

The revolution and its aftermath

The revolutionary government that came to power in Cuba in January 1959 found itself faced with meeting the needs of an underdeveloped country with a population of about seven million people, the majority of whom were poor, ill-housed, ill-educated, and unhealthy. Infant mortality was high—more than 60 deaths per 1,000 live births; maternal mortality was also excessive—125 deaths per 100,000 births. Preventable communicable diseases such as measles, tuberculosis, and acute diarrheal diseases were common. Access to adequate medical care was limited to a minority of citizens, and average life expectancy at birth was only about 62 years (compared with 69.9 years at that time in the U.S.).

According to Milton I. Roemer, a U.S. physician and authority on health systems in other countries, prior to 1959 a strong system of private medical practice existed in Cuba's cities. This private system provided care for those upper- and middle-class people who could afford to pay. Many small private hospitals provided services for the more severely ill in these better-off groups, and the urban poor were served by 46 government-operated hospitals with a total of 9,000 beds. Most medical services were located in Havana, the capital, creating an actual physician surplus there, while practically no medical services were available elsewhere in the country. Medical facilities for the military were well developed, and some major employers operated small private hospitals for their workers.

At the time of the revolution, approximately 20% of the population gained access to health care through a private insurance system that helped to finance medical care for people with steady incomes. This system owned 242 clinics and hospitals and controlled about 12,000 of the approximately 28,500 existing hospital beds. Access to care was determined by social class. The wealthy were treated by private physicians and hospitals; the middle class and skilled workers obtained care through the health insurance program; and the rural peasants and urban poor depended on crowded and understaffed government hospitals and clinics, if they had access to care at all. Preventive services such as immunization were provided quite separately from curative services.

For the majority of the population, the conditions of life were abysmal. Only 38% of Cuban communities had potable water supplies; sewage-disposal systems existed in only about 4%; and garbage collection and disposal were primitive, at best. Safe food storage was difficult in most rural areas because of the lack of electricity and refrigeration. Educational opportunities in health care were limited; there were one medical school, one dental school, and six nursing schools. Tuition at these institutions was relatively high, and few scholarships were available.

Creating the healthiest possible Cuba

There can be no Health for all unless All contribute to health.
—Fidel Castro

The revolution did not originally set out to transform Cuban society. Its goals were more limited and immediate: to overthrow longtime dictator Fulgencio Batista, improve the lot of the average Cuban, and develop a democracy. Castro and his supporters did not come to power with a clear idea of how health services—or, for that matter, any other aspect of society—should be reformed. It was over the first several years of the new regime that concepts of socialism evolved, shaped at least in part by hostile relations with the U.S.

It was not until 1961 that a new Ministry of Public Health was officially established. Its task was clear: to create the healthiest possible population. Castro, who was consistently concerned about and attentive to the health needs of the Cuban people, strongly emphasized the importance of "Health for All" to the success of the revolution. Toward that goal, guiding principles were formulated that remain implicit in the health care system today. These major principles of the Cuban health care system are:

● Health care is a right, available to all equally and free of charge.
● Health care is the responsibility of the state.
● Preventive and curative services are integrated.
● The population participates in the development and functioning of the health care system.
● Health care activities are integrated with economic and social development.

Translating these principles into action was a difficult undertaking. It required substantial changes in organization and philosophy, both within the government and among existing providers of medical care.

During the period following the failed Bay of Pigs invasion, when many in the U.S. Congress continued to advocate overthrow of the Castro regime, the Cubans increasingly turned to the U.S.S.R. and to Soviet-bloc countries for aid and advice. In the area of health, Czechoslovakia, which had strongly integrated health services at the local level, became an important model and consultant. Health systems in other countries were also studied by Cuban health planners.

Accomplishments of the first decade

The goals of the first decade under the revolutionary leadership were ambitious. The evolution of the Cuban health care system has been studied extensively by Margaret Gilpin, an American social worker who lives in Cuba, and Sarah M. Santana, an epidemiologist with an interest in health in Latin America. Their works have been drawn upon in the following summary.

One of the first steps in establishing the new system involved implementation of a plan to nationalize the production, importation, and distribution of pharmaceuticals; strong quality controls and sweeping price reductions were an integral part of this scheme. A similar plan was implemented to provide corrective eyeglasses. Another major initiative aimed at completing new health facilities already under construction, including 7,000 new hospital beds, and eliminating small hospitals of poor quality. Sanitary specialists formed units to travel throughout the country correcting environmental health problems.

A Rural Medical Service was established to take health care, preventive services, and health education to rural areas of Cuba, where most people had never seen a doctor before. This agency constructed 50 local 30-bed hospitals and dozens of outlying med-

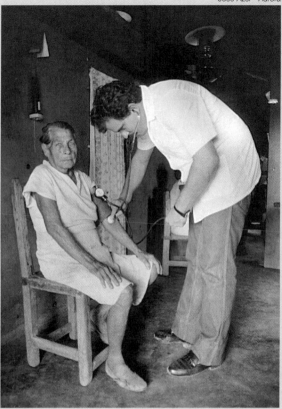

José Azel—Aurora

Under Cuba's innovative Family Physician Program, all Cuban citizens—even those who live in the most remote rural villages—receive regular, twice-yearly checkups from their own family doctors.

ical posts to serve as bases for the hundreds of doctors and dentists from Havana who volunteered their services.

Over a 10-year period, existing private health care facilities were nationalized and incorporated into the Ministry of Public Health; compensation was provided to any owner of property that was confiscated. For the first time, free medical care became available to those who had no means of payment. Treatment of disease was emphasized at first because illness was so widespread and death rates remained needlessly high.

Another important element in this first decade was the development of national programs of infectious disease control and prevention, which targeted in particular malaria, causes of acute diarrhea, and vaccine-preventable illnesses such as diphtheria, tetanus, and polio. Also at this time, local health centers called polyclinics were established as the major component of the system for the delivery of personal health services. As initially envisioned, the polyclinic was to function much like a group practice; the staff consisted of primary care physicians (internists, obstetrician-gynecologists, and pediatricians), dentists, and allied health personnel. Each polyclinic was intended to serve the needs of geographically designated "health areas," comprising 25,000 to 35,000 people. More than 160 such centers were in operation by the end of 1962.

A major setback faced by health planners during this early period was an "epidemic" of physician emigration. Faced with a new political atmosphere and a national health system that promised to change the face of medical practice and limit physicians' incomes, approximately one-third of Cuba's doctors left the country. While the population had grown to more than eight million, by the mid-1960s Cuba was left with only 3,000 physicians and just 16 full-time professors at its medical school.

Nonetheless, as the first revolutionary decade drew to a close, a unified national health system had been established, and plans had been laid to train health personnel in large numbers as quickly as possible. Hygienic and environmental conditions had been improved; infectious diseases were coming under control; and major health indicators such as the infant mortality rate were showing improvement. At the same time, other social and economic initiatives had achieved success; malnutrition had decreased, and full employment and mandatory education had become a reality. A building-construction program had produced new nursing homes and residences for the elderly and the physically and mentally handicapped.

The 1970s: a change of direction

By the early 1970s the concerted effort to increase the number of doctors and dentists in the country was paying off. Infant mortality dropped more than 25% between 1970 and 1975, and maternal mortality more than 15%. During the same period, death rates from diarrheal diseases, tetanus, and tuberculosis were reduced by two-thirds. As part of the effort to assemble

Health status in Cuba: remarkable improvements		
	1960*	1990
population (in millions)	7.3†	10.6
life expectancy at birth	61.8	75.2
infant deaths (per 1,000 live births)	60.0	10.7
maternal deaths (per 100,000 live births)	118.2	29.6
deaths from acute diarrhea‡	58.8†	3.6
measles cases‡	10.5	0.2
tuberculosis cases‡	26.7	5.1
typhoid fever cases‡	17.2	0.6

* some data questionable
† 1962 figure
‡ per 100,000 people

comprehensive public health statistics, almost complete registration of births and deaths was achieved.

In spite of all this good news, however, patients were complaining. A nationwide patient-satisfaction survey indicated that people felt their personal interactions with doctors in the polyclinics to be too brief and superficial and found the waiting time for service too long. The system remained hospital centered, and it lacked sufficient integration of preventive and curative services. Coordination and continuity of medical care were inadequate. The Cuban people, now better educated and more sophisticated, expected more.

Analysis of the system revealed several shortcomings: staff changed frequently; care was often fragmented; and the envisioned team approach to primary care had failed to become a reality, as hospital-based medicine remained more prestigious among health care professionals and physicians were not adequately trained in primary care. In general, the Cuban population was still acting under the old, pre-1959 belief that specialists provided the best care. These findings set the stage for a significant change of direction in Cuba's health system.

The decision was made in 1974 to create a new model of operation for the polyclinics, called "Medicine in the Community." This new approach was based on the idea that health and illness are influenced by the interaction of people with their environment; health care workers must therefore be familiar not only with the health status of the community as a whole (as well as its individual members) but also with the biological, social, economic, and cultural factors that affect it. It was also considered important that health care personnel understand the organization and function of the health services system and know if patients were satisfied with the care they received.

The fundamental objectives of this new health care model were to achieve comprehensive delivery of care to all citizens and to complete the regionalization process. The specific goals included decentralization of administrative functions, establishment of health care teams responsible for all health services provided in a specific area to a specific population, integration of preventive and curative services, encouragement of community participation, especially in the area of health education, and expansion of teaching and research activities. Implementing this shift in emphasis required the redesign of medical school curricula, the revision of residency training programs, and the use of polyclinics as teaching sites.

The new model, introduced in 1976, resulted in broadened health coverage and improved efficiency of health care delivery. The average number of medical consultations increased, and referrals to hospitals diminished. Health educators, sociologists, psychologists, environmentalists, and other nonmedical specialists were included in primary care practice. At the

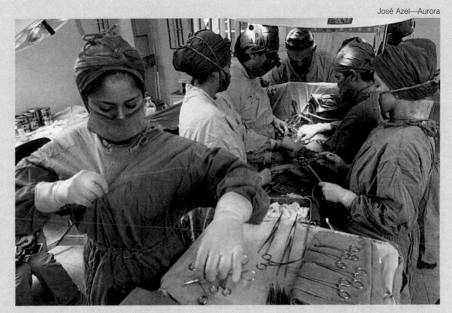

At Havana's Soler Hospital, a surgical team performs lifesaving reconstructive heart surgery on a young child. Cuba's commitment to providing the best possible care for all requires that everyone—rich and poor—have access to state-of-the-art specialty services.

national level there was a better understanding of local needs, and at the local level the response to specific problems improved. The overall health status of the population also continued to improve.

Nonetheless, some problems remained. Busy physicians still had too many patients; continuity of care remained inadequate because specialists' services were not coordinated by a primary care provider; emergency departments were overutilized; and preventive care and curative care still were not adequately integrated. Moreover, patients continued to express dissatisfaction with their interactions with physicians.

"Revolution within a revolution"

In order to meet the continuing health care challenge, Cuban health officials determined that their country would become the first in the world to have every citizen covered by comprehensive family practice. By 1979 the health profile of the Cuban population had changed from one typical of a less developed country—where low-tech measures such as improved sanitation yield dramatic results—to one typical of a developed country—where the population is plagued by chronic ailments such as heart disease and diabetes, which are more difficult to eradicate and require long-term prevention strategies. Public health authorities realized that to address this new reality they would have to devise a program to provide every citizen with a practitioner who could coordinate available services and be responsible for assisting each individual to attain the highest possible level of wellness. Their plan included continued development and refinement of sophisticated technologies and continued modernization of hospitals; at the same time, they sought to counteract the dehumanization that tends to occur with proliferating technology and superspecialization.

The centerpiece of the new plan was the assignment of primary care teams, each consisting of a family physician and a nurse, to serve in communities, neighborhoods, schools, and factories; each team was responsible for improving and maintaining the health status of 600 to 800 people. Specialty backup services were provided to the primary care team through the nearest polyclinic and an increasingly sophisticated hospital system.

This innovative plan, the Family Physician Program, hailed in 1988 as a "revolution within a revolution" by Hiroshi Nakajima, director general of the World Health Organization (WHO), was initiated in 1985. In addition to guaranteeing early diagnosis of disease and comprehensive medical care, the program also emphasized health-promotion activities—health education, lifestyle changes, improvement of hygiene and sanitation. Another goal was to develop community-based rehabilitation for the physically or psychiatrically disabled. The program was also committed to carrying out any medical research that would directly serve the health needs of the population.

Essentially, the role of the family physician was redefined to emphasize health promotion and disease prevention first and diagnosis and treatment of disease second. In an article in the April 1988 issue of the WHO publication *World Health,* Castro described the new family doctor as one who "practises a scientific and humanitarian sort of medicine, with a profound social orientation." Under the Family Physician Program, family doctors were expected to see every resident in the geographic sector for which they were responsible at least twice a year—once in the office and once in the patient's home. Thus, for the first time in Cuba, the well population became part of the physician's mandate.

Primary care: a system that serves the people

Today all Cuban health services are combined in a single integrated system. Every individual is enrolled with a local family physician. Family physician and nurse teams are linked to a polyclinic. Rather than attempting to deliver primary care themselves, as they did in the past, polyclinics accept responsibility for the specialty care needs of patients referred by approximately 30 to 40 family care teams. Each polyclinic, in turn, is associated with a medical school, other health professions schools, and a number of general and specialty hospitals. Responsibility for coordinating the system rests with the Ministry of Public Health.

Family physicians are accountable for their actions to both the Health Ministry and the community in which they work. Individual Cubans are free to visit any family physician if they happen not to like the one located in their neighborhood; if a community is unhappy as a group with "their" physician, they have the option of voting the doctor out. Physicians have office hours every weekday morning, at least one night a week, and one Sunday a month. Afternoons are reserved for making house calls, accompanying patients to specialty consultations, following up on patients who are in the hospital, and carrying out regular inspections of local food stores, pharmacies, and other community facilities that have an impact on health. Physicians are also responsible for initiating educational, environmental, and preventive programs in their communities, working closely with grassroots community groups such as the Federation of Cuban Women and the Committee for the Defense of the Revolution, which participate actively in the work of health promotion and disease prevention.

The role of the Cuban citizenry has been strongly emphasized by Castro. Doctors and other health professionals ought, in his words, "to have confidence in ordinary people and to entrust to their hands the cause of health." Citizens groups are the source of volunteer community health workers who conduct door-to-door public health education campaigns involving such issues as immunization, hygiene, AIDS education (including distribution of condoms), and prenatal care. These volunteer organizations also provide mature female "buddies" for pregnant adolescent women, as well as other services.

Cuban officials expected the Family Physician Program to be fully implemented before the end of 1993, with the placement of 20,000 family physicians in a geographically balanced manner. As of January 1993, coverage of the country's 10.6 million people by family physicians was more than 85% completed. Cuba now boasts 22 medical schools, 4 dental schools, and 34 nursing schools, all producing a steady stream of new health professionals. Tuition is free, but two years of assigned community service are required after graduation. Counting specialists, there is now one physician for every 300 people (the comparable figure for the U.S. in 1990 was one per 463), and there is one dentist for every 1,620 (the U.S. has one per 1,695). By the year 2000, Cuba expects to have 65,000 physicians, of whom 10,000 will be working overseas in international aid programs.

The achievements of the Family Physician Program are well documented. People served by the program report high levels of satisfaction. Access to care is easier than under previous systems; patients are visited at home when ill and have an advocate to oversee their care when they are hospitalized or when consulting a specialist. Emergency room visits have declined, average hospital stays have been reduced, and health indexes show continuing improvement.

Cuba's health status today parallels that of the developed world. Communicable diseases and other conditions related to poverty have been largely controlled. Ninety-five percent of pregnant women receive

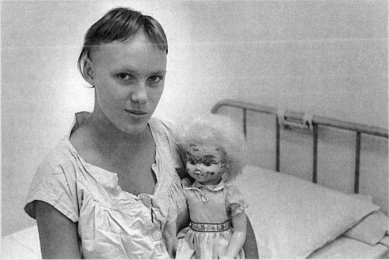

Rick Rocamora

A young victim of the Chernobyl nuclear disaster receives treatment in Havana for radiation exposure. Owing to the quality and sophistication of medical services available in Cuba, patients from many parts of the world are drawn there for care.

prenatal care in their first trimester (compared with 85% in the U.S.), and 98% of two-year-old Cuban children are completely immunized (70-80% in the U.S.). The major causes of death are now the same as in the U.S.—heart disease, cancer, and stroke.

Specialty care: sophisticated and accessible

An important element in the success of Cuba's primary care system has been the concomitant development of its secondary and tertiary care capabilities. The national commitment to providing the best health care possible requires that primary care providers be able to refer patients for high-quality specialty care. Resources have been consistently allocated to support basic biological research, biotechnology and genetic engineering, microsurgery, organ transplantation, artificial heart development, sophisticated medical imaging, lithotripsy, and a national network of immunoassay centers. The country now has 31 neonatal care units, 6 cardiac care centers, a tertiary care ophthalmology hospital, a revitalized mental health care system, and an AIDS sanatorium in nearly every province, to name just a few accomplishments.

Specialist services are available to all Cuban citizens without charge. Unlike people in many other small or poor countries, Cubans do not have to leave their country to receive specialized medical care. In fact, the sophisticated level of treatment available in Cuba draws patients from Latin America and eastern Europe, who go there to obtain medical services not available at home.

Cuba's unique—albeit controversial—approach to AIDS deserves special mention. Unlike their counterparts in most other countries, Cuban public health authorities decided early on in the course of the AIDS epidemic that in order to control the spread of the human immunodeficiency virus (HIV), they would have to isolate all those infected. The result was the creation of a system of regional sanatoriums; these are self-contained communities that provide medical and social support for persons with HIV. Anyone known to be HIV positive is required to live in such a facility. Patients continue to receive their salaries and, where possible, to work. The sanatoriums provide education about transmission of the virus, and when it is clear that the infected person understands how to minimize the risk of infection, conjugal visits and extended travel on the outside are permitted.

Facing an uncertain future

The commitment of the Cuban government to improving the health status of its citizens has been consistent. The two highest priorities of the past 30 years, health and education, have been preferentially funded. The budget allocated to health has grown steadily and now accounts for more than 10% of the national budget.

Perhaps the greatest public health lesson to be learned from the Cuban experience is the importance of asking the right question and then doggedly pursuing the answer. The question Cuban health planners asked was, "What must be done to create the healthiest population possible?" The answer was a system with central control and local accountability, one that provided a mechanism for monitoring its effectiveness and making changes as necessary. Certainly the success of the Cuban health care system belies the notion that strong central control breeds inflexibility.

Today, however, Cuba's remarkable health care system faces a grave threat. The recent political changes in eastern Europe and the loss of economic aid from the former Soviet bloc have led to increasing economic hardship for Cuba, exacerbated by recent tightening of the economic embargo established by the U.S. when Castro came to power. This combination of events has resulted in severe hardships; food is rationed, and energy for transportation and the generation of electricity is scarce, leading to the need for rationing in those areas as well. It is almost impossible for Cuba to import spare parts or other raw materials, including those required for the manufacture of drugs and other medical supplies.

In January 1993 a puzzling epidemic of illness struck in Cuba, leaving thousands of people with visual impairment and other nervous system problems. There was speculation that the symptoms could be related to vitamin deficiencies due to the food shortage gripping the country. The possibility of an infectious agent was also being considered.

Despite the sudden emergence of this disturbing new health problem—which public health authorities were working hard to resolve—the Cuban people are proud of their accomplishments over the past three decades, achieved in the face of tremendous odds. It remains to be seen how their country and its innovative social system will fare in the face of the rapidly changing world order.

Multiple Sclerosis

Multiple sclerosis (MS) is the most common disabling neurological disorder of young adults in the Western world. It seldom occurs before the age of 15 or 16, and it reaches its peak prevalence in persons in their early thirties. The disorder is more common in women than men, afflicting about three females for every two males, and it is typically a disease of exacerbations and remissions.

The French neurologist Jean-Martin Charcot of the Salpêtrière hospital in Paris first gave a good medical account of the disorder in 1857 when he showed that its victims had plaques, or patches of hardening, scattered throughout their brains and spinal cords. He called the disorder *sclérose en plaques*. The plaques are caused by the loss of myelin, the fatty material that makes up the sheath covering the nerve fiber.

Symptoms

Often the first symptoms of MS are caused by patches of demyelination in the optic nerves, resulting in blurring of vision in one or both eyes (known as optic neuritis). This visual disturbance may last for a few days or up to a month or six weeks, after which vision generally returns to normal. Thirty-five percent of men and 75% of women who have an attack of optic neuritis will then go on to develop MS during the ensuing 15 years. That the optic nerve has been affected in the past by demyelination is indicated by a slowing of the conduction of an electrical impulse along the nerve when the test known as the visual evoked response is performed. This slowing occurs in 80% of patients with established MS, although fewer than half can recall having experienced a period of blurred vision.

As the plaques of MS can occur anywhere in the central nervous system, they can cause sensory symptoms, such as altered sensation in part of the body, loss of muscle power, or ataxia (incoordination of movement). When the ataxia is severe, it may result in so-called scanning speech (slow enunciation with a tendency to hesitate at the beginning of a word or syllable).

Those with MS often fatigue easily. A minority may have some problem in controlling urination. Sexual function is usually normal, but sexual activity may be reduced owing to fatigue. Mental functions are generally normal, although depression may occur. It should be emphasized that even after MS has been diagnosed, the majority of those affected are well and able to live a normal or near-normal life. The common stereotype of the MS patient in a wheelchair is inaccurate; probably no more than 5% of those who have the disorder are so seriously disabled.

Life expectancy with MS is more than 30 years after the disease has been diagnosed, which is not much shorter than life expectancy in the general population.

Those with MS do not die from the disorder itself, although the complications, such as immobility, may lead to events that shorten life.

A difficult diagnosis

In the early stages the diagnosis is often in doubt, and the suspicious illness can only be called "possible MS." Typically there is a delay of several years after the first symptoms appear before a firm diagnosis can be made. In autopsy studies it has been shown that plaques characteristic of MS are found in the brains of about 0.2% of the general population over 40 years of age who have had no recognizable symptoms of MS during their lifetime. This means that there are many undiagnosed cases—people with the plaques of MS in their central nervous systems who have not experienced any obvious effects of neurological illness. In societies that do not have well-developed medical services, the diagnosis of MS may be easily overlooked. In North America, which has relatively sophisticated diagnostic services, there are an estimated 200,000 patients with MS, but that number would probably double if "possible" and undiagnosed cases were added.

The criteria that must be satisfied by the doctor to establish a diagnosis of "clinically definite MS" include a reliable history of at least two attacks (*i.e.,* episodes of neurological deficit) as well as objective clinical signs of lesions (demyelination plaques) at more than

Magnetic resonance imaging now provides remarkably clear pictures of the plaques—patches of hardened nerve tissue—that occur in the brains of persons with multiple sclerosis. The white areas around the lateral ventricles of the brain denote the loss of the myelin sheath that covers the nerve fiber.

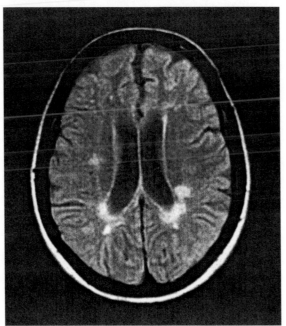

one site within the central nervous system. On the other hand, if a patient has had two attacks but clinical signs of only one lesion or one attack with evidence of two lesions, a diagnosis of MS will be considered only "clinically probable."

Examples of clinical signs are nystagmus, a repetitive to-and-fro movement of the eyes (evidence of involvement of the cerebellar tracts in the portion of the brain that controls coordination of movement), and the "extensor Babinski response," in which the big toe goes up rather than down when the sole of the foot is stroked (evidence of damage to the pyramidal tracts that run along each side of the spinal cord and control the muscles). As already indicated, damage to the optic nerve, or optic tracts, will result in an abnormal visual evoked response. Remarkably clear pictures of actual plaques in the "white matter" of the brain can be seen on magnetic resonance imaging (MRI; discussed below), and laboratory examination of a sample of cerebrospinal fluid (the fluid that surrounds the spinal cord) will reveal whether there are abnormalities in its protein content.

To tell or not to tell?

Often in the past, patients with MS were not told the diagnosis until the disease was well advanced. Perhaps they were told that they had a patch of inflammation in the nervous system or a viral infection. Sometimes patients then discovered that they had been diagnosed as having MS, possibly from a hospital chart or a relative who had been told; this would cause a loss of trust in the doctor—and undue anguish in the patient. It is now the usual practice to tell patients when a diagnosis of MS has been firmly established but to do so with proper emphasis on the good recovery that generally occurs following exacerbations. It should always be stressed that most MS patients have normal or near-normal life expectancy and that only a minority are severely debilitated by the disease. On the other hand, with the first attack of optic neuritis, it is usually sufficient to tell the patient simply that he or she has an inflammation of the optic nerve because at this time a diagnosis of MS has not been made and other symptoms may, in fact, not occur or, if they do, it may be many years later.

Limits of treatments

Many claims for successful treatment of MS have been made over the years, most of which time has shown not to be effective. Among the more recent ones that have been tried is hyperbaric oxygen administered in a compression chamber, a method that had shown some benefits in experimental rodents with central nervous system disorders but not in MS patients. Some patients have undergone plasmapheresis—exchange of the plasma—presumably to remove harmful antibodies that might be destroying the myelin, but

again, while this has helped in some other neurological disorders such as Guillain-Barré syndrome, it does not appear to help in MS. Special diets have also been tried. There is some evidence that a diet low in animal fats is beneficial; such a diet certainly does no harm and will help reduce the risk of coronary artery disease and heart attacks.

Because MS patients often tire easily, it is of importance that they have sufficient rest. Cortisone given by injection or taken orally is often effective in aborting an acute attack, but it cannot be used to prevent attacks. Other drugs are also useful in reducing the spasms and tremors that sometimes occur in MS, and physiotherapy will often help in strengthening muscles and increasing the patient's range of movements.

Clues about cause

The exact cause of MS is still unknown. In recent years, however, medical scientists have greatly increased their knowledge of the underlying factors that lead to MS. Consequently, there is every reason to hope—and, indeed, expect—that this greater understanding of why people get MS will soon lead to specific and effective treatment.

Prevalence patterns—important lessons. The prevalence of MS is not the same in all parts of the world. In the early 1950s Leonard Kurland, professor of epidemiology at the Mayo Clinic, Rochester, Minn., and colleague Knut Weslund showed that MS was three times more common in Winnipeg, Man., than in New Orleans, La. Studies have repeatedly shown that MS is more common in New Zealand than in Australia and that it is very uncommon among the native populations of both Asia and Africa. By the 1950s it had been realized that the prevalence of MS is high in countries that are distant from the equator, that is, in the British Isles, northern Europe, Canada, and the northern U.S., but very low in equatorial regions such as the Indian subcontinent, in China, and in Japan.

In 1949 this author first reported that MS was relatively uncommon among the white South African-born population but relatively common among white European immigrants to South Africa. It was very uncommon among the Asian and Coloured, or mixed race, people of South Africa, and at that time there was no reported MS among black South Africans. In the 1960s epidemiologists Uri Leibowitz, Lipman Halpern, and Milton Alter showed that there was a similar situation in Israel; Jewish immigrants from northern Europe had a much higher chance of developing MS than those from Africa or Asia. However, in both South Africa and Israel, the northern Europeans who immigrated when they were children had a lower risk of developing MS than those who immigrated as adults.

Indications for an environmental cause. In studies conducted in England in the 1970s looking at the prevalence of MS among hospitalized patients in

Greater London and the West Midlands, this author and coinvestigator Marta Elian found that the disease was common among native Britons and immigrants from northern Europe but relatively uncommon among West Indian immigrants and even more uncommon among Asian immigrants from the Indian subcontinent and East Africa. Apparently, the African, Asian, and West Indian immigrants to England had taken with them their low risk of developing MS, which they maintained in their new place of residence. In more recent investigations, however, the same researchers found that the children who were born in England to immigrants from those parts of the world have the same high risk of developing MS as the native English population and not the low risk of their parents. Place of birth and events of early childhood, therefore, appear to have a profound influence on the risk of developing MS—strong evidence that environmental factors are of importance in MS etiology.

In other studies of immigrants to England, it was found that the prevalence of MS in those from the Mediterranean countries of Spain, Italy, and Cyprus was approximately two-thirds of that occurring in natives of England and Wales. This was a much higher prevalence than had been previously reported from the former countries. In sharp contrast, no single immigrant from Malta, another Mediterranean country, was found with MS. Studies then undertaken in Malta confirmed the low MS prevalence there—only four cases per 100,000 population. Studies, however, in four small towns in Sicily, only 96 km (60 mi) away, showed a moderately high MS prevalence, a rate more than 10 times higher than that of Malta. MS had been previously underreported in Italy because studies had been undertaken on large populations, such as that of Palermo (population over one million), where many MS patients would likely be overlooked. Experience has shown that a more accurate reflection of true MS prevalence is derived from studying relatively small populations—of approximately 30,000 to 50,000 people. What then could account for the sudden drop in MS prevalence between two such proximate Mediterranean regions? Clearly it is not climate or ambient temperature. Although the answer is not certain, it has been remarked—only somewhat facetiously—that the clue to the cause of MS "must lie in the sea between Sicily and Malta"!

Curious clusters of disease. That an environmental factor might be responsible for MS was first suggested as far back as 1939, when four of seven veterinary research workers on Bradwell Moor in Yorkshire, England, developed MS. The researchers were studying swayback disease, a disease of the central nervous system affecting young lambs, and it looked very probable that they had been affected by an agent, perhaps a virus, from the sheep's brains, which they were dissecting.

In 1979 John Kurtzke and colleagues at the Veterans Affairs Medical Center, Washington, D.C., described an "epidemic" of MS in the Faeroe Islands of Denmark following the occupation of the islands by British troops during World War II. Kurtzke and others were convinced that there was no MS in the Faeroe Islands before the British occupation—that is, before 1943. Others reject the hypothesis on the grounds that typically patients become predisposed to developing MS early in life—generally before age 15—with the onset of actual MS symptoms occurring many years later. Iceland was also occupied by Allied troops at about the same time as the Faeroe Islands, and John Benedike, Halljrimur Magnusson, and Gunnar Gudmundsen of Reykjavík, collaborating with Charles Poser of Boston, have shown that there was no epidemic of MS in Iceland following the troops' arrival.

Another cluster of MS was reported among seven nurses working at a hospital in Key West, Fla., in 1985, although two of the seven turned out to have a family history of the disease. There are similarities between these and other as-yet-unexplained MS outbreaks.

Despite such clusters, over the years there has been no evidence of any change in overall incidence—*i.e.,* number of cases of MS occurring worldwide—although MS-associated mortality has declined, owing largely to better treatments for complications such as bladder infections. The higher prevalence noted in recent surveys is almost certainly due to these studies' being undertaken in small populations, in which a higher proportion of MS patients is found, and to better diagnostic methods. Moreover, although environmental factors do appear to have a role in MS causation, there is no increased risk of a spouse of an MS patient "catching" MS, nor is the disease more common among doctors and nurses, who in the course of their work are normally more exposed to MS patients than is the general population.

Genetic predisposition. As previously noted, MS is very uncommon among the peoples of China and Japan. Chinese and Japanese immigrants who are born in Hawaii and San Francisco also have a low risk of developing MS, which suggests that they may have a genetic resistance to the disease.

It has long been known that in families where the disease has already been diagnosed, the risk of developing MS for blood relatives is 20 to 50 times higher than for the general population. Even so, in Europe and North America the overall risk for any single family member related to a person with MS is only about two to five per 100 (compared with one to two per 1,000 for the general population). George Ebers and colleagues at the University of Western Ontario have compared the risk of developing MS in monozygotic twins (*i.e.,* those that have developed from a single egg and are therefore genetically identical) and dizygotic (fraternal) twins, who have developed from two separate eggs and are no more identical than any other two siblings. If one monozygotic twin develops MS, there is a 25% likelihood that the other twin will do so also. On the other hand, in 75% of monozygotic twins, the second twin is not clinically affected, although in some cases the plaques that are characteristic of MS can be seen on MRI scans of the second twin's brain.

In the past several years there has been significant progress in identifying genes responsible for a number of disorders, such as cystic fibrosis, Huntington's disease, and Duchenne muscular dystrophy. Diseases that appear to involve a number of genetic factors, which is probably true of MS, have proved more refractory to genetic analysis. It is now possible, however, to undertake comprehensive analysis of the genetic factors in MS; as efforts are under way in the United States and elsewhere to map the entire human genome, medical scientists are taking advantage of the newly available technologies to study families in which some members have MS and others do not. In late 1992 researchers at the National Public Health Institute in Helsinki reported that in a Finnish population group MS was closely linked to the so-called myelin basic protein gene on chromosome 18.

There are, no doubt, other specific genes not yet discovered that convey a predisposition to MS. This author, along with Lefkos Middelton, Hatice Aksoy, Koulis Kyrialis, and Turgay Akalin in Cyprus, is presently studying families in which more than six members have developed MS; detailed knowledge of genetic predisposition will make it possible to identify those individuals at high risk of developing the disorder. If genetic factors turn out to be related to the disease type or severity, this knowledge may also provide prognostic information about the likely course of the disease in individual patients.

Faulty immunity. Other studies are assessing the role of specific genes that control the function of the T lymphocytes, blood cells that play a crucial role in immune responses. MS is, in fact, considered to be an autoimmune disorder, in which the body's defense system reacts to the myelin in the central nervous system as if it were foreign, thus gradually destroying it and causing damage to underlying nerve fibers. MS patients show an increased immune response to a number of diseases of viral origin—particularly to the measles virus—suggesting that a genetic predisposition to MS affects the patient's immunity and that this may be important in the etiology of the disease. The changes that occur in the cerebrospinal fluid in MS, notably an increased production of immunoglobulin in over 60% of patients, also implicate a heightened immune response.

Recent studies of retrovirus infections have shown that a condition similar to MS, known as Jamaican neuropathy, or tropical spastic paraplegia, is caused by the human T-cell lymphotropic virus, type I (HTLV-I).

The research that is presently taking place on the immune response to the human immunodeficiency virus (HIV), the retrovirus responsible for AIDS, may shed further light on the nature of the immune response that occurs in MS.

A clearer picture

New techniques are being used to study the inflammatory process that occurs in MS. For example, it is now possible to grow large numbers of human cells in the laboratory. Genetic engineering has produced large "gene libraries" so that specific immune system cells in persons who develop MS can be compared with those of persons who do not.

With the introduction of the new imaging technique MRI, progress in studying brain inflammation in humans during their life has advanced rapidly. (In the past this could be accomplished only in postmortem studies.) Because MRI works on a magnetic principle and involves no radiation, the examination can be safely repeated at short intervals. MRI reveals the lesions of MS with remarkable sensitivity; therefore, it is of great help in early diagnosis. The earliest detectable change shown by MRI is a breakdown in the barrier that normally exists between the circulating blood and the brain in the area of the plaques, and this typically occurs days before symptoms develop. During the next week or so, the area of abnormality on the image increases quite significantly, probably because of the outpouring of fluid from the brain that occurs with inflammation. After perhaps a month the edema, or fluid accumulation, is absorbed by the brain tissue, leaving a small residual scar. When examined under the microscope, the resulting lesion (demyelination plaque) is found to result from a local allergic reaction around small blood vessels. The insulating myelin sheath is destroyed, but the central part of the nerve fiber, the axon, remains intact, thus offering the potential for repair.

Because the nervous system functions on the basis of the transmission of highly patterned codes of electrical impulses, damage to the myelin interrupts or distorts these patterns, and symptoms result. The cessation of inflammation is associated with the disappearance of the symptoms; thus, complete recovery generally occurs following the early attacks of MS, but repeated damage to the myelin eventually leads to lasting nerve fiber damage and thus potentially debilitating neurological symptoms.

A surprising recent finding is just how often inflammation occurs in previously unaffected areas of the central nervous system. New plaques may appear as often as 10 times more frequently than do changes in the patient's symptoms. This is because of the relatively small size of the inflamed areas and because many of them occur in "silent" areas of the brain—*i.e.,* those that do not control motor or sensory functions.

Recent laboratory studies have provided greater understanding of the allergic reaction involving the blood vessels. First, there is a change in the character of one type of circulating immune cell, the T lymphocyte, which alters the blood-brain barrier, allowing fluid to pass into and out of the brain and causing the local edema described above. The inflammation at this early stage is often completely reversed, but the inflammatory process can also culminate with the arrival of phagocyte cells known as macrophages and microglia, which digest the damaged myelin, and ultimately will lead to progression of the disease.

New therapeutic potential

Such enlightened understanding of the disease process in MS has suggested new strategies for treatment. For example, it may be possible to suppress autoimmunity by removing circulating antibodies or "targeting" monoclonal antibodies—genetically engineered molecules that are prepared in the laboratory—to destroy those cells that migrate to the nervous system and cause inflammation. Much more difficult, but not impossible, would be restoring the capacity for spontaneous nervous system repair, which occurs normally during growth and development but is lost in the mature brain. Another possibility that is being explored is implantation of cells that produce myelin in patients' brains.

Yet a further promising line of treatment is the use of immunosuppressive drugs such as cyclophosphamide, azathioprine, cyclosporin, or antilymphocyte serum. Small-scale trials using such agents are under way. Other trials are testing the potential of interferons (naturally produced antiviral substances) and an experimental drug, Copolymer 1 (COP-1). These are all powerful agents that consequently carry some risk—particularly the risk of subjecting patients to dangerous infections; thus far, none has conclusively shown an ability to prevent attacks.

A new area of investigation has been opened by the findings of Howard Weiner and David Hafler of Harvard Medical School. They have shown in a double-blind study that MS patients who took capsules containing bovine myelin had fewer attacks of MS than a control group (6 out of 15 in the treatment group had attacks, compared with 12 out of 15 in the control group). This is suggestive evidence that the immune system may be induced to tolerate proteins it considers to be foreign.

A solution in sight?

It has now been well established that MS results from some combination of genetic and environmental factors. The environmental factor may well be a reaction to one or a number of viral infections, which are most likely to have their influence during early childhood. Viruses can remain latent in the nervous sys-

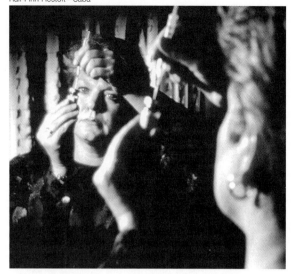

A patient prepares an injection of beta interferon, one of several experimental therapies that may offer promising new treatment for the progressive, though highly variable, damage to the nervous system that occurs with multiple sclerosis.

tem throughout life and cause problems only when, for one reason or another, immunity to the virus is lowered. A good example is the varicella-zoster virus responsible for chicken pox. The virus remains in the nervous system after a childhood chicken pox infection and then, years later, in adulthood, can cause inflammation in a segment of the spinal cord, producing the disease shingles, or herpes zoster. Herpes zoster produces localized vesicles that run along the skin's distribution of nerves and can be very painful; in some cases shingles outbreaks are recurrent. HIV is another example of a virus that persists in the body and can cause neurological symptoms years after the infection has occurred.

An intriguing theory was first proposed by David Poskanzer in 1963. He pointed out that the geographic distribution of MS is very similar to that of poliomyelitis in the years before the Salk and Sabin vaccines became available (*i.e.,* before the early 1960s). In the 19th century poliomyelitis causing paralysis was a disease of infants. It is now realized that with poor hygiene levels, while some babies developed crippling "infantile paralysis," virtually every baby had been infected by the poliomyelitis virus, and most were thereafter immune. By the 20th century, however, with improved hygiene, fewer babies were infected and developed immunity, so many adults became polio victims.

Like polio in adults once was, MS is also uncommon in countries with lower levels of hygiene—especially in the less developed world. It is at least possible that a similar mechanism will explain the low MS prevalence in Asia and Africa as well as its much less common occurrence in South Africa than in Australia and southern Europe, which have comparable climates. Hygienic status may also help to explain why MS is now relatively uncommon in the descendants of European immigrants born in South Africa, where white babies are typically attended by native, nonwhite servants. Although the reason for the low prevalence of MS in Malta is still not clear, perhaps past living conditions, particularly during the World War II years, were closer to those in North Africa than to those in Italy, resulting in acquired immunity in infancy among the Maltese.

The pace of research into the cause and treatment of MS has increased enormously in recent years. These developments owe a great deal to the support received from national MS societies and the International Federation of Multiple Sclerosis Societies. These organizations not only finance research but bring research scientists together to share their findings. In the 1930s U.S. Pres. Franklin D. Roosevelt provided the impetus (through the National Foundation for Infantile Paralysis and the March of Dimes) that resulted in the finding of the solution to the dreaded disease polio. Today a similar sustained effort by governmental and nongovernmental agencies is needed to find the solution to MS, which continues to affect so many people in the prime of life.

—*Geoffrey Dean, M.D.*

Occupational Health

As the world's economy becomes more integrated, occupational health increasingly becomes an international concern. A key area of current debate is the North American Free Trade Agreement (NAFTA), which would lower trade barriers between the U.S., Canada, and Mexico. Many expect that NAFTA will accelerate the trend for U.S. companies to move labor-intensive production processes to Mexico, where labor costs are about one-tenth the U.S. level. In addition, the regulatory climate in Mexico has been more permissive than in the U.S. Advocates of occupational—and environmental—health have called for parallel agreements to NAFTA, which would include strong safeguards for both workers and the environment. Possible initiatives include joint efforts by the U.S. Department of Labor and the Mexican Ministry of Labor and Social Security in training inspectors, assisting companies to comply with regulations, and enforcing standards. Similar concerns have been raised in Europe and Asia, where trade is increasing between nations with widely divergent workplace and environmental standards.

Workers' compensation reevaluated

With health care reform high on the U.S. national agenda, the efficiency and cost-effectiveness of workers' compensation have come under increasing scrutiny. Workers' compensation is a state-based insurance scheme designed to compensate employees for workplace injuries and illnesses. Historically, it has been viewed as advantageous to both employees and employers. It is a no-fault scheme designed to provide rapid compensation regardless of how the injury or illness occurred. Payments are limited to medical expenses and wage replacement, along with some related costs, such as job retraining or even funeral expenses; no punitive damages or "pain and suffering" costs may be paid, and the employee is barred from suing the employer for such damages.

Critics of workers' compensation note that it is inefficient to maintain a separate, parallel insurance scheme for one class of injuries and illnesses. Moreover, it is extremely costly to administer in some states, consuming up to 50% of each premium dollar. Therefore, some have proposed "24-hour coverage" under a national health insurance scheme combining workers' compensation with conventional health insurance (and possibly with automobile insurance as well). Such a plan would significantly change the way occupational medicine services are financed; it might also affect the incentives for physicians to encourage preventive activities.

Disability in the workplace

The Americans with Disabilities Act (ADA), passed by Congress in 1990, took effect in July 1992. This far-reaching law builds on earlier legislation, such as the Rehabilitation Act of 1973, in protecting the rights of disabled people, among them the right to equal treatment in employment. According to Title I of ADA, individuals with disabilities are "qualified" to work if they meet the skill, experience, education, and other job-related requirements of a position held or desired and can perform the essential functions of the job with or without reasonable accommodation.

By prohibiting discrimination against qualified individuals with disabilities, ADA emphasizes job qualifications as the only basis for hiring and advancement. Formerly, through the process of the preemployment physical exam, disabled applicants who were felt to be "bad risks" could be screened out. Now preemployment exams are permissible only after an offer of employment has been made. Moreover, although most medical information collected during this examination remains confidential, the physician is required to collaborate with the employer and the employee in designing necessary accommodations.

The act permits an employer to reject an applicant only if that individual would pose a "direct threat" to self or others on the job. For example, a person with frequent seizures, uncontrolled by medication, could legitimately be excluded from work as a bus driver. Many situations are more ambiguous, however. For example, could a person with sight in only one eye or another who is color-blind be excluded from driving a bus? Many disputes that arise as a result of the new legislation will undoubtedly have to be resolved by means of litigation.

The American workplace: how safe?

The National Safety Council (NSC) estimated that 9,900 U.S. workers were killed on the job in 1991, the most recent year for which statistics were available. A much lower estimate—2,800 deaths—came from the federal Bureau of Labor Statistics (BLS). Most experts, however, believe that the true number of annual workplace fatalities is close to 10,000. The sizable disparity in the NSC and BLS figures reflects the enormous variations in the way different agencies and organizations collect and record workplace health and safety statistics. A similar sort of discrepancy was reported in 1993 by investigators at the University of Michigan School of Public Health, who compared two sets of data—BLS statistics and state workers' compensation records—on the number of workdays missed because of job-related illness and injuries. They found that from 1986 to 1990 state records showed that Michigan workers had missed almost five times the number of days reported in the BLS's National Survey of Occupational Injuries and Illnesses. The Michigan researchers concluded that the government survey "seriously underestimates the magnitude of the problem." These disparities in the statistics continue to confound attempts to evaluate occupational hazards and set priorities for correcting them.

One trend was clear from the 1991 numbers: whereas occupational injuries were declining, work-related illnesses were on the rise. More than 60% of the increase was due to musculoskeletal problems—conditions such as carpal tunnel syndrome and tendinitis, which are especially common in the meat- and poultry-processing, automotive, and textile industries. These disorders now account for more than 50% of all occupational illnesses reported in the U.S., making this the fastest-growing category of occupational ailments—perhaps because of changing work demands or possibly because such disorders are being increasingly recognized and diagnosed.

Hazardous jobs

In 1992–93 the most dangerous job categories continued to be construction (13 injuries per 100 workers), manufacturing (12.7), and agriculture, forestry, and fishing (10.8). Within the manufacturing sector, especially high injury rates were found in meatpacking (45.5 injuries per 100) and shipbuilding and repair (44.1).

Among the most tragic recent occupational disasters were a September 1991 fire in an Imperial Food Products poultry-processing plant in Hamlet, N.C., which killed 25 and injured over 50; a surface explosion at a Blacksville, W.Va., mine in March 1992, which caused the death of 4 miners; a December 1992 methane explosion inside another Virginia mine, in which 8 died; and a January 1993 incident in which 18 construction workers were injured in a building collapse. Although such dramatic incidents account for only a fraction of all workplace fatalities and injuries, they are a constant reminder of the dangers of certain jobs.

Health care workers at risk. Ironically, one field in which workers face numerous hazards is health care. These include exposure to infectious diseases and potentially dangerous chemicals. Currently, the most widely discussed hazard to health care providers is infection with the human immunodeficiency virus (HIV). Public health officials have repeatedly emphasized that HIV is not highly contagious, and the statistics substantiate this: despite the millions of presumed opportunities for transmission, as of July 1993 the U.S. Centers for Disease Control and Prevention (CDC) had recorded only 37 cases of occupationally acquired HIV infection among health care workers.

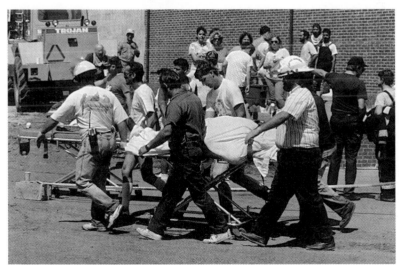

Rescue workers remove the body of a victim from the Imperial Food Products plant in Hamlet, N.C., after a tragic fire in September 1991 that left 25 employees dead and more than 50 injured. Workers trying to flee the blaze reportedly found emergency exits locked. The facility, which had been in operation for 11 years, had never been inspected for safety violations.

Stephen Aldridge

Occupational health

Much more worrisome are the risk of hepatitis B—which may infect as many as 12,000 health care workers annually—and the emerging threat of drug-resistant strains of tuberculosis (TB). In recent TB outbreaks at large public hospitals such as Jackson Memorial in Miami, Fla., and Grady Memorial in Atlanta, Ga., up to half of the staff on some wards tested positive for TB infection. Those at risk include doctors, nurses, nurses aides, dietary and housekeeping aides, and medical technicians; even hospital morgue workers risk infection from cadavers. The National Institute for Occupational Safety and Health (NIOSH) has proposed a number of measures to protect hospital personnel, including strict isolation of TB patients, proper ventilation of isolation rooms, the wearing of personal respirators by workers in close contact with TB patients, TB testing of employees and removal from the job of those found to have active pulmonary TB, and employee education on TB transmission.

Health care workers also face a variety of chemical hazards. Glutaraldehyde, a disinfectant used in the sterilization of medical instruments, causes respiratory and skin irritation and asthma in some people. Occupational exposure to nitrous oxide, the inhalation analgesic also known as "laughing gas," has been linked to cancer, liver diseases, neurological deficits, miscarriage, and birth defects. In 1992 scientists from the National Institute of Environmental Health Sciences and the University of North Carolina School of Public Health published the findings of a large study of female dental assistants exposed to high levels of nitrous oxide, which showed that such exposure adversely affected the women's fertility.

Chemotherapeutic drugs used in the treatment of cancer also pose a risk to health care workers who handle and administer them. These drugs can cause a wide variety of symptoms, including skin irritation, hives, headache, and nausea and vomiting. French researchers reported in 1993 that they had found an association between exposure to anticancer drugs and elevated risk of ectopic pregnancy. In addition, many of these drugs are themselves known to be carcinogenic.

Agricultural workers' ills. Farming, which has always been dangerous work, remains so for a number of reasons. Health care services are often unavailable or inaccessible in remote rural areas. Child labor is still common on farms, placing an especially vulnerable group at risk. Potentially dangerous machinery is used routinely, and "do-it-yourself" repairs may increase the hazard; furthermore, farmers often elect not to use protective equipment. The dangers of farm machinery were highlighted in 1992 by reports from the CDC of four incidents in which women who got their hair caught in hay balers were "scalped" by the machines.

A recent analysis of previous research on cancer incidence among farmers indicated that although they

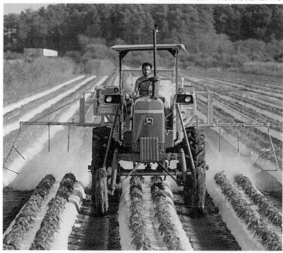

With mounting data indicating that pesticide exposure could be responsible for the higher rates of some cancers among farm workers, the Environmental Protection Agency in August 1992 issued new standards for those who work with these chemicals.

are healthier overall than many other groups of workers, they are at increased risk of a number of cancers, including lymphoma, leukemia, and melanoma and stomach, prostate, and lip cancers. Some of the factors accounting for the risk are well recognized—exposure to sunlight, for example—while others have yet to be identified. Because of concerns that pesticide exposure might be responsible for some of these cancers, in August 1992 the Environmental Protection Agency (EPA) issued more stringent standards for pesticide use by agricultural workers.

Other high-risk fields. Two major studies of the health risks to workers in the semiconductor industry were released in 1992. Both found an increased risk of miscarriage associated with exposure to glycol ethers, the solvents used to etch computer chips.

Other workers at risk are those who clean up environmental hazards and those who maintain and repair bridges and roads. Hazardous-waste-cleanup workers face a variety of toxic exposures; fortunately, however, regulations require careful supervision of such work and the use of protective equipment. Workers who remove leaded paint and asbestos also must be safeguarded; the wearing of protective garments and respirators is required, and work sites must be closely supervised. Still, much abatement work is done by small companies that fail to provide adequate training or protection.

Accounts of lead poisoning among workers who disassemble, repair, or repaint old bridges are not uncommon, and in recent years bridge workers in the northeastern U.S. have also been killed by falls and electrocution. Road-repair workers who labor alongside busy traffic lanes constantly run the risk of being hit by passing vehicles. Nationally, as the U.S. proceeds with repair of its aging infrastructure, many more workers will be facing these kinds of hazards.

Workplace violence: emerging danger

Intentional injury has emerged as an increasing on-the-job risk, especially in some occupations. NIOSH reported that during the period 1980–85 homicide was the third leading cause of death in U.S. workplaces. Employees at highest risk are those who work in 24-hour convenience stores, gas stations, and fast-food establishments. Taxi drivers and law-enforcement officers also face this risk.

The trend toward increased workplace violence reflects the growing epidemic of violent crime in the U.S. Measures to protect workers—such as the installation of Plexiglas shields for taxi drivers, bank tellers, and convenience store clerks—are now common. A parallel development—one for which no protective measures are obvious—is random violence perpetrated by disgruntled employees and former employees. These incidents, too, are becoming more frequent.

Indoor hazards: present but unseen

It is now widely agreed by public health authorities that environmental tobacco smoke (ETS), or "second-hand smoke," is an important indoor air pollutant and a contributing factor in both cancer and heart disease. A major EPA report entitled *Respiratory Effects of Passive Smoking,* published in December 1992, concluded that ETS is a human lung carcinogen and is responsible for approximately 3,000 lung cancer deaths annually in U.S. nonsmokers.

Results from a California survey, reported in 1992 in the *Journal of the American Medical Association,* showed that 2.2 million nonsmokers in California were exposed to ETS at work. Even in workplaces with partial smoking restrictions, nearly half of respondents reported being exposed. Research shows that when nonsmoking policies are implemented in workplaces, those employees who are smokers substantially decrease the total amount they smoke. Therefore, the health of both nonsmokers and smokers benefits from the no-smoking policy.

Another concern in the office environment is the health impact of exposure to video display terminals (VDTs). VDT use has been suspected of contributing to three quite different problems: eyestrain, miscarriages, and musculoskeletal discomfort, especially in the neck, shoulders, and arms. Eyestrain can be minimized with some relatively simple measures—glare filters, proper lighting, adequate work breaks. Miscarriage is both more controversial and more difficult to guard against. And because the vast majority of long-term VDT operators are women, the possible risk of miscarriage is extremely important. A NIOSH study reported in 1991 compared two groups of telephone operators—directory assistance operators who used VDTs and general operators who did not—and found no difference in miscarriage rates. However, a study from the Finnish Institute of Occupational Health, published late in 1992, concluded that certain VDTs—those with high levels of extremely low-frequency electromagnetic fields—did pose a risk of miscarriage. This was the first study to report an association between miscarriage and the electromagnetic fields emitted by VDTs; the investigators cautioned that further research will be needed before any conclusions can be drawn. In the meantime, in 1992 a San Francisco city ordinance aimed at protecting workers who use VDTs—mandating adjustable equipment and adequate work breaks—was struck down by a ruling that held that only the state can regulate workplace safety.

Musculoskeletal disorders: a new epidemic?

As noted above, musculoskeletal disorders constitute the fastest-growing category of occupational hazards.

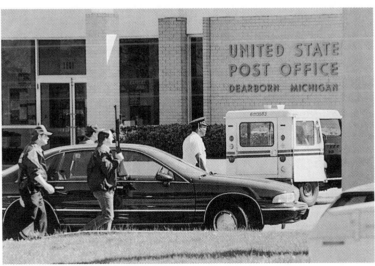

Federal agents surround the Post Office in Dearborn, Mich., in the aftermath of a May 1993 shooting spree by an employee who was upset over his having been denied a promotion. One worker was killed and two injured in the incident. Violence is accounting for an increasing proportion of work-related injuries and fatalities in the U.S.

Occupational health

A 1992 NIOSH study of VDT operators at U.S. West Communications concluded that 21% had potentially work-related musculoskeletal conditions such as shoulder and arm pain and carpal tunnel syndrome. These problems are not restricted to communications workers, however. They have also been reported among electricians, who get "tennis elbow" from repeated use of screwdrivers, packinghouse workers, who are vulnerable to hand and wrist problems from motions used to cut through meat and bone, and automotive workers doing overhead assembly, who experience pain from prolonged arm raising and neck flexion—to name just a few. Recently, studies have documented a high prevalence of upper-extremity disorders among supermarket checkers, keyboard-using newspaper workers, and data entry clerks.

Workers at greatest risk are those whose jobs involve repetitive motions, force, vibration, sustained awkward positions, and mechanical compression of body parts. Consequently, work-related musculoskeletal disorders have been called repetitive motion disorders, overuse syndromes, and cumulative trauma

Workers who use hand-held power tools such as jackhammers are exposed for prolonged periods to mechanical vibration, one of many causes of the musculoskeletal disorders that are now the fastest-growing class of occupational ailments in the U.S.

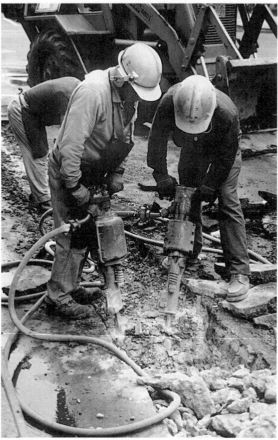

Andrew Dalsimer—Bruce Coleman Inc.

disorders, although the exact cause is unknown in many situations. To measure such factors as force and repetition quantitatively, investigators have videotaped workers on the job and performed computer-based biomechanical analyses of their movements. Defining this group of disorders poses a problem, as there are many distinct ailments of the hands and arms that can cause similar clinical symptoms. Moreover, in many cases symptoms are reported but there are no objective findings, such as physical abnormalities or impaired nerve conduction.

Even though the risk factors and the syndromes themselves are not fully understood, many preventive measures have been tested. One NIOSH study of supermarket checkers found that adopting certain hand positions when passing items over automatic price scanners resulted in decreased hand and arm symptoms. An expert committee of the American National Standards Institute has recommended a range of preventive approaches, including on-the-job surveillance, engineering and design modifications, medical management, and worker education and training.

From the research front

Basic science research continues to clarify the nature of neurotoxicity following exposure to solvents, pesticides, and heavy metals. In a report in the *British Journal of Industrial Medicine,* Swedish scientists described the role of brain cells called astrocytes in brain function. Astrocytes make up over half the cells in the cerebral cortex of higher mammals, serving to maintain the chemical environment of neurons, guide neuron growth, and support immune activity. The Swedish investigators noted that both lead and mercury inhibit the ability of astrocytes to take up the neurotransmitter glutamate, which can derange cell metabolism and may account for the long-term neurotoxicity of these metals.

An important report on radiation health effects was published in the *American Journal of Industrial Medicine* in 1993. A team of investigators led by two British researchers, Alice Stewart and George W. Kneale, reanalyzed the health records of 35,000 people who once worked at the nuclear weapons facility at Hanford, Wash. The investigators reached several important conclusions. First, contrary to earlier reports, many types of cancers—not just leukemias—appeared to have been caused by the radiation exposure. Second, whereas earlier findings emphasized the risk to younger workers, this study found that vulnerability to radiation-induced cancer increases with age. Third, the doses required for causing cancer were far lower than previously expected. These conclusions differed from those based on the health effects observed in Japanese atomic bomb survivors and may revise the thinking about low-dose radiation exposure.

—Howard Frumkin, M.D., Dr. P.H.

Special Report
Work: Dying for It in Japan

by Richard E. Wokutch, Ph.D.

Jun Ishii, an employee of Mitsui & Co., Ltd., spoke Russian. This ability and the surge in trade between Japan and the Soviet Union owing to *perestroika* increased his work load until, pushed beyond endurance, he died. . . . [He] was 47 years old. . . . During the 10 months preceding his death, Ishii had spent 103 days in the Soviet Union as manager of Mitsui's Soviet division. The close succession of business trips had left him almost no opportunity to recover from changes in climate and time zones between the Soviet Union and Japan. Ishii died in a business hotel in Aichi Prefecture, where he had spent five days escorting Russian visitors to local machine manufacturers and conducting business negotiations. . . . As was usual in such cases, Ishii was responsible for seeing to their needs from early morning to late at night.

—Report by Hiroshi Kawahito, secretary-
general, National Defense Counsel
for Victims of Karoshi

In July 1992, two years after he was found dead in his hotel room, Jun Ishii was officially certified as a victim of *karoshi,* or death due to overwork, and his family was awarded compensation. In most such cases, however, the cause of death may not be as apparent as it was in this case. In fact, *karoshi*—its nature, causes, and extent—is one of the most controversy-ridden occupational health issues in Japan today.

Presumed causes

The term *karoshi* is often used rather loosely to refer to a wide range of medical conditions that precipitate death (or serious illness or injury) and are thought to be work related. A more precise definition is provided by Tetsunojo Uehata, a medical authority at Japan's National Institute of Public Health:

A condition in which psychologically unsound work processes are allowed to continue in a way that disrupts the worker's normal work and life rhythms, leading to a build-up of fatigue in the body and a chronic condition of overwork accompanied by a worsening of preexistent high blood pressure and hardening of the arteries and finally in a fatal breakdown.

As this description suggests, *karoshi* usually refers to the fatal or disabling aggravation of cardiovascular disease, most often in the form of heart attack or stroke. However, the term has also been applied to work-related suicides and to circumstances in which work-related stress leads to the fatal exacerbation of other preexisting conditions, such as asthma. Even nonfatal ailments such as ulcers, back pain, and impotence are sometimes mentioned as stress-related problems that may be precursors to *karoshi.*

Karoshi is thought to be a consequence not only of work itself—the fast pace, long hours, and intense pressure typical of the Japanese workplace—but also of various other factors only indirectly related to work. These include the long and tiring commutes that are a fact of life for many Japanese workers, excessive drinking and smoking, cramped living space, and inadequate sleep and exercise. In some cases, like that of Jun Ishii, frequent overseas travel, jet lag, and the toll these take on the body are believed to be contributing factors. In others, psychological pressures caused by job transfers and family separations have been cited. It is precisely because of the many variables involved that establishing the direct relationship of work to a specific *karoshi* case is often very difficult.

Disputes over contested claims for workers' compensation constitute the main forum in which the controversy over *karoshi* is played out in Japan. The primary issue is whether a given death or disability is work related—and therefore compensable under the workers' compensation system—or not work related and thus eligible only for less generous compensation through the Japanese equivalent of the U.S. Social Security system. According to Takanobu Teramoto of the Japanese embassy in Washington, D.C., the Japanese government uses two criteria in deciding whether to accept or reject a *karoshi* claim. First, officials consider whether the worker's job responsibilities were excessively difficult, both compared with his or her normal workload and compared with those of other workers. Second, they consider whether the death occurred within a "reasonable" period of time after the excessive work such that a causal association is likely. Critics of the government's position claim that these criteria have been interpreted too narrowly, with the result that legitimate *karoshi* cases have been disallowed. Workers and families whose claims have been denied have filed appeals, engaged in litigation, and, perhaps most important, generated considerable publicity for their cause.

Extent of the problem

Given the imprecise definition of *karoshi* and the difficulty of determining the cause of death and whether a given case should indeed be considered work related, it is not surprising that estimates of the incidence of *karoshi* vary greatly. At one extreme the National Defense Counsel for Victims of Karoshi, a group of lawyers representing the bereaved families, estimates that excessive work contributes to the death of more than 10,000 Japanese workers each year. Official government statistics are drastically lower. There is, in fact, no category for death due to overwork in official government labor or medical statistics. The first successful workers' compensation claim fitting the *karoshi* profile was approved in 1987. Since then, an average of 620 *karoshi* death and "disability" claims have been filed each year. Of these, an average of 85 are approved.

Because there are no accurate statistics on the incidence of *karoshi,* it is impossible to determine if the increased interest in the phenomenon has been triggered by an actual increase in occurrence. Despite the continued rise in life expectancy in Japan—which is now the highest in the world—there has at the same time been an increase in the percentage of deaths due to cardiovascular disease. A worsening of work-related stress may be the causal factor but, as noted above, other factors—changes in diet, the environment, drinking and smoking habits, or other, non-work-related stresses—may be to blame as well. Also contributing to the attention being paid to *karoshi* is the fact that the Japanese have only recently reached a level of prosperity that has permitted them to focus on the ways in which lifestyle affects health.

The victims

The Japan Karoshi Foundation and the National Defense Counsel for Victims of Karoshi have attempted to gather information on who the victims are and at the same time provide legal advice and publicize the problem through establishing telephone hot lines in major cities. The information on specific cases collected through these hot lines, although subject to the limitations of any self-reported data, nevertheless provides some insight into *karoshi*'s victims.

In their first two years of operation, from June 1988 to June 1990, the *karoshi* hot lines received reports of 1,806 cases. Of these reports, 55% came from women whose husbands had died of stroke or heart disease and who were requesting help in seeking compensation and recognition of the work-related cause of the death; about 17% came from other relatives of deceased or disabled workers. Some 20% of the calls came from individuals seeking help in avoiding health problems due to job-associated stress.

The hot-line calls pertained to individuals from a wide range of occupations; salespeople and office workers were the subjects of 15.4% of the calls, followed by managers (10.9%), manufacturing workers (9.1%), construction workers (7.8%), and truck, bus, taxi, and other drivers (6.7%). The largest category (34.8%) was a miscellaneous classification including a broad spectrum of jobs, from professional to menial. The victims were predominantly male. The largest group of victims comprised those aged 40–54; this was followed by individuals in their late thirties and late fifties. A large number of victims—about 42%—succumbed to strokes. Another 18% had heart failure, and nearly 10% had heart attacks.

Devotion to work and its consequences

The evidence that the Japanese work longer hours than people in many other countries is indisputable. According to the U.S. Bureau of Labor Statistics, the typical Japanese manufacturing worker put in 2,120 hours in 1990, compared with 1,938 hours worked by his or her U.S. counterpart—the equivalent of almost five additional workweeks per year. The extra hours worked by the Japanese take the form of mandatory or strongly encouraged overtime and unused vacation and sick days. Japanese workers on average take only about half of the 15 paid holidays most companies offer each year. In fact, the government runs

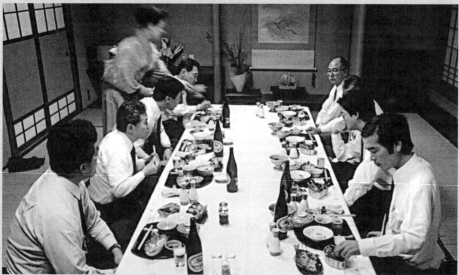

After-hours entertaining is an integral part of the job for many workers in Japan and accounts for a considerable percentage of their overtime. A Japanese executive might be expected to attend business dinners as many as four nights a week.

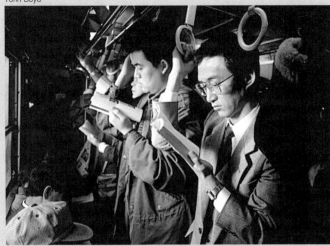

The pressures of work in Japan are not confined to the workplace but extend to many other aspects of daily life. Long, tiring commutes on overcrowded trains are common.

advertising campaigns encouraging workers to take advantage of their vacation time!

Some authorities claim that these official statistics significantly understate the true situation. In the Japanese workplace it is viewed as "disloyal" for a subordinate to leave the office before his or her boss, and it is common practice for workers to be urged to perform "service overtime," which is unpaid—and unrecorded—work time. The practice seems to be especially prevalent among white-collar workers, who typically work well past the nominal end of the working day; moreover, they often are expected to do after-hours entertaining and to participate in weekend company outings.

To what extent is the legendary Japanese dedication to the work ethic to blame for overwork and its adverse effects on health? As one observer commented in the Tokyo newspaper *Mainichi Shimbun:*

Certain Japanese mores are admittedly conducive to an overzealous work ethic. In particular, the high priority placed on group harmony encourages employees to put the good of the company and smooth relations with colleagues and superiors ahead of their own personal needs. There are cases where workers are pushed too far and families are justified in feeling that the employer bears some responsibility. These instances, however, are the exception.

Those who work themselves past the point of exhaustion have made a conscious decision to outshine their peers, presumably in the hope of rapid advancement.

While some view those who die of *karoshi* not as hapless victims but as "creators of their own fate," others point to economic circumstances, especially the high cost of living and declining job security in Japan, as the reasons some workers drive themselves beyond the limits of their endurance.

Addressing the problem—or not?

In the past couple of years, *karoshi* has become a focus of worldwide interest because of the impact of Japanese work practices on international trade rela-

tions. There is no doubt that the Japanese economy has been tremendously successful in the post-World War II era. Now, however, some authorities wonder if this unparalleled progress may not have been achieved at the expense of the Japanese worker. This point of view is frequently invoked by Western critics of the Japanese system, who call on the Japanese to alter their work habits so as not to force their high-pressure business style on others. There is also concern that Japanese companies are exporting stress-inducing work practices to their overseas operations.

Regardless of the various opinions about the extent of *karoshi* in Japan and who is really to blame, efforts are being made to alleviate the problem. There has been considerable emphasis on improving the everyday life of Japanese citizens in recent years, including government-sponsored efforts to reduce the workweek (and the school week for students) and to increase the amount of time spent in leisure activities. The government has also recently established throughout the country 347 regional centers to promote the health of workers employed by smaller companies that have limited facilities for employee medical care. In addition, 47 health research centers are being established to study work-related illness and stress and to train physicians in dealing with these conditions.

Still, critics contend that most of the attempts to remedy the problem are more window dressing for public relations purposes than substantial improvements in the conditions of employment. In fact, statements by Japanese business and government leaders criticizing the work ethic in the West send conflicting signals about the sincerity of efforts to reduce work stress in Japan. In 1989, under pressure from other countries, Japanese banks reduced their workweek to five days. At the same time, however, the workday of bank employees was lengthened, with the result that they were putting in the same number of working hours after the "reform" as before!

Pharmaceuticals

For the 20 million Americans who suffer from migraine headaches (sometimes called "sick headaches"), it came as good news when the first product approved in the U.S. solely as a treatment for migraine became available. In December 1992 the Food and Drug Administration (FDA) approved Glaxo Inc.'s sumatriptan (Imitrex), a drug that can be self-injected by patients at the onset of symptoms. Sumatriptan is marketed in a kit that contains two single-dose (six-milligram) disposable syringes, an autoinjector, and a pamphlet that explains how to load and use the autoinjector and discard empty syringes. A second injection may be administered at least one hour after an initial dose, but no more than two doses should be taken during a 24-hour period. In mid-1993 Glaxo was seeking FDA approval to market an oral version of the drug.

Also new on the market as of December 1992 was paclitaxel (Taxol), an agent derived from the bark of Pacific yew trees, approved as a second-line treatment (*i.e.,* for use after failure of other therapies) of metastatic ovarian cancer. Manufactured by Bristol-Myers Squibb, Taxol may be particularly useful in the treatment of patients with ovarian cancer who are unresponsive to platinum-based anticancer agents; clinical studies indicated that 20 to 30% of such patients experienced a benefit. The drug is also being studied for use in breast and lung cancers.

Among other notable new products approved for U.S. marketing in recent months was the injectable contraceptive medroxyprogesterone (Depo-Provera); it was not a new drug compound, having already been available for treatment of endometrial and kidney

Migraine sufferers can now obtain quick relief with a self-injectable drug, sumatriptan (Imitrex). Within about 10 minutes it generally alleviates not only headache pain but also other symptoms of migraine.

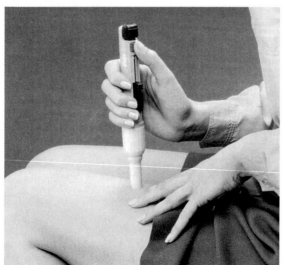

Cerenex Pharmaceuticals

cancers. The newly licensed Tetramune is a vaccine that combines immunizations against four childhood infectious diseases—*Haemophilus influenzae* type B infection, diphtheria, tetanus, and pertussis.

A table listing new drug compounds approved by the FDA in 1992 and the first half of 1993 appears on page 380. The list is broken down into two categories, "priority" approvals and "standard" approvals, designations that replace the A-B-C rating system that had been used by the FDA for more than a decade. Priority drugs—those to treat serious or life-threatening illnesses for which no adequate alternative therapies exist—are given expedited review; the category is reserved for all drugs that would have been A-rated and a portion that would have been B-rated under the former system. The standard category corresponds to the remainder of former B designations (those with some therapeutic gains over products already marketed for the same use) and all drugs that would have received a C rating (with little or no therapeutic gain over other available products).

Pricing: what is "reasonable"?

Taxol, the above-mentioned new drug for ovarian cancer, was developed under a special compact, known as a cooperative research-and-development agreement (CRADA), between Bristol-Myers Squibb and the National Cancer Institute (NCI), a branch of the National Institutes of Health (NIH). Typically, such agreements have a "reasonable price" clause, which requires the manufacturer to set a price that is comparable to that of other treatments for the same condition.

The pricing of CRADA drugs recently received attention on Capitol Hill. Rep. Ron Wyden (Dem., Ore.), chairman of the House Small Business Subcommittee on Regulation, was one of several legislators who wanted to ensure that drugs developed with the help of significant federal funding were priced fairly once they reached the market. In January 1993 the subcommittee held a hearing at which Wyden pointed out that $32 million of taxpayers' money went toward the development of Taxol. Wyden was concerned that Bristol-Myers Squibb had not justified the high price it had set for Taxol to the NCI and that the institute had no accounting of the company's research-and-development costs for the drug. The NCI responded that its responsibility was to measure Taxol's price against that of other approved cancer drugs, not to conduct a cost-based analysis. The NCI insisted that as a biomedical research organization, it is not equipped to perform complex cost analyses. Several proposals were advanced to address the issue of pricing of CRADA drugs, including establishing a price-review panel at the Health Care Financing Administration or within the NIH, negotiating drug prices on the basis of a formula that takes into account development costs and profits, and commissioning an expert panel at

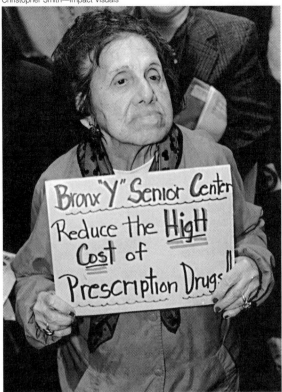

At an April 1993 demonstration, a senior citizen from the Bronx, New York City, lobbies in favor of controls on the escalating cost of medications—expenses that have a disproportionate impact on the elderly.

the NIH that would use manufacturers' data to set drug prices.

In February 1993 Sen. David Pryor (Dem., Ark.), head of the Special Committee on Aging, held a hearing to address CRADA drug pricing as it affects the elderly. The Pharmaceutical Manufacturers Association (PMA), the trade group representing the drug industry, and the Industrial Biotechnology Association proposed that the NIH's royalties from CRADA-developed drugs be increased. However, Pryor quickly concluded that such royalty hikes would create a conflict of interest for the government because of the potential to drive up the cost of drugs to consumers—who, since they had already paid taxes to support the NIH, would in effect be paying twice. Currently, the NIH collects roughly 5% royalties on licenses from products developed with institute funding. Wyden, who was the first witness at the Pryor committee hearing, suggested that commercial drug prices be negotiated at the time the licensing agreement is signed and that several companies be licensed for the same projects in an effort to create price competition.

Another recent research-and-marketing agreement that elicited congressional scrutiny was the contract negotiated by the federally supported Scripps Re-

search Institute, La Jolla, Calif., and the Swiss-based pharmaceutical manufacturer Sandoz. Under the terms of the contract, Sandoz agreed to pay Scripps $300 million, to be disbursed over a 10-year period, in return for the exclusive patent rights to all commercial products developed by Scripps researchers. At a hearing before Wyden's subcommittee, Bernadine Healy, director of the NIH at the time, denounced the agreement, which she characterized as "against the spirit of science and possibly against the law." Wyden requested that the inspector general of the Department of Health and Human Services (HHS) investigate the Sandoz-Scripps deal and audit 130 patents granted to Scripps to determine whether the government's participation in the development of those technologies was properly reported in the patent applications. Prior to the hearing, the NIH asked more than 100 universities and research institutes to provide it with information regarding all commercial agreements with industry. Wyden also requested that all directors of NIH institutes forward to his subcommittee information on their respective CRADAs with private businesses.

In March 1993 Wyden introduced legislation designed to give the NIH more leverage in negotiating commercial agreements. The bill would require the NIH and federally supported research institutions to negotiate a pricing formula for future products prior to entering into a research agreement with a profit-making company. The mandate would take effect in fiscal year 1994. Companies applying to participate in CRADAs would be required to specify the amount of royalties to be paid to the NIH, and those royalties would have to be comparable to the amount spent by the NIH. The bill encouraged colicensing for commercial projects as well as competitive bidding among interested parties.

Why drugs cost so much

The ever increasing cost of pharmaceuticals has exposed the industry to a barrage of criticism from Congress, patient-advocacy groups, consumers, and health care providers. Not only are newly introduced products extremely expensive, the prices of drugs that have been on the market for some time are also raised periodically—sometimes several times per year.

Manufacturers maintain that price increases are needed to fund the considerable costs of research and development. The industry spends 16 to 20% of sales revenues on research and development, for an industry-wide total of approximately $10 billion per year. In the early 1980s the average cost of developing a single drug was estimated at $100 million; by 1993 the cost of bringing a product from the laboratory to market had grown to an estimated $250 million.

Industry critics contend that the increasing cost of research and development does not justify the doubling and tripling of prices that took place during the

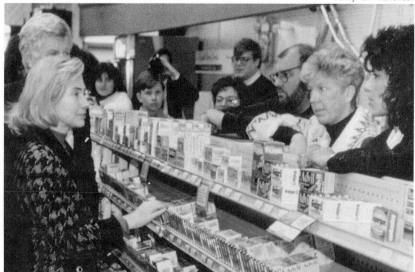

During a March 1993 fact-finding trip, Hillary Rodham Clinton, named by Pres. Bill Clinton to head the federal task force on national health care reform, talks with customers at a Boston drugstore. The pricing policies of pharmaceutical manufacturers are among the most contentious issues in the current debate over how to control health care costs.

1980s. They also point out that the pharmaceutical industry spends approximately $1 billion more each year on marketing than it spends on research and development.

As a result of the Pryor committee's investigations, a number of reports have been produced on apparent inequities in pharmaceutical pricing. One such inequity is that U.S. consumers pay higher prices for drugs than their counterparts in other countries pay for the same medications. A 1992 study by the General Accounting Office found that 121 of the most popular drugs dispensed in identical form and marketed by the same companies in the U.S. and Canada cost on average 32% more in the U.S. The drug industry argued that the study was flawed, pointing out that fewer than 40% of U.S. patients pay the full retail price out of pocket and those who do can request generic products, which cost less. On the other hand, Canada controls drug prices through government-imposed restrictions. The industry maintains that such price controls account for the fact that little drug research and development occurs in Canada.

Another apparent inequity is the vast disparity between the prices that manufacturers charge different customers for the same product. Hospitals, for example, pay less for drugs than do retail pharmacies, and not simply because they get discounts for buying in volume. Drug manufacturers charge lower prices to hospitals in order to increase the likelihood that physicians will use their products, become accustomed to them, and prescribe them outside the hospital setting—where the manufacturers can command higher prices. In addition, hospitals, along with health maintenance organizations (HMOs) and other managed care institutions, have become increasingly cost conscious and have strengthened their price-bargaining power with manufacturers through the establishment of re-

strictive drug formularies (*i.e.,* lists of drug products that health care providers may choose from when prescribing for a given condition).

Although patients, or their insurers, pay for drugs, they do not select the drugs they buy; prescribers do. However, a physician need not have access to every brand of, say, the many antiulcer or antihypertensive drugs on the market; instead, physicians and hospitals or HMOs may decide to purchase only one or two brands in each product category and then seek bid prices from manufacturers. Critics of this system argue that manufacturers compensate for the lower rates of return on products sold to hospitals, HMOs, and other "advantaged" buyers by a process called cost shifting; *i.e.,* charging higher prices to buyers in the retail market.

Hospitals and HMOs have pharmacy and therapeutics (P&T) committees that establish therapeutic categories and then choose certain drug products within each category for inclusion in restrictive drug formularies. In 1990 Pryor sought to save money for the Medicaid program by proposing the establishment of a national P&T committee, whose purpose would be to develop a list of "preferred" drugs within each category. Such a plan, Pryor reasoned, would provide states leverage in negotiating price discounts for pharmaceuticals purchased through the retail market under the Medicaid program. The pharmaceutical industry successfully opposed establishment of a federal P&T committee and a national drug formulary on the grounds that restricting the choice of drug products available under Medicaid would constitute a system of "second-class medicine" for the poor. Pryor then introduced alternative legislation, enacted in 1990, that effectively lowers the price Medicaid pays for prescription drug products. Under this rebate system drug manufacturers are required to pay state

Medicaid agencies rebates on drugs purchased for Medicaid patients.

In its defense the pharmaceutical industry has maintained that it already gives substantial price discounts to a majority of its customers. Approximately 35% of manufacturer sales of prescription drugs are to hospitals, which have price-bargaining power. Of the remaining sales, approximately 45% are covered by health insurance programs, which also have the ability to negotiate prices to varying degrees. A recent study commissioned by Pfizer Inc., for example, found that about 55% of the U.S. pharmaceutical market receives price discounts of 25% or more. Full list price is paid only by "traditional retail pharmacies," which account for about 25% of all pharmaceutical sales.

Helping those who cannot pay

Many pharmaceutical companies have instituted programs to ensure that indigent patients have access to needed medicines. In 1987 Searle became the first major pharmaceutical company to announce such an initiative when it started its "Patient in Need" program for the heart drug verapamil (Calan), a calcium channel blocker. Searle reports that it has distributed $150 million worth of products through the plan since its inception. A more recent example is Bristol-Myers Squibb's Cardiovascular Access Program, which was initiated in March 1992 and within six months had provided free products to more than 1,000 patients. Drugs provided under the program include blood-pressure-lowering agents, a beta blocker, and a drug to reduce cholesterol levels. The Cardiovascular Access Program is one of four Bristol-Myers Squibb indigent-patient programs. The other three—providing free supplies of anticancer agents, the AIDS drug didanosine (ddl; Videx), and an array of other unrelated products—had enrolled a total of 6,400 patients by 1992.

There are conflicting estimates of exactly how many companies have such programs and how many people are helped. Pryor's committee has recommended that the industry establish a panel consisting of professionals and advocates for the elderly that would seek ways to improve dissemination of information about indigent-patient programs; for example, through annual publication of a directory. The PMA has established a toll-free hot line that provides physicians with information about such programs, and it has been suggested that pharmacy and nursing professionals and social service agencies also be made aware of the hot line's existence.

User fees: expediting the review process

To help the FDA further speed the review of new prescription drugs, Congress in 1992 authorized the agency to charge pharmaceutical manufacturers "user fees" for the review of new brand-name products and

to apply the revenues to enhancing the drug-review process. The money was to be used to hire several hundred more chemists and medical officers and to upgrade the agency's computers and other scientific equipment.

Congress authorized the FDA to collect three categories of drug user fees—the most costly being for drug application reviews. Full premarket review of a new drug application (NDA) was set at $100,000 for fiscal 1993, escalating to $233,000 by fiscal 1997. Premarket review of a supplemental NDA (generally, an application to market an existing drug product for a new indication, or use) was $50,000 in 1993, escalating to $116,000 by 1997. The second category is an annual registration fee for prescription drug manufacturers ($60,000 per facility in fiscal 1993, rising to $138,000 by 1997). The third category is for annual registration of prescription drug products ($6,000 for each actively marketed product in fiscal 1993, to reach $14,000 by 1997).

Enactment of the user fee legislation represented the collaboration of the FDA, the pharmaceutical industry, and Congress. Pres. Ronald Reagan first proposed the idea of user fees in the mid-1980s as a tax-cutting measure in the executive branch's federal budget plan. The initial proposals, however, were opposed by all three of the parties concerned. Lawmakers argued that government agencies should be funded by the government. The industry contended that the plan effectively would make drug manufacturers disproportionately responsible for retiring the federal budget deficit. A number of FDA employees saw a potential for conflict of interest in that part of their salaries would be derived from the industry whose products they reviewed.

By 1992, however, two major factors had changed the prevailing attitudes toward user fees. First, because of mounting pressures to reduce the deficit, congressional appropriations to the FDA were not able to keep pace with the growth of the agency's congressionally mandated responsibilities to protect the public. Consequently, FDA resources were being stretched ever thinner. The FDA was dissatisfied with its level of funding; Congress was dissatisfied with the agency's habit of managing crises by shifting personnel from one program to another; and the industry was dissatisfied with the FDA's inability to hire and retain enough reviewers to handle increasing numbers of new product applications.

The second factor was FDA Commissioner David Kessler's impassioned effort to bring the various parties together. Addressing the qualms of Congress and the pharmaceutical industry, Kessler sought to ensure that FDA revenues derived from user fees would add to but not replace funds appropriated by Congress. The law stipulates that total user fee revenues in any given year may not exceed a set percentage of FDA appropriations. Further, fee collection is not authorized until an appropriations bill for that year has been passed, providing FDA funding at a level at least equal to the previous year's appropriations and with an allowance for inflation.

An additional condition of the law is a five-year "sunset" provision to end the user fee program if the FDA does not increase its rate of review of premarket applications and reduce the current backlog of pending applications before 1998. The performance goals for the first five years under the new law are to complete premarket reviews for priority drug products within an average of six months after applications are filed and to complete reviews for standard products within 12 months after filing. If the agency meets these goals, it will effectively cut its review times nearly in half: priority reviews currently average 12 months and standard reviews 20.

New drug compounds approved by the FDA in 1992 and early 1993

generic name	brand name	manufacturer	use
priority approvals			
atovaquone	Mepron	Burroughs Wellcome	*Pneumocystis carinii* pneumonia
cladribine	Leustatin	Ortho Biotech	hairy cell leukemia
enoxaparin (low molecular weight heparin)	Lovenex	Rhône-Poulenc Rorer	prevention of deep vein thrombosis
finasteride	Proscar	Merck	symptomatic benign prostatic hyperplasia
halofantrine	Halfan	SmithKline Beecham	malaria
itraconazole	Sporanox	Janssen	antifungal
mivacurium	Mivacron	Burroughs Wellcome	adjunct to anesthesia
paclitaxel	Taxol	Bristol-Myers Squibb	ovarian carcinoma
rifabutin	Mycobutin	Adria	prevention of *Mycobacterium avium* complex in AIDS patients
sotalol	Betapace	Berlex	ventricular arrhythmia
strontium-89	Metastron	Amersham and Zeneca	pain relief in bone cancer patients with metastases
sumatriptan	Imitrex	Glaxo	migraine
teniposide	Vumon	Bristol-Myers Squibb	lymphoblastic leukemia
zalcitabine	Hivid	Hoffmann-LaRoche	HIV infection
standard approvals			
amlodipine	Norvasc	Pfizer	hypertension and angina
bisoprolol	Zebeta	Lederle	hypertension
cefpodoxime	Vantin	Upjohn	antibiotic
desflurane	Suprane	Anaquest	anesthetic
desogestrel/ethinyl estradiol	Desogen	Organon	oral contraceptive
flosequinan*	Manoplax	Boots	congestive heart failure
gadodiamide	Omniscan	Sterling Winthrop	contrast-imaging enhancement for central nervous system
gadoteridol	ProHance	Bristol-Myers Squibb	contrast-imaging enhancement for central nervous system
lomefloxacin	Maxaquin	Searle	antibiotic
loratadine	Claritin	Schering Plough	allergic rhinitis
masoprocol	Actinex	Block Drug	actinic keratoses
nedocromil	Tilade	Fisons	bronchial asthma
oxaprozin	Daypro	Searle	osteoarthritis and rheumatoid arthritis
paroxetine	Paxil	SmithKline Beecham	depression
terbinafine	Lamisil	Sandoz	dermatologic antifungal
zolpidem	Ambien	Searle	short-term insomnia treatment

* withdrawn from the market, July 1993

Prescription drug interactions: consumer caveats

From time to time, interactions between prescription drugs result in untoward and sometimes very serious reactions. In 1992 two such unusual interactions were reported, implicating two companies' popular nonsedating antihistamines. The products in question were Marion Merrell Dow's Seldane (terfenadine) and Seldane-D (terfenadine with the decongestant pseudoephedrine) and Janssen's Hismanal (astemizole). These drugs have been widely prescribed because they provide relief from allergy symptoms without causing the drowsiness usually associated with antihistamine use. Unlike most prescription drugs, which are advertised only in professional journals, these were promoted directly to consumers, and patients often asked their physicians for these products by name. Furthermore, they were considered safe enough that they would eventually be reviewed for marketing as over-the-counter (OTC), or nonprescription, products. (Both Seldane and Hismanal are already available without prescription in Canada, although they must now be distributed from behind pharmacy counters.)

In July 1992, after reports of numerous cases of arrhythmias (abnormal heart rhythms), including several that proved fatal, resulting from the concomitant use of astemizole or terfenadine and antifungal or antibiotic drugs, the FDA ordered that the labeling for these prescription antihistamines be amended to include prominent warnings about the potential for serious cardiovascular effects. Consequently, the astemizole label now states that "rare cases of serious cardiovascular events" have been observed in persons who exceed the recommended 10-mg daily dose and also take antifungal drugs or antibiotics. The label also advises that patients not take more than 10 mg of astemizole per day. Cardiovascular reactions occurred in patients who had taken daily doses as low as 20 to 30 mg—and some people who used the drug were taking much higher doses. The terfenadine products were ordered to carry a warning specifically contraindicating use of the drugs by patients treated with the antibiotic erythromycin or the antifungal ketoconazole and by persons with hepatic (liver) disease. The warning also advises against exceeding the recommended dose of 120 mg daily. Marion Merrell Dow placed notices in consumer magazines such as *Time* and *People* to warn patients about the possible drug interactions and prepared pamphlets to be distributed in physicians' offices and pharmacies.

OTC drugs: how safe? how effective?

In September 1992 the Nonprescription Drug Manufacturers Association (NDMA) asked the FDA to publish regulations that would improve collection of reports on adverse reactions to nonprescription products. The request followed five months of discussions between the OTC drug industry and the agency and an April 1992 hearing before Wyden's House subcommittee, the latter focusing on whether existing OTC product label warnings were sufficient to alert consumers to potential toxic effects.

The system recommended by the NDMA would require manufacturers to report serious adverse reactions to the FDA within 15 days after they became aware of them. It also would require that the companies annually review both expected and unexpected reactions to their products for any changes in frequency or severity. (A similar reporting system exists for certain prescription products.) The FDA's authority to regulate OTC preparations extends to ensuring their safety and efficacy. Like prescription drugs, some are subject to premarket review and approval. For example, certain topical cortisone creams and the analgesic ibuprofen, both formerly prescription drugs, were approved by the FDA for OTC marketing in formulations that are lower than prescription strengths. Most OTC products, however, do not require product-by-product review, providing they contain active ingredients and are labeled for use in accordance with a series of regulations developed by the FDA. Since 1972 these regulations have been published as part of an ongoing OTC drug review.

In recent years, as part of an effort to streamline the review process, the agency has proposed that numerous ingredients found in a variety of OTC drugs be removed from the market because there is no basis for their use—*i.e.,* they have not been found to be effective. In 1990, 223 ingredients were removed from 19 different product categories, and the following year 111 ingredients were removed from OTC products marketed specifically for weight control.

In August 1992, in its most sweeping action to date, the FDA proposed a ban on 415 ingredients that have no proven efficacy and are found in several classes of OTC products, including digestive aids, topical antifungal remedies, external analgesics, menstruation-related preparations, skin protectants, pinworm treatments, and a broad category comprising internal analgesics, antipyretics (fever-reducing ingredients), and antirheumatics (inflammation-relieving ingredients). The largest number of banned ingredients—86—were in the external analgesic class and included substances used to treat such conditions as diaper rash, insect bites and stings, fever blisters and cold sores, and poison ivy, oak, and sumac. Thus, calamine-containing products would no longer be labeled as anti-itch remedies for poison ivy, oak, and sumac; however, these products could still be marketed as skin protectants. The FDA proposal urged manufacturers of products containing the cited ingredients to reformulate the products or withdraw them from the market within six months.

—Louis A. LaMarca
and Tammy L. Leopold

Special Report
Suing Tobacco Companies: Impact of a Landmark Case

by Leonard H. Glantz, J.D.

- In 1942 Rose Cipollone started smoking.
- In 1981 Cipollone was diagnosed as having lung cancer.
- In August 1983 Cipollone and her husband, Antonio, filed a lawsuit against various tobacco companies, claiming that she developed lung cancer as a result of smoking cigarettes made by the different companies.
- In 1984 Cipollone died. Her husband continued the prosecution of the lawsuit.
- In 1988 a federal district court jury awarded $400,000 in damages to Antonio Cipollone.
- In 1990 the U.S. Court of Appeals for the Third Circuit reversed the judgment of the trial court. Shortly thereafter Antonio died, but the Cipollones' son Thomas continued the lawsuit on his mother's estate's behalf.
- In 1992 the U.S. Supreme Court heard the Cipollone case and ruled on the complex issues regarding the liability of cigarette companies for failure to warn the public of the dangers of smoking.
- On Nov. 5, 1992, the family dropped its suit.

The very complicated and protracted case known as Cipollone v. Liggett Group, Inc. was one of the most closely watched cases in U.S. history. It was the first time that a tobacco company had been found liable for causing a tobacco-related disease. There had been more than 300 unsuccessful attempts of this type prior to this case. As a result, antitobacco advocates and personal injury attorneys hailed the jury verdict as a precursor to a flood of successful lawsuits against tobacco companies. When the Cipollone's dropped the case, they contended they had got what they wanted—to warn and help others and pave the way for other lawsuits by smokers.

The tobacco industry saw things differently. The ultimate outcome was that the cigarette companies were never required to pay the plaintiffs anything, thus continuing the industry's perfect litigation record. The industry viewed this decade-long lawsuit as an expensive annoyance (reports of the cost of defending the lawsuit were as high as $70 million). Although Wednesday, June 24, 1992, the day of the Supreme Court decision, was "bumpy" for tobacco stocks, upon the case's dismissal in November, stocks rose 3–5%, amounting to a vote of confidence from investors.

The Cipollones' lawsuit was initially based on four legal theories. They alleged that the tobacco companies were liable to them on the basis of: (1) "strict liability"—the companies failed to warn consumers of the dangers of cigarette smoking; (2) "express warranty"—the companies promised that cigarettes were safe in their advertising and public statements; (3) "fraudulent misrepresentation"—the companies intentionally misrepresented facts concerning the dangers of cigarette smoking, intending for consumers to rely upon these misrepresentations in making purchasing decisions; and (4) "conspiracy to defraud"—the companies acted together to conceal the dangers of cigarette smoking.

The jury in the 1988 trial court ruled in favor of the tobacco companies on counts three and four and in favor of Cipollone's husband on counts one and two. The jury did not award Rose Cipollone, the smoker and victim of lung cancer, anything. Why? Who ultimately won? What does Cipollone v. Liggett Group mean to future litigants who attempt to sue tobacco manufacturers for damages resulting from their products?

The plaintiff's smoking history

Rose Cipollone started smoking Chesterfield cigarettes in 1942 at the age of 17. She told lawyers in a deposition that she smoked that brand to be "glamorous" and to imitate the "pretty girls and movie stars" who appeared in the advertisements. She also said that Chesterfields were advertised as "mild," which she understood to mean safe. Cipollone also testified that she was an avid magazine reader and frequently listened to the radio. An ad appearing in magazines in 1952 described a "study" in which a "competent medical specialist and his staff" observed people from various walks of life who smoked from 10 to 40 cigarettes per day; 45% smoked Chesterfields from one to 30 years (averaging 10 years). At the beginning and end of a six-month period, each smoker was given a "thorough examination including X-ray pictures" by the "medical specialist," who concluded: "It is my opinion that the ears, nose, throat, and accessory organs of all participating subjects examined by me were not adversely affected in the six-month period by smoking the cigarettes provided." The ad in question carried the headline "PLAY SAFE, smoke Chesterfields."

Cipollone further testified that she regularly listened to the Arthur Godfrey radio show, which was sponsored by Chesterfield. Godfrey had commented on the

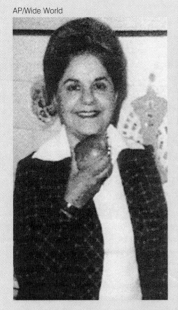

Rose Cipollone filed a lawsuit in 1983 against the various tobacco companies that made the cigarettes she had smoked since 1942, claiming their products were responsible for her developing lung cancer. Though Cipollone died in 1984, her case was continued for another nine years and was among the most closely watched suits in U.S. history.

ad just described: "Now that ought to make you feel better if you've had any worries at all about it. I never did. I smoke two or three packs of these every day. I feel pretty good. I don't know. I never did believe that they did you any harm, and now we've got the proof." Godfrey made many such statements on behalf of his sponsor. At one point he said, "I never recall seeing on anyone's gravestone 'He smoked too much,' did you?" Statements of this sort are alleged to constitute express warranties of safety and fraudulent misrepresentation by the cigarette companies.

In 1955 Cipollone switched to filtered L&M cigarettes. When asked why she changed brands, she said that the "bad stuff would stay in the filter." When asked if the "bad stuff" invoked a concern about health, she replied, "Not really. . . . It was the trend. Everybody was smoking filter cigarettes, and I changed, too." However, Cipollone also testified that through cigarette advertising "I was led to assume that they were safe." Advertising that appeared at that time for L&M stated that the "miracle tip" was "just what the doctor ordered."

In 1968 Cipollone switched to Virginia Slims not for health reasons but because "it was glamorous." In 1970 she switched to Parliaments because she thought the "recessed filter" made it healthier. She again switched in 1974 when her doctor had advised her son to stop smoking; this time she chose the True brand, which was advertised as containing low tar.

Cipollone smoked from one to two packs of cigarettes per day. Since their marriage in 1947, Antonio had continually begged his wife to stop. He told her it was unladylike and bad for her health. Whenever reports were publicized that smoking caused heart disease and cancer, he brought them to his wife's attention. Other members of the family acted similarly.

Understanding the verdicts

There was other evidence that indicated that Rose Cipollone believed that smoking was harmful. Information regarding cigarette companies' advertising claims and whether Cipollone believed them is important to understanding the 1988 jury-trial verdict and is also pertinent to the general difficulties involved in successfully prosecuting similar lawsuits.

The jury found that the companies *did* make express warranties regarding the health aspects of cigarette smoking and should have warned consumers of the risks of cigarette smoking. But the jury also found that Cipollone "voluntarily and unreasonably encountered a known danger by smoking cigarettes" and that she was 80% responsible for her own injuries. In New Jersey, where this lawsuit took place, plaintiffs cannot recover damages if they are more than 50% responsible for their own injury; therefore, Rose Cipollone lost.

Her husband, Antonio, on the other hand, was awarded damages for the loss of his wife because he engaged in no activity that could have contributed to his wife's death. But in 1990 the appeals court reversed the judgment that had been made in his favor owing to errors made by the trial judge in regard to the warranty claim and some other technicalities. Cipollone died five days later, never having received his award. The issue that went to the Supreme Court in 1992, however, had to do with whether the tobacco companies could be liable for failing to warn of the dangers of smoking after January 1966, when a federal law requiring warning labels on cigarette packs went into effect.

The preemption issue

To understand the Supreme Court ruling in this case, one needs to be aware of the development of federal rules regarding smoking warnings and their impact on civil litigation. In 1964 an advisory committee to U.S. Surgeon General Luther Terry issued its now famous report, *Smoking and Health,* which concluded that "cigarette smoking is a health hazard of sufficient importance in the United States to warrant appropriate remedial action." Following that report the Federal Trade Commission (FTC), which is authorized to regulate unfair and deceptive trade practices, promulgated a rule requiring all cigarette advertising and every pack or carton of cigarettes sold in the U.S. to clearly and prominently state that "cigarette smoking is dangerous to health and may cause death from cancer and other diseases." A number of states also began to regulate the advertising and labeling of cigarettes. In July 1965 Congress enacted the Federal Cigarette Labeling and Advertising Act, which mandated warnings on cigarette packs (as of Jan. 1, 1966) but barred such warnings in cigarette advertising. This act superseded the FTC regulations and had two stated purposes: (1) to inform the public of the hazards of cigarette smoking and (2) to protect the national economy from the burden imposed by diverse, nonuniform, and confusing cigarette labeling and advertising regulations. Section 4 of the act required the now well-known warning label on all cigarettes: "Caution: Cigarette Smoking May Be Hazardous to Your Health." Section 5 of the law pertained to "preemption" and stated:

(a) No statement relating to smoking and health, other than the statement required by section 1333 of this title, shall be required on any cigarette package.
(b) No statement relating to smoking and health shall be required in the advertising of any cigarettes which packages are labeled in conformity with the provisions of this chapter.

In 1969 Congress enacted the Public Health Cigarette Smoking Act, which amended the 1965 act in several ways. The required warning was strengthened to say that smoking "is dangerous" to health. The latter act also banned cigarette advertising on radio and television, and the preemption provision was amended to read:

No requirement or prohibition based on smoking and health shall be imposed under State law with respect to the advertising or promotion of any cigarettes the packages of which are labeled in conformity with the provisions of this chapter.

The question presented to the Supreme Court in *Cipollone* v. *Liggett* was: Did these preemption provisions prohibit a person from suing a cigarette company for failing to adequately warn of the risks of cigarette smoking? Preemption is a complex doctrine that involves the allocation of legal authority between the federal and state governments. When the states adopted the U.S. Constitution, creating the federal government, they gave exclusive authority in several areas. For example, only the federal government can raise armies, enter into treaties with foreign governments, or print money. In many other areas the states and the federal government share power. For example, both state and federal governments can tax income, and both can regulate the sale and possession of dangerous drugs. However, under the Supremacy Clause of the Constitution, the federal government may supersede the powers of the states and deprive the state of any authority to regulate a particular matter or industry. For example, if each state had its own air-traffic-control system and rules, it would be virtually impossible to have a nationwide airline industry.

As a general rule, the effect of federal government preemption means that state legislatures and agencies may not enact any laws or regulations in the area that has been "preempted," or overridden. Courts are very cautious about declaring that an area has been preempted by the federal government because such a ruling deprives states of authority to regulate matters they have historically regulated. The Cipollone case presented a somewhat unusual question, as no state legislature or agency had enacted regulations that

required cigarette labeling. Rather, a jury in a civil lawsuit brought by a private individual was being asked to rule that cigarette companies, which had complied with the federal cigarette warning laws, had not done *enough* to warn potential consumers. If a jury decided against the tobacco companies, cigarette manufacturers would then need to change their warnings to avoid future liability. The concern was that juries in all 50 states could require 50 different warnings. Thus, the question was, if state legislatures were preempted from requiring a multiplicity of warnings, could juries or courts require them?

In *Cipollone* the trial court ruled that the preemption doctrine applied only to legislative and administrative rules and did not preempt or prevent lawsuits by private citizens. The federal appeals court ruled that, given the federal cigarette packaging law's goal of uniform labeling requirements, Congress had by implication preempted lawsuits based on the alleged inadequacy of cigarette warning labels. The Supreme Court found this to be a particularly difficult case, and a majority of the justices were unable to agree on an outcome. Four justices found there to be partial preemption so that some lawsuits were permissible; three justices felt there was no preemption; and two justices argued that no lawsuits of any kind could be brought against the tobacco industry.

The four-justice plurality, Justices John Paul Stevens, William H. Rehnquist, Byron R. White, and Sandra Day O'Connor, found that the 1965 law's language prohibiting states from requiring any "statement" relating to smoking and health applied only to affirmative requirements imposed by state legislative or regulatory agencies and did not foreclose lawsuits by private citizens. However, the 1969 federal law, which bans all "requirement[s] or prohibition[s]" imposed under state laws, was broader and prohibited courts and juries from assessing the alleged adequacy of warnings. This means that one may sue a cigarette company for failure to adequately warn consumers of the risks of smoking *prior* to 1969. A tobacco company cannot be sued for failure to warn consumers of risks *after* 1969.

The plurality opinion also held that there are some lawsuits that could continue to be brought. These include lawsuits for breach of express warranty and for fraudulent misrepresentation. The reason these lawsuits are not preempted is that they do not emanate from any state requirement or prohibition regarding smoking and health. Rather, the four justices argued, the claim of breach of express warranty is based on statements and promises *voluntarily* made by the companies—and not on requirements by the states. Likewise, fraudulent misrepresentation claims are derived from the general duty of sellers not to deceive prospective purchasers and are not specifically applicable to smoking and health.

Tobacco on trial: the future

The Supreme Court's decision in *Cipollone* v. *Liggett* was something of a compromise, but its effect was to deprive potential plaintiffs of so-called duty-to-warn claims based on inadequate warnings after 1969. Often such failure-to-warn, or strict liability, claims based on package mislabeling are among the most powerful claims plaintiffs have in product liability lawsuits. In contrast, express warranty and fraudulent misrepresentation claims based on advertising are among the most difficult to win because it must be proved that the plaintiff saw, believed, and relied upon the advertisements in making purchasing decisions. Furthermore, such advertising must contain quite explicit promises, as in the previously mentioned statements made on radio by Godfrey about the harmless nature of smoking. Thus, billboards advertising menthol cigarettes that show young, healthy-looking people playing volleyball on the beach do not constitute an express warranty or fraudulent misrepresentation.

It is well known that advertisements frequently exaggerate or include considerable "puffing." Advertisements for beer and other alcoholic beverages show thin, sober, and healthy young men and women; ads for diet programs present a world of slim and beautiful women; and television commercials for automobiles show the latest model of sports car soaring through the air at top speed, then neatly skidding to a halt on wet roads—without mentioning the thousands of deaths caused by out-of-control motor vehicles each year. Cigarette advertising, by comparison, has become much more restrained over the years.

Since the *Cipollone* decision, the R.J. Reynolds Co. was victorious in a case brought by Charles Kueper of Cahokia, Ill., a 51-year-old former cigarette smoker who was dying of lung cancer. The lawsuit alleged that the tobacco industry had concealed information about smoking's dangers, produced fraudulent and misleading advertisements, and showed "utter indifference to the suffering of others." This is the type of lawsuit that was not prohibited by the Supreme Court's *Cipollone* decision. During the trial the plaintiff, who had started to smoke in the fifth grade and smoked for 40 years, testified that he had some awareness that smoking posed a danger—that his family and doctors had warned him many times over the years to stop smoking. Kueper said he had tried to quit a number of times, but "it's not that easy to quit." As the jury foreman noted in discussing the jury's vote against the plaintiff, the members of the jury concluded that Kueper's smoking was a result of "his free choice."

Ultimately there is a great irony in these cases. The very failure of lawsuits that attempt to prosecute cigarette manufacturers for the harm caused by their products is a direct result of the success of public health initiatives to warn the public of the risks of smoking. The 1969 federal cigarette-labeling law

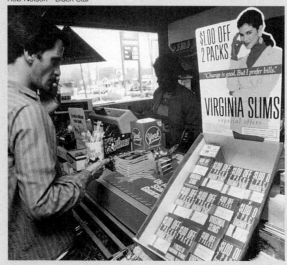

In 1968 Rose Cipollone switched to Virginia Slims because ads made them seem "glamorous." Today it is virtually impossible to win a lawsuit blaming ads for the decision to smoke and then developing smoking-related illness because every ad and every pack state that smoking "is dangerous" to health.

that resulted in every pack of cigarettes sold in the United States carrying the explicit warning that smoking is "dangerous" in effect forecloses lawsuits based on inadequate warnings. Indeed, a 1972 rule of the FTC that requires all print advertising for cigarettes to include warning labels and a 1984 federal law that requires the use of four different, rotating warning messages that describe a variety of risks associated with cigarette smoking increase the public's knowledge of risks and decrease the chance of a smoker's successfully arguing that he or she was ignorant of the risks of smoking.

It is now virtually impossible to convince a jury that a person smoked as a result of cigarette advertising and that he or she did not know smoking presented a risk to health. Moreover, there is not a person who sits on a jury today who does not know of the dangers of smoking. Substantial numbers of jurors will have quit smoking themselves or known someone who has. Indeed, the vast numbers of people who have quit smoking and the ever decreasing numbers of new smokers are a testament to the widespread knowledge of smoking's risks. While there are many who would like to see tobacco companies prosecuted and punished for reaping huge profits from selling a substance that harms and kills so many users, the hazards of smoking are now so well known that such suits are exceedingly difficult, if not impossible, to win. The "glamour" that drew Rose Cipollone to smoking no longer exists—not as a result of successful lawsuits but because public health efforts have been so successful and have led to a remarkable shift in public attitudes (including that of juries) toward smoking.

385

Special Report
France: Fuming over a New Law?

by Alexander Dorozynski

Feu sur les fumeurs ("Open fire on smokers")
La bataille du tabac part en fumée ("Tobacco battle goes up in smoke")
Tout le monde s'en fiche ("Nobody gives a damn")
Pas l'ombre d'une plainte ("Not a shadow of a complaint")

These headlines appeared in the French press when a strict new antismoking law took effect in November 1992. In fact, France's antismoking legislation is similar to measures that have been enacted in many other countries—except that it is not enforced, nor was it intended to be. It is viewed as a first step toward reassuring the French that smoking restrictions do not represent an intolerable deprivation of liberty and at the same time that nonsmokers should be free not to breathe other people's smoke. Hardly a fine has been levied against violators—either individuals who light up in restricted areas, restaurants and cafés that fail to provide adequate nonsmoking areas, or workplaces where the legislation is not respected. Such a low-key approach appears to be prudent and has begun to pay off. People appear to be smoking less in public places; some restaurants have set aside nonsmoking areas, most of them movable according to demand; and the ashtrays placed at the entrances to the Métro (subway) stations are full. And everybody—the government, hotel and restaurant managers, smokers, nonsmokers—is relieved that the new law, which had been equated by some with prohibition, has *not* led to massive demonstrations and violence.

If a long uphill struggle is expected before the French truly turn against smoking, as Americans have, it is not because the French smoke more than others. True, more than a third of French men and women smoke. Although the precise rates are not known, a good way to compare France with its European neighbors is by looking at cigarette sales. If the total number of cigarettes sold in the country is divided by the population, each French man, woman, and child purchases about 1,670 cigarettes a year. This situates the French halfway between "heavy" European smokers (*e.g.,* in Greece, with 3,570 cigarettes purchased per person per year, and Spain, with 2,560) and "light" smokers (The Netherlands, with 1,350 cigarettes, counting the estimated number of hand-rolled cigarettes popular in that country, per person).

Smoking in France increased sharply between 1950 and 1975 but after that appears to have stabilized. However, it is more widespread now among women and youngsters aged 15–20 than it was in the past. Moreover, unlike their counterparts in the U.S. and other countries, French doctors continue to smoke at the same rate as other members of the population.

The Institut National de la Santé et de la Recherche Médicale (National Institute of Health and Medical Research, or INSERM) estimates that smoking in France is the cause of at least 55,000 deaths annually (about 10% of total deaths). Lung and respiratory tract cancers are the principal tobacco-related causes of death, having steadily increased from 14,905 for men and 1,862 for women in 1979 to 18,805 and 2,812, respectively, in 1990. This is followed by cardiovascular diseases (13,000 deaths attributed to tobacco) and chronic bronchitis (10,000 deaths). Added to self-inflicted and preventable deaths are some 40,000 attributed to alcohol, which is also responsible for a significant portion of the additional 10,000 annual deaths from traffic accidents.

The state as tobacco merchant

Even though medical evidence of the harmful effects of tobacco is clear and public consciousness of the risks of smoking is increasing, there are reasons to believe that the struggle for a smoke-free social environment in France will be a long one. One reason is that the French government has a monopoly on cigarette manufacturing and distribution and is not likely to give up this important source of revenue. The monopoly was started more than 300 years ago under the reign of Louis XIV and has continued (with a brief interruption during the French Revolution of 1789) to this day. Its modern version is known as SEITA, or the Société Nationale d'Exploitation Industrielle des Tabacs et des Allumettes, which is the sole producer of cigarettes in the country as well as the distributor of imported tobacco—and which employs some 5,900 people. In France, unlike many countries, one cannot buy cigarettes in supermarkets or from machines. Tobacco products are sold only in some 35,500 licensed stores called *bureaux de tabac* or *débits de tabac,* whose owners, *buralistes,* net about 8% on every pack sold. Many *bureaux* are at the same time cafés, and they also sell government lottery and racetrack-betting tickets, postage stamps, fiscal stamps for paying traffic-violation fines, telephone credit cards, chewing gum and candy, lighters and matches, and newspapers and magazines, among other odds and ends.

In 1992, out of total tobacco products sales of nearly F 50 billion ($9.1 billion), the government's share was F 35 billion ($6.4 billion). Tobacco revenue thus represents at least 2% of the country's budget. In addition, tobacco growers receive agricultural subsidies from the European Community, and the total tobacco sector employs about 50,000 people. Tobacco is included among the commodities that make up the country's price index, and successive governments have opposed tobacco price increases because they push the index up—and make for bad publicity.

It is recognized that the cost of smoking to society is at least twice as high as the government revenue from tobacco. The estimate is about F 60 billion ($10.9 billion) in health costs annually and much more if loss in productivity and such not-so-easily-defined costs as "quality of life" are included. But the health costs are viewed as being more diffused than the cash income. Most of the health expenditures are paid for through the health insurance branch of the social security system, which is financed through contributions by employers and employees. An apocryphal story goes

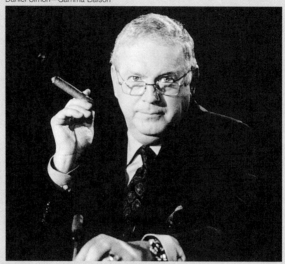

Michel Charasse, former minister of the budget—rarely seen without cigar—was one of several outspoken government officials who opposed the antismoking legislation that took effect in France in November 1992.

A subway rider stubs out his cigarette before boarding his train. Full ashtrays at the entrances to the Paris Métro suggest that the public is complying, at least somewhat, with the country's new restrictions on smoking.

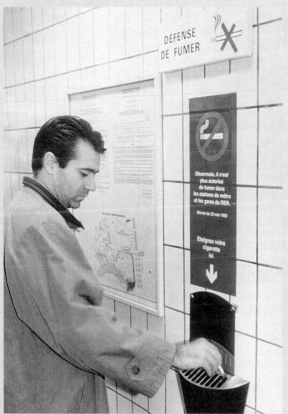

that one finance minister, when told that the country spends three francs in health costs for every franc it takes from tobacco sales, quipped: "I get the one franc. It is my successor who will have to pay out the three francs."

The state thus finds itself in a somewhat duplicitous position regarding laws on smoking. The country's first serious antitobacco legislation was adopted in 1976 when Simone Veil (who then smoked in public) was minister of health. La Loi Veil (the Veil law) restricted smoking in public places and limited the advertising of tobacco products. Madame Veil was again appointed health minister of the new, right-wing government in March 1993 and is expected to actively pursue antitobacco measures. She no longer smokes in public.

In recent years, as a result of epidemiological studies and public health campaigns, awareness of the dangers of both smoking and passive smoking has greatly increased, and in 1990 a group of deputies of the National Assembly pointed out the state's shortsighted policies in trying to reconcile tax revenues from tobacco with its costs in terms of health. The deputies proposed a much more severe piece of legislation, known as la Loi Evin, after Claude Evin, then minister of health. Debates on the proposed legislation once more revealed conflict of interest within the government. The legislation was opposed by Michel Charasse, then minister of the budget (seldom seen without his cigar), but also by the minister of culture, the minister of youth and sports, and the minister delegate for communications (who probably had in mind the significant tobacco subsidies that go to the movie industry, to sporting events—particularly automobile racing—and, through advertising, to the press).

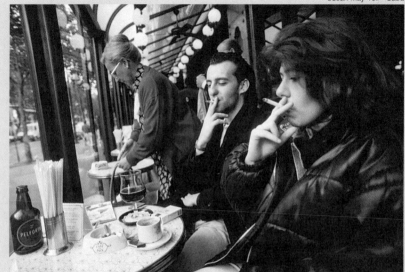

Susan May Tell—Saba

At Paris' popular bistros, smokers continue to puff away with little apparent restraint. Though all restaurants and cafés in France are now supposed to provide adequate areas for nonsmokers, smoking and nonsmoking sections are movable upon demand. All in all, the approach to the new law restricting smoking in public places has been notably low key, and few fines have been levied against violators.

The bill passed in the parliament nevertheless and was published in the official parliamentary gazette (*Le Journal Officiel*) in January 1991. A month later SEITA attempted to bypass not only the pending legislation but the earlier (1976) law, according to which no product could be marketed or offered for free if it bore the name or the emblem of a tobacco product. SEITA then launched a new brand of cigarettes bearing the name Chevignon, a maker of jackets and other fashionable items of clothing that enjoy popularity among the young. The Ministry of Health promptly protested, while that of the Budget (which has authority over SEITA) argued that the new brand was not launched to incite young people to smoke but rather to persuade tobacco users to buy SEITA products rather than foreign brands. In two months' time Chevignon cigarettes were taken off the market. The Evin law was finally passed in January 1992, to become effective in November of the same year.

Tough to enforce

The law is hard, but its enforcement is even harder. The Evin law describes in great detail restrictions on smoking in public places. It stipulates that there be no smoking in those parts of offices and workplaces that are used by all employees—hallways, cafeterias, conference and waiting rooms—but that smoking areas with sufficient space and good ventilation be provided. An individual with his or her own office can chose to smoke or to abstain. The law provides for negotiation and arbitration in cases of conflict and states that employers cannot decide unilaterally to ban smoking in their enterprises.

Nonsmoking regulations in bars and restaurants were, from the start, known to be inapplicable in most cases. They specify that in all public places where food and beverages are served, whether closed (in-

doors) or open (France's famous sidewalk bistros), smoking and no-smoking areas should be designated at the discretion of the management but can be rearranged at will. No physical partitions are required, but adequate ventilation (seven liters of circulating air per minute per occupant, the same as for smoking areas in offices) should be provided.

Smoking is also restricted in schools, colleges, and universities, even in open spaces such as courtyards. However, designated smoking areas should be provided for teachers and students over 16 who wish to smoke—a directive known from the start to be impracticable, as educational establishments in France are notoriously short of space.

The law is quite strict for public transportation facilities. Smoking had already been prohibited in suburban commuter trains (since January 1991), and the Evin law also proscribed smoking in bars and snack bars of long-distance trains and in corridors and spaces between cars. About one-third of the nation's railway cars are reserved for smokers. Smoking is forbidden on the platforms of subway and railroad stations, except uncovered ones, and in railroad stations and airports (although the latter have designated smoking areas). The French airline Air Inter had already forbidden smoking on all of its national flights, but Air France allowed for smoking areas. In 1993 some nonsmoking "medium-range" flights (*e.g.,* to Switzerland, Italy, Germany, and other neighboring countries) were inaugurated.

Individual fines for smoking in nonsmoking places range from F 135 to F 1,300 (about $25 to $235). Employers and managers who do not comply with the new rules can be fined up to F 6,000 (nearly $1,100).

When the law went into effect on the first day of November, a Sunday, it had been heralded by national television programs that emphasized its *non-*

388

repressive nature in its attempt to protect nonsmokers from inhaling other people's smoke. It was widely known that police officers and inspectors in public transportation and other facilities were instructed not to mete out fines. Treading with caution on the thin ice of Gallic susceptibility was no doubt encouraged by the memory of a monstrous gridlock throughout the country inflicted three months earlier when truck drivers protested en masse against the introduction of punitive measures for violators of driving laws, forcing the government to back off and ease the rules.

Predating the enactment of the law, horror stories about antismoking legislation in the United States abounded. These included stories about the firing of employees after the clandestine detection of nicotine in urine tests. Then there was the shock experienced by Gerard d'Aboville, who became a national hero when he rowed his way alone across the stormy Pacific (from Japan to the United States) in July–November 1991. Upon landing in Ilwaco, Wash., the Frenchman was chastised for having done something socially unacceptable and "un-American" when he lit up a cigarette at his press conference. D'Aboville wondered what he had done and, when told, was quick to point out that the cigarette he smoked was made in America. He has since been awarded the honorary title of "premier fumeur de pipe de France" ("number one pipe smoker") by the Pipe-Club de France. (The sportsman occasionally smokes a pipe but claims to be a "reasonable smoker" who respects nonsmokers' rights.)

When the Evin law took effect, the daily and weekly press as well as television leaped on the newsworthy occasion to editorialize and poke fun at the legislation. A few prophesied "grumbling," "violence," and "a new apartheid" between smokers and nonsmokers. Others protested against government interference with privacy and liberty and in one case wondered when a similar breach would reach the bedroom. One magazine noted the ironic situation in America: "In the United States, where nicotine is synonymous with dismissal, divorce, the electric chair, everybody should know that in the face of the British Stamp Act, Virginians shot first. George Washington, Thomas Jefferson, James Madison, James Monroe were planters. Tobacco paid for powder . . . and gave independence. . . . What ingratitude!"

Just before a total ban on tobacco advertising in France went into effect on Jan. 1, 1992, the tobacco industry sponsored "special editions" of two national newspapers, *Le Figaro* and *Libération:* a smokers' edition on tobacco-colored paper and a nonsmokers' edition in blue. This advertising "coup" was paid for by Rothmans International, makers of Peter Stuyvesant cigarettes, which rank among the top five cigarettes in France, preceded by Marlboro, which accounted for one-fifth of sales in 1992, Gauloises *brunes* (referring to their dark brown tobacco), Gitanes *brunes,* and Camel. The nonsmokers' edition carried the prominent and ironic notice "This copy does not carry advertising for Peter Stuyvesant cigarettes." The advertising ban was a blow to the daily and particularly the weekly press; it was followed by a partial ban of alcohol ads. Apparently, both tobacco and alcohol manufacturers have switched their emphasis from advertising expenditures to price reductions, and newspapers complain of as much as a 30% loss in advertising revenues.

At the Université de Paris X (Paris-Nanterre), Sylvie Redin, head of medical services, said: "The decree is simply inapplicable. We can't create space for smokers; we don't have enough as it is. And we can't discipline half of the students." Nonsmoking signs had existed in amphitheaters well before the Evin law, and they do not appear to be having any more effect

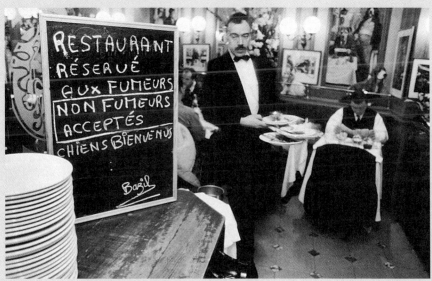

Some French restaurant owners are going out of their way not to offend their smoking patrons. The sign in this establishment reads: "Restaurant reserved for smokers. Nonsmokers accepted. Dogs welcome."

Sipa

now than they did then, which was not much. Unions protested against "the increased disciplinary power of management."

Café owners would not dream of excluding smokers who light up when they order their *petit noir*—the traditional tiny cup of espresso coffee served in the thousands of cafés and bistros, bastions of French conviviality. Most restaurants, as required, acquired smoking and nonsmoking signs but move them about to accommodate clients. Thus, if smoking clients appear to dominate, there may be little breathing space for the random client who does not. A few establishments, however, defiantly posted a notice that "nonsmoking clients are welcome."

A crucial enforcement difficulty stems from the traditionally rebellious Gallic attitude toward authority. Anarchic parking, littering, and dog droppings on the sidewalks are widespread in many French cities (in Paris special motorcycle squads have been instituted to handle the canine feces). Pedestrians typically exhibit a cavalier attitude, seeming to avoid designated crossings and dashing at will across streets and through intersections. *Le Monde,* the respected national daily, ran an article about the Evin law under the headline: "The glorious indiscipline of the smoker."

Tobacco's enduring mystique

Ultimately, perhaps the greatest obstacle to French antismoking efforts is the deeply entrenched aura of romance surrounding tobacco. This "love affair" started around 1561 when Jean Nicot, the erudite French ambassador to Portugal, extolled the medicinal virtues of tobacco and gave some to Catherine de Médicis, the illustrious queen consort of Henry II and regent of France, to treat her migraine headaches. The story goes that she was cured and subsequently encouraged the planting of tobacco in France. The plant was first known as *nicotiane,* after Nicot, and when the tobacco alkaloid was isolated in 1828, it was called "nicotine."

James I of Scotland condemned tobacco as being "repugnant to the eye, detestable to the nose, dangerous for the brain, appalling to the lungs"; popes excommunicated people for snuffing tobacco in churches; and in Russia a tribunal formed in 1634 could order smokers' noses to be cut off. But in France, Louis XIII took great pleasure in snuff tobacco, while d'Artagnan and musketeers animated the streets of Paris with the clanging of their swords and the smoke of their pipes.

Tobacco certainly has its place in France's literary tradition. In Molière's 1665 play *Don Juan,* the eponymous protagonist and ultimate French libertine proclaims: "There's nothing like tobacco: it is the passion of honest people, and he who lives without tobacco is not worthy of living. . . . Not only does it rejuvenate and purge the human brain, but it instructs souls

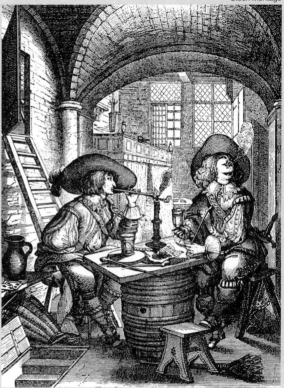

Aristocrats during the reign of Louis XIV take great pleasure in a full pipe. The French love affair with tobacco, which began in the mid-16th century when the substance was extolled for its medicinal properties, has flourished ever since.

with virtue." A contemporary of Molière, the dramatist Pierre Corneille, considered tobacco "divine." The early 19th-century Romantic poet, novelist, and critic Petrus Borel wrote: "Fortunately, as a consolation, we have adultery and Maryland tobacco."

During World War I, French citizens were urged to use tobacco sparingly so that the soldiers on the front line would receive their rations. Until recently tobacco was distributed to recruits in the French armed services as part of their pay. At the end of World War II, American cigarettes (notably, "the Lucky Strike that went to war") became symbols of liberation and were used as currency.

Indeed, many of France's postwar luminaries and heroes were admired by the public through a heavy cloud of cigarette (or pipe) smoke. The pipe of Jean-Paul Sartre; the cigarette of André Malraux, who chain-smoked through inspiring talks on television; the dark Gauloise glued to the lower lip of Jacques Prévert, whose favorite interpreter, Yves Montand, was also rarely seen without a cigarette—all consecrated the smoking habit as a symbol of the intellectual and the poet. Smoking's romantic image was and continues to be perpetuated by artists—the "new wave" of French actors, led by Jean-Paul Belmondo, whose entrance on the scene was usually preceded by the glowing end of his cigarette. Of course, such American actors as Humphrey Bogart and John Wayne, ever popular among French audiences, certainly did their part to reinforce the French love of smoking. More recently, the popular French composer and singer Serge Gainsbourg not only chain-smoked through television talk shows but paused during his songs to take deep draws.

Until 1975 tobacco was accepted as a completely licit product. According to Albert Hirsch, a pneumologist, and sociologist Serge Karsenty in their recent book, *Le Prix de la fumée* ("The Cost of Smoke"), "It was even recommended by the government: free distribution during military service, thus reinforcing its image as a masculine product of first necessity, together with wine, shaving cream and shoe polish." The same authors, looking at the evolution of the smoking habit, note: "Twenty or 30 years ago, you were initiated to tobacco during military service. Now it happens on school benches, sometimes as early as at the age of 10 or 11."

Cheap smokes

Another highly controversial measure to discourage smoking is an increase in the price of cigarettes. From many a politician's viewpoint, price increases not only affect the cost-of-living index but are a poor reflection of the government's effectiveness. Moreover, such increases are unpopular with the electorate. In May 1993 the average price of a package of cigarettes in France had jumped to F 13 ($2.40), up from F 11.30 ($2.09). Still, cigarette costs remained among the lowest in Europe (about half the price of a pack in Denmark or Norway but still twice as high as in Greece and four times higher than in Spain).

Whether as a result of the price hikes or not, the

volume of tobacco sales in France decreased by 5.1% during the first four months of 1993 in comparison with the same period a year earlier (from 24,840 to 23,750 tons). At the same time, price increases of April 1992 and January 1993 pushed sales for that period from F 11,110,000,000 ($2 billion) to F 12,450,000,000 ($2,270,000,000), an increase of 12.1%.

According to Robert Molimard of the Société Française de Tabacologie at the Hôpital Salpétrière in Paris, a group that studies the chemistry and health effects of tobacco: "Studies have shown that when prices go up, butts get shorter, which is more toxic." Molimard believes that the Evin law has the merit of making people conscious that smoking must not constitute a norm but thinks that the fiscal windfall it has generated could be put to better use than subsidizing automobile and motorcycle racing (which was done to compensate for the loss of tobacco advertising). He has suggested that research could focus on ways of minimizing the harmfulness of cigarettes. For instance, novel genetic engineering approaches could diminish the carcinogenic nitrates in tobacco plants. The Société believes that the neurochemical and psychosocial mechanisms of tobacco dependence deserve more thorough study and that they should be financed by SEITA profits.

French doctors: doing their part?

A survey carried out among physicians by the European Medical Association of Tobacco and Health in February 1993 found that the number of physicians in France who smoke has decreased somewhat (21% smoke regularly and an additional 11% occasionally) but, surprisingly, two out of three physicians consider that tobacco addiction, unless it poses a specific risk to their patients, is not relevant to their professional activity. In addition, it appears that physicians who smoke minimize the pathogenic role of tobacco, except in the two very obvious tobacco-related diseases, lung cancer and chronic bronchitis. When patients complain of an ailment that is not obviously related to tobacco, three out of four smoking doctors do not even question them about their smoking habits.

A breath of fresher air

In spite of anecdotal evidence to the contrary, the Evin law appears to be a significant stepping-stone toward protecting the rights of nonsmokers and making smoking somewhat less fashionable in the land of Gauloises. The results of the first survey of more than 300 large companies in or near Paris, carried out by the National Committee Against Tobacco Addiction, indicated that the air, at least in the workplace, is a bit fresher, that most companies abide by the new rules, and that smoking on the job has started to decrease. Whether the French will ever truly abandon their "glorious indiscipline" remains to be seen.

Cigarettes: cost of the habit (January 1993)	
selected countries	price per pack (dollars)
Norway	4.87
Canada	4.34
Denmark	4.33
United Kingdom	3.41
Hong Kong	2.78
New Zealand	2.67
France	2.09
United States	1.89
Japan	1.75
Spain	0.60
Thailand	0.59
Philippines	0.44
Brazil	0.42

Sources: Worldwatch Institute and Non-Smokers' Rights Association of Canada

Women's Health

In recent years many health care providers, when assessing the gains and losses in matters related to women's health, have found the balance to be heavily weighted on the loss side. In recent months, however, there have been indications that the scale is beginning to tip in favor of gains. Two such progressive recent developments are the long-delayed U.S. Food and Drug Administration (FDA) approval of Depo-Provera as a contraceptive and the potential approval of RU-486 for abortion and other medical indications. Another favorable change during the past year: the FDA announced that women will no longer be banned from participation in trials determining the safety of new drugs (a policy based on the rationale that their exclusion protected against possible fetal damage in women who became pregnant during the trial) and that drug companies will henceforth be required to analyze gender differences in determining appropriate drug dosages as well as the efficacy and side effects of new pharmaceutical agents.

On the negative side, however, are the continuing debate and some mounting concerns over the safety of silicone gel breast implants and the ever increasing incidence of breast cancer. In addition, of continuing uncertain significance for the health and well-being of women is the use of tamoxifen in the prevention of breast cancer. And although there has been some relaxation of constraints on freedom of choice, what those ultimately bode for women's health is far from certain. Attempts to deny poor women free access to abortion continue and, in the view of some observers, have taken on more pronounced racial overtones.

Depo-Provera: a "new" contraceptive option

On Oct. 29, 1992, an event occurred that had been 25 years in the making—the FDA gave the Upjohn Co. the go-ahead to market medroxyprogesterone acetate (DMPA; Depo-Provera) as a contraceptive. The story behind Depo-Provera's approval offers instructive insights into the impact that the political process can have on the practice of medicine.

Deliberation and delay. Although often referred to as a new contraceptive method, Depo-Provera is, in fact, many years old. DMPA, a synthetic form of the natural hormone progesterone, was originally licensed in the U.S. in 1960 for the treatment of habitual and threatened spontaneous abortions and the gynecologic condition endometriosis. Because subsequent reviews showed the drug to be ineffective when used to treat these conditions, FDA approval for these uses was withdrawn in the early 1970s. In 1972, however, the drug was approved as adjunctive treatment for patients with endometrial cancer, and in 1978 it was approved for treatment of renal cancer.

The first two events in a long series of attempts to obtain approval for the *contraceptive* use of DMPA came in 1967, when Upjohn filed a request to this effect, and in April 1973, when the FDA's Obstetrics and Gynecology Advisory Committee unanimously recommended that approval be granted. Six months later the proposed labeling for the contraceptive use of the drug (*i.e.,* the dosage recommendations and listing of indications, contraindications, and side effects) was published in the *Federal Register,* and in April 1974 the FDA wrote a final approval notice. This notice was never published, however, because a violent controversy over Depo-Provera had already begun to erupt. In October 1974, Rep. Lawrence H. Fountain (Dem.-N.C.), in response to intense pressure from various consumer and women's advocacy groups concerned about reports linking DMPA with cancer, successfully petitioned to stay the drug's approval, an action that was sanctioned by Caspar Weinberger, then secretary of health, education, and welfare (HEW).

In December 1975 the FDA advisory committee again reviewed the Depo-Provera data and recommended approval, this time under specific conditions previously laid out in the *Federal Register.* Once again, no approval was forthcoming, and one year later Sydney Wolfe of the Public Citizen Health Research Group, a Washington, D.C.-based consumer advocacy organization, requested that HEW refuse to approve DMPA, citing several remaining concerns about its safety. The pressures on the FDA to withhold approval were continued, and in August 1977, Upjohn was requested to withdraw its application. The following month, however, Upjohn notified the FDA that it would not withdraw the application. Then in August 1978 the House Select Committee on Population held public hearings on DMPA.

In the meantime, in March 1978 the FDA had informed Upjohn that DMPA was not approvable as a contraceptive. The company responded by requesting an opportunity for a hearing in the form of a public board of inquiry (PBI) rather than having the matter adjudicated in a hearing by an administrative law judge. Donald Kennedy, then FDA commissioner, approved the formation of a three-member PBI, and five days of open hearings were finally held in January 1983. After another long delay, the PBI recommended in October 1984 that DMPA not be approved for general marketing as a contraceptive. Two members of the board, while recognizing the drug's high rate of effectiveness and its safety record over a short term, were opposed to approval. They cited an alleged lack of long-term safety data, particularly regarding the drug's potential to cause cancer. The remaining member of the board voted for approval, filing a minority report. Upjohn filed exceptions to the report and in August 1986 asked that additional new and relevant data be added to the PBI record and that the case be reopened. However, then FDA commissioner Frank Young denied

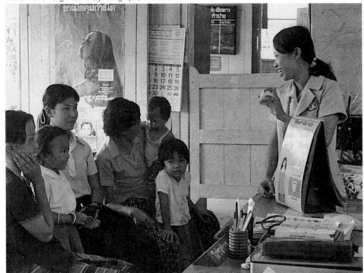

A community midwife in northern Thailand teaches local women about the different forms of contraception available to them. Injectable contraceptives are a popular option in that country. With the Food and Drug Administration's approval of Depo-Provera in October 1992, American women too now have access to such a method of birth control.

this request, suggesting that the company withdraw the original application and submit a new one that included the new data.

A new submission was prepared and was sent to the FDA in April 1992. Two months later the agency's Fertility and Maternal Health Drugs Advisory Committee, after careful review, unanimously recommended approval of DMPA as a contraceptive. This time the recommendation was accepted by the FDA, and formal approval was granted on Oct. 29, 1992.

Throughout the 1970s and '80s, the opponents of DMPA kept up an aggressive campaign against it, as did certain segments of the media. In 1987, for example, a highly publicized controversy erupted when it was revealed that the Indian Health Service (IHS) was using DMPA for family-planning purposes. At a Senate hearing Everett R. Rhoades, director of the IHS, defended his agency's policy.

At the same time, many groups of health care professionals, including the American College of Obstetricians and Gynecologists, declared themselves in favor of DMPA for birth control. Several influential international organizations also recommended that the drug be approved for use as a contraceptive. The first of these was the World Health Organization (WHO), which conducted a review and concluded in 1979 that there was no reason to discontinue Depo-Provera in the many countries where it was already in use. In 1980 an advisory panel of the U.S. Agency for International Development (AID), the organization responsible for administering U.S. foreign aid programs, recommended that DMPA be made available as a contraceptive option in countries receiving American assistance. (This was not done, however, because AID policy prohibits the distribution abroad of drugs for indications that are not FDA approved.) Finally, the International Planned Parenthood Federation re-

evaluated DMPA in 1980 and concluded that it would continue to make the drug available, as had been its practice since 1971.

In the meantime, despite the absence of FDA approval, many U.S. physicians were already giving patients DMPA as a contraceptive agent. Not all doctors recognize that once a drug has been approved in the U.S. and is being marketed for use in certain specific conditions, it is entirely legal for a practitioner to use it in another, as-yet-unapproved but medically sound way, provided that patients are adequately informed. On the other hand, many physicians refrained from prescribing Depo-Provera as a contraceptive because of fears of potential legal liability.

Safety concerns: data and documentation. During all the years of FDA delay, although unapproved in the U.S., DMPA was being used as a contraceptive by more than 30 million women in more than 90 countries around the world. What prevented its approval in the U.S. was a concerted effort on the part of certain women's and consumer advocacy groups to publicize the reputed health risks of the drug. In fact, these safety concerns were mainly the result of the consistent misinterpretation of both human and animal data from studies on Depo-Provera carried out by Upjohn in the 1960s and '70s. In particular, the opponents cited data derived from tests involving dogs (beagles) and rhesus monkeys. In the canine studies animals that were given high doses of DMPA for a number of years developed breast tumors. Unfortunately, the beagle was a poor choice for these experiments inasmuch as it has a high rate of spontaneous breast tumors and will develop such tumors when given virtually any hormone. This fact was belatedly recognized by regulatory agencies in the U.K. and then finally by the FDA, which now consider the beagle to be an inappropriate test animal for evaluating hormones.

393

The Upjohn data also showed that two rhesus monkeys developed endometrial cancer when given 50 times the human dose of DMPA. However, in another, unrelated study, endometrial cancer occurred in a control animal. Moreover, these tumors occurred in an anatomic structure found in the monkey but not in women. The relevance, if any, to the human female of these particular animal studies was debated for many years, and it was concluded that there is little, if any.

At the June 1992 meeting of the FDA's advisory committee, with the contraceptive effectiveness of DMPA and the earlier animal studies no longer at issue, the committee members focused their attention on safety concerns involving the human female, particularly the possible association of the drug with certain malignancies. In the years since the PBI, a large body of new data on Depo-Provera had been gathered and reported, particularly by WHO. The malignancy of greatest concern was carcinoma of the breast. The WHO data showed that if there was indeed an increased risk of breast cancer in women using Depo-Provera, there was only a weak association, approximately equivalent to that noted with oral contraceptives. Furthermore, breast cancer risk was minimally increased only during the first four years of use and was present mainly in women under 35 years of age. Moreover, the risk did not increase with increasing duration of use, nor was it greater in women who had used DMPA for more than five years.

These findings suggested that Depo-Provera was not a cause of breast cancer but rather may have stimulated the growth of preexisting malignant tissue, causing it to become clinically apparent. In addition, the WHO studies did not show any increased risk for cervical, ovarian, or liver cancers. In fact, they indicated a decreased risk of endometrial cancer at least as great as and probably greater than that observed in women who took oral contraceptives.

Two issues were raised at the June hearings that had not been considered at earlier meetings. The first of these was based on data from New Zealand showing that bone density was decreased after five years of Depo-Provera use. However, the bone loss observed was less than that seen in postmenopausal women, did not reach the levels associated with fractures, and was reversible with cessation of DMPA.

The other concern was stimulated by two reports suggesting, first, that accidental pregnancies occurring one to two months after an injection of DMPA might result in increased risk of infants' being born at low birth weight and, second, that the risk of neonatal deaths might be increased. However, because Depo-Provera is virtually 100% effective when the first injection is given as recommended (in the first five days of a normal menstrual period), these risks were not believed to be of any great clinical significance. More-

over, although concerns had been raised in the past about the possible induction of birth defects by progestogens, these have been proved groundless, and no such associations have been found in DMPA users.

Another claim erroneously made in the past was that Depo-Provera induces permanent sterility. The evidence to date indicates that while there is a well-documented delay in the return of fertility, it is only temporary; 70% of women who discontinue DMPA to try to become pregnant conceive in the first year, and more than 90% conceive by the end of two years. This two-year delay is comparable to that seen in prior oral contraceptive and intrauterine device (IUD) users, as well as in women trying to become pregnant who have used no contraception at all. Further, there is no evidence of any relationship between the duration of administration of DMPA and the length of time that it takes a woman to become fertile again. However, it has been found that women of lower body weight tend to become pregnant sooner than women of higher body weight.

How the drug works. Depo-Provera is similar in structure to the hormone progesterone, which is produced normally by the ovaries. The synthetic product is an aqueous suspension of microcrystals, which, because of their low solubility, have a prolonged period of effectiveness. DMPA for contraception is injected intramuscularly, usually in the arm or buttock, every three months in a dose of 150 mg.

DMPA blocks ovulation and also produces thinning of the lining of the uterus. The combination of these two actions makes it one of the most effective contraceptive agents ever developed. Pregnancy rates with the drug range from 0 to 0.22 per 100 women-years of use. The only other comparably effective methods are Norplant (subdermal hormonal capsules that are left in place for up to five years, approved for use in the U.S. in 1990), the newer copper and hormone-bearing IUDs, and female sterilization.

The only side effects of DMPA that occur with predictable frequency are changes in menstrual patterns. In the first three to six months, many women experience irregular bleeding, which may be extremely heavy in rare cases but lessens with time. At the end of one year, 57% of women have stopped having menstrual periods; the rate increases to 68% after two years. Many women look forward to this event, and most are not disturbed by it once they understand that it is normal, they are not pregnant, and there is no threat to their health. In fact, DMPA reduces the risk of iron-deficiency anemia associated with bleeding.

This form of contraception is appropriate for the majority of women of reproductive age. Depo-Provera offers particular advantages to women unable or unwilling to use other forms of contraception: those who have difficulty taking (or remembering to take) oral contraceptives; those who are unable to use estrogen;

those who have contraindications to IUDs; and those who, for whatever reason, are unable or unlikely to use barrier contraceptives effectively. It may have special advantages for sexually active teenagers, whose compliance with methods requiring consistent use is often poor.

Depo-Provera is also very useful at the end of the reproductive years, allowing older and premenopausal women who wish to retain their childbearing potential to do so without fear of unintended pregnancy. The potential long-term efficacy of this form of birth control makes it an ideal option for a woman who believes that she has completed her family and yet does not want to undergo surgical sterilization. In addition, women for whom other contraceptive methods are contraindicated—those who are postpartum, lactating, or have sickle-cell disease—can use Depo-Provera. In fact, sickle-cell disease is often improved with DMPA use.

Many health care providers believe that DMPA is an ideal form of contraception for those women who have no contraindications to its use and who find it an attractive option. It is unquestionably a significant addition to the choices currently available to American women.

RU-486: an option thus far denied

RU-486 (mifepristone), a drug developed by the French pharmaceutical company Roussel Uclaf and its parent company, Germany's Hoechst A.G., as a medical abortifacient, is available in France, Britain, Sweden, and China but has thus far been denied to American women. Nonetheless, there are a number of compelling reasons why it would be advantageous for them to have access to a safe and effective non-surgical method for early termination of unwanted pregnancies. For one thing, it would enable a woman to make the choice to terminate her pregnancy and have the procedure carried out in the privacy of her doctor's office, with the assurance of confidentiality.

Abortion: legal but increasingly inaccessible. With the Supreme Court's 1973 decision in *Roe* v. *Wade,* the abortion picture changed dramatically in the United States. Although women of means had always been able to obtain safe abortions either at home or abroad, this option had been denied to less affluent women. As a result, before 1973 many thousands of illegal abortions were performed each year, resulting in hundreds of deaths and unknown numbers of cases of severe hemorrhage, infection, and permanent injury. With the granting of freedom of choice, however, all this began to change. New surgical techniques such as suction abortion were developed and increasingly utilized, leading to safe and effective first-trimester outpatient procedures. Also, once abortion was legalized, women learned to seek this option early in pregnancy rather than postponing the decision to terminate the

pregnancy until a later and riskier stage. These factors combined to reduce the rates of deaths and medical complications in these instances to close to zero. Allowing women to choose whether to continue an unplanned (and frequently unwanted) pregnancy gave them a new kind of control over their lives and enabled them to plan for the future with a new sense of freedom and confidence. Finally, the societal costs of illegal abortion began to abate.

Why, then, given the successful record of surgical abortion, is there a need for a medical method of terminating early pregnancy? The reasons are multiple and interrelated and fall into three categories—personal, medical, and societal. Despite the ease and safety of suction abortion, a medical method of abortion—one using a chemical agent—obviates the need for surgical intervention and is therefore an approach preferred by many women. In addition, a medical option, as already noted, would allow greater confidentiality for both women and their health care providers. Given the increasing and often violent harassment of patients and physicians, their families, and co-workers; the burning, bombing, and vandalizing of abortion clinics; and, recently, the brutal murder of a physician in Pensacola, Fla., by an antiabortion extremist, the need for privacy is becoming ever more evident and urgent.

Quite predictably many doctors, faced with harassment and death threats, have reluctantly stopped performing abortions. In some cases doctors are wearing bulletproof vests and carrying guns. Some clinics have installed alarm systems and bulletproof windows. Under these circumstances access to abortion has understandably continued to decline. The number of U.S. hospitals offering terminations dropped from 1,654 in 1977 to 1,040 in 1988. And today more than two-thirds of obstetrician-gynecologists will not do these procedures. Also contributing to decreased availability is the fact that only 13% of U.S. medical residency programs currently require training in early-abortion techniques, and only 7% require instruction in second-trimester methods. In 1985 almost one-quarter of the programs required both.

Another factor limiting financial support of and freedom of access to abortion is increasingly restrictive legislation. Such legislation has a major impact on low-income, minority, and rural women in particular, often preventing them from obtaining a medical service that is ostensibly legally available to them. It is also creating an increasingly untenable situation for medical professionals who are trying to offer women safe, effective, and compassionate health care.

The "moral property" of women. It was recognized in 1982 that RU-486 would interfere with the action of the hormone progesterone, which is essential to the continuation of early pregnancy. After extensive testing in 15 countries, the agent was approved for

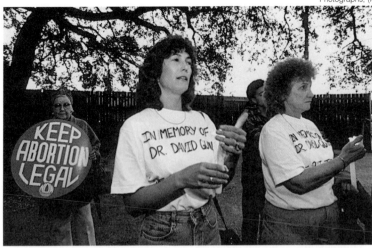

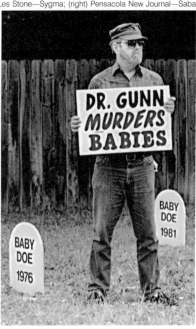

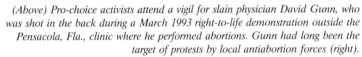

(Above) Pro-choice activists attend a vigil for slain physician David Gunn, who was shot in the back during a March 1993 right-to-life demonstration outside the Pensacola, Fla., clinic where he performed abortions. Gunn had long been the target of protests by local antiabortion forces (right).

use as an abortifacient in France in 1988. Then, only one month later, as the result of tremendous political pressures—including threats by U.S. antichoice activists of boycotts against the drug's manufacturer—it was withdrawn from the market in France. Two days later, however, declaring that RU-486 was "the moral property of women, not just the property of the drug company," French Minister of Health Claude Evin ordered Roussel to resume distribution.

The World Congress of Obstetrics and Gynecology fortuitously happened to be meeting in Rio de Janeiro at the time, and the conferees, upon hearing the news from France, signed and sent to Paris a petition for the resumption of RU-486 distribution. Similar actions were taken by the American Medical Association, the Institute of Medicine of the National Academy of Sciences, and other groups all over the world. As a result, RU-486 continues to be used in France and is now approved in Britain, Sweden, and China. It may soon be available in India, The Netherlands, Hungary, Italy, Chile, Hong Kong, and Singapore, and elsewhere—where clinical studies of the drug are either under way or scheduled.

Attempts to conduct studies in the U.S. that would lead to FDA approval have been consistently thwarted. Fearing commercial reprisal, Roussel has steadfastly refused to make RU-486 available to U.S. researchers. In addition, political pressure brought to bear on the FDA led to a ban on importation of small quantities of RU-486 for personal use, although other unapproved drugs are allowed into the country for individual use. In a widely publicized event, in July 1992 U.S. customs agents seized a single dose of the drug being taken into the country by a pregnant woman who

had obtained it in London for the purpose of inducing an abortion.

A proven record. RU-486 is taken by mouth up to the seventh to ninth week of gestation, followed 36–48 hours later by an injection of a prostaglandin. Recently it was shown that an oral prostaglandin, misoprostal—which has already been approved as a treatment for peptic ulcers under the trade name Cytotec—may work just as well and thus may eliminate the need for a follow-up office visit. However, antichoice groups are currently attempting to drive this drug off the market.

More than 120,000 women in France, Sweden, and Great Britain are estimated to have used RU-486. Roussel has reported that half of the 160,000 abortions performed annually in France have been induced by RU-486. In general, it has been proved to be extremely safe and effective—safer in fact than first-trimester surgical abortion. Most women complete their abortions in 1–1½ weeks after use of the two drugs, very few needing follow-up surgery. Only one death has been reported, and this was due to the injectable prostaglandin—not RU-486—given, moreover, to a poor candidate, a woman who was hypertensive and a heavy smoker. Following this occurrence, doctors in France switched to the oral prostaglandin.

Outlook for the future. While many U.S. medical professionals are concerned because access to a proven safe and effective medical abortifacient is being blocked by a vocal and aggressive minority, the clinical interest in RU-486 is not limited solely to its use in reproductive medicine. The drug has shown considerable promise in the treatment of a number of major medical problems, several of great potential importance to women: it appears to be effective in the

396

treatment of breast cancer and endometriosis; it helps to soften the cervix to facilitate childbirth, avoiding the necessity of cesarean delivery in certain instances; and it shows considerable promise as a contraceptive and a morning-after pill. Other possible uses of RU-486 are not limited to women; they include treatment of glaucoma, inoperable brain tumors, Cushing's syndrome, burns, and obesity. The ban on RU-486 as a medical means of abortion has also stopped virtually all research into these other potentially important areas, leaving many investigators both frustrated and angry.

With the start of the administration of Pres. Bill Clinton in January 1993, however, it appeared that this picture might change. The FDA agreed to lift its import ban on RU-486 and to permit testing in the U.S. Roussel agreed to license the drug and the manufacturing technology to the Population Council, a nonprofit research organization based in New York City. Still, no American company has yet been authorized to carry out the studies necessary for FDA approval. It is believed that a small company with few products would be the most likely to undertake the testing, as it would be far less vulnerable than a large company to threats of boycotts. Given the number of unresolved issues, it seems unlikely that RU-486 will soon be available to American women.

Breast implants: controversy continues

The debate about silicone gel breast implants, which began in 1991, continues to rage and to escalate. Concern about the safety of these devices has not abated, and the repercussions of the FDA hearings on the implants in 1991 and 1992 continue to be felt. Perhaps the foremost of these repercussions has been a large number of requests for removal of implants, some prompted by symptoms believed to be

due to the implants but many triggered simply by fear and anxiety. At the same time, there has been a sharp decline in the number of implant procedures. Moreover, only one company is currently still making the devices. According to 1992 FDA-imposed restrictions, patients who have had mastectomies for breast cancer or have major deformities can get implants for breast reconstruction but must be enrolled in a study protocol approved by the FDA. A research protocol for the use of implants for cosmetic breast enlargement is under development, but enrollment will be limited to only the number of subjects needed to answer questions about implant safety.

Another repercussion of the FDA hearings is an acceleration of clinical evaluations and laboratory studies in an attempt to resolve lingering safety issues. Of greatest concern is the association between implants and autoimmune or connective tissue disease, antibodies to silicone having been reported in a number of women. Attempts are also being made, with magnetic resonance imaging and ultrasound as well as standard X-ray mammography, to determine the true incidence of complications such as contracture (the formation of a tight capsule of scar tissue around the implant), bleeding, leaking, and rupture.

Questions about the safety of the still-available saline implants continue to be asked and will be the subject of future FDA hearings. Understandably, this prospect has led to attempts to find innovative—and theoretically safer—materials. Devices made of non-silicone materials are now beginning to be evaluated.

The final, most inflammatory, and most predictable result of the FDA's 1992 ban on implants has been the rapid increase in lawsuits by women seeking compensation for harm alleged to have been caused by the devices. The first implant trial resulted in a multi-million-dollar verdict for the plaintiff; it is unclear how

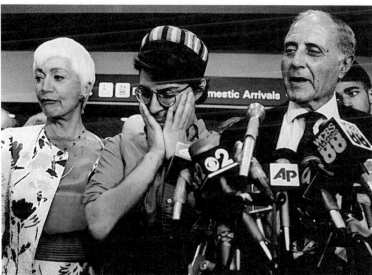

Rebecca Cooney

Accompanied by her physician (left) and an abortion rights activist (right), a woman who attempted to bring a single dose of RU-486, the French abortion pill, into the the U.S. faces news cameras after the drug was seized by customs officials at New York's Kennedy International Airport.

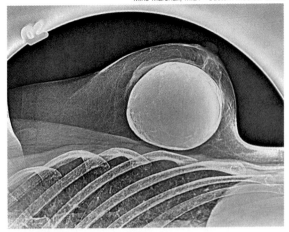

A mammograph reveals a silicone gel implant within a woman's breast. Owing to continuing safety questions about the devices—particularly whether they cause autoimmune reactions—many women have sought to have them removed.

many such cases will ultimately be tried, but it is clear that this case is only the tip of a litigious iceberg.

Breast cancer: treatment and prevention

The fear of breast cancer looms large in the minds of many women. For women in the U.S. the risk of developing breast cancer ranges from one in 20,000 at age 25 to one in 8 at age 95. The most recent data published by the American Cancer Society predicted 183,000 new cases in 1993—representing 32% of cancers in women—and 46,300 deaths. Moreover, between 1980 and 1987 the incidence of breast cancer in the U.S. rose from 85 to 112.4 per 100,-000—a 32.2% increase. Breast cancer mortality has not changed since 1930, despite the increased use of mammography. However, lesions are being found earlier, and long-term data are expected to show a decrease in the death rate that will confirm the advantage of early diagnosis and treatment.

The treatment of breast cancer has undergone tremendous changes in the past 20 years. In the 1970s the treatment of choice was the Halsted radical mastectomy and axillary lymph node dissection. This left many patients not only with deformity but also with a permanently swollen and poorly functioning arm. By the 1980s many surgeons had switched to a modified radical procedure and later to partial mastectomy and then lumpectomy. This change was due in part to the discovery of estrogen and progesterone receptors in tumor tissue, enabling doctors to more accurately determine the stage of the disease and to better estimate the prognosis of individual tumors. Therapy used in conjunction with surgery (adjuvant therapy) also underwent considerable change, moving from radiation in the 1970s to chemotherapy in the '80s.

Two new drugs are now being used in the treatment of breast cancer. The first of these is Taxol (paclitaxel), a drug approved by the FDA in 1992 for treatment of ovarian cancer. This agent has received extensive media coverage. It is, in fact, very effective in breast cancer, with partial remission of symptoms in more than half the women treated and about 10% showing complete remission. However, Taxol has considerable toxicity and, owing to its limited supply, is very expensive. The other drug, the subject of even more publicity, is tamoxifen. It has been shown that with long-term use this drug increases survival rates, and it is now considered a treatment of choice for women with invasive breast cancer. However, although generally well tolerated, it too can have significant side effects, the most disturbing of which are endometrial cancer, blood clots, irreversible damage to the retina, and possibly liver cancer.

Because of tamoxifen's proven effectiveness against breast cancer, it was proposed by the National Institutes of Health that clinical trials be conducted to determine whether it could prevent breast cancer in women with known risk factors. Thus, in 1992 the National Cancer Institute began trials to test the prophylactic potential of the drug in 16,000 "high-risk" healthy women. While this approach is conceptually attractive, it is also controversial, and many people have questioned whether healthy women should be subjected to such a powerful and potentially toxic agent with unproven benefits.

Reproductive freedom: expanding?

In the U.S. the change in political administrations offered hope to those suffering as a result of limitations on reproductive choices and cutbacks in funding of family-planning programs, which were felt both domestically and internationally. Shortly after taking office, President Clinton announced that five of the most restrictive actions of previous administrations were being overturned: (1) the "gag rule," which prohibited abortion counseling in government-funded clinics; (2) the so-called Mexico City policy, which cut off U.S. aid to any international family-planning programs involved in abortion-related activities; (3) the blocking of fetal tissue research, which had effectively thwarted important research initiatives; (4) the ban on importation of RU-486 for personal use; and (5) the prohibition of abortions in overseas military hospitals.

Since that time other changes have been proposed that would increase women's health choices. These include an end to the ban on federal support of abortions for indigent women and the return of funding for vital international family-planning programs. How many of the proposed changes will actually be effected and what their combined impact will be—whether they will result in truly greater reproductive freedom—remain to be seen.

—*Elizabeth B. Connell, M.D.*

Special Report
Music and the Mind: Scientific Musings
by Gail McBride

Can the eye of science *feel* the true character of music, and its unique power to animate the person?
　　　　　　　　　　　　　　—Oliver Sacks, *Awakenings*

As neurologist and author Oliver Sacks observed, listening, playing, singing, or just moving to music often has dramatic effects on patients with profound neurological impairments, such as stroke or Parkinson's disease. Like Sacks, many neurologists, psychologists, musicologists, and others for years have been fascinated by music's role in human behavior and its effects on the functioning of the brain and nervous system. Equally compelling are the brain processes that are involved in producing and responding to music.

The scope of this interest has ranged from ponderings on the creative impulse to intensive scientific study, such as using the highly sophisticated imaging technique of positron emission tomography (PET) to record the metabolic activity of the brain while it is engaged in a musical task. Yet despite many intriguing observations and clear evidence that music therapy can be effective in rehabilitating some neurologically impaired patients, because of the brain's awesome complexity, very little is known with certainty. In fact, some things that were once accepted—for example, that the "music center" of the brain is located in the right hemisphere—no longer are. As one leading scientist in the field put it, investigators are only beginning to "tame" the "wilderness of [their] ignorance."

Recent developments in the neurosciences have led to wide-ranging neuroanatomic research and exploration of the brain's organization and mental processing as they relate to music. As a testament to this work, in November 1992 a symposium, "Music and the Brain," was held in Chicago. The conference was organized and directed by Andrea Gellin Shindler, founder and executive director of the newly established Foundation for Human Potential of Chicago, with assistance from the Chicago Symphony Orchestra and the School of the Art Institute of Chicago and funding from, among others, the National Institute of Mental Health and the National Institute on Aging. The symposium brought together neurologists, psychiatrists and psychologists, musicians, music therapists, educators, cultural anthropologists, and others for three days of lectures and discussions. The spectrum of topics covered was as diverse as the backgrounds of the participants.

Among the many questions posed at the conference were: What is the basis of musical creativity? Why does music pervade all cultures? Can brain areas involved in musical ability be localized? How can the genius of a Mozart be explained? What makes the musical savant so exceptional? Why do people vary in their perceptions of music? What is the role of the auditory system in music? How are music and language related? And what has been learned from studying well-known musicians with known or suspected neurological deficits? The following provides a glimpse of some of the recent insights into this broad and fascinating field of study.

The nature of creativity

One of the topics addressed at the Chicago conference was whether musical creativity is unique and independent of other mental processes or whether creativity in music and in other disciplines is the product of common mental processes. In the book *Frames of Mind: The Theory of Multiple Intelligences* (1983), the Harvard University psychologist Howard Gardner made a case for the former view, proposing that there are multiple and distinct types of intelligence, such as visual, verbal, and musical.

Among those who have explored the latter possibility is Robert S. Root-Bernstein, professor of physiology at Michigan State University. Specifically, he has looked at scientists (including mathematicians) who have been musicians (or other kinds of artists) as well, often of high caliber. Indeed, many scientists (past and present) have been or are virtuoso performers, and some have even designed and made musical instruments as well as composed. Albert Schweitzer, Aleksandr Borodin, and the contemporary scientists Solomon Snyder and Stephen Jay Gould are just a few examples of scientist-musicians.

Although music and science are seemingly disparate fields, Root-Bernstein has concluded that common mental processes underlie the creative activities in each. In his words, the "coincidence of abilities" is not "by chance." By studying the mental processes involved in the scientific and musical endeavors of these "doubly gifted individuals," Root-Bernstein has found that they rely on precise "tools of thinking"— analogizing, pattern forming, abstracting, and kinesthetic thinking, among others. The main talent of creative people, he believes, is the ability to transfer between modes of thinking and to make connections between insights and ideas—be they of a scientific, musical, or other nature.

Music and neuroanatomy

Because of the many associations that have been observed between music and specific anatomic structures in the brain, the belief persists that certain brain areas must be more involved with music than others. Many scientists have attempted to identify such potential brain centers by studying people with brain dysfunction or damage.

In a type of epilepsy called musicogenic epilepsy, susceptible people may have seizures upon hearing specific passages or types of music—for example, a portion of the second movement of Beethoven's Fifth Symphony or salsa music. The abnormal electrical activity associated with this type of seizure (seen on an electroencephalogram, or EEG) is usually in the right or left temporal lobe of the brain, the portion generally associated with acoustic (auditory) sensations.

In contrast, patients who have what are called musical partial seizures spontaneously "hear" (i.e., hallucinate) sounds in their minds. Those sounds can be music, speech, or noises (such as whirrs, clicks, or single tones). Such hallucinations produce EEG activity that is also focused in the temporal lobe but more often in the brain's left hemisphere.

The Montreal surgeon Wilder Penfield triggered hallucinatory seizures in 20 patients during neurosurgery by stimulating certain areas of the cortex (the brain's outer layer). One patient could "hear" a male chorus and orchestra performing "White Christmas"; another "heard" a jingle from a radio commercial. Other patients heard words rather than music, but Penfield found there was no apparent separation between brain areas that precipitate hallucinated words or music. Other scientists have found that some elderly persons who are becoming deaf may have so-called release hallucinations; i.e., they "hear" music, often from their distant past. The mechanism is unclear but does not appear to be epileptic.

Another way to relate music to certain brain areas has been to study persons whose brains have been injured or impaired through illness or who have undergone brain surgery. Sometimes these people lose certain musical abilities that they had previously (known as amusia). The location of the injury or disorder offers clues to the specific brain area that was the presumed source of that lost musical ability.

Some people with damage to the brain have aphasia—a language disturbance that often involves the inability to speak or write—but no amusia. That is, they can no longer speak, but they can "sing" words and/or compose music. Commonly these people have damage to the left hemisphere, which, in most right-handed people, is the brain's language center. One example is a composer who suffered a severe aphasia—could neither comprehend what was said to him nor read nor write—but he was still able to compose quite well and, despite his aphasia, wrote songs, quartets, choruses, and a symphony.

Another group of patients that have been studied—the largest group—have both aphasia and amusia. A well-known composer, Maurice Ravel (discussed below), is an example. A third group have amusia without aphasia, a condition that is probably not widely diagnosed because language skills remain intact and victims do not seek treatment. These patients may have normal language function and may be able to recognize a melody, but they cannot sing or whistle. Most have been found to have lesions in the brain's right hemisphere; thus, investigators believe that the right side of the brain may affect musical pitch more than rhythm. On the other hand, some patients with lesions in the left hemisphere have problems reading or writing music.

Individual patients, however, present almost endless variations within each of these three groups. Thus, at least for the present, firm conclusions about specific locations of unique musical skills cannot be drawn.

Music and language

The defects of aphasia and amusia highlight the relationship between music and language. One investigator of this relationship is John C.M. Brust, professor of neurology at Columbia University College of Physicians and Surgeons, New York City. Brust points out that there are well-recognized musical aspects of everyday speech—rhythm, pitch, and inflection, known collectively as prosody—and that prosody can be intrinsic (the sound of speech—e.g., whether it sounds German or French), emotional, or propositional (conveying meaning).

A type of music therapy based on prosody has helped some patients who have aphasia without amusia. Over two centuries ago it was observed that a young man rendered speechless after a major blow to the head was still able to sing in a church choir. This intriguing preserved ability, in spite of a severe aphasia, prompted therapists to investigate the potential of music therapy for aphasia.

About 20 years ago Nancy Helm-Estabrooks, a speech pathologist at Boston University School of Medicine, and colleagues Robert Sparks and Martin Albert developed the technique called melodic intonation therapy. As Helm-Estabrooks described the therapy at the Chicago symposium, a patient first is instructed to sing short phrases and sentences as simple sing-song melodies containing only high and low tones—the pitch pattern resembling as closely as possible how the phrase or sentence would be spoken. Next, the phrase or sentence is sung with an exaggerated stress pattern in more of a monotone, much like choral speaking. Gradually the melodic content is faded, and the patient "speaks" rather than sings the phrase or sentence; finally, he or she responds to questions by using normal speech.

Melodic intonation therapy is used to draw out language function, presumably from the right hemisphere. It is particularly useful for restoring acceptable speech in patients with left hemisphere strokes that impair articulatory agility but spare auditory comprehension.

Perception of music

In addition to studying patients with brain dysfunction, such as epilepsy or brain injuries, there are newer ways of investigating the relationship between music and the brain. One such technique is called dichotic listening. In these investigations earphones are used to feed different messages, tones, or music into a person's two ears simultaneously. If the left hemisphere is dominant, the person will primarily describe what was fed into the right ear, and vice versa. The technique is controversial, however, because it is not difficult for the tester to unwittingly increase one ear's advantage over the other—for example, by decreasing the duration of noise fed into one ear or manipulating the acoustic features of the sounds. Furthermore, what may appear to be differences and asymmetries between the two cerebral hemispheres can reflect internal auditory pathway delays or other kinds of information loss that affect what is heard. Hence, results of such studies have varied greatly depending on how the technique is set up; the subject's age, aptitude, and training; and whether recognition of melody, pure tones, timbre, pitch, or rhythm is used as the criterion. Differences also occur depending on whether only a basic tone or the basic tone plus its overtones (tones whose frequencies are multiples of the frequency of the basic tone) is played.

Nonetheless, some useful information has emerged from dichotic listening studies. For instance, as neuropsychologist John J. Sidtis at the University of Minnesota has found, complex pitch perception (timbre, involving overtones) appears to be a right-hemisphere ability, whereas basic speech perception is focused in the brain's left hemisphere. Others have suggested that the right hemisphere is especially concerned with emotional aspects of music, whereas the left hemisphere is more concerned with analytic aspects. Reflecting on the evidence for cerebral localization of musical processing at the symposium, Brust quipped, "I probably listen to Tchaikovsky with my right hemisphere, Haydn with my left, and rock with my brain stem."

Diana Deutsch, professor of psychology at the University of California at San Diego, has been a pioneer of music-perception studies and is the discoverer of what is now dubbed the "Deutsch illusion."

Her discovery came about when she used a dichotic listening situation in which subjects were presented simultaneously with single alternating notes an octave apart—the lower note first in the left ear and the higher note first in the right ear. Subjects, however, reported always hearing the high note only in the right ear, alternating with a low note only in the left ear—the Deutsch illusion. Later, however, another investigator showed that although most nonmusicians report the illusion, most musicians do not, suggesting perhaps that musical experience can change the brains of musicians.

Deutsch and her colleagues have extended their analyses to more complex situations. They have found, for example, that the perception of certain patterns of tones—whether melodies are perceived as ascending or descending—not only varies among subjects but also is distinctly affected by shifts in key, a phenomenon that no one had expected and that remains unexplained.

In the past few years, many neuroscientists, using the newer imaging techniques of PET and magnetic resonance imaging (MRI), have begun taking a new look at the brains of people involved in musical tasks and are questioning some of the older views. These studies, proceeding from the premise that music is a unique human attribute—a type of communication system distinct from but possibly on a par with verbal skills—may shed important new light on cerebral topography and a great deal else.

Ravel's musical brain

The inspiration for a very intriguing recent study conducted by neuroscientists at McGill University, Montreal, was the French composer Maurice Ravel. Ravel developed a degenerative brain disease in 1929, and his final years of life were clouded by a mild type of aphasia and to some extent by amusia; he died in 1937 at age 62. His aphasia led to difficulty in finding the correct words to express himself (although he could usually make himself understood, and he was still able to comprehend language satisfactorily). Soon after the disease's onset, he became unable to read or write words but, for a time, he was able to commit his compositions to paper, although words on his scores (to indicate dynamics and tempo) were poorly written and often misspelled.

Part of the tragedy of Ravel's illness was that although he could still listen to and enjoy music, play scales on the piano as before, and perceive pitch, rhythm, tempo, and pace, as well as detect any errors made when his own compositions were played, he could not read a score and then play or sing it himself. In the end, though he could still compose melodies and harmonies in his mind, he could not write them down or play them.

At the Chicago symposium Justine Sergent, director

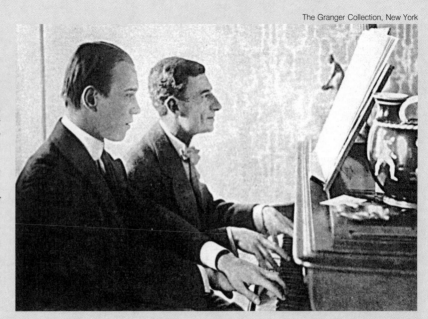

The French composer Maurice Ravel—in his prime in 1912—plays his score for the ballet Daphnis and Chloe *with Russian dancer Nijinsky (seated on his right). Later Ravel developed a degenerative brain disease that left him unable to play the piano, read a musical score, or write down music and also affected his ability to express himself with words. Although much about the composer's illness remains a mystery, it raises intriguing questions about the functional organization of musical functions in the brain— particularly whether musical and verbal abilities derive from the same cerebral structures.*

of the cognitive neuroscience laboratory at the Montreal Neurological Institute and associate professor of neurology and neurosurgery at McGill, reported on the results of brain-imaging studies of 10 highly skilled right-handed pianists made while they were sight-reading and listening to themselves play an unfamiliar piece of music with the right hand on a keyboard.

It was the musical abilities that Ravel lost that Sergent and her colleagues were attempting to assess. They wanted to know what brain areas are involved in the translation of musical notation or ideas into patterns of sounds. They knew musicians rely primarily on spatial information—the notes' position relative to one another on a staff—in order to read and play.

While the 10 subjects were performing their task, PET scans were made of their cerebral blood flow (an indication of brain activity) over the span of one minute. PET scans of brain areas activated during performance of more familiar, "control" tasks (such as playing scales) were also made. Using a sophisticated computer processing method, the researchers were able to "subtract" the latter images from the former and then superimpose the "remaining" PET scans over an MRI scan of each musician's brain. This enabled them to see what brain structures were specifically activated during the experimental task.

What they found was that the sight-reading/playing/ listening task recruited a neural network involving all four of the brain's main lobes (frontal, parietal, occipital, and temporal) in both hemispheres as well as the cerebellum, which is concerned with movement. Sight-reading and listening, without playing, specifically activated certain brain areas, such as the inferior parietal lobules of both hemispheres, leading the researchers to believe that these areas play a key role in the ability to connect notes on a musical score

with their corresponding sounds—a facility that Ravel lost. These areas are next to but separate from those involved in the linking of visual and auditory representations of words.

The results also indicated an important role in the three-part task for the superior parietal lobule, which normally is not activated when subjects play notes they are reading. The researchers believe this portion of the brain may underlie translation of what the eyes see (*e.g.,* a score) to what the fingers play. In other words, that brain region accommodates the processing of spatial information from the score into the brain's motor cortex and then into a motor "program" that directs the patterning, timing, and positioning of fingers on the keyboard.

Sergent and colleagues were surprised by their results, although Sergent herself has always maintained that the brain works as a whole. There is much more, of course, to learn about the complex neuroanatomic aspects of music making. As Sergent wrote in *Science* in 1992, the acts of "sight-reading and playing are only a fraction of musical experience, and we are still far from understanding the pleasure and emotions elicited by music, as well as the composer's mind."

Emotion in music

In fact, other studies done in Sergent's laboratory bear on the emotional side of music and indicate that possibly a component of the brain's limbic system may be activated when a musician listens to music or plays from memory. Other research suggests strongly that the limbic system—comprising a number of structures located deep in the brain, including the amygdala and hippocampus—is active in emotion. In the last several years, it has become evident that emotions are generated by the amygdala, whereas the hippocampus is crucial for forming memories of life events and storing them in the brain. Neurologist Elliott Ross at the University of North Dakota School of Medicine, Fargo, believes, on the basis of recent studies, that the right hemisphere's limbic system is the source of primary emotional content in the performance of music.

Among other relevant studies of the brain using PET scans were those done some years ago by researchers John C. Mazziota and colleagues at the University of California at Los Angeles, involving both musicians and nonmusicians listening to music. In this case glucose metabolism (another indicator of brain activity) rather than cerebral blood flow was measured. On hearing music, the musically unsophisticated subjects—who said they tended to just enjoy listening to music or to "sing along" with it—showed more activity in the right side of their brains, whereas the musicians—some of whom said they visualized the notes they heard on a score or in other ways—showed greater activity in the left hemisphere. According to Ross, this seems reasonable because the written notes, chords, and scales that musicians work with are a form of "language" that symbolically represents music, and symbolic aspects of language processing are ordinarily handled best by the left hemisphere, whereas the nonverbal affective aspects of language are handled by the right hemisphere.

How do musicians play?

How the neuromuscular system controls musical performance and the development of musical skill is another fascinating focus of study. A number of researchers are now studying the role of the basal ganglia deep in the brain with respect to the playing of music and that of the cerebellum in the timing of skilled movements. "The experience of learning music involves, for the nervous system, transforming this eager enthusiastic chorus of somewhat clumsy activity into something more coordinated," neurologist Frank R. Wilson of the University of California at San Francisco told the symposium audience. "But what actually happens in the brain? We don't yet know."

In one study, Wilson statistically analyzed four different performances by a pianist who was connected to a computer that measured motor activity while he was playing the fourth movement of Chopin's *Sonata in B Minor,* a piece with numerous right-hand descending runs. The performances were almost identical. Moreover, there was great similarity between the performances of this pianist and those of another playing the same piece. Wilson theorizes that for the musician practice converts playing into an automatic and unconscious activity.

Music: a language for savants

So-called musical savants are people who generally are mentally retarded but show unusual musical skill. These individuals are most often male; they often have congenital blindness or very poor vision; and most have language delay and difficulty in verbal communication.

A complement to the lectures at the Chicago symposium was a special performance by Tony DeBlois, who at age 18 is blind, mentally retarded, and possibly autistic and is an accomplished pianist. In 1991 DeBlois received the Itzhak Perlman Award from Very Special Arts of the John F. Kennedy Center for the Performing Arts in Washington, D.C. At the conference he played both classical music and jazz (his favorite).

Tony was a premature child with a host of physical problems. Oxygen therapy at birth for treatment of neonatal jaundice led to destruction of his retinas and thus blindness. When he was three years old, his mother noticed that he responded particularly to sounds in his environment. By the time he was of preschool age, he clearly had language difficulties and attention and motor-coordination problems, but these were accompanied by obvious musical abilities. His mother encouraged his musical abilities from an early age, and his involvement in music, despite his severe retardation, seems to have fostered some development of his verbal and social skills. Currently Tony is a special student at Boston's Berklee School of Music.

Leon Miller, associate professor of psychology at the University of Illinois at Chicago, has studied musical savants and is the author of the book *Musical Sa-*

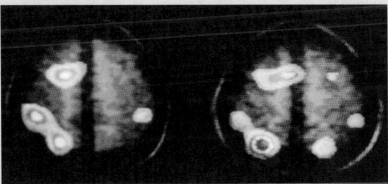

"Averaged" brain images of 10 professional pianists sight-reading and playing a Bach partita show the localized activation of cerebral structures for component operations of the sight-reading task. Lower bright areas reflect the brain's involvement during reading of the score and translation of the notes into finger patterns; uppermost bright areas indicate activation of the frontal cortex, responsible for the organization of the motor movements of playing.

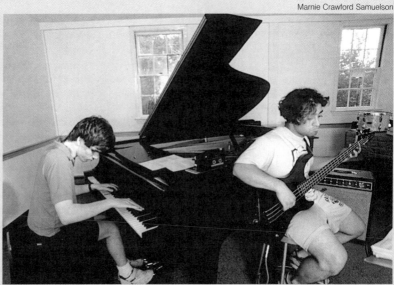

Practicing with a member of his jazz ensemble group, Tony DeBlois plays up a storm at the piano. Tony is blind and mentally retarded but at a very young age demonstrated remarkable musical ability. He has since become an accomplished pianist, playing both classical music and jazz, and is now a student at a Boston music school. Professionals who have studied musical savants like Tony believe that music becomes a "language" that offers them a way of understanding and relating to the world.

vants: *Exceptional Skill and Mental Retardation* (1989). Miller has found that, as in DeBlois' case, the intense musical interest of savants appears very early in life. Among their many unusual traits, he has found, is their remarkable "ear" for new musical material; they can usually play a piece of music with uncommon mastery of melody, harmony, and tonal structure after a single hearing. They also tend to have perfect pitch.

Music may offer savants a method of communicating with the world—one that links them to their families and the rest of their environment. Miller points out that both music and language rely on the auditory system and thus have important similarities. But whereas in most children the language function becomes predominant as they grow up, this does not happen with savants.

Because many musical savants are blind, Miller speculates that normal visual input to the occipital lobe is lacking and, thus, cortical areas typically dedicated to processing this information have nothing to do; there may then be a rededication of these portions of the cortex to other functions. In support of this, Tedd Judd, a neuropsychologist at the Pacific Medical Center in Seattle, Wash., says that in many cases savants have suffered oxygen deprivation during birth, which would preferentially damage the cerebral areas that are actively developing at the time. Moreover, many savants have a pattern of language development that resembles the type of aphasia known as transcortical aphasia, in which the speech centers seem to be isolated from other cortex areas where most semantic connections are made. While this may inhibit the development of some abilities, such as abstract reasoning and linguistic processing, it may allow other functions, such as repetition skills (which many savants possess), acoustic sensitivity, and musical memory to develop quite fully.

Current theories of brain organization hold that specific brain areas are dedicated to certain functions but are connected with each other. Recent experiments with developing primates show that when damage occurs to a specific brain area that is closely connected to another, the neural network is altered in such a way that a "competing" brain area may enlarge, essentially to fill a gap. Thus, as Ross and other neurologists, such as the late Norman Geschwind of Harvard Medical School, have speculated, normally less-prominent intellectual functions could become more prominent—often to an extraordinary degree. This type of functional reorganization could occur in the developing brain of a child, giving rise to the extraordinary skills observed in savants.

Miller suggests that there is a special relationship between music and language early in human development. Before they can understand words, infants use a combined music-language system; they clearly derive emotional information from the "melodic line" of their parents' speech as well as from other sounds in their environment. Furthermore, Miller points out that, as in the case of the savant, "music can emerge as a special way of understanding and relating to the world."

Although broad differences exist between the two cerebral hemispheres, with much of the language function tending to be served by the left, there are many links between the two hemispheres—as seen, for example, in the melodic intonation therapy described above. Increasingly, scientists are finding that some plasticity in the brain may be quite common. Ross and Sergent are among those who believe that the neurology underlying musical and artistic creativity is a very complex one that involves the participation of the whole brain rather than just the right hemisphere, as had been so commonly assumed and accepted.

Contributors to the World of Medicine

Caron Chess
Environmental Health (coauthor)
Director, Center for Environmental Communication, Rutgers, the State University of New Jersey, New Brunswick

James I. Cleeman, M.D.
Special Report Cholesterol Counts (coauthor)
Coordinator, National Cholesterol Education Program, National Heart, Lung, and Blood Institute, National Institutes of Health, Bethesda, Md.

Edward P. Cohen, M.D.
Special Report The Promise of Gene Therapy
Professor, Department of Microbiology and Immunology, University of Illinois College of Medicine, Chicago

Miriam Cohen, Ph.D.
Special Report Mind, Mood, and Medication in Later Life
Psychologist, New York City

Elizabeth B. Connell, M.D.
Women's Health
Professor, Gynecology and Obstetrics, Emory University School of Medicine, Atlanta, Ga.

Francis H.C. Crick, Ph.D.
Special Report Reflections on Solving the DNA Puzzle
Kieckhefer Distinguished Research Professor, Salk Institute for Biological Studies, La Jolla, Calif.

Geoffrey Dean, M.D.
Multiple Sclerosis
Emeritus Director, the Medico-Social Research Board of Ireland, Dublin

Alexander Dorozynski
Special Report France: Fuming over a New Law?
Science Writer and Editor, Recloses, France

Adam Drewnowski, Ph.D.
Diet and Nutrition
Professor of Community Health Programs and Director, Human Nutrition Program, University of Michigan School of Public Health, Ann Arbor

Howard Frumkin, M.D., Dr.P.H.
Occupational Health
Director and Associate Professor, Division of Environmental and Occupational Health, Emory University School of Public Health, Atlanta, Ga.

George A. Gellert, M.D., M.P.H., M.P.A.
Special Report Health Care Reform in Eurasia: The Next Revolution
State Epidemiologist and Assistant Director, Disease Prevention Services, Arizona Department of Health Services, Phoenix

Ray W. Gifford, Jr., M.D.
Hypertension (coauthor)
Senior Physician, Department of Nephrology and Hypertension, and Senior Vice-Chairman, Division of Medicine, the Cleveland Clinic Foundation, Cleveland, Ohio; Chairman, Joint National Committee on the Detection, Evaluation, and Treatment of High Blood Pressure

Leonard H. Glantz, J.D.
Special Report Suing Tobacco Companies: Impact of a Landmark Case
Professor of Health Law, Boston University School of Medicine/School of Public Health

Robert A. Goepp, D.D.S., Ph.D.
Special Report Dental Implants: On the Cutting Edge
Professor, Departments of Pathology and Surgery, University of Chicago

Philip M. Hanno, M.D.
Men's Health
Professor and Chairman, Department of Urology, Temple University School of Medicine, Philadelphia

Donald R. Hopkins, M.D., M.P.H.
Disease Eradication
Senior Consultant, Global 2000, Carter Center, Atlanta, Ga.

C. William Keck, M.D., M.P.H.
Special Report Health for All: A Dream Realized in Cuba
Director, Akron Health Department, Akron, Ohio; Director, Division of Community Health Sciences, Northeastern Ohio Universities College of Medicine, Rootstown; Past President, American Public Health Association

Louis A. LaMarca
Pharmaceuticals (coauthor)
Capitol Hill Editor, *F-D-C Reports: "The Pink Sheet,"* and Senior Editor, *Weekly Pharmacy Reports: "The Green Sheet,"* F-D-C Reports, Inc., Chevy Chase, Md.

Joyce C. Lashof, M.D.
Special Report Public Health in the U.S.—Not Making the Grade
Dean Emerita and Professor of Public Health, University of California at Berkeley School of Public Health; Past President, American Public Health Association

Claude Lenfant, M.D.
Hypertension (coauthor); *Special Report Cholesterol Counts* (coauthor)
Director, National Heart, Lung, and Blood Institute, National Institutes of Health, Bethesda, Md.

Tammy Leopold
Pharmaceuticals (coauthor)
Managing Editor, *"The Blue Sheet,"* F-D-C Reports, Inc., Chevy Chase, Md.

Stephen Lock, M.D.
Special Report John Snow Gets His Monument: London's Tribute to a Medical Pioneer
Research Associate, Section of History of 20th Century Medicine, Wellcome Institute for the History of Medicine, London; Editor Emeritus, *British Medical Journal*

Wendy K. Mariner, J.D., LL.M., M.P.H.
Health Care Law
Associate Professor of Health Law, Boston University School of Medicine/School of Public Health

405

Gail McBride
Special Report Music and the Mind: Scientific Musings
Freelance Medical Writer and Editor, Chicago

Charles-Gene McDaniel, M.S.J.
AIDS
Professor and Chair, Department of Journalism, Roosevelt
University, Chicago

Beverly Merz
Genetics
Editor, *Harvard Women's Health Watch,* Boston

Ralph W. Moss, Ph.D.
Alternative Medicine
Cochairman, Panel on Pharmacological and Biological Treat-
ments, and Member of the Ad Hoc Advisory Board, Office of
Alternative Medicine, National Institutes of Health, Bethesda,
Md.; Author, *Cancer Therapy: The Independent Consumer's
Guide to Non-Toxic Treatment & Prevention* (1992)

Thomas H. Murray, Ph.D.
Medical Ethics
Professor and Director, Center for Biomedical Ethics, Case
Western Reserve University School of Medicine, Cleveland,
Ohio; Editor, *Medical Humanities Review*

David B. Reuben, M.D.
Aging
Associate Professor of Medicine and Interim Director, Multi-
campus Program in Geriatric Medicine and Gerontology,
University of California at Los Angeles School of Medicine

Edward J. Roccella, Ph.D., M.P.H.
Hypertension (coauthor)
Coordinator, National High Blood Pressure Education Pro-
gram, National Heart, Lung, and Blood Institute, National
Institutes of Health, Bethesda, Md.

Mukti H. Sarma, Ph.D.
Cancer
Adjunct Professor of Chemistry, State University of New York
at Albany; Editor, *Cancer Watch,* Schenectady, N.Y.

Patricia T. Schloesser, M.D.
Child Care
Clinical Associate Professor, Department of Pediatrics, Uni-
versity of Kansas School of Medicine, Topeka

Richard Stone
Infectious Disease
Staff Reporter, *Science,* Washington, D.C.

Daniel Wartenberg, Ph.D.
Environmental Health (coauthor)
Associate Professor, Department of Environmental and Com-
munity Medicine, University of Medicine and Dentistry of
New Jersey—Robert Wood Johnson Medical School and the
Environmental and Occupational Health Sciences Institute,
Piscataway, N.J.

David G. Whiteis, Ph.D.
Health Policy
Assistant Professor of Public and Environmental Affairs
(Health Policy), School of Public and Environmental Affairs,
Indiana University at Fort Wayne

Richard E. Wokutch, Ph.D.
Special Report Work: Dying for It in Japan
Professor of Management, the R.B. Pamplin College of
Business, Virginia Polytechnic Institute and State Univer-
sity, Blacksburg

What's Your Nutrition IQ?

The editor and senior editor of the *Medical and Health Annual* are always "hungry" for nutritional edification and so eagerly await their issues of *Nutrition Action Healthletter*—a perpetual source of sound and enlightening information. When they received the October 1992 issue, with its "Food Facts" quiz, they learned just how much they did *not* know. Both editors (who had considered themselves more or less nutritionally in-the-know) were, to their chagrin, stumped by many of the questions. Their respective scores were 19 and 21 (of a possible 42), which ranked them at the high end of "not too shabby"—and a long way from being "nutrition whizzes."

Because the editors were so challenged by the quiz, they felt the *Annual*'s readers would be too. The quiz, along with our detailed answer section, appears on the following pages. So, turn the page and good luck!

—The Editors

Questions

1. *About how many teaspoons of sugar (or corn syrup) are there in a 12-oz can of cola?*

   a. 5   b. 7   c. 10   d. 13

2. *A cup of whole milk has eight grams of fat. How many grams of fat does a cup of 2% "low-fat" milk have?*

   a. 2   b. 3   c. 4   d. 5

3. *Which of these cereals has less than 25% added sugar?*

   a. Honey Nut Cheerios   c. Bran Buds
   b. Frosted Flakes   d. Life

4. *Which of these cereals is low in fiber?*

   a. Wheatena   c. oatmeal
   b. Cream of Wheat   d. oat bran

5. *Which of these cereals is not low in fiber?*

   a. shredded wheat   d. granola
   b. Rice Krispies   e. all of the above
   c. corn flakes

6. *Which of these fruit juices is a source of vitamin C (assuming none has been fortified)?*

   a. grape   c. prune
   b. apple   d. pineapple

7. *Which of these fruits is low in beta-carotene?*

   a. nectarine   d. cantaloupe
   b. papaya   e. tangerine
   c. grapes

8. *Which of these fruits is low in potassium?*

   a. banana   d. watermelon
   b. grapefruit   e. honeydew
   c. cantaloupe

9. *About how many teaspoons of added sugar are there in one cup of fruit yogurt?*

   a. 1   b. 2   c. 3   d. 5   e. 6

10. *Which of these is not a whole grain?*

    a. bulgur   d. grits
    b. millet   e. oatmeal
    c. popcorn

11. *Which of these is rich in complex carbohydrates?*

    a. pretzels   d. rye crackers
    b. pasta   e. all of the above
    c. biscuits

12. *Which of these is lowest in beta-carotene?*

    a. zucchini   d. brussels sprouts
    b. broccoli   e. winter squash
    c. kale

13. *Which of these cookies usually has the least fat?*

    a. chocolate chip   c. sandwich
    b. peanut butter   d. oatmeal

14. *If you eat 2,000 calories a day, your daily saturated fat intake should be less than how many grams?*

    a. 20   b. 25   c. 30   d. 35

15. *How many grams of saturated fat are there in two slices of a Pizza Hut medium hand-tossed cheese pizza?*

    a. 8   b. 12   c. 14   d. 18

16. *Which of these meats has the least fat?*

    a. extra-lean ground beef
    b. ground turkey
    c. ground turkey breast
    d. ground chicken

17. *Which skinless chicken or turkey part has the most fat (assuming that the serving sizes are equal)?*

    a. breast   c. wing
    b. thigh   d. drumstick

18. *Which has the least cholesterol?*

    a. skinless chicken breast
    b. skinless turkey breast
    c. trimmed top round steak
    d. flounder
    e. all have about the same

19. *Which has the least saturated fat?*

    a. flounder
    b. skinless chicken drumstick
    c. trimmed veal loin
    d. trimmed top round steak

20. *Which has more than two grams of saturated fat in a four-ounce cooked serving?*

    a. skinless chicken breast
    b. skinless turkey wing
    c. trimmed beef top round (select grade)
    d. trimmed beef bottom round (select grade)
    e. pork tenderloin

21. *Which has less than 500 mg of sodium per serving?*

    a. Campbell's Healthy Request vegetable soup
    b. Dorito Thins
    c. turkey roll
    d. V8 juice
    e. Lean Cuisine Zucchini Lasagna

22. *Which has more than 150 mg of cholesterol in a four-ounce serving?*

    a. shrimp   d. lobster
    b. scallops   e. crab
    c. clams

23. *True or false? Children aged two to five years should not drink 1% low-fat or skim milk.*

24. *Which of these vegetables is not a source of calcium?*

    a. kale   d. collards
    b. broccoli   e. bok choy
    c. green beans

25. *Which is low in folic acid?*

    a. leafy greens   d. finfish
    b. orange juice   e. beans
    c. wheat germ

26. *Which of these foods from McDonald's has the fewest calories?*

    a. large french fries
    b. Quarter Pounder
    c. chicken salad with blue cheese dressing
    d. biscuit with sausage
    e. all have about the same

27. *True or false? Most people need the iodine in iodized salt.*

28. *True or false? Most Americans get more than enough phosphorus in their diets.*

29. *Which is not a source of vitamin E?*

    a. wheat germ   c. leafy green vegetables
    b. nuts   d. vegetable oils

30. *Which of these sandwiches has the most saturated fat?*

    a. Swiss cheese   d. sliced turkey breast
    b. tuna salad   e. peanut butter and jelly
    c. chicken salad

31. *True or false? Vegetarians often get too little protein.*

32. *Which has less than 300 mg of calcium per serving?*

    a. yogurt   d. cheddar cheese
    b. cottage cheese   e. none of the above
    c. skim milk

33. *Which of these vegetables is a source of vitamins A and C?*

    a. mushrooms   d. cucumber
    b. green peas   e. celery
    c. eggplant

34. *Which is not a source of zinc?*

    a. wheat germ   d. broccoli
    b. sirloin steak   e. lentils
    c. turkey

35. *Which breakfast item has the least fat?*

    a. bagel with cream cheese
    b. danish
    c. English muffin with jam
    d. doughnut
    e. all have about the same

36. *True or false? A 12-oz wine cooler has more alcohol than a 12-oz beer.*

37. *Which is not a good source of iron?*

    a. clams
    b. black beans
    c. round steak
    d. raisins

38. *Which bread typically contains the most fiber?*

    a. raisin
    b. rye
    c. pumpernickel
    d. oatmeal
    e. all have about the same

39. *An ounce of whole-milk mozzarella has six grams of fat. How many grams of fat does an ounce of part-skim mozzarella have?*

    a. 2   b. 3   c. 4   d. 5

40. *Which of these has less than 1,000 mg of sodium per serving?*

    a. Stouffer's Beef Pie
    b. Pizza Hut Supreme Pizza
    c. Campbell's Pork & Beans
    d. Burger King Whopper with cheese
    e. Taco Bell Bean Burrito with red sauce

41. *Which of these is low in fiber?*

    a. artichoke
    b. green pepper
    c. strawberries
    d. sweet potato (no skin)

42. *True or False? It would be nice if at least the last question on this quiz were easy!*

"Food Facts" quiz from Nutrition Action Healthletter, *October 1992, adapted with permission from the publisher, the Washington D.C.-based Center for Science in the Public Interest, a nonprofit organization that advocates improved health and nutrition policies.*

Answers

1. c. There are 10 tsp of sugar in the average 12-oz can of cola. This adds up to 160 "empty" calories that squeeze out more nutritious foods in the diet and promote tooth decay. Diet sodas, which replace the sugar with artificial sweeteners such as aspartame or saccharin, have one calorie per serving, but none of the artificial sweeteners has been shown to be perfectly safe.

2. d. The government says that a low-fat food can contain no more than three grams of fat per serving. Because of a loophole, however, 2% milk, with five grams of fat per cup, can call itself "low-fat" even though it is not. One-percent milk, on the other hand, is truly low-fat, with less than three grams of fat per cup. Buttermilk has two grams of fat per cup, and skim milk has almost none.

3. d. Life cereal contains 21% sugar, Bran Buds 29%, Honey Nut Cheerios 36%, and Frosted Flakes 39%. Many cereal makers add large amounts of unwanted sugar in the form of cane sugar, corn syrup, honey, brown sugar, and molasses. Sugar is listed under "Total Carbohydrate" on the food label. Recommended cereals would be those with no more than five grams of sugar in a one-ounce serving.

4. b. White-flour Cream of Wheat is low in fiber (one gram in a one-ounce serving). Wheatena and oatmeal (three grams per ounce) and oat bran (four grams per ounce) are low-fat fiber sources and help put a dent in the 20–35 g of fiber that the National Cancer Institute says people should eat every day from a variety of grains, fruits, vegetables, and beans. (The average American eats only 11 g of fiber a day.) Insoluble fiber (*e.g.,* wheat bran) helps prevent constipation and diverticulosis and may protect against cancer. Soluble fiber (*e.g.,* oat bran) may help lower blood cholesterol.

5. a. Whole grain cereals—such as shredded wheat, Wheaties, or Grape-Nuts—generally have at least three grams of fiber per serving. Many popular ready-to-eat cereals are made from refined flour and have little fiber (one gram of fiber per ounce or less). That includes Rice Krispies, granola, and corn flakes.

6. d. Vitamin C (ascorbic acid), a water-soluble vitamin, is an antioxidant. It is essential for healthy bones and blood vessels and aids in the absorption of iron. Most people know orange and grapefruit juices are good vitamin C sources, with 97 and 83 mg, respectively, in eight ounces. They may not know pineapple juice (27 mg in eight ounces) is also a good choice. Prune juice has just 11 mg, while eight ounces of apple juice have only two milligrams, and grape juice contains no vitamin C at all. The Recommended Dietary Allowance (RDA; established by the Food and Nutrition Board of the National Academy of Sciences, National Research Council) for vitamin C is 60 mg a day for a healthy adult. Children need somewhat less, but pregnant women need about 70 mg, and women who are breast-feeding need 90 mg or more.

7. c. Beta-carotene is found in plant foods, mainly dark green and deep yellow vegetables and fruits. Some studies strongly suggest that beta-carotene helps prevent certain cancers. Other research is under way to determine if beta-carotene in amounts of 25,000 to 50,000 IU (international units) reduces the risk of heart disease or cataracts. In the body beta-carotene is converted into vitamin A (retinol), an essential fat-soluble vitamin that aids in the prevention of night blindness and promotes healthy hair, teeth, gums, bones, skin, and mucous membranes. The U.S. Recommended Daily Allowance (U.S. RDA) for vitamin A is 5,000 IU. Canteloupe is a good source of beta-carotene (8,610 IU in half a melon), as are nectarines (1,000 IU each), tangerines (770 IU), and papaya (2,820 IU per cup). Apricots are also high (three have 2,770 IU; a cup of dried apricots has 9,410 IU). A high beta-carotene intake can cause the skin to turn orangish.

8. b. Bananas are a good source of potassium, with 450 mg in a single medium-size banana. Melons are another good source; canteloupe has 413 mg in ¼ melon, watermelon has 560 mg per slice, and honeydew has 350 mg per slice. Half a grapefruit has 167 mg. Potassium, along with sodium and chloride, are electrolytes that together regulate the balance of water and dissolved substances

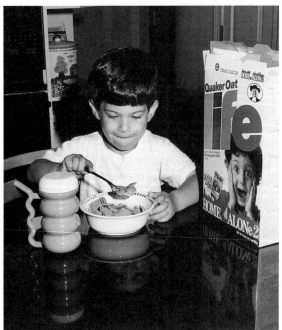

Karen Wollins

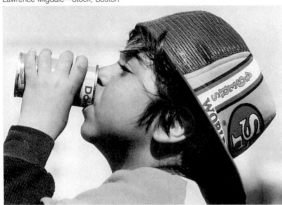

Lawrence Migdale—Stock, Boston

in the body's cells. Diuretic drugs can deplete the body of potassium—the mineral is lost in the urine—so patients who take them may need supplemental potassium in addition to potassium-rich foods.

9. e. The problem with most fruited yogurts is their added sugar, corn sweetener, or fruit-juice concentrate. Fruit-blended and fruit-on-the-bottom yogurts have about six teaspoons of sugar per eight-ounce serving. Flavored yogurts (vanilla, lemon, or coffee) typically have a third less sugar than the other two varieties. Calorie-conscious consumers should go for plain low-fat or nonfat yogurt and add fresh fruit.

10. d. Whole grains have not had their protective outer layer (bran) and central germ removed. The bran and germ are sources of fiber, vitamins (B vitamins, E, folic and pantothenic acids), and minerals (chromium, copper, iron, magnesium, manganese, and zinc). Refined grains, with the bran and germ removed, are low in fiber and nutrients—even when "enriched" (a few B vitamins and iron added back). Oatmeal, bulgur, popcorn, and millet are whole grains, while grits are made from refined corn.

11. e. All grains are rich in complex carbohydrates (starch and fiber). Starch is called a complex carbohydrate because it consists of a long chain of sugars. Both short-chain and single sugars are called simple carbohydrates (or just sugar). Grains can be either whole or refined. Brown rice is the entire grain. White rice is refined—that is, its outer layer has been removed. The same holds true for wheat. Whole wheat flour—the key ingredient in whole wheat breads, pastas, and crackers—is made from the entire wheat kernel. White flour is refined—the bran and germ have been removed. Whole grains contain more fiber, vitamins, and minerals. But even refined complex carbohydrates (such as many pastas and white rice) are good for you because most of the alternatives—foods with fat and saturated fat—are worse. Diets high in fat increase the risk of heart disease or cancer.

12. a. Zucchini is very low in beta-carotene, with the equivalent of 216 IU in a ½ cup. The beta-carotene in cooked broccoli is 1,100 IU per ½ cup. Other good cooked vegetable sources include kale (4,810 IU), and brussels sprouts (561 IU), and winter squash—ranging from 86 IU in spaghetti squash to 7,140 IU in butternut squash. Carrots are especially high in beta-carotene (20,250 IU in a medium-sized raw carrot).

13. d. Cookies, even the fat-free ones, are high in sugar and low in nutrients and far from being a health food. Still, some will not do as much damage as others.

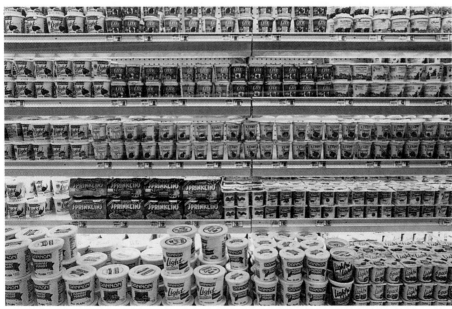

Karen Wollins

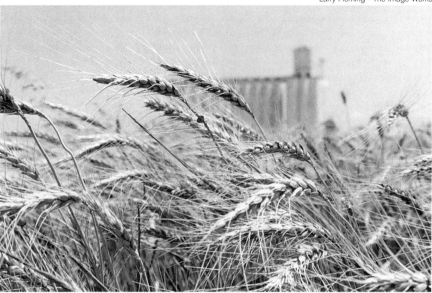

Peanut butter cookies are the fattiest, averaging three teaspoons of fat in a one-ounce serving. Chocolate chip cookies have about half that much fat, while sandwich cookies are slightly less fatty than chocolate chips. On average, oatmeal cookies are the lowest in fat, averaging less than a teaspoon of fat per one-ounce serving.

14. a. Health authorities recommend that to cut the risk of heart disease, people get less than 10% of their calories from saturated fat—about 20 g a day for a 2,000-calorie diet. A more ideal diet gets 7–8% of calories from saturated fat (15 g). To cut back on saturated fat, eat less meat and dairy products (the largest sources of saturated fat in most Americans' diets).

15. c. Pizza is usually high in saturated fat, supplying half a day's worth in just two slices. To reduce the saturated fat, order pizza with "half the cheese" and skip the fatty meats such as pepperoni, sausage, and ground beef. Or, better yet, make your own pizza at home with low-fat cheese and top it with vitamin-rich vegetables such as spinach or broccoli.

16. c. Ground beef, even when labeled "extra lean," is high in fat, averaging over four teaspoons of grease in a four-ounce broiled patty. Ground turkey or chicken averages about 20% less fat but is still fatty. Ground turkey breast is the lowest-fat choice, averaging less than one teaspoon of fat in four ounces.

17. b. Not all poultry is low in fat. The breasts are lowest, averaging one teaspoon per four-ounce skinless chicken breast. Drumsticks have one and one-half times more fat. Wings have twice as much fat as the breast. And thighs, which are the fattiest, have three times more fat than the breast.

18. e. Poultry, meat, and fish all contain about 75 to 100 mg of cholesterol in a four-ounce cooked serving. (Health authorities recommend no more than 300 mg per day—ideally no more than 250 mg.) The amount of saturated fat that these foods contain, however, varies widely. On average, fish contains the least amount of saturated fat, while red meat contains the most.

19. a. Many fish (except fatty fish such as mackerel or herring) are low in saturated fat, averaging one gram or less per four-ounce serving. Examples are flounder, trout, sole, snapper, haddock, and scallops. Skinless chicken drumsticks and well-trimmed top round steak have twice that amount in a four-ounce serving. Trimmed veal loin has three times as much.

20. d. A four-ounce serving of beef bottom round has slightly more than two grams of saturated fat. The others all have less than two grams.

21. b. While most people expect salty-tasting snack foods such as potato, corn, or tortilla chips to be high in sodium, a one-ounce serving of Dorito Thins has only 135 mg. Healthy Request Soup, processed turkey roll, and Lean Cuisine Zucchini Lasagna have four times that amount; V8 juice has five times more. The average person gets three-fourths of his or her sodium from processed foods (*e.g.,* luncheon meats, hot dogs, ham, cheese, soups) and one-fourth from the salt shaker. The National Academy of Sciences recommends no more than 2,400 mg of sodium per day and ideally no more than 1,800 mg.

22. a. Not all shellfish are high in cholesterol. Most average between 60 and 120 mg in a four-ounce serving—as much as or less than chicken or turkey. Shrimp, how-

412

ever, is loaded with cholesterol. A four-ounce serving of cooked shrimp contains 218 mg, more than two-thirds the daily maximum.

23. False. Children under the age of two should not be on low-fat diets. They need whole milk, and their fat and calorie intake should not be restricted. Because infants are growing so fast, they require three to four times more calories per pound of body weight than adults. But their stomachs are small, so they need to get many calories in the little they eat. Fat has the most calories. After two years of age, children should be switched to 1% low-fat or skim milk.

24. c. Calcium is one of the most important minerals in the diet. It builds strong bones and teeth, promotes proper muscle and nerve function, and aids in blood clotting. There is evidence that women who do not get enough calcium when they are young are more prone to osteoporosis (a progressive loss of bone mass) in later years. The RDA for children aged 1–10 and adults aged 25 years and older is 800 mg, while those aged 11–24 and pregnant or lactating women need 1,200 mg. The easiest way to get calcium is from milk and other dairy products (a cup of milk has about 300 mg). Some nondairy sources of calcium include one cup of cooked kale (90–180 mg) or broccoli (72 mg) or three ounces of canned salmon with bones (203 mg).

25. d. Folic acid (folacin or folate), a B-complex vitamin, can prevent spina bifida and other devastating birth defects that occur when the neural tube (which becomes the spinal cord and brain) fails to close in the developing embryo. The trouble is that the defect occurs before a woman knows she is pregnant, so by the time her obstetrician prescribes folic acid supplements to meet the increased needs, it is too late. Therefore,

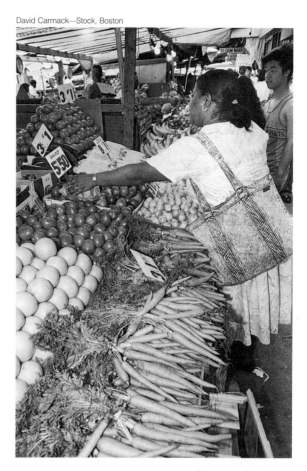

it is recommended that any woman who might become pregnant take a daily 400-µg (microgram) supplement; this should be increased to 800 µg when she becomes pregnant. Foods rich in folic acid include leafy green vegetables such as spinach (131 µg in a ½-cup cooked serving), chicken livers (655 µg in three ounces), brewers

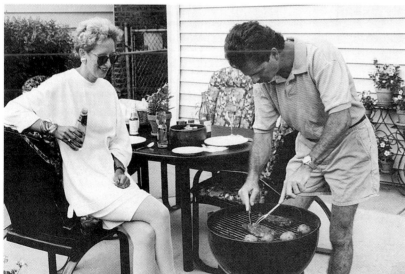

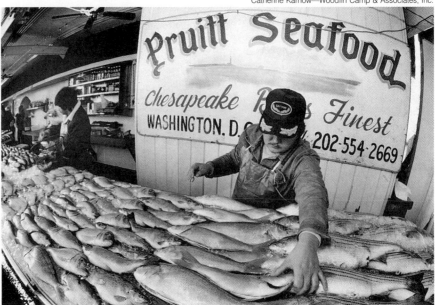

yeast (313 μg per tbs), orange juice (109 μg in an eight-ounce glass), wheat germ (100 μg per ¼-cup serving), and dried beans, notably lentils (358 μg per cup) and black beans (256 μg per cup). Folic acid is easily destroyed in cooking and is more readily obtained in raw fruits and vegetables.

26. e. All of these popular McDonald's fast-food items have about 400 calories. Depending on what dressing is chosen, a low-calorie, low-fat chicken salad can be one of the best or worst alternatives to a fatty Quarter Pounder or greasy fries. For example, a packet of Lite Vinaigrette adds 50 calories and ½ tsp of fat to the salad, while a packet of Blue Cheese dressing adds 250 calories and 4½ tsp of fat.

27. False. While iodine deficiency used to be a problem, today most Americans get too much iodine in their diets. Iodine is essential for maintaining a healthy thyroid gland and for normal metabolism of the body's cells. Iodine deficiency causes goiter, an enlargement of the thyroid gland resulting in a prominent swelling at the front of the neck. Before the 1920s, when iodine was first added to salt, goiter was a problem in the Midwest, where the soil is low in iodine. Today most Americans should not use iodized salt because they get enough iodine from seafood, processed foods containing iodized salt, and dairy products processed in facilities that use iodine to disinfect equipment.

28. True. Phosphorous is an essential mineral that combines with calcium to promote strong bones and teeth. Red meats, beans, nuts, and whole grains are all good sources of phosphorous, and most Americans consume far more than the 1,000-mg U.S. RDA.

29. c. Vitamin E comprises a group of fat-soluble compounds known as tocopherols—the most common form being alpha-tocopherol. Vitamins E, A, and C are antioxidants—nutrients that block oxidation in the body's cells and may help prevent some forms of cancer. Recent studies have shown a possible decrease in the incidence of heart disease with the use of supplements containing 100 IU of vitamin E. Vitamin E is commonly found in foods rich in polyunsaturated fats, particularly nuts (*e.g.*, almonds, with 2 IU per oz), wheat germ (4 IU per oz), vegetable oil (sunflower oil has 6 IU per tbs), and margarine (1–8 IU per tbs).

30. a. Cheese is high in artery-clogging saturated fat; in fact, the average deli Swiss cheese sandwich contains an entire day's allotment. Peanut butter, chicken salad, or tuna salad sandwiches (although high in total fat) have about 80% less saturated fat. To limit all fat, stick to sliced turkey breast without the "mayo."

31. False. Many Americans get at least 50% more protein than the RDA, and young children get over three times the RDA. Protein is not found only in meat and milk. Bread, rolls, and crackers constitute the third largest source of protein in the average American diet. Vegetarians who eat dairy products and eggs need not worry about mixing complementary proteins. The proteins in milk and eggs have a complete array of the amino acids that the body cannot produce. Even strict vegetarians who avoid milk and eggs can get enough protein by combining legumes and whole grain products that are rich in complementary amino acids. Typical high-protein vegetarian meals include red beans and rice, baked beans and brown bread, hummus (a chickpea dip) with pita bread, and corn tortillas with refried

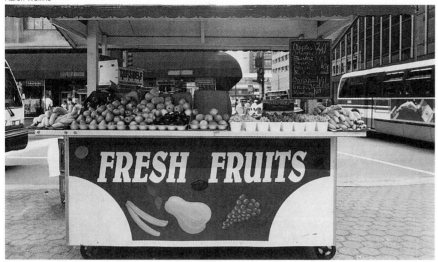

beans. Tofu, made from soybeans, has nine grams of protein per serving and can be used in many recipes in place of meat.

32. b. Not all dairy products are created equal. Cottage cheese has only 68 mg of calcium in a four-ounce serving (7% of the U.S. RDA). A one-cup serving of plain low-fat yogurt has 415 mg (50% of the U.S. RDA). An eight-ounce glass of skim milk has 302 mg (30% of the U.S. RDA), and a one-ounce portion of cheddar cheese has 200 mg (20% of the U.S. RDA).

33. b. Mushrooms, eggplant, cucumbers, and celery have less than 10% of the U.S. RDA for vitamin A or C per half cup. Peas, on the other hand, are an excellent source of both. A half cup of cooked peas contains 8 mg (13% of the U.S. RDA) of vitamin C and 534 IU of vitamin A. Cooking, canning, and freezing deplete the vitamin C in peas somewhat (as in all fruits and vegetables), but the vitamin A remains high.

34. d. Zinc is a trace element that is essential for proper growth. Zinc is particularly prevalent in seafood (cooked eastern oysters contain 204 mg per four-ounce serving), sirloin steak (7 mg per four-ounce serving), and wheat germ (4.7 mg per ¼-cup serving). Zinc is available to a lesser extent in chicken (1.1 mg per serving), turkey (1.9 mg per serving), and dried beans such as lentils (2.5 mg per cup) but is almost nonexistent in green vegetables (broccoli, for example, has 0.3 mg in a half cup).

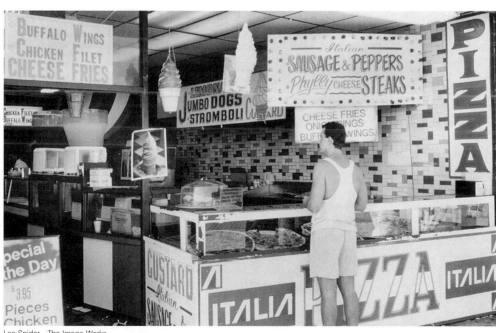

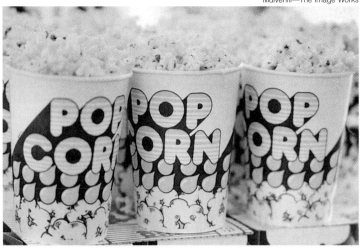

35. c. Although bagels and English muffins are both low in fat, a two-tablespoon smear of cream cheese adds over two teaspoons of fat. Fat-free jams and jellies are a much better choice, whether spread on an English muffin or on a bagel. Doughnuts and danish are fatty, averaging three or more teaspoons of fat each.

36. True. Wine coolers have slightly more alcohol (6%) than regular beer (4%). Table wines, on the other hand, have about 10–14% alcohol.

37. d. Iron is an essential part of hemoglobin, which carries oxygen in the red blood cells. Iron-deficiency anemia can be a serious problem for young children or for women who are pregnant or who menstruate heavily. The U.S. RDA for iron is 18 mg. Pregnant women generally cannot meet their iron needs by diet alone and therefore usually receive supplemental iron of up to 60 mg per day. Good sources of iron are cooked clams (31 mg in a four-ounce serving), black beans (4 mg per cup), and round steak (3 mg in four ounces). Raisins are a very poor source of iron, with only 0.8 mg in ¼ cup. While liver is rich in iron, its high cholesterol count makes it a poor choice. Iron-deficiency anemia is no more common among vegetarians than nonvegetarians because vegetarians get adequate amounts from beans, nuts, and fortified grain products and because the less iron one eats, the more efficiently the body absorbs it. Eating iron-rich foods with vitamin C-rich foods also increases the absorption of iron.

38. e. Just because a bread is labeled "multigrain," "stone-ground," "wheat," "rye," "pumpernickel," or "oatmeal," that does not mean it is made with much whole grain flour and is rich in fiber. Consumers should read the label and make sure the bread they buy lists whole wheat flour as the first ingredient.

39. d. Part-skim mozzarella cheese sounds much lower in fat than it really is. It averages five grams of fat per ounce, about the same as the whole-milk version.

40. c. A one-cup serving of Campbell's Pork & Beans has 740 mg of sodium, compared with a Stouffer's Beef Pie (1,130 mg), two slices of Pizza Hut Supreme Pizza (1,363 mg), a Burger King Whopper with cheese (1,177 mg), and a Taco Bell Bean Burrito with red sauce (1,148 mg)—each of the latter having about half a day's allowance of sodium.

41. b. Sweet bell (green) peppers contain almost no fiber (one gram in half a pepper). Half a cooked artichoke or a cup of strawberries has three grams of fiber. An average sweet potato (even without the skin) has three grams. Other good fiber sources include bananas (three grams), apples (four grams), pears (four grams), popcorn (four grams in a three-cup serving), and kidney beans (six grams in a half cup).

42. True!

Scoring

0–10 What happened? Give yourself a lifetime subscription to *Nutrition Action Healthletter.*

11–21 Not too shabby. But forget that appearance on "Jeopardy."

22–32 Pretty darned good. Consider yourself a "source" of nutrition knowledge.

33–42 You're a nutrition whiz! Ask your friends to take the quiz so you can gloat.

Answers prepared by Melinda C. Shepherd, Associate Editor, Encyclopædia Britannica Yearbooks, with assistance from Jayne Hurley, R.D., Associate Nutritionist, Nutrition Action Healthletter.

HEALTHWISE

sound information about matters of health

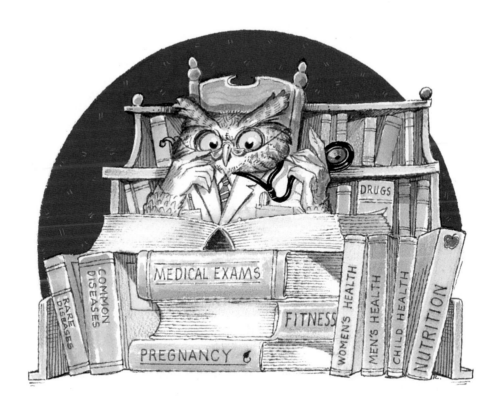

Fruits, Vegetables, and Health

by Gladys Block, Ph.D.

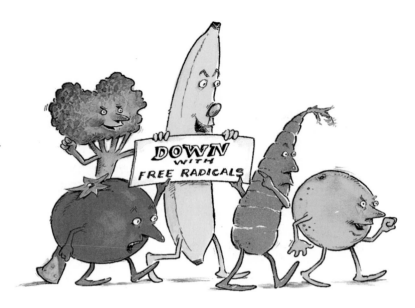

Mothers have been telling children for generations, perhaps millennia, to "eat your vegetables." Too many people have ignored that advice. Now, though, there is a wealth of scientific evidence that mother was right—that vegetables (and fruits) not only are important components of a well-balanced diet but are actually associated with better health and a lower risk of major disease.

The evidence for such benefits comes both from epidemiological studies and from laboratory studies. Epidemiologists typically study the dietary causes of disease by comparing the food consumption patterns of people who do develop a particular disease (such as cancer) with the dietary intake of people who do not develop that disease. For example, they might ask: Are persons with a low fruit intake more likely to develop cancer in subsequent years than are people who eat a great deal of fruit? Or they might look at people who have cancer to see if they were more likely to have had a low vegetable intake in prior years than people who are now cancer-free. "Prospective" and "retrospective" studies such as these are done with very large numbers of persons and can take into account other risk factors, such as smoking, which might also be related to the development of the disease in question.

While epidemiologists attempt to determine the effect on health of specific foods or components of food, laboratory scientists approach the question of what causes a disease such as cancer from a different angle—through the investigation of precise mechanisms occurring at the cellular level. Today epidemiological research and laboratory research are converging as a result of recent scientific insights into the importance of so-called free radicals and the "oxidative" damage they cause—specifically the role that such damage plays in causing many diseases—and, indeed, in the process of aging itself.

What are free radicals?

In Earth's environment oxygen is both essential for most life and a source of damage to biological systems. While metabolism converts most oxygen into stable molecules such as water and carbon dioxide, some small amount inevitably escapes and is converted into a highly reactive form called a free radical. A free radical is a molecule that has an unpaired electron. Such a molecule is extremely unstable and seeks to stabilize itself by grabbing an electron from another molecule. This attack can be directed at many different molecules, including DNA (the basic genetic material), proteins, carbohydrates, and lipids (fats such as cholesterol).

In the human body a free radical attack on DNA can cause damage to the cell's genetic instructions, leading to a loss of cell function, uncontrolled cell growth, mutation (a relatively permanent change in the cell's genes), and even cancer. When free radicals attack proteins, cell damage and decreased enzyme activity result. Enzymes are made up of proteins, and they drive the body's biochemical processes. Carbohydrate damage by free radicals can alter cell receptors so that the cell cannot "receive" biochemical and hormonal messages; carbohydrate damage also breaks down, or depolymerizes, the intercellular "glue"—the substances between the cells such as hyaluronic acid and collagen—that provides structure and allows cell-to-cell communication. Free radical attacks on lipids can damage cell membranes, alter crucial lipids such as low-density lipoprotein (LDL) cholesterol, and cause self-propagating chain reactions that keep generating more free radicals.

Sources of free radicals are ubiquitous in the environment as well as within people's bodies. Oxygen itself is one source, as was noted above. Cigarette smoke is undoubtedly the chief external free radical source to which most people are exposed; cigarette

418

smoke contains not only large numbers of free radicals but other toxic substances as well. Still other external free radical sources are alcohol and air pollutants such as ozone and nitrogen dioxide. Even aerobic exercise contributes to the body's free radical burden.

Surprisingly, however, unless one is a cigarette smoker, the majority of oxidative damage a person is subjected to probably comes not from external but from internal sources. Normal—indeed essential—bodily biochemical reactions produce highly reactive, oxygen-containing radicals. Certain enzyme systems and electron-transport systems are vital and continuous sources of these oxidants. Moreover, specific white blood cells known as neutrophils perform part of their infection-fighting function by releasing a burst of free radicals.

Antioxidants: the body's defense

Organisms on Earth have developed a host of biological mechanisms, including an array of enzyme systems, to block, or protect against, free radicals and to repair damage once it has occurred. In addition to these protective enzyme systems, most animals (but not humans) also synthesize their own supply of antioxidants, such as vitamin C. Humans, on the other hand, must depend on an adequate dietary intake of foods that provide antioxidants and other nutrients involved in DNA synthesis and repair.

Fruits and vegetables are foods that provide not only vitamin C but a host of carotenoids, the best known of which is beta-carotene; folic acid; vitamin E; and numerous other, less well-investigated factors, all known or suspected to be involved in the prevention and repair of oxidative damage. At present, scientists are unsure of the relative importance of these various nutrients, nor do they know their precise individual mechanisms of action. What is abundantly clear, however, is that all such nutrients have a powerful antioxidant effect and that a diet rich in fruits and vegetables provides many if not all of them.

In response to the evidence supporting the health benefits of a high fruit and vegetable intake, the National Cancer Institute (NCI) and the U.S. Department of Agriculture (USDA) have issued specific recommendations for Americans: every day people should consume two or more servings of fruit or fruit juice and three or more servings of vegetables—i.e., "five a day." In 1992 the national Five-a-Day for Better Health program promoting increased consumption of fruits and vegetables was launched. This ambitious effort, the largest-ever industry-government joint public health campaign, aims to educate the public about the benefits of consuming more fruits and vegetables and to assist consumers in making choices through advertising and store displays. (Produce growers and marketers as well as some 30,000 supermarkets nationwide are participating.)

Cancer protection

Over the past two decades, nearly 200 epidemiological studies have examined the role of diets that are both high and low in fruits and vegetables and the risk of developing cancer. The studies have been carried out in some 17 countries as diverse as Turkey, China, The Netherlands, and the United States. In the U.S. investigations into the potential of these foods to prevent cancer have been conducted in places as remote from each other as upstate New York and rural Louisiana. Some 18 different types of cancer have been examined; for almost every cancer site, studies have found reductions in cancer risk among people with a high fruit and vegetable intake.

The lungs are one example—perhaps a surprising one—of a cancer site in which the evidence for cancer protection from fruits and vegetables is strong. In 30 of 32 studies, significantly reduced lung cancer risk was associated with a higher intake of fruits, vegetables, or both. A study in The Netherlands obtained detailed dietary information from close to 900 men and then kept track of their health over the next 25 years. The results showed that those men who ate the least fruit had a risk of developing lung cancer more than three times higher than that of study subjects who consumed fruit in plentiful quantities. The beneficial effect of fruit consumption was seen even after the risk factors of age and cigarette smoking were taken into account.

Other studies have found a reduced lung cancer risk among people with a high intake of vegetables. Diets that are rich in beta-carotene and other carotenoids, as well as in vitamin C, appear to be particularly beneficial.

Of course, the single most effective way to lower one's chance of becoming a victim of lung cancer is to stop smoking. However, evidence is strong that for people who have stopped smoking and want to reduce their risk even further, as well as for people who are exposed to others' tobacco smoke, a diet that is rich in fruits and vegetables, because of its powerful antioxidant nutrients, is likely to significantly reduce their risk of developing lung cancer.

Studies conducted in the U.S., Italy, France, Brazil, Uruguay, India, China, and elsewhere have shown that the risk of oral and esophageal cancers is reduced by a high fruit intake. Even after smoking and alcohol consumption (two important risk factors for those cancers) had been taken into account, persons who regularly consumed fruits with a high vitamin C content had a lower cancer risk. Studies have also found that a low intake of fruits and vegetables (especially fruits) is associated with increased risk of developing stomach cancer.

Cancers of the colon and rectum are among the major cancers of developed nations. Because a low intake of dietary fiber is thought to be a risk factor, a

Fruits, vegetables, and health

high-fiber diet has been widely studied and promoted as a way to reduce the risk of colorectal cancer. Fruits and vegetables are major sources of fiber, and in the U.S. they actually provide much more of the population's total fiber intake than do whole grain products. Thus, many studies that have estimated the beneficial effects of fiber have usually calculated fiber consumption from study subjects' intake of a long list of fruits and vegetables and usually just a few grain products. While fiber itself may indeed play a role, it is likely that other components of fruits and vegetables also offer protection against colorectal cancer. In the early 1970s Eric Bjelke, a Norwegian investigator, studied cancer risk in Norway and Minnesota. Bjelke concluded that "for colorectal cancer, the large majority of the population may be at increased risk compared to the minority with very high vegetable intakes." Other studies, conducted in the U.S., Australia, Belgium, Italy, and Israel, among other places, have also found that both vegetables and fruits appear to lower the risk of these bowel cancers.

A recent study compared the dietary histories of men who had bladder cancer and men without cancer. The former had consumed significantly fewer fruits and vegetables, especially those high in vitamins A and C, than had the cancer-free subjects.

Investigators in Canada conducted a "meta-analysis" in which they pooled the results of 12 studies of the role of dietary factors in breast cancer. The results indicated that saturated fat was a risk factor, which had been suggested by a number of observational studies. But they also indicated that a diet high in fruits and vegetables (represented by dietary vitamin

C intake) was as strong and statistically significant a factor in the protective direction as saturated fat was in the harmful direction.

Good for the heart

In addition to the impressive evidence about a beneficial role in cancer prevention, exciting new research suggests that the antioxidants found in fruits and vegetables may have an important role in reducing heart disease. Evidence for this effect exists at the biochemical level as well as coming from animal and human studies. Atherosclerosis begins with a series of early changes in the artery walls. At the earliest stage, the endothelium that lines the arteries is damaged, and laboratory evidence indicates that oxidation has a role in that damage. Cultured endothelial cells have been shown to change both their appearance and their function when oxidized LDL cholesterol (the "bad" cholesterol) is added to the culture; this does not occur when unoxidized LDL is added. The damaged endothelium allows macrophages (a type of scavenging white blood cell) to enter the arterial wall, attracted by the oxidized LDL. The macrophages ingest the oxidized LDL much more readily than they do normal LDL; in the process, they become "foam cells," building up to form artery-clogging plaque.

Considerable evidence indicates that antioxidants block these processes at each stage, scavenging for free radicals *before* they can attack other biomolecules and thereby breaking the chain reaction of lipid oxidation and buildup of artery-clogging plaque. Recent research has shown that vitamin C and vitamin E in particular prevent LDL from being oxidized.

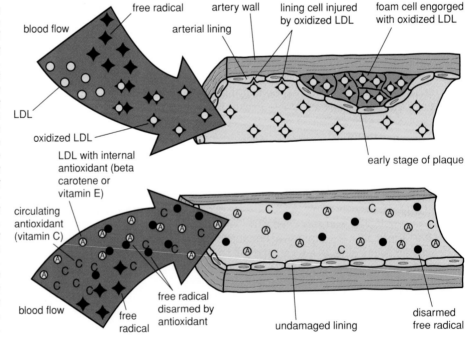

LDL cholesterol particles moving through the arteries become altered (oxidized) by circulating free radicals (top). Research suggests that oxidized LDL can injure the arterial lining, leading to heart disease. When repair cells arrive at the injured site, they absorb LDL and bloat into foam cells, which lodge under the lining, forming atherosclerotic plaque. Antioxidants such as vitamin C, beta-carotene, and vitamin E from fruits and vegetables disarm free radicals (bottom). Vitamin C circulates in the blood, while the latter two compounds are carried within the LDL particles themselves.

Karen Wollins

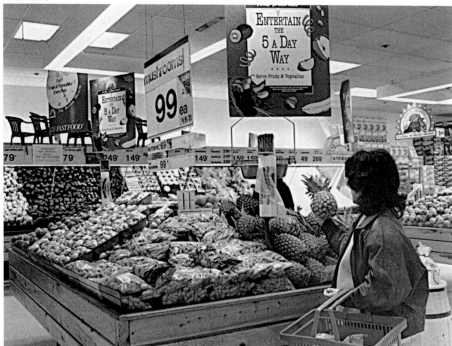

Surveys indicate that when it comes to eating their fruits and vegetables, Americans have a lamentable track record. In an effort to encourage them to make more sensible dietary choices, the National Cancer Institute and the Produce for Better Health Foundation initiated the Five-a-Day for Better Health program. Some 30,000 supermarkets nationwide are providing in-store health and nutrition information and mounting special displays that encourage shoppers to consider the cabbages and carrots and cantaloupes—before rushing on to the snack and soda aisles.

Laboratory studies in rabbits, rats, and monkeys have shown that when the animals were fed a high-fat, atherogenic diet, the arterial damage was substantially lower if their diet was also high in antioxidants. In human studies a high antioxidant intake has been associated with lower cholesterol levels and lower blood pressure.

In a study of men who had suffered a first heart attack before the age of 45, the susceptibility of the patients' LDL to oxidation correlated highly with the severity of the coronary atherosclerosis. Vitamin C has been shown in laboratory experiments to be of the first line of defense against LDL oxidation in plasma. A 12-month investigation in India found that heart attack patients who were put on a diet that included high intake of fruits and vegetables suffered fewer cardiac events (subsequent heart attacks or sudden death) than those who followed a conventional reduced-fat diet. And in a placebo-controlled intervention study in which U.S. physicians were the subjects, those who had angina pectoris (paroxysmal chest pain precipitated by deficient oxygenation of heart muscle) or had had previous coronary bypass surgery and were given beta-carotene had many fewer major heart attacks and cardiovascular deaths than did those in the study who had not received beta-carotene supplementation. These and other results have led some researchers to suggest that dietary micronutrients such as vitamins C and E and beta-carotene and perhaps other carotenoids could have a major role in future strategies for atherosclerosis prevention.

Nutrients against eye disease?

A relatively new finding—that the antioxidant nutrients that are found in fruits and vegetables may have protective roles in age-related ocular disorders—could have very important implications for the prevention of cataracts, which are the third leading cause of blindness in the U.S., and age-related macular degeneration, a sight-robbing deterioration of the retina. In the presence of oxygen, ultraviolet light generates free radicals or precursors that produce oxidative damage to proteins in the eye's lens, leading to increasing opacity. In the young, repair mechanisms exist, but these become progressively less effective as people age. It has been hypothesized that oxidation may be involved in most types of cataract and in age-related macular degeneration. This hypothesis is supported by animal as well as human studies.

Animal studies have evaluated the protective potential of many nutrients in the development of cataracts. In those studies vitamins C and E delayed or prevented cataracts in animals. Some antioxidant enzymes also seem to have protective mechanisms. Several large epidemiological studies have found that persons who had age-related eye diseases consumed significantly less of the antioxidant nutrients vitamins C and E and beta-carotene than did persons who did not develop those degenerative eye conditions. A leading investigator recently concluded that "cataractogenesis is causally related to photooxidative stress" and that "the consensus is impressive" for a protective role for antioxidants.

Antioxidants and fiber: selected fruit and vegetable sources	
vitamin C	% of U.S. recommended dietary allowance (RDA)
1 navel orange	133
1 raw kiwifruit	125
6 oz grapefruit juice	104
¼ cantaloupe	94
¼ c (4) cooked brussels sprouts	80
½ c strawberries	70
½ c cooked frozen broccoli	62
6 oz tomato juice	55
½ c cooked frozen cauliflower	47
beta-carotene*	
½ c canned pumpkin	538
1 baked sweet potato	498
1 medium carrot	405
½ c cooked frozen spinach	148
½ c cooked butternut squash	143
¼ cantaloupe	86
½ c cooked frozen kale	83
½ c cooked frozen mixed vegetables	78
3 raw apricots	55
fiber	grams[†]
½ c turnips	4.8
½ c brussels sprouts	3.8
1 c spinach	3.5
1 small pear or orange	2.9
1 small apple	2.8

*no RDA set for beta-carotene; percentage is calculated on the basis of conversion of beta-carotene to vitamin A
[†]National Cancer Institute recommends 20–35 g of fiber a day; fiber also available in whole grain foods and dried beans and peas

Because epidemiological studies cannot completely resolve uncertainties about causation, the National Eye Institute of the National Institutes of Health is presently conducting a major investigation, the Age-Related Eye Disease Study, which is expected to run for 10 years and will involve close to 5,000 male and female subjects ranging in age from 60 to 75 years. The development of cataracts in those subjects who are given supplements containing vitamins C and E and beta-carotene will be compared with cataract risk in subjects given a placebo. The provocative questions about whether vitamins and nutrients have a preventive role in cataract development and age-related macular degeneration are among those that will be investigated in the course of the clinical trial. It may be that eating carrots is good for eyesight after all!

Still more benefits

Finally, some data exist suggesting that general health and well-being are improved with increasing intake of fruits and vegetables. In a large national survey, Americans were asked to rate their health as excellent, very good, good, fair, or poor. Investigators then looked at the blood levels of vitamin C in those people. The researchers limited the sample just to those who were not taking vitamin supplements because people who take supplements might be biased toward reporting their health as better. The results were impressive. Within each age group, persons with low blood levels of vitamin C were much more likely to have reported their health as poor or fair, and people with high levels were more likely to have reported their health as excellent or very good.

Diets around the world

Despite the exhortations of parents and grandparents, and despite decades of advice from nutritionists, many people's diets are astonishingly poor in terms of quantity of fruits and vegetables consumed. In the United States large national surveys of dietary practices are conducted by the USDA and the National Center for Health Statistics. Such surveys have been examined to determine how many servings of fruits and vegetables are typically consumed by Americans on a daily basis.

One analysis looked at the Second National Health and Nutrition Examination Survey (NHANES II), conducted over the years 1976–80. That survey had collected information on every bit of food and drink that some 12,000 adults had consumed in a single 24-hour period. Almost half the population (45%) had consumed no fruit or fruit juice on the day of the survey; only 43% had consumed any "garden vegetables"— that is, vegetables other than potatoes and salad; and fewer than 25% had eaten fruits or vegetables rich in vitamin C or carotenoids. Finally, the investigators found that only 9% of the population had consumed five or more servings of fruits and vegetables in one day—the amount recommended by the USDA and the NCI; among black Americans consumption was even poorer—only about 5% had had the recommended five daily servings.

It might be suspected that dietary habits have improved since 1980. Thus, data on approximately 1,500 women interviewed in the 1986 USDA Continuing Survey of Food Intakes by Individuals (CSFII) were also examined. In that survey dietary information on each participant was obtained for four to six independent days over an entire year. The results were no better. The proportions of respondents consuming fruit and vegetables on any given day were about the same as the proportions seen in the 1976–80 survey. Almost 20% reported having consumed no servings of fruit or fruit juice on any of four nonconsecutive days; 43%

had no citrus fruit or juice; and 70% had no dark green or deep yellow vegetables.

It is quite evident that consumption of fruits and vegetables in the United States falls far short of recommended levels and is inconsistent with the strength of the evidence on the health benefits of those foods. How does this compare with fruit and vegetable intake in other countries? For many countries the situation is similar, and in some instances it is even worse. In a study in India, the "high fruit intake" category consisted of persons who ate fruit at least once a week! In a large study in Lin Xian (Lin Hsien), China, an area with an extremely high esophageal cancer incidence, the high fruit intake category consisted of persons who ate fruit at least 35 times per year. And in a dietary survey in Puerto Rico, 75% of the study group reported that they never had fresh fruit in their diet, and 87% had no more than two portions of vegetables per week. Clearly, there are some populations with extremely low fruit and vegetable intake, and typically these populations are ones with very high cancer rates.

Many northern European countries have high cancer and heart disease incidence and low intake of fresh fruits and vegetables. Scotland, for example, has among the highest rates of these diseases of any industrialized nation—and is famous for its "meat and potatoes" diet, with fruits and vegetables infrequently consumed. The same is true of many eastern European countries.

In contrast, countries of the Mediterranean tend to have higher intakes of fruits and vegetables and a lower prevalence of cancer and heart disease. In Italy, for example, per capita consumption of fresh fruits is 130 kg (286 lb) per year, compared with only 40 kg (89 lb) in the United States. And Italians consume about twice as many tomato products—sources of vitamin C and carotenoids—than do Americans (63 kg per capita, compared with 32 kg).

The Mediterranean diet in general has been the subject of considerable interest and research. Many Mediterranean cuisines include whole grains and olive oil (both good sources of the antioxidant vitamin E), wine, and many fruits and vegetables. Other factors may, of course, be important, such as a healthy level of physical activity. But it would appear that a Mediterranean diet is both delicious and health-promoting.

A recently observed phenomenon that has been much discussed is the so-called French paradox—namely, that the French tend to have high intakes of fat, largely from cheese and creamy sauces, but a low incidence of heart disease. Moreover, the French are heavy smokers. One explanation for this paradox is that the French have a high intake of fruits and vegetables. There is also some speculation that antioxidants in red wine may be associated with a reduced heart disease risk.

Getting your "five a day"

Does "five a day" sound like an impossible amount? Think again. Any of the following are considered "one serving":

- one cup of raw leafy greens, such as lettuce or spinach
- one-half cup of raw or cooked vegetables of most types, such as broccoli, cauliflower, peas, green beans, etc.
- one average carrot
- one large celery stalk
- one medium potato
- one-half acorn squash
- one medium apple, orange, banana, or similar-sized fruit
- one-third of a cantaloupe or other melon
- one-half grapefruit
- one-half cup of a small fruit, such as grapes, or cut fruit, such as diced pineapple
- one-quarter cup of dried fruit, such as raisins
- three-quarters cup of pure fruit juice or vegetable juice

A typical day's menu might look like this: fruit or juice with breakfast, a salad with lunch, a piece of fruit for a snack, and a potato and one green or yellow vegetable with dinner—five servings! In fact, the possibilities for incorporating fruits and vegetables

"It's kohlrabi, the next hot vegetable."

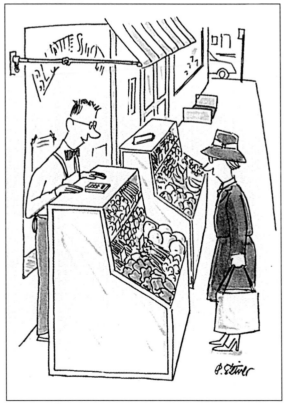

into nutritious and delicious dishes are endless: a vegetable omelette (for breakfast, lunch, or dinner), a vegetable-topped pizza, a hearty vegetable soup, a sliced banana or berries on cereal. Moreover, such a diet can be accommodated even with the busiest of modern lifestyles. It just requires a commitment to including fruits and vegetables on a daily basis—and, of course, remembering to put the banana in the lunch sack.

Does it matter which foods one eats or in what form? With current intakes so low, the primary goal for each individual should be getting the number of servings up to five a day. The NCI recommends at least one vitamin C-rich food a day and at least one vitamin A (carotene)-rich food a day. Examples of vitamin C foods are the citrus fruits and juices, melons, tomatoes or tomato juice, and broccoli; carotene-rich foods are deep-orange-colored and dark green leafy vegetables and fruits (see Table). But all fruits and vegetables contain valuable nutrients, and probably all contain antioxidants. For example, while apples are not rich in either vitamin C or carotene, they and their juices do contain bioflavonoids, which are antioxidants; they are also a good source of fiber. Most people can easily meet the recommendations by choosing their favorites.

What about the effects of cooking? A few studies have found that raw vegetables are particularly effective in reducing cancer risk. However, this does not mean that cooked vegetables have lost all their value. Storage and cooking do reduce the vitamin C content of foods somewhat, but they do not eliminate it altogether (unless the food is boiled for hours). In fact, cooking has even been found to improve the availability of beta-carotene to the body. And in some cases, canned or frozen food may even be superior since it is usually picked at optimal ripeness and preserved rapidly. A prudent recommendation would be to eat fresh or raw vegetables if it is convenient and if one likes them (in a salad, for example) and cooked vegetables—fresh, frozen, or canned—if that is most convenient or desirable.

The vitamin supplement question

What about taking vitamin supplements? Such supplements, of course, contain many of the well-established nutrients of which fruits and vegetables are the natural sources (e.g., beta-carotene, vitamins C and E, folic acid, iron, magnesium, calcium, and zinc). For some people, given the sorry state of their intake (as the evidence presented above so clearly suggests), taking supplements might be a prudent step to ensure adequate intake of all nutrients. Further, some recent studies have suggested that supplement use in addition to an adequate diet may confer additional benefits. For example, the large national NHANES I

Follow-up Study found that persons who had above-average intakes of vitamin C from fruits and vegetables and also took supplements had significantly lower total mortality, from cancer and other diseases, over 10 years than the group who had above-average intakes from diet and did not take supplements. This study controlled for education, income, smoking, and a variety of other risk factors. Thus, it may be that the extra insurance provided by supplements is beneficial.

While dietary supplements may provide a potential safeguard, it is important to realize that it is not appropriate to take supplements instead of improving intake of fruits and vegetables. This is for the very practical reason that there are hundreds of beneficial compounds in fruits and vegetables that cannot be obtained from a vitamin pill—such things as bioflavonoids, isothiocyanates, phenols, literally hundreds of carotenoids other than beta-carotene, and, of course, fiber. Nature packaged them together; they enhance each other's absorption or action and perform independent biological functions, and those components cannot be put into a pill.

Mother was right—after all

In conclusion, the evidence is strong that a diet rich in fruits and vegetables and the antioxidant nutrients they provide not only is generally healthful but actually reduces the risk of many types of cancer, probably heart disease, and perhaps certain age-related eye diseases and other, as yet uninvestigated, aging-associated conditions. Increasing fruit and vegetable consumption is a dietary recommendation that may be easier to achieve than most people think. In fact, it may be more easily followed than are admonitions to reduce the percentage of calories from fat or increase fiber intake; yet, at the same time, increasing fruit and vegetable consumption will move toward those goals as well.

The fact that people do not eat enough of these important foods has been a largely unrecognized but serious problem. That, however, is changing. Americans' inadequate consumption of fruits and vegetables was a subject that the New York Times recently deemed worthy of an editorial:

Millions of Americans can still remember what it was like to have to eat a mess of overcooked carrots because they were good for their eyesight. They can also remember what it was like to consume spinach . . . because Popeye owed his muscles to it. . . . Until they found their champion in a President . . . who announced to the world that he didn't like broccoli. . . . But how misplaced that hate! How wrong those millions of Americans! Because it is from stuff like broccoli . . . that they may gain a brighter, healthier future.

Will "five a day" keep the doctor away? Very probably!

Strep Infections

by Rafael E. Campo, M.D.,
and Alan L. Bisno, M.D.

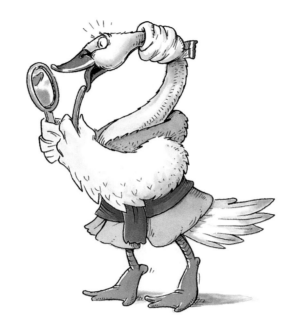

The streptococci, a common and ubiquitous group of bacteria, are among the many microbes that normally inhabit the human body; they are also capable of causing serious, even life-threatening infections. The name is derived from two Greek words, *streptos,* meaning "twisted," and *kokkos,* "berry." Under the light microscope, streptococci appear as round, berrylike balls strung together in chains. Strep bacteria were first identified as agents of human disease in the latter years of the 19th century as a result of the pioneering investigations of such distinguished microbiologists as Louis Pasteur and Robert Koch.

Classifying the streptococci

The systems currently used to classify the streptococci are imperfect and somewhat confusing. Clinical microbiologists employ three different and overlapping schemes. The simplest depends upon the way the streptococci appear when grown in the laboratory in a culture medium containing sheep's blood. In this scheme the organisms are classified on the basis of whether they destroy (hemolyze) the red blood cells in a circular zone surrounding the bacterial colonies growing on the culture plates.

A more precise approach to classification is based upon certain biochemical characteristics of the organisms, such as their ability to digest certain sugars. While this approach divides streptococci into a variety of different species, not all streptococci can be differentiated by this technique.

A third and highly useful form of classification relies on differences between the antigens in certain constituents (mainly carbohydrates) of the bacterial cell wall. (Antigens are substances capable of stimulating an immune response.) These antigenic differences form the basis for the differentiation of streptococci into so-called serogroups—groups A through H and K through T. As with biochemical classification, not all streptococci can be typed according to serogroup.

Strep organisms: many and varied

The streptococci include many bacteria that may harmlessly colonize the skin or mucous membranes of humans but, under appropriate circumstances, are capable of causing serious disease (*see* Table, p. 427). One such organism is *Streptococcus pneumoniae,* also known as the pneumococcus, the most common cause of contagious acute bacterial pneumonia. *S. pneumoniae* may also cause sinusitis, middle ear infections, and occasionally infections of the central nervous system (meningitis), joints, and heart valves.

S. mutans, a common bacterium found in the mouth—and a major cause of dental caries (tooth decay)—can initiate serious illness if it is able to establish residence in normally sterile body sites such as the heart valves. *S. sanguis* and *S. bovis* also can cause heart valve infection. The enterococci, *Enterococcus faecalis* and related organisms, normal inhabitants of the lower gastrointestinal tract, commonly cause urinary tract infections and can infect heart valves.

S. agalactiae, also known as the group B streptococcus, frequently colonizes the female genital tract and is a major cause of life-threatening and often lethal infections of the bloodstream and central nervous system in newborns. Infants who survive group B strep infection may have impaired vision or hearing; some are developmentally delayed. To prevent such congenital defects, the American Academy of Pediatrics recommended in 1992 that all expectant mothers be tested for the presence of group B streptococci in the birth canal between the 26th and 28th weeks of pregnancy. Women who test positive and who have complications of pregnancy (*e.g.,* premature labor, fever before and during labor, early rupture of the fetal membranes) may require intravenous antibiotic therapy during labor and delivery to ward off infection in the newborn. Like virtually all streptococci, the group B organism is highly susceptible to penicillin.

Among all the streptococci, the most important human pathogen is *S. pyogenes,* also known as the group A streptococcus. *S. pyogenes* is a highly complex microorganism, significant both because of the

425

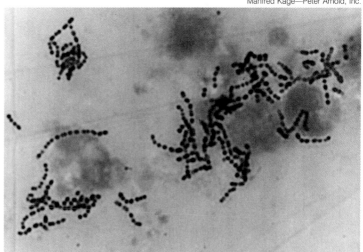
Manfred Kage—Peter Arnold, Inc.

Streptococcus pyogenes, *also known as the group A streptococcus, seen through a light microscope, is typical of the strep bacteria in appearance—chains of round, berrylike structures that resemble beads on a string.* S. pyogenes *is one of the most important human pathogens in the strep group, causing streptococcal pharyngitis, or "strep throat."*

acute infections it causes and because of two serious diseases—rheumatic fever and glomerulonephritis—that may occur in the aftermath. The principal source of its virulence is believed to be a substance known as M protein, a filamentous molecule that protrudes through the cell wall into the external environment, preventing white blood cells of the immune system from recognizing and ingesting the organism. M protein molecules vary in their structure, and such variations allow group A streptococci to be divided into over 80 M protein types. When humans are infected by group A streptococci, they develop antibodies that counteract the effect of M protein. Such immunity, however, is type specific, so a person who has become immune to one type of group A streptococcus still can be infected by others. Streptococci are also enclosed in a slimy capsule that provides additional defense against ingestion by white cells but is less effective in this regard than is M protein.

During the course of their growth, group A streptococci produce a number of substances that assist them in invading and spreading through human tissues. They also produce certain toxins. Of particular note are substances called streptococcal pyrogenic exotoxins, which are responsible for the characteristic rash of scarlet fever. These toxins also cause high fever, suppression of immune responses, and, in experimental animals, organ damage. The discussion below focuses on infections associated with group A streptococci.

Strep throat

The group A streptococcus is the causative agent of streptococcal pharyngitis, commonly known as "strep throat." This illness occurs worldwide, showing no predilection for any race. It occurs with equal frequency in males and females. Although in the past it was believed that streptococcal throat infection was less common in the tropics than in the temperate

zone, the high incidence of rheumatic fever seen in many tropical areas suggests that this is not the case. Strep throat is primarily, but not exclusively, a disease of children aged 5 to 15 years. In temperate climates it occurs more frequently in the colder months of the year. Thus, among school-age children during the winter, strep throat is common and occasionally epidemic. Most children will experience one or more episodes during childhood or adolescence.

Group A streptococci are present in large numbers in the noses and throats of children who have strep throat, and 15% or more of asymptomatic children may also carry the organism in smaller numbers in their throats during the winter. The infection is spread from person to person by respiratory secretions and is favored by close contact. Acutely ill persons are much more likely to spread the organism than are those who are carrying the bacterium but have no symptoms. Contaminated bedding, clothing, and house dust are not important means of transmission.

The patient with strep throat typically experiences the rather sudden onset of sore throat, manifested particularly by pain on swallowing, along with headache and fever, usually in the 38.3°–40° C (101°–104° F) range. These symptoms may be accompanied by abdominal pain, nausea, and vomiting, particularly in children. The patient's throat is markedly reddened (pharyngitis), and the tonsils are red and enlarged (tonsillitis). Characteristically, there are small patches of pus on the throat, especially the tonsils. The lymph nodes at the angles of the jaw are enlarged and tender. Patients with strep throat do not have diarrhea, nor do they have the runny nose, red eyes, and cough typical of the common cold.

The clinical manifestations of strep throat overlap broadly with those of acute sore throat caused by viruses—the latter being a considerably more common condition. Distinguishing these two kinds of sore throat has important implications for treatment. Antibiotics are required in the patient with strep throat to prevent complications such as spread of the infection into the sinuses and ears and, most important, development of rheumatic fever. On the other hand, antibiotics are usually both unnecessary and inadvisable in the treatment of viral sore throat. For this reason, patients with sore throat and fever *not* accompanied by symptoms of the common cold should consult a physician. This is especially crucial for children, who have a higher incidence of both strep throat and rheumatic fever than do adults.

In most instances the physician will want to swab the patient's throat to test for the presence of group A streptococci by means of either a throat culture or a newer, faster immunologic process. The culture requires at least overnight incubation, and the physician may well elect to withhold antibiotic therapy until the culture results are available. This delay does not increase the risk of rheumatic fever in a child with strep throat. On the other hand, rapid immunologic tests make it possible for group A strep to be detected almost immediately, the results often being available while the patient is still in the doctor's office. Because the rapid test is slightly less sensitive than the culture, however, most authorities suggest that a negative rapid test be confirmed with a culture. In such a case antibiotic treatment should not be instituted unless the confirmatory throat culture is positive.

If the throat culture indicates the presence of group A streptococci in the throat of a patient with acute sore throat, therapy will be administered in the form of a single injection of long-acting penicillin or a 10-day course of oral antibiotics (usually penicillin or, in one who is allergic, erythromycin). Either with or without antibiotic therapy, in most cases the symptoms of strep throat abate in about three days. Many patients taking oral antibiotics—particularly children—discontinue their medication once they begin to feel better. However, parents should make certain the full 10-day treatment is followed to provide optimal protection against rheumatic fever.

The course of strep throat is shortened by about 24 hours if therapy is started within the first day of onset of symptoms. Patients who have symptoms are highly contagious—they can easily infect schoolmates and family members. Children are considered noninfectious and may return to school or day care after having been under treatment for at least 24 hours, provided their temperature has returned to normal.

Scarlet fever

Scarlet fever may develop one to two days after the onset of strep throat. It is characterized by a red rash that first appears on the chest and spreads to the rest of the body, sparing the area around the mouth. The rash resembles a sunburn in color but is distinguished by tiny red raised spots that give the skin a sandpaper-like feel. The patient's tongue is covered with a whitish coat at first but later becomes intensely red ("strawberry tongue"). The rash fades after about a week, and the skin begins to peel off in flakes, a process that may go on for another one or two weeks. Treatment is the same as for strep throat without the rash.

Scarlet fever is caused by a toxin produced by the streptococcus. As with strep throat, the great majority of cases occur in school-age children. However, only a minority of patients with strep throat will develop scarlet fever. Its occurrence depends in part on the infecting strain of streptococcus and in part on the patient's immunity to the toxin. In rare instances scarlet fever may occur after streptococcal infection of the skin or of a surgical or traumatic wound.

At times scarlet fever occurs in epidemic waves. In the preantibiotic era, such epidemics were greatly feared; patients experienced raging fevers, extreme prostration, and even death. Their homes were often placed under strict quarantine. Nowadays the disease is much milder, usually amounting to no more than a typical strep throat with a rash. Undoubtedly, the advent of this milder form of the disease is due in part to the effect of antibiotic therapy, but it may also be attributed to changes in the virulence of the prevalent streptococcal strains.

Streptococci frequently involved in human disease	
classification	type of infection
group A	strep throat; middle ear infections; sinusitis; scarlet fever; pneumonia; "childbed fever"
	infections of skin, including impetigo, erysipelas, cellulitis
	acute rheumatic fever; acute glomerulonephritis
group B	meningitis and bloodstream infections in newborns
group C	sore throat*
group D (including enterococci)	infections of urinary tract, heart valves, wounds, and bedsores
group G	sore throat* infections of skin, soft tissues, and bloodstream
S. pneumoniae	pneumonia; middle ear infections; sinusitis; meningitis; heart valve infections
S. mutans	dental caries; heart valve infections
S. sanguis	heart valve infections
S. bovis	heart valve infections
*infrequent	

Impetigo

Impetigo is a skin infection characterized by single or multiple lesions, usually on the face and extremities. The lesions appear initially as small bumps filled with pus (pustules), but these soon rupture and form thick, flaky, yellowish crusts. Facial lesions are often due to the spread of strep infection from the upper respiratory tract.

Impetigo that develops on the exposed areas of the trunk and the extremities is also known as *pyoderma* and often occurs in preschool-age children as a result of minor cuts, abrasions, or insect bites that become infected. Such infections usually occur in the summer in temperate climates, but they may be seen throughout the year in tropical parts of the world, particularly in circumstances in which personal hygiene is poor.

Although children with impetigo do not generally run a fever or feel ill, the skin infection may be a precursor of a serious kidney disease, glomerulonephritis (*see* below). Treatment is similar to that for strep throat, but in some cases of impetigo, topical antibiotics may be effective.

It is important to note that not all cases of impetigo are due to *S. pyogenes.* Staphylococcal organisms are frequently the culprit, and some cases are due to coinfection with both strep and staph organisms. The presence of staphylococci in the lesions may alter the choice of antimicrobial therapy.

Invasive infections

In addition to impetigo, group A streptococci sometimes cause more serious and extensive infections of the skin, soft tissues, and muscles, including cellulitis, erysipelas ("Saint Anthony's fire"), necrotizing fasciitis, and myositis. *S. pyogenes* may invade virtually any tissue or organ in the body, with potentially life-threatening consequences. Of special note are infection of the lung (pneumonia) and infection of the uterus at childbirth, or puerperal sepsis (the dreaded "childbed fever" of the preantiseptic era).

Complications of group A strep infections

Poststreptococcal complications—those developing in the aftermath of infection—have the potential to be serious or even fatal. The two most dangerous are rheumatic fever and glomerulonephritis.

Acute rheumatic fever. Undoubtedly, the most feared complication of streptococcal infection is rheumatic fever. It usually occurs within one to five weeks after a strep throat, at which time the affected individual develops one or more of the following: (1) severe and painful arthritis, involving a number of joints and associated with fever and malaise; (2) involuntary movements of the face and extremities, known medically as Sydenham's chorea and popularly as Saint Vitus' dance; (3) inflammation of all layers of the heart muscle (carditis). Other manifestations may include a distinctive red rash and pea-sized nodules under the skin. The arthritis, movement disorder, rash, and nodules eventually resolve completely. In a minority of patients, however, inflammation of the heart may lead to chronic scarring of one or more heart valves. Scarred valves may become leaky or obstructed (or both), leading eventually to heart failure that can be fatal or necessitating surgical removal of the valves and replacement with artificial ones.

Despite decades of intensive investigation, the exact biological mechanisms responsible for the development of rheumatic fever remain unknown. The disease does not result from infection of the heart, joints, or other tissues by group A streptococci. Indeed, it does not manifest itself until *after* all evidence of the acute infection has subsided. Because the group A streptococcus has many constituents that are structurally and antigenically similar to human tissues, most authorities believe that rheumatic fever results when the immune response to the streptococcal infection inadvertently attacks the body's own tissues.

The epidemiology of rheumatic fever mirrors that of strep throat; thus, the disease is most common among school-age children. The etiologic agent and site of infection in rheumatic fever are specific—that is, only group A streptococcal infection of the upper respiratory tract results in rheumatic fever. Neither throat infection with other groups of streptococci nor group A streptococcal infections of the skin or other sites cause the disease. The streptococcal infection that precedes rheumatic fever need not be symptomatic. Thus, many patients diagnosed with rheumatic fever have no history of recent strep throat. However, recent infection may be documented by a throat culture or by a blood test for antibodies to the group A streptococcus.

Historically, the risk of developing acute rheumatic fever after an episode of untreated symptomatic strep

Symptoms and signs of strep throat	
symptoms (subjective findings)	signs (objective findings)
sudden onset of sore throat with pain on swallowing	temperature of 38.3°–40° C (101°–104° F)
nausea, abdominal pain*	red throat
headache	enlarged, red tonsils with visible pus
prostration	tender, enlarged lymph nodes at the angles of the jaw
	skin rash†
*particularly in children †infrequent	

throat has varied from as high as 3% in severe epidemics of acute sore throat among military recruits to considerably less than 1% in sporadically occurring infection among schoolchildren. At least one of the factors influencing this risk is the nature of prevailing streptococcal strains. Group A streptococci vary widely in their potential to elicit the disease, with certain strains being highly rheumatogenic. A second factor may be the existence of conditions favoring rapid transmission of streptococci from person to person, as may occur in crowded households or military barracks. Appropriate antibiotic treatment of symptomatic strep throat is highly effective in preventing rheumatic fever—underscoring the importance of accurate diagnosis and early and proper treatment.

People who have experienced an attack of rheumatic fever are much more susceptible than others to developing rheumatic fever after subsequent bouts of strep throat. Susceptibility to recurrence is greater in patients with residual valvular heart disease, but the risk of recurrence wanes with increasing age and the length of time since the most recent rheumatic fever attack. All individuals who suffer a bout of rheumatic fever should receive prophylactic antibiotic therapy to guard against recurrences. The most effective form of prophylaxis is a single injection of long-acting penicillin every four weeks (or possibly every three weeks in countries with an extremely high incidence of the disease). Though less effective, daily oral prophylaxis may also be used. The decision about when—if ever—such preventive therapy may be discontinued will vary from case to case and thus should be made on an individual basis.

Acute glomerulonephritis. Glomerulonephritis is an inflammation of the portion of the kidney (the glomerulus) that is involved in filtering fluid from circulating blood into the renal tubules. Clinical manifestations include facial puffiness (particularly around the eyes), swelling of the legs and feet, blood in the urine giving it a smoky or rusty appearance, and high blood pressure. The retention of fluid in the lungs may cause shortness of breath. The group A streptococcus is only one of a number of causes of such inflammation.

As with rheumatic fever, poststreptococcal acute glomerulonephritis is not due to direct tissue infection by the streptococcus. Rather, it occurs a few days to weeks *after* infection with certain nephritogenic (kidney-damaging) streptococcal strains. The damage to the kidney results from the interaction of streptococcal antigens with antibodies produced by the patient, but the exact identity of the offending streptococcal antigen remains uncertain.

The strains of group A streptococci that cause glomerulonephritis appear for the most part to be distinct from those that cause rheumatic fever. A major difference between rheumatic fever and glomerulonephritis is that the former occurs only after strepto-

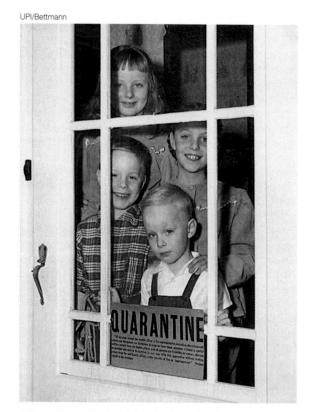

Like millions of U.S. children in the 1940s, these Wisconsin youngsters were quarantined when another sibling came down with scarlet fever. This disease, common in the preantibiotic era, occurs less often today and in a much milder form.

coccal throat infection, while the latter may follow a strep infection of either the throat or skin. Indeed, some of the largest reported epidemics of poststreptococcal glomerulonephritis have occurred in tropical countries among underprivileged children whose pyoderma lesions contained highly nephritogenic streptococci. Another difference between the two illnesses is that antibiotic therapy is not as effective in preventing poststreptococcal glomerulonephritis as it is in preventing acute rheumatic fever. And unlike people recovering from rheumatic fever, those who have experienced an attack of acute glomerulonephritis are not at increased risk of recurrence of the kidney infection.

Strep returns—with a vengeance

Rheumatic fever is an extremely common disease in the Indian subcontinent, the Arab Middle East, and many countries of Africa and South America. In these less developed regions it remains among the major causes of cardiovascular disease and death. In marked contrast, the incidence of acute rheumatic fever has been declining in the industrialized nations of North America and western Europe since the early years of the 20th century. By the late 1970s the incidence of rheumatic fever had reached unprecedented lows in the U.S.; the disease had virtually disappeared

429

from the affluent suburbs of U.S. cities, persisting primarily in low-income inner-city neighborhoods where the population was predominantly African-American or, in some instances, Hispanic. The reasons for the decline are uncertain but are presumed to relate to improved living standards—as reflected in better nutrition and hygiene, improved access to medical care, and decreased household crowding—as well as to the effectiveness of penicillin in preventing the disease.

However, during the period from 1985 to 1989, a stunning resurgence of rheumatic fever took place in the U.S. An epidemic of some 200 cases occurred in Salt Lake City, Utah, and environs, and smaller clusters of cases were reported in Columbus and Akron, Ohio; Pittsburgh, Pa.; Nashville and Memphis, Tenn.; New York City; Morgantown and Charleston, W.Va.; Kansas City, Mo.; and Dallas, Texas. A number of these outbreaks involved white children from middle-class suburban families. Moreover, recalling a scenario that was common up until the early 1960s, outbreaks of rheumatic fever occurred at the Ft. Leonard Wood (Missouri) Army Training Center and the naval training center at San Diego, Calif.

Another remarkable development beginning in the late 1980s was the appearance of extremely severe, rapidly progressing, and life-threatening forms of invasive group A streptococcal disease, primarily affecting adults. This phenomenon has by no means been limited to the United States or Canada; similar cases have been reported in Great Britain, Scandinavia, eastern Europe, and Australia. (The phenomenon was brought to public attention in 1990 by the sudden death at age 53 of Jim Henson, creator of the beloved Muppets, from group A streptococcal pneumonia.) Among those most vulnerable to these devastating infections are elderly persons, those with chronic diseases, pregnant women, intravenous drug users, and people taking immunosuppressive medications. In many such cases the initial focus of the infection is the skin and underlying soft tissues, with subsequent spread of infection to the bloodstream (bacteremia) and, in some cases, the development of areas of gangrene.

A number of cases have been reported in which patients have gone into shock, experienced major organ failure (kidney, liver, heart, and brain), and often developed a generalized rash. This constellation of findings is reminiscent of those associated with the better-known staphylococcal infection toxic shock syndrome (TSS). The latter is a disorder caused by a bacterial toxin and is often associated with the use of superabsorbent menstrual tampons. While the toxic-shock-like syndrome caused by the group A streptococcus is not related to tampon use, it may well be due to streptococcal toxin similar to the staphylococcal toxin that causes TSS. Even with appropriate antimicrobial therapy, approximately one-third of patients who develop this streptococcal toxic-shock-like

syndrome have died. These fearsome strep infections are not unprecedented—similar overwhelming infections were well described in the 19th century and in the preantibiotic years of the current century.

Scientists have not yet been able to explain the recent resurgence of rheumatic fever and the increased incidence of life-threatening group A streptococcal infections. For unknown reasons the strains of streptococci currently circulating in the U.S. are more virulent than those that prevailed over the preceding three decades. At least three characteristics of the streptococci, not all of which are expressed in the same bacterial strains, may be responsible for the enhanced virulence. First, certain types of group A streptococci that are preferentially associated with rheumatic fever and invasive disease have become more prevalent. Second, some of the strep organisms have been found to exhibit extremely prominent capsules, a feature that is associated with enhanced virulence and rheumatogenic potential. Finally, many of the strep bacteria currently causing the toxic-shock-like syndrome produce a particularly potent form of the pyrogenic toxin that has been quite rare in recent years.

Preventing strep-related illness

The most important measures for preventing group A streptococcal infections are accurate diagnosis and prompt and effective treatment of strep throat. Fortunately, all group A streptococci remain exquisitely susceptible to penicillin, and there are a variety of effective options for the penicillin-allergic patient. As noted above, those who have experienced an attack of rheumatic fever must continue to take antibiotic drugs for many years, sometimes indefinitely, to prevent recurrences. Streptococcal skin infections, particularly impetigo or infected insect bites or cuts in children, should be treated by a physician to minimize the possibility of the development of glomerulonephritis.

Unfortunately, little can be done in most circumstances to prevent life-threatening streptococcal infections such as the toxic-shock-like syndrome, which develop quite suddenly. However, significant local skin and soft-tissue infections, particularly when accompanied by fever, should receive prompt medical attention. Patients who develop life-threatening invasive infections need to be hospitalized without delay, usually in an intensive care unit equipped to support vital organ functions.

Several groups of researchers are attempting to develop a safe and efficacious vaccine for prevention of group A streptococcal infection. Advances in the understanding of the structure of group A streptococci, and of the mechanisms by which these organisms combat the body's immune defenses, provide a basis for optimism.

Infant Crying

by **Philip Sanford Zeskind, Ph.D.**

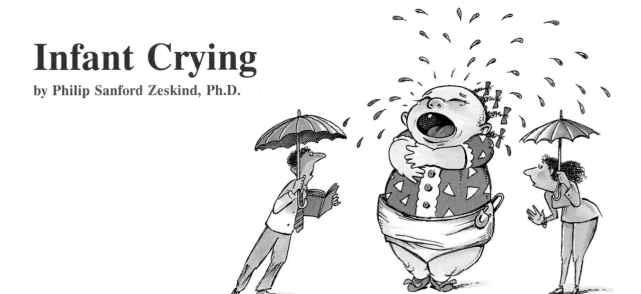

And when I was born, I drew in the common air, and fell upon the earth . . . and the first voice which I uttered was crying, as all others do.

—Apocrypha, "The wisdom of Solomon," 7:3

Infants do not cry without some legitimate cause.

—Ferrarius (16th-century physician)

Perhaps no single behavior is as uniquely critical to the survival and development of the newborn as its crying. The very first cry burst, and subsequent gasp for air, dramatically increases the infant's ability to breathe and assists in reorganizing the cardiorespiratory system from that of a fetus to that of a neonate. In the first six to eight weeks of life, crying is a reflexive behavior primarily under endogenous (internal) control, reflecting such conditions as hunger or the need for stimulation. As part of a major reorganization of the nervous system at two to three months, crying becomes more exogenously (externally) controlled as the infant learns to attract the attention of parents and other caregivers. A second biobehavioral shift occurs at approximately seven to nine months, characterized by major changes in cognitive abilities and affective states (the baby's capacities to think and express feelings). At this stage crying may be caused by fear of strangers or separations from the caregiver.

Because of the complex and changing meaning of this seemingly simple behavior, it is important for parents to appreciate its contribution to the health and development of their infants. In recent years scientists have learned a great deal about the role and the meaning of infants' cries. Indeed, they have discovered there is more to crying than meets the ear.

The cry sound: whimpers to wails

Crying is the as-yet-inarticulate newborn's way of communicating with the world at large. The vocifer-

ous, urgent, imploring sound of crying is a "biological siren" that alerts parents about conditions that disrupt the physiological well-being of the infant. In addition to establishing proximity and initiating contact between parents and infants, the sound of crying, which behavioral scientists typically describe as being "aversive," elicits such responses as feeding, holding, and rocking, which ameliorate the immediate causes of crying. These same responses of parents to the cry sound also provide the types of stimulation that facilitate the infant's physical, emotional, social, and cognitive development. Thus, the cry sound serves as a superb teacher; it yields essential information about the infant's needs and the kinds of behaviors that will terminate its distress (as reflected by the cry). Unfortunately, there is also increasing evidence that the determination of some parents to stop the sound of crying may lead them to physically abuse their young infants.

Understanding what and how the cry communicates has long been a subject of study for scientists interested in the natural history and adaptive significance of early behavior. As new technologies have become available, researchers have utilized these to investigate the meaning of this universal yet unique behavior. Both aural and visual aspects of the cry have been the focus of their studies.

The first known attempt to objectively quantify the sound of crying came in 1838 when the naturalist William Gardiner used musical notation to describe the melody and rhythm of crying. In 1872 the famous evolutionary theorist Charles Darwin used photographic plates and line drawings to illustrate facial expressions that depicted different emotions, including different patterns of infants' crying. The German researchers T. Flatau and H. Gutzman are credited with making the first recordings of the sound of crying in 1906, us-

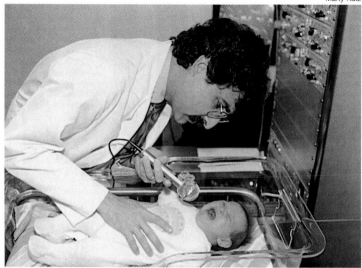

Using sophisticated sound spectroscopy analysis, psychologist Philip Zeskind at Virginia Polytechnic Institute measures the frequency of an infant's cries. Such measurements can provide important information about the baby's general health and well-being as well as its subsequent course of development; extremely high-pitched, or "hyperphonated," cries may signal underlying damage to the developing nervous system.

ing wax cylinders of Thomas Edison's newly invented phonograph. In 1927 the psychologist Mandel Sherman used silent motion pictures to examine whether adults could identify the specific causes of infants' crying. With the development of the sound spectrograph in the 1940s, the harmonic structure and temporal (durational) components of crying were measured objectively from a visual image of the cry sounds burned onto carbon paper. The use of digital technology and high-speed computers has enabled today's psychologists, linguists, and physicians to use sophisticated sound spectroscopy techniques to obtain precise measurements of the pitch, loudness, and length—in fact, of over 80 different elements—of crying.

The first sound spectrograph measurements of crying showed that it is a rhythmic repetition of an expiratory sound followed by a brief pause and then by an inspiratory period and a second brief pause before the next cry expiration. The pause between the expiration and inspiration is typically shorter than the pause between the inspiration and the beginning of the next cry expiration. This pattern of sounds and pauses results in a rhythm that is perceived (by the listener) as an expiratory sound followed by an inspiration. Variations in the duration of these elements are associated with different conditions of arousal, such as hunger or pain. The "hunger" (or basic) cry has a steady rhythmic sound with an expiratory phase that lasts about 0.9 second and first and second pauses that last about 0.09 and 0.2 second, respectively. In contrast, the initial segments of a "pain" cry are characterized by a sudden onset, a long expiratory component often lasting four or more seconds, and long pauses that sound as if the infant is holding his or her breath.

Sound spectrograph analyses can also be used to measure the level, or frequency characteristics, of the sound. Sound waves are caused by the vibration of the vocal folds in the larynx as the infant exhales. The rate of vibration is called the "fundamental frequency" and is perceived as the basic pitch of the cry sound. If the vocal folds work in coordination, they produce a complex, periodic sound, which consists of harmonic components at various multiples of the fundamental frequency. The harmonic that has the greatest amplitude—or loudest sound—is typically called the "dominant frequency." The cry sound that most infants emit when they are least stressed is typically "phonated." A phonated cry has a symmetrical pattern of harmonics and intensity and a fundamental frequency that ranges from 250 to 600 cycles per second, or hertz (Hz). An ordinary cry of an infant has a frequency of about 440 Hz, which would register on the musical scale at about the note A (below middle C).

In contrast, "hyperphonated" cries have an unusually high-pitched sound with a fundamental frequency that ranges from 1,000 to 2,000 Hz or higher. The hyperphonated cry is associated with medical and biological conditions that reflect damage to the nervous system and adversely affect the newborn's ability to regulate his or her level of arousal. A third pattern of cry sound occurs when the infant's vocal folds are overstimulated and work in an uncoordinated manner, again reflecting poor ability to regulate the level of arousal. In the "dysphonated" cry pattern, the lack of coordination of the vocal folds results in an aperiodic (or irregular) sound wave that produces turbulence, which obscures part or all of the harmonics of the basic cry pattern. The dysphonated cry has a raucous sound, as if the infant is angry.

Cries during the first two to three months of life comprise variants of the durational and frequency characteristics described above. Although, as already noted, there are common duration patterns for the so-called hunger and pain cries, contrary to popular notions that specific cry sounds result from discrete causes, such as being wet or tired, there is wide scientific acceptance that the sound of crying at this age reflects a continuum of infant arousal. Research shows that the acoustic characteristics create a graded signal that changes as the level of arousal increases or diminishes. For example, the longer expiratory sounds and pauses of a cry stimulated by pain become increasingly shorter as the discomfort, and consequently the level of arousal, subsides. As the infant is soothed, the characteristics of the pain cry eventually resolve into the moderate durations characteristic of the basic, so-called hunger, cry. Conversely, the moderate durations of expiratory sounds and pauses in the hunger cry become increasingly shorter as the infant's hunger and arousal increase.

The face of crying

While the actual *sound* of crying can communicate the infant's needs across great distances, there are also aspects of crying that serve as a more proximal form of communication. Following the pioneering work of Darwin, others have continued to explore the communicative value of the facial expressions associated with crying. Facial expressions can serve as a warning signal that the infant is about to cry and thus needs to be attended to in a manner that will prevent further distress. The baby's expression immediately before crying usually comprises a grimace, furrowed brows, squinting eyes, and fleeting pout of the lips. Once a full-blown cry has begun, however, the infant's jaws gape open, the lips are pulled back horizontally, and the upper lip is raised across the gums.

In response to audio tapes of infant crying, adults typically show decelerations in heart rate, a sign of attention and concern. When the baby's facial expression is coupled with the sound of crying, however, adults respond with increases in diastolic blood pressure and skin conductance, both of which are indexes of increased autonomic arousal in response to a perceived aversive situation.

Current debates among developmental psychologists center on whether the facial expressions of newborn and young infants communicate discrete emotions such as fear, pain, or sadness. While newborns show discriminable facial expressions to such stimuli as different tastes, the facial expressions associated with crying most likely vary along a continuum of distress, much like the variations in cry sounds. Differences in the degree of distress are seen in the facial expressions during crying of infants with colic (discussed below), and parents' perceptions that greater facial activity is associated with greater distress and pain are usually quite accurate.

How much do infants cry?

In contrast to the relative serenity of the womb, the postnatal environment barrages the infant with a vast array of novel sensory conditions, including changes in illumination, sounds, humidity, and temperature—all of which affect the regulation of the newborn's arousal. Changes in the infant's ability to manage these sensory conditions result in parallel changes in the amount of time the baby cries.

Crying occurs when internal or external conditions, such as hunger or changes in temperature, upset homeostatic balance, resulting in stimulation of the sympathetic nervous system (the part of the regulatory, or autonomic, nervous system that expends energy). In order to restore a more efficient level of metabolic activity, the infant's parasympathetic nervous system (which conserves energy) inhibits the level of arousal, and crying stops.

On average, the newborn cries less than one hour per day. The amount of crying increases to a peak of 2–2½ hours per day at six to eight weeks and then, at about three months of age, typically decreases to one hour. Although this developmental curve is similar across many cultures, the amount of crying varies widely from infant to infant.

As noted above, most infants respond to changes in stimulation with a surge in sympathetic nervous system activity and disruption of homeostatic balance, resulting in a bout of crying. Regaining homeostasis is aided by caregivers' holding, rocking, and softly talking to the infant. Parents may attempt to soothe an infant who is crying because of such overstimulation by vigorous rocking; this, however, is likely to increase the stimulation and thus prolong the bout of crying.

On the other hand, some infants continue to respond to the factors that disrupt homeostasis with a strong parasympathetic surge that suppresses arousal and crying. These infants tend to sleep for long periods and typically are hard to arouse, often startling at changes in sights and sounds. While they may appear to be "easy babies," their lack of crying may actually reflect an inability of the nervous system to incorporate the stimulation that accompanies being awake and alert.

Differences in the amount of crying among infants may also result from the ways they are raised. For example, infants who are breast-fed cry more often than infants who are fed formula from a bottle. Although a traditional view is that breast-fed infants cry more because they tend to be hungrier, studies have suggested that their crying is more likely to result from normal, healthy regulation of arousal, which, in bottle-fed infants, may be suppressed by the nutritional content of formula.

Another important factor that affects the amount of crying is the extent of rhythmic stimulation. Infants who are raised in cultures where they are routinely carried on the mother's body cry less than infants raised in cultures where they are often left in cribs or child seats for relatively long periods of time. Some

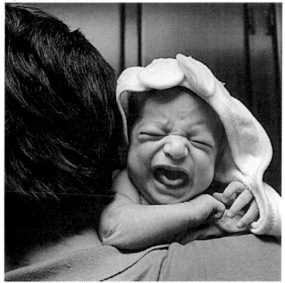

Crying is the newborn's way of communicating. The imploring sound of the cry alerts others to conditions that disrupt the baby's physiological well-being, usually eliciting a response—holding, rocking, comforting—that will restore homeostasis and end the crying.

studies suggest that carrying the infant decreases the amount of crying because the rhythmic motions intrinsic to the carrier's movement provide vestibular stimulation. (The vestibular system contributes to the infant's sense of balance and orientation.) In the absence of other forms of stimulation, infants may provide self-stimulation by crying. One study showed that increasing the amount of time that infants were carried by two hours a day (when they were not crying) decreased crying by as much as an hour.

Interestingly, there has been little systematic research into the effects of giving infants a pacifier to quell their crying. Some pediatricians believe that pacifiers hinder self-regulation and thus cause over-reliance on external sources for relieving arousal and distress. Others believe that pacifiers will lead to "nipple confusion" in breast-fed infants. Neither of these suppositions has been confirmed. On the other hand, giving premature infants pacifiers has actually been shown to provide beneficial stimulation and promote the development of regulatory systems.

Of course, a major concern of parents is what to do when an infant does cry. Many parents are concerned that they will spoil their youngster if they always respond with urgency to cry sounds. Most research shows, however, that rapidly responding to the infant in the first few months of life is actually related to *less* crying over time. Crying during this period is primarily reflexive, and the amelioration of the endogenous causes of crying is thought to be more potent than the possibility that the infant is learning to "manipulate" his or her parents' behavior. For many

infants, simply being held close to the shoulder and gently rocked will provide the perfect combination of the vertical position and rhythmic stimulation. Recent research also suggests that giving a crying infant 0.1 milliliter (a drop) of a 14% sucrose solution (sugar and water) may stop a sustained bout of crying for up to five minutes. One hypothesis currently being tested is that such a sucrose solution calms infants by activating the production of natural opioids in the brain.

Excessive crying: is it colic?

Sometimes excessive crying is considered a clinical syndrome, known as infant colic. While there is no universally accepted definition for this well-known condition, it is often defined by the "rule of threes"—in which infants show paroxysms of extreme fussing and crying lasting for a total of more than three hours a day, at least three days a week, for at least three weeks. The cry sound tends to be piercing and monotonal, and the infant is usually unresponsive to any soothing. Some clinicians believe that colic is gastrointestinal in origin and reflects intestinal distress (often excessive gas) resulting from an immature digestive system. Others believe that cases of excessive crying may be a normal response to the kinds of stimulation to which infants must adapt. Although the distinction between colic and excessive crying remains unclear, colic is one of the most commonly diagnosed pediatric conditions in the United States and other Western countries, with estimates of about 700,000 cases a year in the U.S. alone.

Parents are usually very alarmed by excessive crying; they are often concerned that their infants are suffering from some sort of pain. Sometimes they are right, but other times they may overreact. Knowing what to do when their baby seemingly cries unceasingly can be very difficult. Parents need to develop an appropriate strategy, but different approaches must be tailored to the individual situation.

Parents often complain that excessive crying causes *them* to suffer from a lack of sleep, that it increases their level of frustration and general irritability, and that it causes family disruption. They also report that the sound associated with excessive crying is unusually aversive. In the past few years researchers have found that the distinctive cries of infants with presumed colic in fact have a higher fundamental frequency, a higher-pitched and louder dominant frequency, and/or greater proportions of dysphonation than cries of noncolicky babies. These findings provide an objective basis for why parents experience these cries as so distressing.

Cries as a diagnostic aid

Recognition of the potential for the sound of infant crying to communicate important information about the health and well-being of an infant has a long history—dating as far back as Hippocrates. In the past three decades or so, listening for abnormalities in the cry sound has become a formal part of the standard pediatric examination. In the early 1960s physicians and psychologists began to systematically study differences in the cry patterns in a wide range of disorders that were known to affect the integrity of the infant nervous system. These early studies showed that in infants with various forms of neurological dysfunction, (1) sustained cries were delayed or slow to be elicited, (2) overall bouts of crying were relatively short, and (3) the sound itself had an abnormal fundamental frequency. Infants with Down syndrome, for example, were found to have a hoarse cry with a low fundamental frequency, averaging about 250–300 Hz. Most adverse biomedical conditions, however, are characterized by the presence of hyperphonated cry sounds. Thus, newborns with hyperbilirubinemia (severe jaundice), bacterial meningitis, encephalitis, and birth asphyxia as well as preterm and low-birth-weight infants typically have high-pitched cries. These hyperphonated cry sounds are in fact so distinctive that one genetically caused form of brain damage is called *cri du chat* ("cry of the cat"), on the basis of the characteristic high pitch of the cry.

More recently, studies have shown that crying can provide crucial information about the neurological health of the infant in the *absence* of other abnormal clinical signs. Neonates whose births are marked by a high number of obstetric difficulties, for example, are more likely to show signs of nervous system damage later in infancy than are babies who have normal, uncomplicated births. In extreme cases the damage may have fatal consequences. Importantly, these infants show no abnormal signs on routine physical and neurological examinations at birth.

Now, however, infants who may be at such risk can be distinguished at or soon after birth by specific measures of their crying. Even when only one or two days old, these seemingly healthy infants manifest the same characteristics in their crying that early researchers noted in youngsters with neurological damage—*i.e.,* a higher-than-normal threshold for elicitation of a sustained cry, shorter-than-normal overall bouts of crying, and a distinctive cry sound that is short and hyperphonated. Several studies have shown that these particular cry features occur in infants with a subtle form of prenatal malnutrition that adversely affects the developing nervous system. This condition may result from poor prenatal care, maternal metabolic disturbances, or such common practices as mothers' smoking cigarettes, drinking alcohol, or consuming inadequate amounts of protein during pregnancy. While the subclinical effects of this condition often go undetected, these infants are at risk of developing problems that range from early death to exceptionally poor intellectual and social development.

The ability to detect damage to the developing nervous system from early crying behavior has led researchers to investigate the potential subclinical effects of the mother's use of toxic substances. For example, it has been shown that women who smoke marijuana during pregnancy, even in very small amounts, may cause damage to their developing fetus, but at birth this damage often goes undetected. Even though infants whose mothers smoked marijuana may be born at full term, have a normal birth weight, and be considered healthy by routine postnatal examinations, these babies may exhibit cries with a shorter duration, an increased amount of dysphonation, and a higher and more variable fundamental frequency than infants whose mothers did not use marijuana during their pregnancies.

The analysis of crying has also helped clarify some apparently inconsistent effects of prenatal cocaine exposure. Some infants so exposed seem overly "excitable," while others are found to be "depressed." Cry analysis has shown that the easily excited infants have cries that are of longer duration and that have a higher fundamental frequency, whereas depressed infants' cries have longer latencies and greater amounts of dysphonation. Using complex statistical models, researchers have been able to determine that the former measures are directly related to the neurotoxic effects of cocaine, while the latter measures are related to signs of intrauterine growth retardation, which is an indirect effect of cocaine on fetal growth. The significance of these findings is that they reflect the functional state of the infant's brain stem and autonomic nervous system.

Measuring infant crying in the absence of other abnormal signs may have important ramifications for many other prenatal conditions that have previously been thought to be inconsequential. For example, infants whose mothers drink alcohol during pregnancy may not show any of the severe physical signs of fetal alcohol syndrome—a group of congenital abnormalities ranging from distinctive facial features, malformed joints and limbs, and upper airway and cardiac defects to mental retardation. In the absence of such signs, many physicians have advised that small amounts of alcohol can be safely consumed by women during their pregnancies. A recent study suggests that cry analysis at birth may prove to be a way to detect adverse effects of prenatal exposure to even small amounts of alcohol—effects that may become manifest later.

Because the brain stem and autonomic nervous system are responsible for the integration of many sensory-motor functions, including the acoustic characteristics of crying, abnormal variations in the cry sound may be highly related to other "soft" signs of neurological insult—*e.g.,* lack of alertness and inability to integrate sights and sounds or demonstrate smooth motor coordination. Infants with abnormal thresholds for crying also have problems regulating their level of arousal in a way that may be seen in unpredictable sleeping patterns, digestive disturbances, and difficult temperaments. The combination of these reduced capabilities detrimentally affects the infant's interactions with parents and his or her capacity to learn. Consequently, the analysis of crying can be predictive of an infant's subsequent social and intellectual development. In one study, for example, the fundamental frequency of newborns' cries was found to be highly predictive of their mental and physical development during the first two years of life and of their cognitive skills at age five.

One condition whose causes have long eluded physicians and that might be predicted by early crying patterns is sudden infant death syndrome (SIDS). SIDS is characterized by the sudden and inexplicable death of a seemingly healthy infant during the first year of life. SIDS incidence peaks between three and six months of life. In the United States, where there are approximately 5,400 cases each year, SIDS is the leading cause of death of infants between the ages of one month and one year. While there are many possible causes of SIDS, abnormal brain stem development appears to be a common finding. Over the years a number of studies of infants who died suddenly have shown that their cries as newborns were marked by hyperphonation. One large study used very detailed spectral analysis of the cries of 24,000 normal, full-term newborns to predict which infants might later succumb to SIDS. The frequency characteristics of the cries, including the number of times within a single cry segment the sound changed its acoustic structure, from phonated to hyperphonated, correctly predicted approximately half of the infants who later died suddenly. False-positive predictions—*i.e.,* the cry suggested that the infant was at risk, but the infant did not die during the first year—occurred in only 3% of cases. The study found that infants were 32 times more likely to die of SIDS if they had these abnormal cry features than if they did not.

Parental responses: the best and the worst

As previously indicated, variations in the fundamental frequency of crying not only reflect the biological condition of the infant but have a significant impact on the parents' response: as a baby's cry increases in pitch, so does the urgency parents feel to respond. Humans are generally more responsive to higher-pitched sounds, especially those above 800 Hz; sounds that reach the 2,000-Hz level have been shown to increase the production of urinary corticosteroid, a physiological indicator of stress. Studies have shown that both men and women experience high levels of stress when they hear the hyperphonated cries of infants. Physiological reactions may include increases

in muscle tension, blood pressure, and breathing and heart rates. Across cultures, mothers find the high-pitched cry sounds of their infants more arousing than phonated cries, and both mothers and fathers indicate that they are more likely to react to hyperphonated cries with behaviors that would immediately terminate the noxious cry sound.

The arousing effects of such cries can be a two-edged sword. In most cases the distinctive hyperphonated cry sound, which typically shifts in and out of a falsetto screech, leads to the perception that the infant is unwell. Even young adults with no children of their own perceive the sound of a hyperphonated cry as a signal for special nurturing care. As a biological siren, hyperphonation alerts parents to attend to the immediate needs of their infant, usually by picking the child up and cuddling and comforting him or her, thereby providing the kinds of social and vestibular stimulation that restore homeostasis. The adult's response to the cry thus is usually beneficial to the baby's health and well-being.

The other edge of the sword, however, may be particularly sharp. In some cases parents become so irritated by the noxious and oppressive sound of hyperphonated cries that they withdraw from their infants both emotionally and physically. Studies show that these parents do not play with and talk to their newborns. Such neglect can have profound consequences. Without the social interaction and other forms of stimulation that attentive parents provide, the child's social and mental development suffers. Moreover, because these infants are typically frustrating and unrewarding, parents become even more likely to withhold stimulation and attention over time. Such neglect may further stifle the infants' intellectual and social development—even beyond that caused by any neurological problems.

In extreme cases parents may react to the aversive sound of the cry by physically abusing the infant. Abusive parents tend to complain that their infants' excessive and unquellable wailing became intolerable and that this ultimately led to their abusive acts. Recent investigations have shown that parents who abuse their infants in fact have a lower physiological tolerance to cry sounds than do other parents, as indicated by measures of muscle tension, blood pressure, and breathing and heart rates.

Of course, all parents have the ultimate responsibility of nurturing and providing loving care for their children—and *not* resorting to abuse—no matter how irritating a child's crying may be. However, in some sad cases, personality characteristics of the parents make them unable to cope with infants whose only way of communicating is to cry, and this unfortunate circumstance may have the worst consequences on these infants' health and development.

Congestive Heart Failure

by Marc K. Effron, M.D.

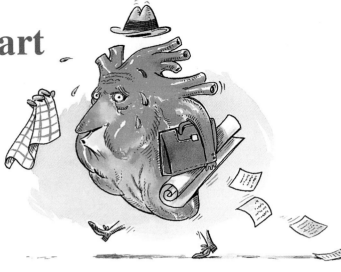

The heart is a remarkable organ. Each day the human body depends upon this powerful muscle to pump approximately 7,600 liters (2,000 gal) of blood rich in oxygen and vital nutrients to meet the metabolic needs of its diverse organs, muscles, and tissues. Congestive heart failure is a serious medical condition resulting from the inability, or failure, of the heart to adequately pump blood through the circulation. The symptoms result directly from this ineffective pumping action as well as from a panoply of secondary changes that occur throughout the body. When the heart is not doing its job effectively, the circulatory system gets backed up, causing the lungs and peripheral tissues as well as the heart itself to become *congested* with fluid. Patients may complain of fatigue, shortness of breath, and swelling (edema) of the feet and legs.

Congestive heart failure is an unfortunately common illness with major social and economic consequences. Both men and women are affected, although the proportion of male patients is larger. In the United States alone there are over 2.5 million sufferers including 3 to 5% of the population aged 65 years and over. Their illness leads to approximately one million hospitalizations each year. There is a 50% chance of dying during the first five years after the onset; in severe cases mortality is over 50% in the first year.

Multiple causes

A variety of injurious processes can cause the heart to fail. In industrialized countries coronary artery disease is the major cause. In less developed regions of the world with less access to modern medicine, rheumatic fever leading to heart valve damage continues to add many new cases of heart failure each year. In the majority of cases, congestive heart failure involves an impaired ability of the heart's left ventricle to contract and eject blood, known as systolic dysfunction.

Myocardial infarction. In the U.S. and most industrialized societies, myocardial infarction (heart attack) is the single most frequent cause of congestive heart failure. A heart attack occurs when a blood clot forms in a coronary artery at the site of a cholesterol-laden plaque. This obstructs the flow of blood to part of the ventricular muscle, and permanent damage ensues. Although there is a risk of death with this acute event, most patients survive an initial myocardial infarction, the area of damage forming a ventricular scar. If the injury is sufficiently large, congestive heart failure appears quite early. In other cases the symptoms of heart failure may appear years later as the remaining heart muscle gradually fatigues and is unable to compensate for the damaged segment.

Heart failure due to myocardial infarction is a late manifestation of coronary artery disease. Elevated blood cholesterol, hypertension (high blood pressure), diabetes, cigarette use, and familial factors can all set the stage for the chronic process of atherosclerosis, in which the buildup of cholesterol and proliferating cells over many years creates obstruction in the wall of a coronary artery.

Hypertension. Chronic high blood pressure subjects the heart to an excessive workload; the higher the blood pressure, the harder the heart must work to pump the blood. The left ventricle initially hypertrophies (thickens) to permit the forward pumping of blood against the increased resistance. However, this hypertrophy can make the ventricle too stiff and not allow adequate relaxation of the chamber for passive filling, a condition known as diastolic dysfunction. Later in the disease process, the left ventricle may dilate and fail in its forward pumping action as well (systolic dysfunction). Early detection and treatment of hypertension prevent this type of congestive heart failure.

Valvular disease. Malfunction of one or more of the heart's valves is another common cause of congestive heart failure. Valves malfunction by becoming stenotic (too narrow) or regurgitant (leaking backward), or they display a combination of both defects. Stenosis of a

437

valve obstructs the forward flow of blood, elevates the pressure in the chamber behind the valve, and eventually exhausts the heart's ability to eject blood forward. Valvular regurgitation reduces the effective output of the heart, as a portion of the ejected blood leaks back across the valve and into the chamber. In an effort to compensate for such a leak, the chamber enlarges and ejects greater and greater volumes of blood until the heart muscle is overly dilated and fatigued.

Rheumatic heart disease remains common in populations lacking adequate public health programs and ready access to antibiotics. Rheumatic fever is initiated by a streptococcal sore throat. A past infection extensively scars and distorts the cardiac valves. The mitral valve is the most commonly affected, followed in order of susceptibility by the aortic, tricuspid, and pulmonary valves.

There are many other causes of valvular disease. These include: a congenital defect of a valve that causes the heart to fail in infancy or much later in life; infective endocarditis, a serious bacterial infection that destroys portions of the valve tissue; spontaneous rupture of the supportive chords of the mitral valve, which causes acute regurgitation; and, in the elderly, degeneration of the aortic valve leaflets resulting from fibrosis (fibrous tissue buildup) and calcium deposition, which eventually leads to aortic valve stenosis.

Cardiomyopathy. Diffuse deterioration of the cardiac muscle is known as cardiomyopathy. The condition can result from exposure to certain toxins. Chronic consumption of alcohol leads to cardiomyopathy and is an important cause of congestive heart failure; if detected at an early stage, the condition may improve with abstention. Anthracycline drugs used in cancer chemotherapy injure the myocardial cells in a cumulative manner; in some patients the amount and dosage of chemotherapeutic drugs that can be tolerated may be limited by this toxic effect.

Although genetic and environmental factors are occasionally implicated, most cases of cardiomyopathy are idiopathic (without an identifiable cause). A patient typically complains of congestive heart failure symptoms; when he or she is examined by a physician, the left ventricle is found to be dilated and very weak.

Myocarditis. Viral infection of the heart muscle, known as viral myocarditis, is a sporadically occurring but fulminant (coming on suddenly with great severity) cause of heart failure. Patients may recover fully or be left with a chronically impaired left ventricle that is indistinguishable from that of idiopathic cardiomyopathy. In South America, Chagas' disease, a parasitic infection of the myocardium transmitted by an insect vector, is a major cause of heart failure.

Right heart failure. When the heart's right ventricle fails, it is usually secondary to the stress imposed by left ventricular failure. Cases of isolated right ventricular failure are much less common, occurring in

patients with chronic lung disease, pulmonary emboli (blood clots), certain congenital heart defects, or primary disease of the pulmonary arteries. The condition is provoked by high blood pressure in the lungs (pulmonary hypertension). In some cases acute right heart failure is the result of a heart attack in the right ventricle (right ventricular infarction).

Other causes. For some patients heart failure is provoked by use of medication with a myocardial depressant effect. Beta-blocking drugs and the calcium channel antagonist verapamil are effective treatments for hypertension and angina but can induce congestive heart failure if there is a preceding abnormality of ventricular function. Heart function returns to normal when the culprit medication is withdrawn.

Occasionally, a very slow or very fast heart rate provokes congestive failure. Treatment of the abnormal rhythm often successfully treats the failure.

The disease process

This discussion of the disease process, or pathophysiological mechanisms, in congestive heart failure pertains primarily to heart failure caused by systolic dysfunction, or impaired contractility of the left ventricle. The term *inotropy* refers to the state of myocardial contractility. A positive inotropic effect is one that enhances the power of cardiac contraction; a negative inotropic effect depresses contraction.

Calcium plays a central role in the contractile action of heart muscle. Normally, calcium ions are stored in the sacroplasmic reticulum, specialized compartments of the myocardial cells, until the heart muscle receives a signal to contract. The calcium then rushes to the myofilaments—the key contractile elements of the heart muscle cells—and facilitates the biochemical steps of muscle contraction.

When the heart's left ventricle is dysfunctional, various mechanisms—hemodynamic (relating to the blood circulation), neurological, hormonal, and renal—are activated to compensate for a loss of functioning myocardial cells and to maintain an adequate cardiac output. However, these same mechanisms later lose their effectiveness or even worsen the condition.

Compensatory changes. When the left ventricle cannot eject blood effectively, there is an increase in wall tension as the chamber becomes dilated and overfilled during its filling stage. The remaining myocardial cells contract with increased vigor, a positive inotropic response. This action is known as the Frank-Starling mechanism (after the physiologists Otto Frank and Ernest Starling, who accounted for these changes in 1918). The biochemical basis of the mechanism appears to be an augmented sensitivity of the myofilaments to calcium.

Diminished cardiac output is detected by specialized sensors in the aorta and carotid arteries, which send a signal to the central nervous system. The sympathetic nervous system is then activated. Myo-cardial cell receptors for adrenaline (beta-adrenergic receptors) are stimulated by direct sympathetic nerve pathways to the heart and an increase in circulating adrenaline. This boosts calcium delivery to the myofilaments. Beta-adrenergic stimulation drives the heart to beat faster and exerts a strong positive inotropic effect.

These compensatory steps ironically add to the workload of an already weak left ventricle. Cardiac work increases with chamber dilation and elevated wall stress. Sympathetic nerve activation also stimulates the body's alpha-adrenergic receptors, leading to constriction of the veins and arteries. An increase in venous tone reduces the reservoir-like capacity of the veins and overfills the heart. An increase in tone of the peripheral arterioles (tiny branches of arteries that terminate in the capillaries) raises resistance to the forward ejection of blood from the heart.

Other counterbalancing steps then come into play. In response to increased ventricular wall stress, more muscle protein is synthesized. The wall thickens, and the stress is distributed to more muscle tissue. New contractile proteins are synthesized, which increase energy efficiency. So-called stretch receptors in the atria send an inhibitory signal to the sympathetic nervous system. The neurohormonal substance atrial natriuretic peptide is secreted into the bloodstream and counters excessive sympathetic stimulation and also promotes excretion of sodium by the kidneys, countering the expansion of blood volume that accompanies dilation of the ventricle.

Loss of compensatory balance: a vicious cycle ensues. These hemodynamic and neurohormonal changes facilitate adequate pump function early in the course of left ventricular disease, but this balance cannot be maintained indefinitely. In time, the beneficial effects are lost, as there is a limit to the heart's ability to favorably alter its structure and contraction. Consequently, the body becomes less responsive to certain neurohormonal signals. It is at this stage that clinically overt congestive heart failure intervenes.

Sustained ventricular wall stress eventually causes loss of myocardial cells, leaving the chamber wall thinned and fibrotic (composed of fibrous tissue). With

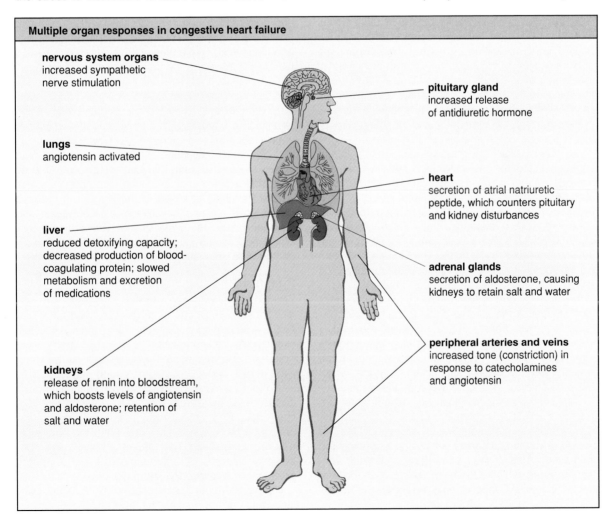

Multiple organ responses in congestive heart failure

nervous system organs
increased sympathetic
nerve stimulation

lungs
angiotensin activated

liver
reduced detoxifying capacity;
decreased production of blood-
coagulating protein; slowed
metabolism and excretion
of medications

kidneys
release of renin into bloodstream,
which boosts levels of angiotensin
and aldosterone; retention of
salt and water

pituitary gland
increased release
of antidiuretic hormone

heart
secretion of atrial natriuretic
peptide, which counters pituitary
and kidney disturbances

adrenal glands
secretion of aldosterone, causing
kidneys to retain salt and water

peripheral arteries and veins
increased tone (constriction) in
response to catecholamines
and angiotensin

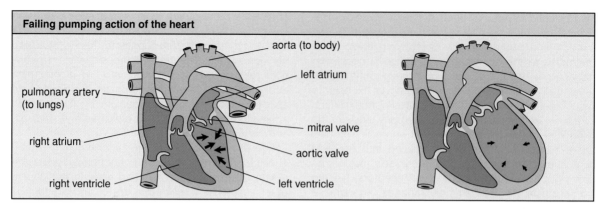

(Left) Normally the heart's left ventricle ejects 60–70% of its blood volume forward with every beat. In congestive heart failure (right) this pumping action of the heart is reduced, and the dilated and thin-walled left ventricle ejects less than 40%, and in some cases as little as 15%, of its contents.

the loss of compensatory changes, atrial natriuretic peptide becomes depleted, and the body becomes resistant to what limited amounts are still released into the circulation. Vasoconstricting hormones now act without opposition, further increasing wall stress.

As this vicious cycle continues, the ventricle dilates more and more and its inotropic state further deteriorates. The Frank-Starling mechanism cannot continue at extremes of ventricular distension, so the heart no longer responds to increases in chamber volume with increases in contractility. The failing ventricle loses its positive inotropic response to sympathetic nervous system activity—the ventricular beta-adrenergic receptors becoming less numerous and effective.

As heart failure progresses, the body's renin-angiotensin system is activated. The sympathetic nervous system provokes the release of the neurohormonal substance renin from the kidneys; renin facilitates the activation of angiotensin, a potent vasoconstrictor (*i.e.,* a substance that induces narrowing of blood vessels). Angiotensin exerts its effect on peripheral arterioles; it also alters the kidneys' ability to handle sodium and water. This renal action is of pivotal importance, causing sodium to be reabsorbed in the kidney tubules and retained in the body. Angiotensin then stimulates the adrenal gland to secrete aldosterone, a steroid hormone that regulates the body's sodium-water balance, thus enhancing the kidney's retention of sodium. Angiotensin also stimulates the pituitary gland to release antidiuretic hormone, which further promotes retention of water by the kidneys.

The excessive accumulation of salt and water becomes manifest as congestion of the lungs and peripheral tissues. Left-sided heart failure elevates the pressure in the pulmonary veins and congests the lung tissue. This is often followed by right-sided ventricular failure, which elevates the pressure in the systemic veins and congests both the lower extremities and the internal (visceral) organs.

At this stage the lungs become stiffer and their expansion more difficult. Consequently, the work of breathing increases. Fluid in the alveoli (air sacs) and lung tissue limits the transport of oxygen from inspired air into the bloodstream. Shortness of breath and falling blood oxygen levels ensue. Fluid may also accumulate in the pleural space between the lungs and chest wall. These pleural effusions further restrict the lung volume and the patient's ability to breathe.

The liver, too, is affected. It becomes distended and cannot carry out its usual functions. It is less able to detoxify body "poisons" and produces less of the protein that enables blood coagulation. Medications are metabolized and excreted at a slower rate.

In the most advanced stage of congestive heart failure, the cardiac output is exceedingly low. Despite tremendous vasoconstriction, the blood pressure also is low. Perfusion of blood to the kidneys is reduced to the point where renal filtration is inadequate and chemicals from the urine accumulate in the blood. Blood flow to the brain is also reduced, and brain centers that control respiration begin to malfunction.

Symptoms

Fatigue and shortness of breath (dyspnea) are usually the first symptoms of congestive heart failure. At first, dyspnea may occur only during heavy physical exertion. As the congestive heart failure progresses, however, dyspnea occurs with minimal activity and even at rest, and a bothersome cough may appear.

At night so-called paroxysmal nocturnal dyspnea, a sudden awakening from sleep with difficult breathing, may occur. This is caused by a shift of fluid from the peripheral tissues into the lungs when the body is in a horizontal position. The patient generally prefers to sit up or stand up during this distress, as the upright position helps relieve the shortness of breath.

Congestive heart failure causes the feet and lower legs to become swollen. This lower-extremity edema

440

recedes slightly overnight, but fluid again accumulates in the feet and legs when the patient is upright during the day. With severe retention of fluid, the abdomen swells as well.

Extensive lung congestion (pulmonary edema) may develop suddenly and cause severe respiratory distress. The patient typically coughs up copious amounts of frothy sputum, which in some cases may be tinged pink with blood.

In advanced congestive heart failure, when cardiac output is extremely low, there is muscle wasting and loss of appetite, strength, and energy. Ultimately, the patient's mental alertness and cognitive functioning are hampered, and ambition and drive wane.

Diagnosis

There are several steps in the diagnosis of congestive heart failure. The physician starts by obtaining a detailed medical history. The patient may describe a particular pattern of dyspnea that specifically suggests the cause of his or her complaints. The symptom pattern is all the more important when abnormal physical findings are not present or obvious at the time of initial evaluation.

The doctor will check the pulse and respiratory rate; these may be elevated, particularly when pulmonary congestion is severe. Listening to the lungs with a stethoscope may detect rales, crackling sounds characteristic of excess lung fluid.

An exaggerated cardiac impulse is both seen and felt at the overlying chest wall. Auscultation (listening to the heart with a stethoscope) may reveal an abnormal heart sound known as a gallop. If there is underlying valvular disease, heart murmurs can be heard as well.

Palpation of the abdomen may reveal a distended and tender liver. There may also be signs of excess fluid in the abdomen. The lower-extremity edema typically results in "pitting"; the skin over the affected areas readily yields to finger pressure, leaving a temporary depression, or "pit."

Tests that are likely to be done in the diagnostic process are an electrocardiogram and a chest radiograph (X-ray). The electrocardiogram can give clues to the underlying cause of congestive heart failure. It can show evidence of myocardial infarction as well as ventricular enlargement or hypertrophy. The chest radiograph reveals an enlarged heart, congestion of the pulmonary veins, and excess fluid in the lungs and pleural space.

Echocardiography, which uses high-frequency sound to create a sonar image of the heart, enables the cardiologist to view the size and contractility of the heart's chambers. The echocardiographic image also shows the state of the heart's valves; Doppler ultrasound is then used to measure the abnormal blood flow at stenotic or regurgitant valves.

A detailed and invasive test that may be performed is cardiac catheterization, requiring the threading of narrow catheters from the femoral vessels of the thigh up into the heart. Such testing is usually not needed for the basic diagnosis of heart failure but is used in some cases to find the underlying cause. It is also used to measure and confirm the extent of valvular dysfunction if surgery is contemplated.

Treatment

Like the diagnosis, the treatment of congestive heart failure is individualized, depending on the extent and chronicity of the illness. A number of measures may be used; the doctor will determine which are appropriate. In general, therapy is aimed at reducing the workload of the heart, increasing the heart's ability to contract, and decreasing the amount of salt and water the body retains.

Diet. The diet for patients with congestive heart failure must be very low in sodium because the body will attempt to retain any sodium that is consumed. Two grams (2,000 mg) of sodium is a reasonable daily limit. Salt should not be added to food in its preparation or at the table. It is best to prepare foods using fresh and pure ingredients rather than relying on factory-processed foods—unless a low-sodium content is specified on a product label. (As of May 1994, all prepackaged foods sold in the U.S. must display their sodium content on the label. "Sodium-free" or "salt-free" will refer to foods having less than 5 mg of sodium per serving, "very low sodium" to foods containing 35 mg of sodium or less per serving, and "low sodium" to foods having no more than 140 mg.) Table 1 provides the sodium content in selected food items.

With careful salt restriction, there is usually no need to limit the intake of water. Restriction of fluid intake is more difficult for the patient than limitations on sodium and can compromise nutrition. Nevertheless, in severe cases a patient may be asked to limit daily fluid consumption temporarily or permanently.

Pharmacological therapy. Therapeutic drugs (*see* Table 2) are the mainstay of treatment for most patients with heart failure. These medicines are grouped into three main classes: diuretics, inotropes, and vasodilators. Drugs within each class show individual patterns of absorption, metabolism, and duration of action and may have different side effects.

Diuretics. The diuretics are usually the first drugs used to treat newly diagnosed congestive heart failure. They act directly on the kidneys to reverse the process of sodium and water retention. The urinary excretion of salt and water (diuresis) draws the excess fluid out of the lungs and peripheral tissues and reduces the blood volume. A lower blood volume decreases ventricular wall stress.

Most diuretics deplete the body of potassium as well. The potassium lost in the urine must be re-

Table 1. Sodium in selected foods		
	amount	sodium (mg)
cooked cereal, rice, pasta (unsalted)	½ c	trace
ready-to-eat cereal		
corn flakes	1 oz	250
shredded wheat	1 oz	trace
bread	1 slice	varies
most vegetables (fresh or frozen, no salt)	½ c	less than 70
vegetables (canned, frozen with sauce)	½ c	140–460
tomato juice (canned)	¾ c	660
vegetable soup (canned)	1 c	820
fruit (fresh, frozen, canned)	½ c	trace
milk	1 c	120
yogurt	1 c	160
processed cheese (American)	1 oz	405
mozzarella cheese (part skim)	1 oz	130
Parmesan cheese (grated)	1 tbs	95
fresh meat, poultry, fish	3 oz	less than 90
tuna (canned, water-packed)	3 oz	300
bologna	2 oz	580
ham (lean, baked)	3 oz	1,020
Italian salad dressing (store-bought)	1 tbs	115–370
vinaigrette dressing (homemade, no salt)	1 tbs	trace
catsup, mustard	1 tbs	180
soy sauce	1 tbs	1,030
salt	1 tsp	2,000
dill pickle	1 medium	930
mixed nuts (dry roasted)	1 oz	trace
mixed nuts (dry roasted, salted)	1 oz	190

placed so that hypokalemia (low serum potassium) can be avoided. Severe hypokalemia causes muscle weakness and potentially life-threatening heart rhythm abnormalities. Although potassium stores can be bolstered by intake of potassium-rich foods, such as bananas and raisins, most patients taking diuretics require regular doses of concentrated supplemental potassium. This dietary supplement, either a liquid or a pill, is formulated for delayed release in order to prevent irritation of the stomach and intestines.

The "loop" diuretics, furosemide and bumetanide, are the major diuretics used to treat congestive heart failure. They are known as loop diuretics because they inhibit resorption of sodium and water at a specific site (the loop of Henle) along the kidney tubules. These agents have a prompt and potent diuretic action. Patients with uncontrolled or recent-onset heart failure sometimes receive a drug orally; for faster action the drug may be given intravenously. The ensuing diuresis can quickly relieve symptoms of pulmonary congestion. Once stabilized, patients take furosemide or bumetanide orally on a daily basis to prevent reaccumulation of salt and water.

The beneficial effects of furosemide and bumetanide must be balanced against the potential for overdiuresis and dehydration. Elderly patients are particularly susceptible to these complications. Excessive reduction of the blood volume may cause low blood pressure and compromise the function of the kidneys. Long-term therapy may result in hyponatremia (low serum sodium), which, if severe, leads to delirium, seizures, and coma. Magnesium depletion also can occur, causing disturbances of the heart rhythm. In order to prevent these potential side effects, it is important that blood pressure, renal function, and electrolytes be closely monitored on a regular basis.

The distal tube diuretics constitute the other important group of diuretic drugs used for heart failure. Hydrochlorothiazide and metolazone are among the most commonly used, but there are many other drugs in this group as well. They act at the distal convoluted segment of the kidney tubules, where they promote diuresis by interfering with the resorption of sodium and chloride. These diuretics are less potent than the loop diuretics and can lose their effectiveness with chronic use. They are best used in combination with loop diuretics when an additive effect is needed.

Inotropic drugs. Plant derivatives known as cardiac glycosides are among the oldest drugs used in medicine. The 18th-century English physician William Withering studied the popular folk remedy for dropsy (edema). He discovered that an extract of the foxglove plant, *Digitalis purpurea,* had a beneficial effect on dropsy; this had been suggested to him by an old Shropshire woman who used the concoction herself. In 1785 Withering published his famous account of the trials he conducted with foxglove. The modern drug purified from digitalis, digoxin, is the most commonly used cardiac glycoside, and it continues to play a major role in the treatment of congestive heart failure.

As an inotropic agent, digoxin augments the force of contraction of the diseased ventricle. The molecular basis of the digoxin effect originates at the surface membrane of the myocardial cells. Digoxin alters the balance of sodium and potassium across the cells' surface and forces a shift of calcium into the myofibrils. A boost in muscle fiber contraction follows, resulting in greater force of the ventricular chambers. Whereas digoxin does not appreciably increase the output of a normal heart, the weak and failing heart may be significantly aided by this positive inotropic action.

The initial oral or intravenous dose (loading dose) of digoxin is determined by the patient's body mass. The drug is then distributed throughout various body tissues. Because digoxin is eliminated from the body primarily via the kidneys, patients with renal failure should receive lower doses in order to prevent high concentrations of the drug from building up in the bloodstream and tissues of the body.

Despite its well-recognized benefit, digoxin is a potentially dangerous substance. A narrow margin of safety exists between therapeutic doses and toxic amounts. Digoxin toxicity is manifested by loss of appetite, nausea, vomiting, mental confusion, disturbances of vision, and seriously abnormal rhythms of the heart (either extremely fast or extremely slow). Elderly patients and those with renal failure or potassium depletion are particularly prone to these toxic effects. Certain other drugs, such as the antiarrhythmic drug quinidine, can impair the elimination of digoxin from the body, causing a toxic accumulation. Even if an effective and safe dose is established for an individual patient, subsequent changes in gastrointestinal absorption or in renal function may precipitate digoxin toxicity. Regular measurement of a patient's serum digoxin level enables the physician to adjust the dose and avoid such a toxic level.

Other inotropic drugs, administered intravenously, stimulate the beta-adrenergic receptors of the heart, providing a powerful inotropic effect. Dopamine and dobutamine (sympathomimetic amines) are used for this purpose in severely ill patients. They supply short-term support and may be used as a temporary treatment to permit recovery of cardiac function or transition to oral medication.

Dopamine is used in cases of acute low cardiac output (known as cardiogenic shock) in patients who have survived an extensive heart attack. At its upper dose range, dopamine also stimulates the alpha-adrenergic receptors, which leads to constriction of arterioles and thereby helps support the blood pressure. High-dose infusion of the beta-adrenergic drugs requires close monitoring of heart rate, blood pressure, and cardiac rhythm.

The so-called phosphodiesterase inhibitors constitute another group of positive inotropes. In the U.S. amrinone and milrinone are drugs of this class that are currently available. By inhibiting activity of the enzyme phosphodiesterase, these agents raise the intracellular levels of cyclic adenosine monophosphate, which in turn stimulates contractility of the heart muscle. Use of both drugs is currently limited to short-term intravenous treatment of severely ill patients. Orally administered phosphodiesterase-inhibitor therapy has not been shown to yield sustained benefits, and one long-term study revealed an increased mortality for patients treated with oral milrinone.

Research efforts are currently under way to develop new inotropic drugs. A promising candidate is vesnarinone (OPC-8212), which potentiates cardiac contraction by altering the flux of sodium and potassium across the myocardial cell membranes. In two research trials the agent reduced symptoms, improved cardiac function, and increased survival in patients with chronic heart failure.

Vasodilators. The advent of vasodilator therapy has significantly altered the treatment of congestive heart failure over the last two decades. Whereas previous treatments directly targeted either the weak heart mus-

drug class	common examples	form	side effects
diuretics			
loop	furosemide bumetanide	oral or intravenous	potassium depletion
distal tube	hydrochlorothiazide metolazone	oral or intravenous oral	potassium depletion potassium depletion
positive inotropes			
digitalis glycosides	digoxin	oral or intravenous	cardiac and gastrointestinal toxicities
beta-adrenergic agents	dobutamine dopamine	intravenous	arrhythmias
phosphodiesterase inhibitors	amrinone milrinone	intravenous	decreased survival if used long term
direct vasodilators	nitroprusside flosequinan	intravenous oral	cyanide toxicity low blood pressure
neurohormonal agents with vasodilator action angiotensin-converting enzyme inhibitors	enalapril catopril	oral	low blood pressure, kidney dysfunction, and cough

Table 2. **Drugs for congestive heart failure**

cle (positive inotropes) or the retained fluid (diuretics), vasodilator drugs act at the peripheral blood vessels to interrupt the severe peripheral vasoconstriction that overloads the heart. This approach recognizes that congestive heart failure is a systemic condition. Since it results from an interplay of cardiac and peripheral changes, reversing the peripheral changes can help the performance of the heart.

Vasodilators relax the smooth muscle cells in the walls of veins and arterioles. Vasodilator treatment increases venous capacity, which shifts the blood volume away from the overfilled heart chambers. Arterial resistance decreases, enabling the left ventricle to pump the blood forward more efficiently.

The vasodilator nitroprusside sustains cardiac output in the most severe stages of congestive heart failure, acting on both veins and arteries. Because this potent form of therapy must be given intravenously by continuous infusion and requires careful monitoring of the blood pressure, it is reserved for critically ill patients. If cardiac function has deteriorated to a state of shock, nitroprusside can be used in conjunction with dopamine or dobutamine.

Flosequinan, an orally administered vasodilator that was approved for use in the U.S. in 1993, directly dilates both veins and arteries and provides sustained cardiac output and exercise capacity improvement. Its long-term effect on survival requires further study.

The most effective oral agents with a vasodilator action are the angiotensin-converting enzyme (ACE) inhibitors. In recent years the prospect of prolonging life with ACE inhibitor drugs has moved this class of drugs to the forefront of congestive heart failure therapy. ACE inhibitors block the activation of angiotensin. Less activated angiotensin leads to less vascular tone. The high degree of effectiveness of these drugs may also be due to their ability to attenuate the diverse neurohormonal changes that are associated with heart failure.

Patients treated with ACE inhibitors show improvement in symptoms, exercise performance, and specific indexes of heart function; they also require fewer hospitalizations for heart failure and have a prolonged survival. The ACE inhibitor enalapril may even prevent the development of congestive heart failure in asymptomatic patients with mild to moderate degrees of ventricular impairment.

There are many drugs available in this category. Enalapril and captopril are two of the most commonly used. Considering the far-reaching actions of the ACE inhibitors, side effects are surprisingly infrequent. Symptomatic low blood pressure, deterioration of renal function, angioedema (sudden localized tissue swelling), and cough are among the occasional reasons to stop therapy.

Other treatment modes. In cases where congestive heart failure is brought on by slow or fast heart rate, treatment is directed at the abnormal rhythm per se. An electronic pacemaker can overcome the slowest rates. Drug therapy is usually used to suppress rapid rhythms, such as atrial fibrillation.

In cases of heart failure brought on by valvular heart disease, surgical repair or replacement of the abnormal valve can improve cardiac performance. This is particularly true for patients with stenosis of the mitral or aortic valve.

Cardiac transplantation has proved to be an effective treatment method in patients with severe congestive heart failure unresponsive to other measures. This dramatic surgical procedure has become better accepted with the availability of cyclosporine, a very effective suppressor of the immune system that is used to prevent organ rejection. The use of transplantation remains limited, however, by its high cost and a lack of donor hearts.

Ancillary therapies. Patients with severe congestive heart failure face an increased risk of stroke. Blood clots can form along the wall of the dilated left ventricle, dislodge, and travel to the brain. The anticoagulant drug warfarin can prevent this serious complication.

Patients with severely diminished left ventricular function also are faced with the risk of cardiac arrest due to ventricular arrhythmias. Prevention of sudden arrhythmic death remains a difficult challenge. Some antiarrhythmic drugs have a significant negative inotropic effect and can clearly worsen congestive heart failure. These drugs also have what is known as a proarrhythmic potential; in some patients receiving antiarrhythmic drug therapy, the arrhythmias get worse rather than better.

The automatic implantable cardioverter-defibrillator is a more dependable treatment for life-threatening ventricular arrhythmias. This device automatically detects and terminates dangerous arrhythmias by acting as a pacemaker or by delivering a strong shock to restart the heart. Surgeons implant the newest version of the cardioverter-defibrillator by threading the electrical leads to the heart via the subclavian vein, accessible just under the clavicle (collarbone). Unfortunately, it is still difficult to predict which patients with heart failure are in greatest need of this aggressive antiarrhythmic therapy.

Research directions

In addition to an ongoing program to develop new inotropic drug compounds, there is a resurgence of effort to study the basic cellular mechanisms of heart muscle activity. It is hoped that such research efforts will offer a better understanding of myocardial cell processes and that this knowledge ultimately will help prevent what is so often an inexorable deterioration of heart function.

If the Shoe Fits . . .

by Dean Stern, D.P.M.

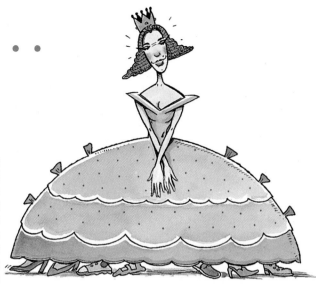

Humans began to walk upright at least 1.5 million years ago, and ever since that time, people have had problems with their feet. And this started even before there were shoes! Nowadays, as people try to meet the demands of an active lifestyle and at the same time maintain a stylish image, the feet are often a battleground where fashion and functionality fight it out. No one can afford to be slowed down by sore feet due to poorly fitting or inappropriate shoes. It is essential, therefore, to know how to choose comfortable, well-fitting footwear.

Feet: complex and adaptable

The human foot is a complex, dynamic anatomic structure that encounters many stresses in the course of an average day. The foot contains 28 bones, 30 joints with numerous ligaments, 19 muscles, and a multitude of tendons that extend around the ankle joint from the 12 muscles in the leg. Numerous blood vessels and nerves also enter and exit the foot.

The foot serves three primary functions: support, propulsion, and shock absorption. It is also an excellent adaptor, capable of conforming to a variety of different terrains. This is made possible by means of complex biomechanical interactions between the many joints and muscles within the foot and leg. With the advent of shoes, the feet gained in adaptability, becoming able to withstand greater demands and to expand the range of human activities. Even with their feet cushioned and protected, however, people continued to experience problems. In time, many of these difficulties came to be blamed on footwear rather than on the lack of it.

Foot problems: blame the shoe?

To what extent do shoes cause foot problems? This question has been debated for many years and has been the focus of some scientific study. The majority of researchers now agree that, while shoes can exacerbate foot problems they rarely cause them. In fact, investigators have found that sore, aching feet are no more prevalent in societies where people wear shoes all the time than in those where the majority of the population goes unshod. So what is the main factor in the development of foot problems?

Genetics plays a major role. Most people who have foot deformities such as bunions or hammertoes have inherited these problems from parents and grand-parents who suffered from similar conditions. In many instances structural abnormalities of the foot are inherited directly—that is, the individual is born with the problem. An example is so-called intoeing, or juvenile hallux valgus (a condition in which a newborn's great, or big, toe angulates toward and sometimes even overlaps the second toe). In other instances it is the tendency for developing a deformity that is passed on, so the problem does not become evident until later in life. In such cases shoes can—and often do—play a part in the exacerbation or progression of the problem.

One exception to the general rule that shoes do not in themselves cause foot problems is in the case of women who regularly wear high-heeled (i.e., over five centimeters [two inches]) shoes and experience a variety of problems. A condition particularly associated with high heels is Achilles tendinitis—inflammation of the tendon that joins the muscles of the calf to the calcaneus, or heel bone. When the heel of the foot is elevated, the Achilles tendon contracts. In a woman who wears high heels every day, the tendon eventually becomes shorter and loses its elasticity. If she then changes to low-heeled shoes, the tendon is overstretched and can become irritated and inflamed.

The ideal shoe: what to look for

If a person were to go shopping for the "ideal" shoe, what qualities and features would he or she look for? To begin with, such a shoe would provide excellent support and shock absorption; it would also be durable and comfortable. Loafers, sandals, and, in the case of women's shoes, low-heeled slip-on pumps are *not* ideal shoes. While they may not be the most fashionable, oxfords (i.e., low-heeled laced shoes), more than any other shoe style, offer the greatest support for the instep and arch, the best fit with the least slippage in the heel, and the best all-around construction—all of which are important factors for

445

people who are on their feet for long periods. By comparison, a slip-on shoe with a moccasin-style design provides less arch support, allows more slippage in the heel and instep, and also tends to stretch out of shape more readily. These characteristics, along with a usually thinner, less resilient sole, make this style of shoe less suitable than the oxford for long periods of standing and walking.

Several aspects of shoe structure and function should be taken into consideration when one is choosing a new pair. These include the amount of cushioning, degree of flexibility, size and shape of the toe box, composition of the sole, and height and width of the heel. The following are some guidelines for evaluating these features.

Cushioning. A shoe must have adequate cushioning in several places, including the heel counter (the cuplike support around the bottom of the heel), the collar of the shoe (upper edge around the ankle), the inside of the tongue, and the arch area. Some shoes come with built-in insoles that provide extra cushioning and support to the forefoot (ball of the foot and toes) and arch. In others this insole is removable, giving the wearer the option of replacing the insole when it wears down, rather than having to replace the entire shoe. It is important to note, though, that there is such a thing as too much padding on the inside of a shoe; excessive padding can cause the feet to overheat, resulting in excess perspiration. Dampness due to perspiration sets the scene for the development of tinea pedis ("athlete's foot"), a common fungal infection that can cause itching and painful blisterlike eruptions on the side of the foot and can lead to even more troublesome bacterial infections.

Flexibility. A good shoe is flexible in the forefoot, allowing for a certain amount of give in this area when the toes bend upward (dorsiflex) during walking. It is a simple matter to test a shoe's flexibility; one does this by placing the widest point of the sole on a firm surface, holding on to the heel, and pressing downward on the front of the shoe. The toe area should bend with ease, while the rest of the sole should remain firm in order to provide maximum support to the arch of the foot. If the sole is overly flexible, the shoe will not provide adequate control and support for the foot. On the other hand, if the sole is too firm, the wearer may develop pain and discomfort in the ball of the foot or possibly even a stress fracture (*i.e.,* small crack) in one of the metatarsal bones.

Toe box. The toe box (the front of the shoe enclosing the toes) is a particularly important part of the shoe and one that people typically overlook. The toe box of the ideal shoe is long enough to allow approximately 1¼–2 cm (½–¾ in) between the longest toe and the tip of the shoe. The toe box should also be roomy enough to allow the toes to wiggle freely, and its shape should correspond roughly to the outline of the forefoot.

Sole. To reduce the chance of premature wear to the sole—which can alter one's gait—the sole of the shoe should be made of a durable material. This material should allow for evaporation of perspiration; as noted above, shoes that retain moisture promote fungal as well as bacterial growth, causing both skin infections and unpleasant foot odor. (A helpful hint for minimizing these moisture-related problems is to use cedar shoe trees; the cedar wood absorbs excess moisture and helps reduce odor, while using shoe trees helps to maintain the shape of the shoe.) The sole should also have enough of a tread to provide good traction during walking, thus decreasing the chance of injuries due to falls.

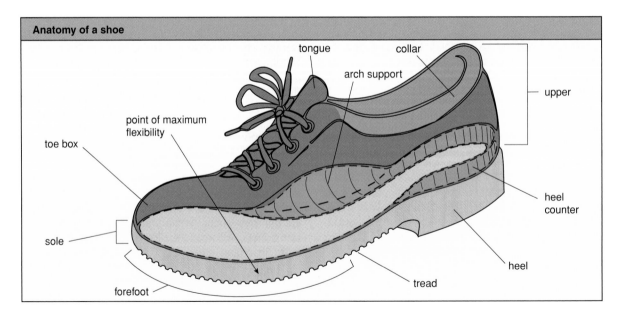

Anatomy of a shoe

tongue · collar · arch support · upper · point of maximum flexibility · toe box · heel counter · sole · heel · forefoot · tread

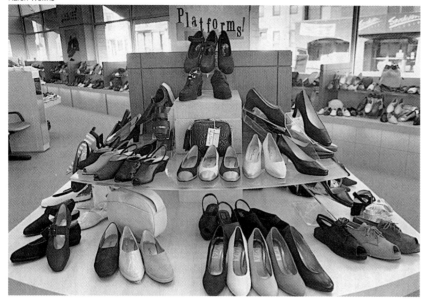

Despite the enormous variety of shoes available, many people find that shopping for a comfortable pair can be a frustrating experience. Finding the "right" shoe takes time, patience, and an understanding of what constitutes a proper fit.

Another function of the sole is to absorb shocks to the foot on impact with the ground, especially in the forefoot and heel areas. Many innovative materials are now being used to provide enhanced shock absorption. Some shoe companies have developed sophisticated air chambers or springy, rubberlike cushions, which are built into the sole of the shoe to reduce the shock transmitted to the wearer's feet, legs, knees, and even lower back.

Heel. Both the height and the shape of the heel are important. Average heel height for men should be 2⅘–3⅘ cm (1⅛–1½ in); women should wear heels no more than 3⅘–5 cm (1½–2 in) high. The width of the heel should be equal to or slightly larger than the width of the foot. This prevents instability at the ankle joint and helps decrease the chance of ankle turns and sprains.

In general, all of the above considerations apply to the purchase of both walking and athletic shoes. Most of these guidelines are also relevant when shoes are purchased for everyday wear. However, since the latter are the shoes people wear 90% of the time, their comfort and durability are paramount. The ideal work (or school) shoes should have all-leather soles and uppers. In addition to facilitating evaporation, leather uppers have many other advantages over synthetics such as vinyl. Leather is less likely than a synthetic to contain chemicals and dyes that could cause allergic reactions and so-called contact dermatitis (an inflammatory skin reaction due to "contact" with an irritant). Synthetic materials tend to be more rigid than leather and are therefore more likely to rub against the skin, creating blisters and calluses, and to exert pressure on existing corns and calluses. Synthetics also tend to split and crack more readily than leather and thus are less durable.

Tips for the smart shoe shopper

Despite the choice of different types of shoes available to today's consumer, finding the right pair can be a frustrating experience. The following are some tips to make shoe shopping easier and more rewarding.

• It is always best to buy shoes at the end of the day, after one has been up and about for some hours. During the day the feet can swell as much as a half to a full size in width, length, or both; thus, a shoe that fits well in the morning could be uncomfortably tight by evening.

• For the best fit, shoes should always be tried on with the same type of socks or hose that will be worn with them.

• The feet should be measured regularly. One should be sure to have *both* feet measured (most people have one foot that is larger than the other) and choose a size that will fit the larger foot.

• The shopper should stand during the fitting process so that all of the body's weight is on the feet. There should be at least 1¼ cm between the tip of the longest toe and the end of the shoe.

• It is important to walk around the store in the shoe to see if it feels comfortable. If shoes are not comfortable in the store, it is unlikely that they will feel any better on the street. One should not buy shoes that are too tight or that rub and hurt the feet, assuming that they will stretch and become more comfortable as they get broken in.

Poor fit . . . poor feet!

No matter how expensive or well made the shoe, if it fits the wearer poorly, pain and discomfort are sure to develop. Different parts of the feet will be affected, depending on the nature of the fit problem. When shoes are too narrow, for example, problems tend to

447

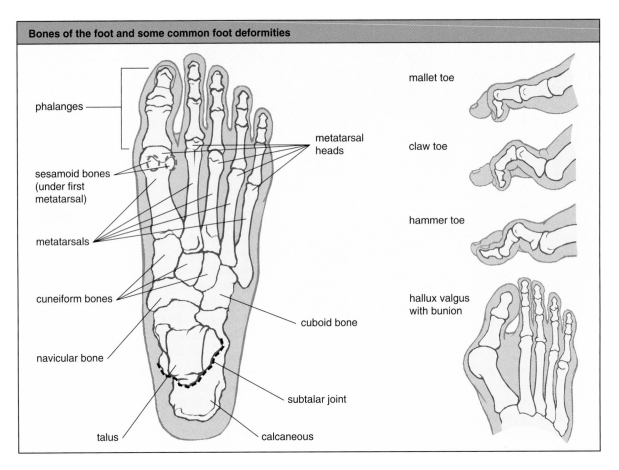

develop in the instep or forefoot, especially the toes. These can be minor—a friction blister—or major—disabling pain in the metatarsal bones and the formation of a bunion (a protuberance on the side of the foot at the base of the great toe, due to enlargement of the joint at the base of the great toe).

If, on the other hand, a person wears shoes that are too short, the heel counter may rub against the back of the heel, causing bursitis (inflammation of a small sac that lies between a tendon and bone). In time, the repeated irritation may lead to a characteristic deformity at the back of the heel known as "pump bump," or Haglund's deformity (bony enlargement of the posterior portion of the calcaneus and the development of bursitis in the region of the Achilles tendon). Another common problem that can be made worse by shoes that are too short is the development of contractures of the toes, caused by the toes' jamming against the end of the shoe. These conditions are known as hammertoe, mallet toe, and claw toe deformity (*see* diagrams, above). They are often accompanied by calluses on the tops of the toes (*i.e.,* corns) and on the balls of the feet under the heads of the metatarsal bones. Claw toe in women may also be caused by habitual wearing of nylon hose that are too short in the toe.

Worst of all, however, are the problems that develop or are made more severe when a person wears shoes that are *both* too narrow and too short. In this case the majority of the problems will arise in the forefoot, contributing to the development of a bunion, a tailor's bunion (a prominence on the outside edge of the foot just behind the small toe), and contractures of the toes.

When feet need special attention

While properly fitting shoes are important for all busy people, some circumstances call for extra care in buying and fitting shoes. Three special cases to be considered here are the footwear needs of older people, pregnant women, and people with diabetes.

Aging. As people age, many things about their bodies change, not least their feet. The aches and pains of degenerative arthritis (osteoarthritis) are frequently felt first in the small joints of the feet. With advancing years people may also note that their shoe size increases. This is due to spreading out of the joints of the foot as the ligaments and tendons stretch. A gain in weight may have a similar effect.

Pregnancy. Changes in foot size and structure are commonly seen in women during and after pregnancy. In the normal course of a pregnancy, as the

448

body prepares for delivery, a hormone called relaxin is released that allows the cartilage of a woman's pelvis to become more elastic. This same substance also affects the ligaments that help support the long arch of the foot, allowing the foot to lengthen and causing the arch to fall slightly in some women, a great deal in others. This process is often a cause of foot pain during or just after pregnancy.

Diabetes. Approximately 20% of hospitalizations in persons with diabetes are for foot problems. The two main causes of these problems are poor circulation and neuropathy (loss of sensation). These conditions make people with diabetes more likely than others to develop sores on their feet—a simple blister, for example, instead of healing normally, may become infected—and less likely to experience the pain that signals a foot problem. In extreme situations the person with diabetes may develop gangrene of the feet or toes, and amputation becomes necessary. Well-fitting shoes that do not rub or irritate the feet are crucial to minimizing complications of diabetes. People with diabetes should always choose shoes made of leather rather than synthetic materials. They should check to see that new shoes have a soft, smooth lining with no protruding stitching or seams that could rub and cause irritation. Thickly cushioned soles and a wide forefoot allowing adequate toe room are also important. New shoes should probably be worn for only a few hours at a time, and the feet should be inspected regularly to make sure that no sores are developing.

When orthoses can help

Most people, if they shop with care, should be able to find a shoe that suits their needs. For some people, however, no matter what type of shoe they buy or how many pairs they own, foot pain and discomfort

are ever present. In these cases orthoses, also called orthotic devices, may be the answer.

Orthoses are devices that go inside the shoe and change the way it fits the foot. Orthoses may be made of rigid, semirigid, or flexible materials, depending on the problem they are meant to solve. They function in three ways: they control the motion of the foot during walking, running, or standing; they accommodate a foot deformity such as a bunion; and they relieve pain. Among those who may benefit from orthoses are athletes, people with diabetes, people with arthritis that affects their feet, and children with foot deformities.

Athletes and others who participate in sports that involve running commonly complain of problems such as arch fatigue, heel pain, plantar fasciitis (inflammation of the plantar fascia, a band of tissue that runs along the plantar surface, or sole, of the foot), and pronation syndrome (pain associated with flattening of the arch and inward rolling of the foot). These problems occur because the main joint of the foot, the subtalar joint, becomes unstable and allows for excessive pronation of the foot. Pronation is a rotation of the foot in which the sole faces laterally (*i.e.,* away from the midline of the body); its opposite is supination, turning of the foot so that the sole faces medially (toward the midline of the body). An orthotic device can correct overpronation by preserving the normal range of motion of the foot while at the same time supporting the arch and restricting inward rolling of the foot.

In persons with diabetes the use of orthoses can reduce friction at pressure points on the feet and alleviate pressure on prominent bones and painful joints. These are important functions, as repeated rubbing may ulcerate the skin and eventually cause infection. Orthoses are also used to add extra cushioning, pro-

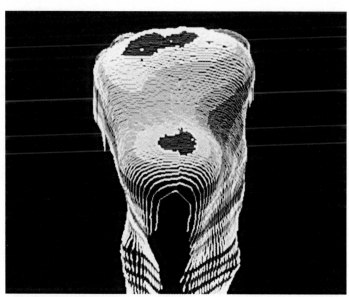

John N. Bergmann, D.P.M., Bergmann Orthotic Lab

Recent technological advances make it possible to create highly precise orthotic devices. In just seven seconds a three-dimensional image of the patient's foot is captured by an optical scanner; the image is then converted into digitized data that can be displayed on a computer screen as a height-contour map (left). The map can also be used to diagnose foot problems and to determine proper shoe size.

viding a greater measure of shock absorption to reduce trauma to feet numbed by neuropathy. In people suffering from arthritis, orthoses help reduce excess motion of the foot, another source of pain.

Children with normal feet do not need orthoses. However, those with congenital foot problems such as juvenile hallux valgus or other orthopedic abnormalities—for example, having one leg that is shorter than the other—can benefit from orthotic devices. Children outgrow their orthoses as rapidly as they outgrow their shoes, so new devices have to be made periodically.

There are three basic kinds of orthotic devices: functional, dynamic, and accommodative. Functional devices allow a normal range of motion in the joints of the feet while preventing overpronation. These devices are used mainly by athletes, children and adolescents with foot problems, and very active people who are on their feet a great deal. Functional devices are usually made from rigid to semirigid materials such as polypropylene, Rohdur (a kind of plastic), and fiberglass, all of which provide control but also have some shock-absorption qualities.

Dynamic devices serve to restrict motion, absorb shock, and support the arch. They are used mostly by people with diabetes or arthritis, less active people, and those with large foot deformities. They can be made to fit around and protect lesions such as calluses, ulcers, and bony outgrowths. Dynamic devices are made from softer materials such as cork, leather, foam rubber, and moldable materials.

Accommodative devices are usually used in cases where there is a very painful area on the foot, such as a neuroma (a tumor or mass growing on a nerve). They are made with any of the above-mentioned materials in a variety of combinations.

Orthoses are "prescribed" by a podiatric physician (foot doctor) or an orthopedist after an examination of the patient's feet, which includes an evaluation of the feet when the individual is both standing and walking. If the doctor thinks an orthotic device is warranted, he or she then makes plaster casts or impressions of the person's feet. Some foot specialists are now using computer-assisted design to create highly accurate models of the foot. The impressions are sent to an orthotist—one who fabricates orthotic devices. New orthoses are usually worn for a two-week break-in period, after which time the individual should be seen again by the doctor, who checks to see that the orthoses are functioning properly and makes any necessary adjustments.

Not all orthotic devices fit into just any kind of shoe.

Patients should consult a specialist about the proper footgear to wear with orthoses. New shoes should always be tried on with the orthoses.

Finally, it should be noted that most people probably do *not* need orthoses. Often one can relieve minor foot problems and make shoes more comfortable by using soft, cushionlike insoles or other ready-made devices available at local medical supply and sporting goods stores. These products may be adequate for a person with minor foot fatigue or foot pain. Still, it is a good idea to consult the foot doctor before purchasing such devices.

A word about athletic shoes

With the proliferation of different kinds of shoes for different sports and activities, many people are confused about which type of athletic shoe to buy and how many pairs they really need. The notion that a walking shoe provides different benefits from a running shoe is not merely a gimmick devised by shoe manufacturers to boost sales; there *are* some important differences—in walking, running, aerobics, and other athletic shoes. However, this does not mean that a shoe that is appropriate for one activity cannot be worn for another. For example, running shoes generally have added cushioning, a feature that some walkers find desirable. However, walking shoes are usually more rigid in the forefoot than running shoes, and the extra flexibility afforded by the running shoe may not be appreciated by all walkers. Cross-trainers, as the name implies, combine the features of different kinds of specialty shoes—e.g., the flexible forefoot of a running shoe and the control of sideways (lateral) motion of an aerobics shoe. In general, if a person engages in a particular sport or fitness activity several times a week, it is a good idea to have the right shoes for that activity. An exception is the shoe designed to be used on certain surfaces, such as a basketball court, which can also be worn for other sports played on the same surface, such as handball.

When buying athletic shoes, people should follow the same basic guidelines used when shopping for everyday-wear shoes; e.g., going shopping after a workout rather than before, wearing the same kind of socks that will be worn with the shoe, and making sure there is sufficient toe room. While the most expensive athletic shoes probably are no better than average-priced shoes, cheap shoes are usually made of inferior materials and will wear out faster. The best bet is probably a moderately priced brand-name shoe.

Overweight Children

by Alvin N. Eden, M.D.

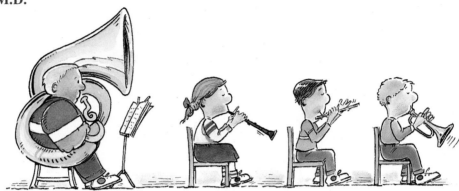

Obesity in the U.S. continues in epidemic proportions; it is estimated that as much as 60% of the population is obese—that is, 20% above ideal weight for height. Moreover, the problem seems to be getting worse with time. In a 1987 report Steven L. Gortmacker and colleagues at the Harvard School of Public Health analyzed data from four large national surveys and concluded that American children were actually fatter than they had been 20 years earlier. A decade ago, speaking before the Senate Select Committee on Nutrition and Human Needs, Sen. Edward Kennedy (Dem., Mass.) observed, "While children in West Africa melt away from starvation, America stands in ironic contrast as a land of overindulged and excessively fat. In many ways, the well-being of the overfed is as threatened as that of the undernourished." Today famine and hunger remain facts of life in much of Africa and in many Third World countries, while in the U.S. overeating is an established national pastime. Meanwhile, data continue to accumulate documenting the adverse consequences of obesity.

Adult obesity: origins in childhood

Most practicing pediatricians can vouch for the fact that the problem of obesity often begins early in life; young children, overfed and underexercised, are started on the road to a lifelong battle with obesity and its many associated health risks. Like their adult counterparts, a large percentage of U.S. children are overweight, and many of these obese kids will grow up to be obese adults. Further, it is clear that the longer a child stays fat, the greater the risk of his or her remaining fat throughout life.

What is so bad about being fat? As far as adults are concerned, the answer is obvious: obesity shortens life. The incidence of such serious problems as high blood pressure, heart attacks, stroke, kidney disorders, diabetes, and arthritis among obese individuals is extremely high.

Obesity that begins in childhood (early-onset obesity) is much more difficult to treat than adult, or late-onset, obesity. In addition, the obese child is likely to suffer from the psychologically damaging consequences of distorted body image, low self-esteem, and impaired interpersonal relationships—problems that, like obesity itself, often continue into adulthood. In contrast, people with late-onset obesity have not been shown to manifest this combination of personality traits or to suffer from severe adjustment disorders.

Not only is the treatment of adult obesity extremely difficult, too often it fails. Even those adults who *are* successful in reducing have a difficult time keeping the weight off; the relapse rate in this group is well over 90%. The medical literature is filled with reports of treatment regimens that fail to produce lasting "cures." The dismal results of such programs make it clear that the best solution to the problem of obesity is to prevent it from developing in the first place, and the logical time to start is in childhood. Children who are thin from the start will have a much better chance of remaining thin for the rest of their lives.

Special complications of childhood obesity

Many parents and grandparents—and even some health professionals—still mistakenly believe that fat toddlers or preschoolers are just as healthy as normal-weight or thin ones. This is simply not true. There is, in fact, an extremely high correlation between childhood obesity and the incidence of a variety of childhood medical problems. For example, children who are markedly overweight consistently suffer more from respiratory illnesses than children who are not fat. And because fat children are more likely to consume large amounts of sugary snack foods, they are prime candidates for tooth and gum problems. Studies also show that overweight youngsters suffer more injuries than their thinner counterparts. The reason is not hard to understand, considering that they make larger tar-

451

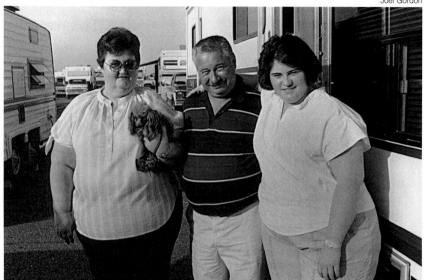

That genetics plays an important part in obesity is well recognized today. Offspring of two obese parents have an 80% risk of being overweight themselves. These children can achieve a normal weight, although they may have to struggle harder to maintain it than do their counterparts who have no genetic predisposition for obesity.

gets, are not as well coordinated, and simply cannot move as fast as their thin peers. In school athletic programs the fat child has been shown to have a comparatively higher incidence of sports- and activity-related injuries.

Cardiovascular risks. The greatest single danger of childhood obesity is its association with risk factors for coronary heart disease. Many fat school-agers and teens already have higher cholesterol levels and blood pressure than their normal-weight peers. Several recent studies add to the evidence that these conditions go hand in hand with obesity in predisposing these youngsters to developing heart disease.

In 1988 M. Daniel Becque and colleagues at the University of Michigan Medical School found that by adolescence obese youngsters already have multiple high-risk factors for the development of coronary heart disease. They examined a group of teenagers for the following indicators: levels of total cholesterol and high-density lipoprotein cholesterol (HDL, the so-called good cholesterol), serum triglyceride levels, systolic and diastolic blood pressures, maximum work capacity (a measure of endurance, or aerobic fitness—assessed by the measurement of oxygen consumption during exercise), and family history of coronary heart disease. Of the obese subjects studied, 97% had four or more risk factors for heart disease. An exercise program, along with moderate dietary restriction for only 20 weeks, resulted in a significant reduction in the high-risk status of these teens.

Further evidence of the dangers of being overweight comes from the Muscatine Study, a long-range investigation involving more than 4,000 schoolchildren in Muscatine, Iowa. In a report in *Pediatrics* the researchers concluded, "It is likely that persistent obesity in children indicates an increased risk

of cardiovascular disease for those children in their adult life, especially when accompanied by elevated blood pressure." The Muscatine Study demonstrated, among other things, that excess body weight relative to height is associated with increased blood pressure and decreased levels of HDL.

Long-term health effects. A report published in the *New England Journal of Medicine* in November 1992 underscored the importance of preventing obesity in childhood rather than trying to reverse it later on. The researchers examined the long-range effect of obesity on more than 500 adolescents who had been enrolled in a Harvard University study in the 1920s and '30s. They found that men who were overweight as teenagers had nearly twice the death rate of those who had been slender during adolescence. Among the female participants, no increase in death rates was found, but being overweight in adolescence was linked to an eight-fold subsequent increase in problems with activities of daily living, such as climbing stairs, lifting heavy objects, and walking one-quarter of a mile. The conclusion of this investigation was that overweight in adolescence predicted a broad range of adverse health effects later in life—independent of adult weight.

Psychological consequences. The risks of childhood obesity are not limited to physical problems. Fat youngsters are often unpopular with their peers. They are viewed as "different," and frequently their behavior sets them apart because they cannot keep up with more active and athletic playmates. In addition, obese children manifest personality traits very similar to those of minorities and other groups that are targets of discrimination. These traits include withdrawal, depression, and a tendency to be overly concerned about social status. The overweight adolescent is especially

452

vulnerable. At the very time when he or she needs to be building self-confidence and self-esteem—when the body is changing, emotions are in turmoil, and both boys and girls are highly conscious of their appearance—to be overweight is often a tragedy.

Moreover, it is an unfortunate but well-documented fact that society discriminates against fat people. Studies have shown that prejudice against the obese cuts their chances of college acceptance in half. When it comes to employment, all other things being equal, a thin job applicant will almost always be chosen over a heavy one because most people associate fatness with ill health, lack of self-discipline, and even lack of ability. The intractable nature of childhood obesity, combined with the very serious physical, psychological, and social problems associated with it, makes it clear that *prevention* is the best course.

Causes of obesity: today's thinking

Before the 1950s it was commonly thought that obesity was caused by an endocrine disorder. Today, however, it is known that childhood obesity is rarely caused by a hormonal imbalance. The so-called sluggish metabolism or sluggish thyroid that formerly was blamed for the extra pounds carried by an overweight youngster has now been shown to be almost nonexistent, and most of the pediatricians who treat childhood obesity very rarely see youngsters who have endocrine dysfunction. A parent thus can be almost 100% certain that obesity is *not* the result of an endocrine disorder if the overweight child is of normal height for his or her age.

The consensus today is that obesity has not one cause but many. Certainly, there is a strong genetic component. If both parents are overweight, their offspring have at least an 80% chance of being obese, although scientists do not know why this is the case. There are many theories about the genetics of obesity but no clear answers. One recent study suggests that infants born to overweight mothers have a low level of energy expenditure—are physically inactive—during the first year of life and that this is an important factor in their rapid, early weight gain. In fact, these infants were found to burn calories less efficiently and thus have a lower physical capacity than those infants born to normal-weight mothers. However, even these "high-risk" children need not grow up to be fat if proper measures are instituted early on (though they may have a somewhat greater struggle to achieve and maintain a normal weight).

Environmental factors also play an important role in the development of weight problems. There is little question that the combination of a sedentary lifestyle and a high-calorie diet (usually high in sugar and fat)—rather than genetic predisposition—explains the continuing increase in the prevalence of pediatric obesity in the United States. In the past 20 years, among 6- to 11-year-olds, there has been a 54% increase in the prevalence of obesity (defined as body fat amount above the 85th percentile) and a 98% increase in the prevalence of superobesity (defined as body fat above the 95th percentile). In the next oldest age group, 12- to 17-year-olds, the prevalence of obesity has risen 39% and superobesity 65%. This was found to hold true for both sexes and for both blacks and whites. One important factor behind this significant increase in obesity is that children today spend more time watching television and less engaging in physical activity than their counterparts in the 1960s and '70s. Another contributing factor is that kids now eat out more often than before, especially in fast-food establishments, where what they eat is usually high in both fat and calories (and also high in salt).

Strategies for prevention

Basically, there are two keys to preventing childhood obesity: learning proper eating habits early in life and developing proper exercise habits early in life.

Establishing good eating habits. What infants eat—and how much—sets a pattern for later years. Studies

Snacks: how they stack up	
popular—but poor—choices (serving size)	calories
orange soda (8 oz)	126
fruit drink (8 oz)	110
vanilla milkshake (10 oz)	345
frozen fudge bar	110
ice cream, premium (½ cup)	270
candy-coated chocolate candies (1 oz)	130
peanut brittle (1 oz)	125
potato chips (1 oz)	158
french fries (small order)	220
pecan brownie (2 oz)	224
chocolate chip cookies (5 small)	250
coconut cookies (5 small)	390
peanut butter cookie (1 large)	205
some healthier alternatives	
carrot (medium)	40
apple (medium)	81
orange (medium)	62
banana (medium)	60
nonfat yogurt, plain (8 oz)	120
ice milk (½ cup)	140
graham crackers (2)	60
gingersnaps (5 small)	125
air-popped popcorn (1 cup)	23
grapefruit juice, unsweetened (6 oz)	70
tomato juice (6 oz)	32

Fighting the "SOB"* syndrome	
activity	number of calories burned in 30 minutes
strolling	70
vacuuming	120–150
bowling	120–150
mowing lawn (power)	120–150
making beds	150
tennis (doubles)	150–170
brisk walking	175
jogging	225
mowing lawn (manual)	230
folk dancing	230
cycling	250
tennis (singles)	250
basketball	275
roller skating	325
cross-country skiing	330
swimming laps	340
running	450

*"sitting-on-the-behind"

show that breast-fed babies are less likely to develop into obese children than infants who are bottle fed (just one of a great many advantages of breast-feeding). This may be because breast-feeding mothers are less anxious than bottle-feeding mothers about introducing solid foods early, a practice that simply adds calories that are not required nutritionally. Also, bottle-feeding mothers tend to be more concerned about amounts—for example, making sure the infant drinks a certain number of ounces of formula—while women who breast-feed cannot measure the amount of milk consumed but rather stop feeding when the baby seems satisfied, a more natural situation. The breast-fed baby is therefore rarely overfed.

Although not directly related to obesity, it is important that a baby *not* be started on regular cow's milk before one year of age. This is the current recommendation of the Committee on Nutrition of the American Academy of Pediatrics. Cow's milk has much more salt and protein than either breast milk or formula and thus puts an added strain on the infant's kidneys.

The challenge: conquering the American way of eating. Far too many children grow up never having learned how to eat properly. Overstuffed from the moment they are born, they not only get fat but are often poorly nourished as well, despite the large amounts of food they consume. Added to the ingrained American habit of eating too much for the body's energy needs is the preference for eating the wrong foods. So-called junk foods—high in calories, low in nutrition—seem to be the order of the day. This trend is aided and abetted by the advertising industry, whose television commercials, especially during children's programs,

promote the wrong types of foods. Kids are bombarded with ads for sugarcoated cereals, drink mixes, and snack cakes, but how often do they see a commercial for carrots, broccoli, or apples?

Unfortunately, it is becoming increasingly difficult for families to eat meals together. Many people grab a quick breakfast, high in sugar and calorie content, such as a doughnut or a Danish. Lunch is eaten on the run or often skipped altogether or replaced by a series of snacks. Dinner may be eaten as a family, but even these meals are becoming rare events in many households. What is more, they too often consist of convenience foods with dubious nutritional value. In between these so-called mealtimes, there is continuous snacking. It has been estimated that between 30 and 50% of all calories consumed in the U.S. are eaten as snacks.

Since the burden of preventing childhood obesity rests with the parents, they must take responsibility for teaching children proper nutrition and helping them adhere to it despite outside pressures. Junk foods must be eliminated from the house, and children must be served three well-balanced, nutritious meals each day. Between meals, fruits and vegetables should take the place of candy, cookies, and soda. Children learn by example, so parents must take the lead.

Guidelines for parents. The best ways to put a child on the road to achieving and maintaining normal weight are summed up in the following simple guidelines.

● Emphasize low-fat, low-cholesterol foods. Getting into the low-fat, low-cholesterol habit will give children a head start in fighting atherosclerosis and heart disease later in life. Guidelines endorsed by the National Cholesterol Education Program and the American Academy of Pediatrics recommend that anyone older than age two get no more than 30% of calories from fat. It is estimated that the current average is 35% or higher.

● Cut down on the use of salt. If children learn to enjoy less salty foods now, chances are they will continue with a low-salt diet later on, when high salt intake and high blood pressure are linked.

● Hold the line on sugar. Parents need to curb a child's "sweet tooth" in order to ensure that he or she gets enough of the basic nutrients found in non-sugary foods.

● Include enough iron. An iron-rich diet can prevent fatigue, anemia, and misbehavior. (Recent reports linking too much iron with heart disease are preliminary and inconclusive—and do not, in any case, apply to children.)

● See that the child's diet includes fiber. Not only does fiber aid digestion, it helps protect against a number of gastrointestinal diseases, including appendicitis, diverticulosis, and cancer of the colon and rectum in adulthood.

454

• Fight the SOB ("sitting-on-the-behind") syndrome. If parents encourage children to exercise instead of watching television, they will develop good exercise habits that will last throughout life and protect them from high blood pressure, heart disease, and non-insulin-dependent diabetes.

Parents can help prevent their children from ever becoming fat—with all its attendant health consequences—by planning and serving meals that include: whole-grain breads, cereals, and pasta; low-fat meat, fish, and poultry; fruits and vegetables; and low-fat dairy products. It is also important to "fat-proof" the house. This means getting rid of all high-calorie, low-nutrition items such as cookies, cakes, doughnuts, chips, and sweet drinks (soda, Kool-Aid, sugar-added juices, etc.) and stocking the refrigerator with healthier choices, such as a variety of fresh fruits and raw vegetables, low-fat yogurt, low-fat cheeses, and unsweetened fruit juices.

Getting into the exercise habit. There is little question that, along with overeating, lack of exercise is a primary reason for the continuing epidemic of childhood obesity. Food puts the pounds on—but only if the calories consumed are not expended in activity. There must be a balance of calorie intake and energy output. The equation is simple: if children take in more calories than they burn, or expend in exercise, they will gain weight.

It may seem surprising, but many fat school-agers and adolescents actually eat less than their thinner friends. It is their inactivity that accounts for the extra calories, which, in turn, result in excessive fat deposition. Psychiatrist Hilde Bruch, a leading authority on obesity and other eating disorders, studied overweight children extensively. In one of these studies, she found that out of 160 obese youngsters, 76% of the boys and 88% of the girls were almost totally inactive. Thus, the crux of the problem is not that overweight kids eat too much but that they eat too much for the energy they expend. Increased activity is therefore an essential element of any regimen for the prevention and control of childhood obesity.

The problem of inactivity and weight gain begins early in life. From birth, most babies born in industrialized nations are "protected" from exertion. They are pushed around in strollers, confined in playpens, and driven about in cars. With increasingly overcrowded urban areas, growing street traffic, and less open space, parents often must make "appointments" for their children to play with each other. And too often this "play" consists of sitting in front of the television set munching cookies and chips.

It is absolutely essential that parents make every effort to encourage exercise, and the earlier this is started the better. Even before they are walking, infants and toddlers can be encouraged to move around and to play actively. All children must be taught to participate regularly in physical activities (suitable to their level of development) because once ingrained, these habits, like eating habits, are hard to change. A child who does not move around much will undoubtedly turn into an inactive adolescent and then a sedentary adult. Aerobic exercises such as brisk walking, jogging, cycling, running, lap swimming, and dancing burn up calories efficiently; these activities should be particularly encouraged.

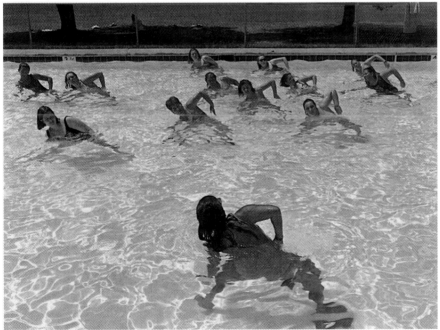

Youngsters at a weight-loss camp in Pennsylvania engage in a vigorous water-aerobics workout. Experts believe that obesity that begins in childhood is even harder to treat than adult-onset obesity—and a large percentage of U.S. children are overweight. These campers gain an advantage by learning proper eating habits and, equally important, adopting an active lifestyle.

Marilynn K. Yee—The New York Times

Overweight children

Unfortunately, owing to budgetary restraints, many schools across the U.S. have had to reduce or even eliminate physical education programs. Schools are not sharing the burden of instilling the importance of exercise in youngsters. In 1993 only five states required physical education classes for grades one through 12, and only 36% of schools had daily physical education sessions. Illinois is the only state that still requires physical education on a daily basis. The average grade-school child participates in only 30 minutes of physical education per week, and studies show that even during much of that time he or she may not be expending energy.

Making exercise a family affair right from the beginning is extremely helpful. Bicycle riding, ice skating, skiing, bowling, hiking, badminton, and swimming are all excellent activities for the entire family. Children should be encouraged to become proficient at a sport because once they do, they are more likely to enjoy it and stick with it. Thus, activities that can be continued throughout life are ideal. While team sports such as football, hockey, and baseball may provide fine exercise, it is not always easy to organize a team. Sports that require just one partner or no partners have obvious advantages.

Losing weight: what works, what doesn't

While limiting calorie intake and encouraging exercise are the keys to preventing childhood obesity, what can parents do if their child is already overweight? The earlier an overweight youngster's weight is brought back to normal, the better off he or she will be. The age of onset of the obesity and its severity are the most important determinants of its persistence. Thus, if a child becomes very fat early in life and remains fat through adolescence, it becomes extremely difficult to lose the weight and keep it off in adulthood.

Appetite suppressants, injections, and hormones such as thyroid can be dangerous and are contraindicated in children; besides, they generally do not work. Crash or fad diets should never be used; it is dangerous for a child (or anyone else) to lose weight too rapidly. Instead, the overweight youngster and his or her parents should see a physician who can help them map out a plan to get rid of the extra fat slowly. The doctor will probably provide a specific program that includes both diet and exercise components. Meals must be tailored to meet the individual needs of each child. For example, a growing adolescent requires more calories than a two-year-old. However, certain guidelines can be followed for all overweight children over two years of age:
- Serve only skim milk.
- Eliminate rich desserts.
- "Fat-proof" the house.
- Serve less red meat and more chicken and turkey (without skin), veal, and fish.

- Eliminate foods with added sugar such as cereals and drink mixes.

For providing healthier meals for the entire family, including the overweight child, the following five general principles of food preparation will be of use:

1. Avoid recipes that call for deep-frying; dishes prepared in this way always contain large amounts of fat.

2. Reduce fat when sautéing or stir-frying; try using half the amount of oil or butter called for in the recipe. The family probably will not miss the extra fat, and 120 calories are saved for every tablespoon of fat that is eliminated. When packaged foods are prepared, the same practice can be followed: if, for example, the directions on the box call for two tablespoons of butter or margarine to be added to a powdered sauce mix in a casserole dish, try adding only one or two teaspoons.

3. Use a nonstick skillet to avoid the use of fat in cooking.

4. When thickening a white sauce, try mixing the flour with the cold liquid (instead of combining flour with butter) and simmer for five minutes over low heat. Use two tablespoons of Parmesan cheese for a low-fat cheese sauce.

5. Substitute low-fat salad dressings for those containing oil, mayonnaise, or sour cream. Low-fat dressings can be made with low-fat buttermilk, blended cottage cheese, or yogurt—garlic, vinegar, lemon juice, herbs, and spices added to taste.

The other key to a child's successful weight loss—exercise—cannot be overemphasized. The table on page 454 lists a number of recreational activities and active household chores that are appropriate for children and will expend calories and promote weight loss over time. The body must burn 3,500 calories in order to lose a single pound (0.454 kg) of fat. Thus, a regular daily period of increased physical activity—whether exercise or chores—is vital to a program for conquering childhood obesity.

Normal weight: an achievable goal

With rare exceptions, a child should never lose more than one to two pounds per week. Weight loss by dieting and exercise should be a slow and steady process. A little simple arithmetic will demonstrate how easy it can be to lose one pound each week: if 3,500 calories equals one pound of fat, a reduction of 500 calories per day will do the trick ($500 \times 7 = 3,500$). A child can eliminate 500 calories per day by eating 250 fewer calories and burning up an additional 250 calories in exercise. Therefore, by simply eliminating five small chocolate chip cookies a day and by riding a bicycle for 30 minutes, he or she can lose a pound in a week.

It really is not that hard. Parents *can* help their child to achieve the goal of normal weight—now and for life!

Exercise and Weight Loss: The Myths, the Facts

by Barry A. Franklin, Ph.D.

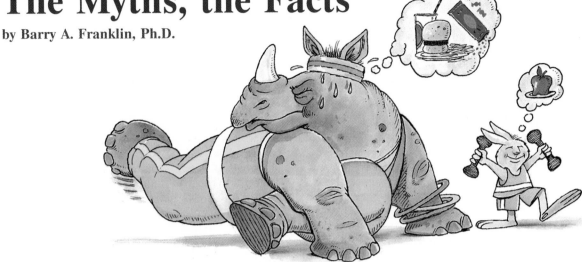

Approximately 25% of . . . men and 40% of women . . . reported that they were currently trying to lose weight. . . . The average man wanted to lose 30 pounds and to weigh 178 pounds; the average woman wanted to lose 31 pounds and to weigh 133 pounds.
—*American Journal of Public Health,* September 1992

I can't exercise because I'm too fat. . . . Exercising makes me ravenous and then I eat too much. . . . I'd look ridiculous in a jogging suit. . . . I'm too tired to exercise.
—arguments against exercise

Obesity is a serious medical concern for a large percentage of the population. Being overweight has been directly or indirectly linked to several chronic health problems, including coronary heart disease, diabetes, certain types of cancer, osteoporosis, and gallbladder disease. Consequently, weight reduction is often prescribed in the prevention and medical treatment of many cardiorespiratory, metabolic, and musculoskeletal conditions.

The simplistic views that obesity is due solely to overeating or that it can be effectively treated through caloric restriction are not valid. While it is true that some obese persons eat prodigious amounts of food, many eat less than their leaner counterparts. What often distinguishes those who are significantly overweight from their leaner counterparts is that they are far less physically active.

The role of physical activity in weight-reduction programs has generally been minimized, particularly when compared with dietary intervention. However, exercise, with or without caloric restriction, offers several important advantages over caloric restriction alone. Regular physical activity improves musculoskeletal and cardiorespiratory fitness. Moreover, many forms of exercise offer enjoyable leisure-time activities, whereas dieting for most people is difficult and unpleasant. Finally, weight lost through exercise consists primarily of fat loss, whereas dieting (especially crash or fad dieting) is more likely to lead to the loss of water and vital lean tissue.

Unfortunately, overweight people are often confronted with myths and misconceptions regarding the role of exercise in reducing body weight and fat stores. They may also be easily deceived by an overwhelming number of gimmicks, gadgets, and fads that are promoted as "miracle" methods of reducing—few of which are legitimate and many of which may be dangerous.

Caloric cost of exercise: many theories

The effectiveness of exercise in the control of body weight has been discounted by many who claim the amount of activity required for caloric output to be significantly affected is prohibitive. To support this, they often point to energy equivalent tables that present the rates of caloric expenditure for various physical activities (usually in kilocalories burned per minute per kilogram of body weight). On the basis of such tables, it would seem that to work off one pound (0.454 kg) of fat, one would have to walk for 14 hours or split wood for 7 hours or play volleyball for 11 hours.

Exercise proponents, however, may argue that the calorie-expending effects of physical activity do not depend on a single bout of exercise but are cumulative. If one chops wood for one 20-minute period a day or walks for 40 minutes a day, one could lose a pound of fat in 21 days and reduce body weight by about 7.7 kg (17 lb) in a year. Still others would counter that the true caloric effect of exercise must consider the "net energy cost" of each exercise bout (calculated as the total energy cost of the exercise minus the energy cost of normal activity during the same time period). For most individuals such a net cost is about two kilocalories per minute less than the gross cost. Thus, if one walks 60 minutes and expends 300 kcal, the net cost of the exercise is 180 kcal, not 300 kcal. Because a pound of fat equals 3,500 kcal and losing weight requires a negative caloric balance, it is apparent that if net energy expenditure alone is considered, a substantial amount of exercise is required for facilitating a significant weight loss.

Fortunately, the caloric expenditure associated with exercise is *not* limited to the time of the activity alone. It is well documented that in the postexercise recovery period more oxygen is consumed than is normally required for sustaining resting metabolism. Because each liter of oxygen consumed is equivalent to approximately five kilocalories, this results in an additional energy expenditure subsequent to the cessation of physical activity. The delayed postexercise return of oxygen consumption to resting levels has been attributed to numerous factors, including the biochemical replenishment of adenosine triphosphate, which serves as the "fuel" for all the energy-requiring processes within the body's cells; augmented cardiopulmonary metabolism; increased body core temperature; and elevation of certain hormones, especially epinephrine and norepinephrine.

Physiologists have quite clearly demonstrated that exercise *is* beneficial in the control of body weight. This is so not only for the energy losses incurred during the exercise but because a considerable additional caloric expenditure occurs following exercise.

Walking versus running versus bicycle riding

It is worthwhile to consider the comparative energy expended by three common forms of exercise. The caloric cost of walking as opposed to running has been the subject of considerable controversy. Some claim that the longer exercise duration involved in walking a given distance results in approximately the same caloric expenditure as running that same distance over a shorter period of time. The laws of physics would appear to support this hypothesis in that a given weight moves a given distance by both methods.

On the other hand, numerous studies have demonstrated that running a given distance expends more calories than does walking the same distance. The gross caloric costs of walking and running are approximately 1.15 kcal per kilogram of body weight per mile (1 mi = 1.61 km) and 1.7 kcal/kg/mi, respectively. Unless an individual walks at a very slow pace or runs at an extremely fast pace, the caloric cost for a given distance is relatively independent of speed. Although many obese persons may be unable to run, a substantial energy expenditure can result if they walk a longer distance.

Outdoor bicycling is an energy-efficient method of covering distance. Although the energy cost of bicycle riding varies with the type of bicycle, the mechanical efficiency of the rider, and his or her body weight, the gross caloric cost approximates 0.6 kcal/kg/mi. But again, as with walking and running, the caloric cost for a given distance is relatively independent of speed. The cyclist thus expends approximately one-half the kilocalories of the brisk walker and one-third those of the runner covering the same distance. Expressed another way, the energy cost of bicycling three miles

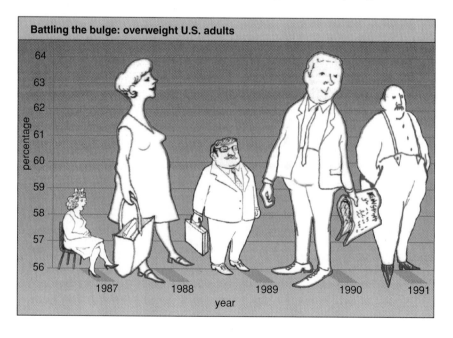

Battling the bulge: overweight U.S. adults

is the approximate equivalent of walking one and a half miles or running one mile. The table provides a comparison of the gross caloric expenditure per mile at various body weights for walking, running, and outdoor cycling.

Exercise: effects on appetite

A common excuse for not exercising is that physical activity always increases appetite and caloric intake, negating the energy expenditure of the exercise itself. Although it is true that an increase in food intake generally parallels an increase in physical activity, this relationship appears to hold only within a certain activity zone.

In a classic experiment conducted several decades ago, researchers demonstrated that at extremely high or low levels of daily energy expenditure, appetite no longer worked as a guide to balancing food intake and the amount of energy used. Rats that were exercised daily for up to one hour decreased their food intake and body weight in comparison with sedentary control animals. When the exercise duration was increased beyond one hour, food intake increased but only to the extent that body weight was maintained. At exhaustive levels of exercise (*i.e.,* six hours a day), both food intake and body weight decreased.

More recently, investigators measured caloric intake and physical activity in industrial workers. Five different occupational activity categories were determined: sedentary, light work, medium work, heavy work, and very heavy work. The researchers found that there was a linear relationship between activity level and caloric intake in those in the middle three categories (the light-to-heavy activity range), but those in the sedentary range tended to weigh more and consumed a greater number of calories, while those engaged in very heavy work consumed more but weighed less. The results thus substantiated the earlier findings in animals.

In humans most research indicates either no change in food intake with moderate exercise of extended duration or slight decreases with vigorous exercise of shorter duration. This latter effect (appetite suppression) is attributed, at least in part, to the increased level of catecholamines evoked by strenuous exercise. Catecholamines include adrenal hormones (*e.g.,* epinephrine and norepinephrine) that may have a role in appetite-control mechanisms.

Shrink those hips: the myth of spot reduction

In the U.S., where the health and aesthetic disadvantages of excess adiposity are well recognized, "spot reducing" is a multimillion-dollar industry, with health spas and personal trainers promising that people can "take inches off the waist, thighs, or buttocks—without dieting and in just minutes a day." The concept is based on the belief that it is possible to selectively

Calories burned: running, walking, cycling				
body weight		kcal/mi*		
(lb)	(kg)	running	walking	bicycling (outdoors)
110	50	85	58	30
132	60	102	69	36
154	70	119	81	42
176	80	136	92	48
198	90	153	104	54
220	100	170	115	60
242	110	187	127	66
264	120	204	138	72

*one mile = 1.61 km

"burn off" fat from a particular part of the body by exercising that body area. However, considerable research casts doubt on the validity of spot reduction.

In the early 1970s researchers first tested the proposition that one can selectively reduce fat in one part of the body. They compared the circumferences and amounts of subcutaneous fat in both arms of accomplished tennis players. It was hypothesized that if exercise of a particular body part selectively reduced fat tissue in that area, then the racquet (playing) arm should have less fat than the inactive (nonplaying) arm. Although circumference measures in the playing arm were greater than in the nonplaying arm (owing to muscular hypertrophy), measures of skin-fold thickness revealed no difference between the two arms in subcutaneous fat deposits.

Perhaps the most convincing evidence against spot reduction comes from more recent studies of the effects of localized abdominal exercise training on regional fat, or adipose cell size. Fat biopsies were taken from the abdomen, buttocks, and upper back in 13 male subjects before and after a rigorous 27-day abdominal exercise (sit-ups) training program. Fat-cell diameter decreased significantly at all three sites, with no significant differences in the rate of change between sites. Although conventional sit-ups are commonly promoted as a way to reduce abdominal fat, this experiment demonstrated that such exercise does not preferentially reduce the amount of subcutaneous fat in the abdominal region alone.

The physiological explanation behind spot reduction is that exercising a muscle causes fatty acids (a primary energy source in muscular exercise, particularly exercise of mild to moderate intensity) to diffuse into the muscle in the "target" area from its overlying fat pad. Instead, it appears that fatty acids from adipose tissue stores *throughout the body* are mobilized during exercise to supply the needed energy fuels. Perhaps one reason why spot-reducing exercise sometimes appears to work is that if the exercise intensity is sufficiently strenuous and the exercise duration long enough, fat from the entire body, including the target area, will be reduced.

Effortless exercise

Passive exercise that "does the work for you" has been touted as an effective way to reduce or redistribute body fat. Do these approaches have any merit?

Let a machine do the work. Several years ago researchers investigated the validity of the weight-reducing claims made for the mechanical vibrating machines commonly found in health clubs and gymnasiums. It was hypothesized that if the devices oxidized or "massaged away" body fat, as their promoters say they do, then the individual's oxygen uptake and/or blood fat levels should be increased during the "workout."

Thirteen men, some considerably overweight, were subjected to a 15-minute period of abdominal vibration. During and after the exercise bout, oxygen consumption was measured (as a reflection of caloric cost). In addition, venous blood samples were drawn before and shortly after the exercise and again several hours later. Results showed that blood fats remained essentially unchanged as a result of the vibration. Av-

The desire to melt away fat effortlessly is not new; this "vapor bath" contraption from earlier times differs little from the rubberized "sweat" suits and heated belts on the market today. The temporary dehydration that occurs only creates the illusion of fat loss—and can be dangerous.

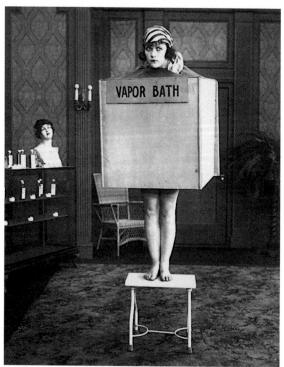

Culver Pictures

erage caloric cost of the 15-minute exercise session, including the postvibration recovery period, was only 11.4 kcal more than each man would have expended had he remained just sitting for an equivalent period of time. This "net cost" represents approximately $\frac{1}{19}$ of an ounce of fat. Thus, losing a pound of fat (3,500 kcal) would require 307 such 15-minute periods of abdominal vibration, or roughly six exercise sessions per week for a year! The investigators concluded that "the vibrator is not to be taken seriously as a device to assist in fat reduction or shifting of fat deposits within the body." Such devices are, at best, capable of moving fatty tissue, not *removing* it.

Sweat it off. Special weight-reducing exercise garments, including heated belts and rubberized suits, are semipermeable or impermeable to moisture, and their promoters claim that by wearing them one can lose weight more rapidly—through increased sweating but without increasing exercise intensity or activity level. In other words, the clothing does all the work.

Most such garments promote excessive dehydration (loss of body water) by heat, localized pressure, or tissue compression. Although circumference measures of various body areas (*e.g.,* waist, thighs, upper arms) as well as scale weight may in fact decrease until rehydration occurs, these losses are unrelated to any actual or lasting reductions in body weight or fat stores. Nevertheless, manufacturers capitalize on the short-lived, or apparent, losses to highlight the supposed benefits of their products.

In fact, impermeable or semipermeable exercise clothing acts to increase water losses and restrict evaporative cooling. The loss of water causes a reduction in effective circulating blood volume and a subsequent drop in blood pressure. As a result, the heart rate increases disproportionately to keep up with increasing metabolic demands during exercise. Rubberized sweat suits worn during exercise trap sweat between the suit and the skin. Trapped sweat cannot evaporate to cool the body, and convective heat loss is also inhibited, thus depriving the body of its normal mechanisms for cooling. The increased metabolic rate from exercising, coupled with the added burden imposed on the body's temperature-regulating mechanism, may result in a severe rise in body core temperature and potentially serious heat-related disorders.

The ideal garment for reduction of body fat would be clothing that promotes energy expenditure, caloric restriction, or both. Unfortunately, no material has yet been found that effects these necessary lifestyle changes. It is not surprising that some manufacturers have modified their advertising to include the recommendation (in small print, of course) that a diet or exercise program accompany wearing of their garment to maximize its effectiveness.

Reduce horizontally. The late Robert M. Hutchins, former chancellor of the University of Chicago and

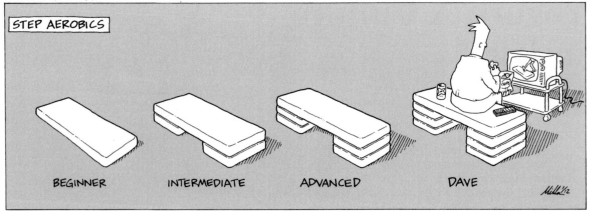

chairman of the Board of Editors of *Encyclopædia Britannica,* once said: "Whenever I feel like exercise, I lie down until the feeling goes away." Promoters of some electrical muscle stimulators (EMS) would have people believe that such behavior can actually result in a workout. Advertisements in supermarket tabloids tout these devices for everything from weight loss to body shaping and toning to spot reducing to the removal of cellulite (dimpled fat that often appears on the hips, thighs, and buttocks). For example, ads claim that "microelectroimpulses" provide the same figure-toning results as "3,000 sit-ups without moving an inch" or "10 miles of jogging while lying flat on your back."

Unlike many gimmicks, EMS units have a legitimate basis. They are often used by physical therapists in the treatment of certain medical conditions—*e.g.,* decreasing pain and swelling, enhancing strength in atrophied muscles, promoting healing after certain injuries or some kinds of surgery, and relaxing muscle spasms. These purposes are a far cry from the sensational claims for EMS products for effortless weight loss or body shaping. The only reduction emanating from advertised EMS devices occurs in the consumer's billfold.

The Food and Drug Administration, the federal agency that regulates the marketing of "medical devices" and evaluates their safety and effectiveness, considers muscle stimulators that are promoted or used for "body shaping and contouring" to be misbranded and fraudulent. Accordingly, the agency has recently banned the sale and distribution of many devices whose manufacturers have failed to substantiate their advertisements.

In addition to the deceptive claims, EMS devices can be dangerous if improperly used. There have been numerous reports of electric shocks and burns resulting from the products, and they can be especially hazardous to pregnant women, patients with cardiac pacemakers, and people who have epilepsy. Like most other effortless-exercise products, EMS units, at the very least, may be worthless; on the other hand, they can be quite dangerous.

To exercise or not to exercise?

While it is doubtful that long-term compliance with any sort of exercise program will be easy for the dedicated "couch potato," exercise (alone or in combination with caloric restriction) is an important, and probably the best, way to achieve lasting and meaningful weight loss. The balance between intensity and duration of exercise should be regulated to yield a high total caloric expenditure, approximating 300 to 500 kcal per exercise session, amounting to 1,000 to 2,000 or more kcal per week. Exercise should be engaged in at least three days per week and should include sustained large muscle activities that are maintained continuously and are rhythmic and aerobic in nature. The exerciser needs to choose an appropriate form of exercise that is enjoyable and suitable for his or her lifestyle—an activity he or she will stick with. Reductions in body weight and fat stores can even result from brisk walking programs, provided that the walking duration is sufficient (exceeds 30 minutes several times a week).

Long-term treatment of obesity that relies chiefly on caloric restriction is successful in as few as 5% and probably no more than 20% of all cases. Drastic dietary changes often lead to recidivism and concomitant fluctuations in body weight—a phenomenon known as the "rhythm method of girth control." Recent studies suggest that long-term compliance with exercise therapy may be no better. Clearly, misinformation is a big part of the problem.

Sensible caloric restriction coupled with an enjoyable exercise program nonetheless offers the greatest potential for success. Until these simple tenets are realized, many will continue to embrace the opinion voiced so eloquently by Shakespeare's Hamlet, Prince of Denmark: "There's a divinity that shapes our ends" (Act V, scene 2).

Yogurt: A Culture in Itself

by Susan M. Kleiner, Ph.D., R.D., L.D.

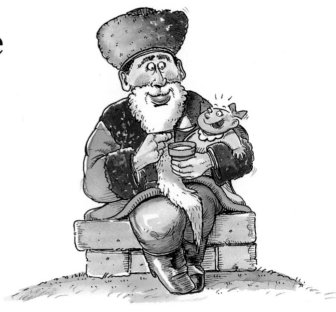

Yogurt (also spelled yoghurt, yoghourt, or yourt), a food made of milk fermented by bacterial cultures, has been eaten throughout the world for at least 4,000 years. Asians, Middle Easterners, Europeans, and Scandinavians all have their own names for this time-honored dietary staple. In certain languages the word for yogurt means "life"—*e.g.,* the ancient Assyrian *lebeny* and the Middle Eastern *laban*—reflecting a strong belief in its life-giving properties. Today scientists are actively investigating the possible health benefits of yogurt—its contribution to good nutrition as well as its potential for preventing and treating certain diseases.

The "discovery" of yogurt has been traced to an accident. According to this probably apocryphal story, a nomad carrying a goatskin bag of milk on a long journey across the desert opened the bag to find not the liquid he had started out with but a tart custard instead. The heat and bacterial cultures inside the bag had transformed the milk into a new food. Over the centuries many kinds of milk, including milk from sheep, goats, yaks, cows, buffalo, and even horses, have been used to make this cultured product.

In certain central Asian societies where yogurt has been eaten for centuries, many people reportedly live to be 100 years of age or older. Their long lives are often attributed to the fact that they consume yogurt on a regular basis. Even the bacteriologist Élie Metchnikoff, a 1908 Nobel laureate, attributed the longevity of the self-proclaimed centenarians of the Caucasus region to their regular consumption of yogurt. (Today it is believed that most of these venerable elders exaggerated their ages.)

In demand

In the United States yogurt was virtually unknown half a century ago. Then in 1942 Daniel Carasso, an immigrant from Spain, arrived in New York City with his father's recipe for yogurt and the dream of becoming an entrepreneur. He founded the Dannon Yogurt Co., the country's first commercial yogurt manufacturer. Since that time, yogurt has become an increasingly popular American food. According to one market-research survey, U.S. consumption of yogurt has grown from less than 0.45 kg (one pound) per person in 1970 to nearly 2 kg in 1990 and was predicted to reach 2.1 kg in 1993. The amount of refrigerated cup yogurt

sold in the country is forecast to grow by nearly 12% by 1996. Still, this does not even come close to the demand for yogurt in France, Switzerland, and many other European countries, where people eat 6.8 kg or more a year.

In comparison with the plain, cultured yogurt eaten in much of the world, the varieties of yogurt available to Americans seem virtually endless. These include whole-fat, low-fat, and nonfat; plain and flavored; unsweetened and sweetened; with fruit, nuts, or granola; thick, thin, and in drinkable liquid form; and with or without live bacterial cultures. And now, of course, there is the popular alternative to ice cream: frozen yogurt.

Part of yogurt's appeal is that it contains the important nutrients found in other dairy products such as milk and cheese, but its flavor and texture can be manipulated to please almost any palate. Yogurt is particularly well suited to today's fast-paced American lifestyle because it provides a high-protein, high-calcium, low-fat food that can be a meal or a snack, is convenient to eat, needs no preparation, and is not too filling.

What is yogurt?

Yogurt is milk that has been coagulated by lactic acid fermentation; it may also contain a variety of additional ingredients such as powdered or skim milk, sweeteners, or fruit. Lactic acid fermentation is stimulated by one of two species of bacteria, *Lactobacillus bulgaricus* and *Streptococcus thermophilus*. Some yogurts contain cultured strains of both of these organisms. According to the food standard set by the World Health Organization and the Food and Agriculture Organization, in Europe and other countries yogurt culture organisms must be alive, active, and numerous in the final product. The U.S. Food and Drug Admin-

462

istration (FDA) definition of yogurt, however, permits treatment with heat after culturing is complete. This type of heat processing destroys a significant number of the bacterial cultures. Under FDA regulations, the word *live* on the label indicates that living bacteria are present in the yogurt. *Active* means that the bacterial cultures have the ability to ferment milk into yogurt.

All yogurt sold in the U.S. is made from pasteurized milk. The fermentation cultures of *L. bulgaricus* and *S. thermophilus* are added to the milk after pasteurization (a heat sterilization process) to produce yogurt with live and active cultures. This cultured milk then incubates at about 44° C (112° F) for four to five hours until curd (thick, coagulated milk) forms. Heat-treated products are made by this same process, but the yogurt is heated once again after fermentation, which kills and deactivates the cultures—and thereby eliminates their potential health benefits. In the U.S. heat-treated yogurt products must be labeled "heat-treated after culturing." All yogurts containing live, active cultures have such wording on the label as "with active yogurt cultures," "contains living yogurt cultures," or "contains active cultures." On the other hand, some yogurts advertise "made with active cultures," a statement that is true for all yogurt and does not mean that the product actually *contains* active cultures. Only yogurts that are not heat-treated retain their active cultures in the final product. (In many European countries strict regulations prohibit heat-treated products from being labeled as yogurt.)

Yogurt manufacturers use additional processes and ingredients to make the large variety of styles available in the U.S. Some yogurt products contain a third bacterial culture, *L. acidophilus,* which is added at the same time as the other cultures. Flavoring and fruits are added after the bacterial cultures. Low-fat and nonfat varieties often contain stabilizers such as gelatin and pectin to produce a firmer texture. Nonfat milk solids (milk proteins that have been extracted from the liquid) may also be added as a way of thickening the product. The natural sour taste of lactic acid can be masked by the addition of sweeteners such as sugar, honey, aspartame, or fruit. Fruit can be added sundae style (on the bottom) or Swiss or French style (blended throughout).

Frozen yogurt, the newest yogurt product on the market, is in many cases "yogurt" in little more than name only. Frozen yogurt is a blend of milk, sweeteners, and stabilizers, along with a bit of "yogurt mix." Yogurt mix is dry milk and inactive bacteria; therefore, the bacteria never actually ferment the milk. There are no federal guidelines for the identification of frozen yogurt. Although it has more in common with ice cream than with true yogurt—albeit with only half as much fat—frozen yogurt owes much of its popularity to the mistaken belief that it offers the same health benefits as yogurt that contains active cultures.

A nutrient-wise choice

All dairy foods are excellent sources of protein, calcium, phosphorus, magnesium, riboflavin, vitamin B_{12}, and niacin. Yogurt, however, is a unique source of nutrients and is superior to milk in several important respects. For example, a single cup of yogurt serves up 30 to 45% of the recommended daily dietary calcium (about which more is said below). Thus, yogurt provides three times more calcium than an equal amount of milk. Moreover, the specific combination of nutrients in yogurt actually enhances the intestinal absorption of many of the other minerals, such as phosphorus and iron. And because yogurt is often fortified with nonfat milk solids, it may contain more protein than milk.

The culturing, or growing, of the bacteria that make yogurt also affects the nutrient content. As part of their metabolic process, the yogurt bacteria produce folic acid, giving yogurt a folic acid content that is nearly twice that of milk. On the other hand, the culturing process uses up vitamin B_{12}, so there is less of this vitamin in yogurt than in milk.

Protein. Protein is essential for maintaining and repairing the body's tissues; for the optimal functioning of the immune system; for healthy growth during gestation, infancy, childhood, and adolescence; and for muscle building in adults. Both milk and yogurt are good sources of protein. But because of the unique culturing process that creates yogurt, the protein in yogurt is more easily digested than that in milk. While this does not make a great deal of difference for adults, it can make the transition from breast milk or formula to dairy products easier for infants and young children. Yogurt is therefore an excellent protein source for these age groups.

As mentioned above, nonfat milk solids are added to many low-fat and nonfat yogurts to give them a thick, custardy consistency. This processing technique offers the added benefit of raising the protein content of these yogurts, as well as enhancing the content of lactose (milk sugar), minerals, and vitamins.

Calcium. Ninety-nine percent of the body's calcium is stored in the bones and teeth. The skeleton is continuously undergoing a remodeling process in which it loses and gains bone minerals throughout life. When bone loss is much greater than gain, however, the bones can become brittle and weak and more susceptible to fracture—the condition osteoporosis. Having an adequate calcium intake is an important step in preventing osteoporosis. And, as noted above, yogurt is an excellent natural source of calcium. Depending on the type of yogurt, one can obtain anywhere from 274 to 452 mg of calcium by consuming a cup of yogurt. (The U.S. recommended dietary allowance for calcium is 800 mg per day for children and adults and 1,200 mg per day for young people 11 to 24 years old and pregnant and lactating women.)

Yogurt: a culture in itself

Lactose. Lactose, the natural sugar found in milk, enhances intestinal absorption of calcium. When digested, lactose is broken down into two simple components, glucose and galactose. But in order for lactose to be reduced to its smaller parts, the enzyme lactase is required. Unfortunately, many people lack this enzyme in their digestive tracts. This condition, called lactose intolerance or lactase insufficiency, causes gastrointestinal upset when a food containing lactose is eaten. People with lactose intolerance tend, therefore, to avoid milk products. This situation can lead to a calcium deficiency for some people.

Cultured yogurt offers a solution for many individuals who have mild lactose intolerance. The live, active cultures contribute lactase that predigests much of the lactose in yogurt, reducing the absorption problem. Additionally, the lactase-producing live cultures appear to be able to survive passage through the stomach to the small intestine, where they are able to help digest whatever lactose is left in the yogurt. Thus, cultured yogurt products allow lactose-intolerant individuals to enjoy all the benefits of milk without suffering the discomfort.

Fat and cholesterol. The fats in yogurt are the same as those found in milk. In its official standards for fat content, the FDA recognizes three main categories of yogurt:

- whole-milk yogurt—contains at least 3.25% fat and at least seven grams of fat per cup
- low-fat yogurt—0.5 to 2% fat, with one to six grams of fat per cup
- nonfat yogurt—less than 0.5% fat, with one gram or less of fat per cup

Very creamy yogurts may contain more than seven grams of fat per cup, and custard-style yogurts are more similar in fat content to low-fat yogurts. The cholesterol content of yogurt is generally low, ranging from 0 mg per cup in some nonfat yogurts to 29 mg per cup in whole-milk yogurt.

Today's dietary guidelines recommend that all adults reduce the amount of fat and cholesterol in their diets to help prevent chronic diseases such as heart disease and cancer. Since they are low in fat and cholesterol and packed with important nutrients, low-fat and nonfat yogurts are perfect choices for those trying to eat a healthful diet. Yogurts without added sugar are low in carbohydrate and are not considered a primary carbohydrate source. Yogurts with added sugar contain more carbohydrate simply because of the added sugar.

A yogurt a day . . .

A great deal of scientific interest is currently focusing on the possible health benefits of the live, active cul-

Nutrient content of yogurt: what's in a cup*								
type of yogurt	calories	fat (g)	calories from fat (%)	carbohydrate (g)	protein (g)	cholesterol (mg)	calcium (mg)	sodium (mg)
plain								
whole-milk	139	7.4	48	10.6	7.9	29	274	105
low-fat	144	3.5	22	16.0	11.9	14	415	159
nonfat	127	0.4	3	17.4	13.0	4	452	174
flavored (vanilla, lemon, etc.)								
low-fat	194	2.8	13	31.3	11.2	11	389	149
nonfat								
fruit-added								
low-fat	225	2.6	10	42.3	9.0	10	314	121
nonfat	165	<1.0	<5	34.0	8.0	0	200	150
nonfat with aspartame	100	0.4	4	17	9.0	<5	240	150
breakfast-style	228	3.7	15	40.6	8.0	na†	na†	91
frozen‡								
regular (whole-milk)	220	6.0	24.5	36	6.0	20	160	90
low-fat	200	4.0	18	36	6.0	10	240	100

*per 8-oz cup

†not available

‡single serving usually averages 3–4 oz

Sources: Jean A.T. Pennington, *Bowes and Church's Food Values of Portions Commonly Used*, 15th ed., New York: Harper & Row, 1989, and manufacturers' data

tures in yogurt. Specifically, researchers are seeking to determine whether the bacteria themselves, and the lactic acid that they produce, have protective effects against disease. The finding that the live, active cultures in yogurt can survive digestion in the stomach and pass into the small intestine—and possibly the colon—intact has led scientists to investigate age-old notions about this food's reputed and potential health benefits. The following is a summary of recent findings.

Gastrointestinal infections. Diarrhea is usually caused by the invasion of the digestive tract by disease-causing organisms. The organisms, ingested in food or water, survive digestion and multiply in the intestine, producing pathogens that cause gastro-intestinal infection and its uncomfortable symptoms. Many laboratory studies have shown that active yogurt cultures (*L. bulgaricus, S. thermophilus, L. acidophilus*) can destroy common food-borne disease-causing organisms, such as salmonella, shigella, *Escherichia,* staphylococcus, *Listeria,* and *Campylobacter.* The lactic acid bacteria of the yogurt culture fight these disease-causing organisms in several ways. For one, the yogurt cultures produce acids that are able to enter and inactivate the harmful organisms. In addition, within the digestive tract the active bacterial cultures compete with the disease-causing organisms for essential nutrients and therefore essentially "starve out" the injurious bacteria. Finally, it is likely that the cultured bacteria of yogurt produce by-products of metabolism that are damaging to the disease-causing bacteria. Ultimately the organisms are destroyed, thereby preventing infection.

It has also been observed that the cultured bacteria of yogurt can protect against antibiotic-induced diarrhea that can occur with certain of these drugs, e.g., the tetracyclines, which can destroy the digestive system's natural antagonists to disease-producing organisms. Yogurts containing the *L. acidophilus* culture appear to be the most effective for this purpose, perhaps because this organism may be better able than the other two lactic acid cultures to survive digestion in the stomach.

Yeast infections. Medicinal folklore has long held that acidophilus (*i.e.,* containing *L. acidophilus*) milk and yogurt can help prevent vaginal yeast infections. The first study that finally put this long-held notion to the test was done in 1992. Researchers at Long Island (N.Y.) Jewish Medical Center monitored a group of women who suffered from chronic yeast infections over a six-month-period, during which the women consumed a cup of plain yogurt a day. Then the investigators asked the same group to refrain from eating yogurt for a six-month period. They found that consuming one cup of yogurt with live, active *L. acidophilus* every day did indeed reduce the incidence of infections by as much as a third. Thus, women who ordinarily had three vaginal yeast infections in six

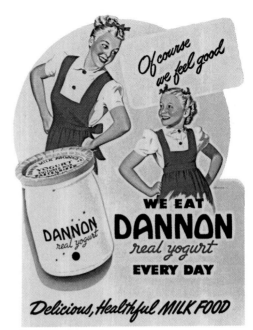

The Dannon Company, Inc.

months suffered only one. Because *L. acidophilus* apparently survives digestion better than the other lactic acid cultures and is believed to be able to colonize the gastrointestinal tract, it is theorized that the organism may somehow migrate from the intestines to the vagina; there it produces hydrogen peroxide, which inhibits the growth of yeast. It is important to note that all yogurts do not contain *L. acidophilus.* Those that do contain this culture say so on the label.

Cancer. There is some scientific evidence that the live, active cultures in yogurt, especially *L. bulgaricus* and *L. acidophilus,* may help prevent or manage some forms of cancer. The conclusions of the studies are limited because research on the effect of yogurt in cancer has been conducted only in animals; the

A calcium counter's guide	
food source (serving size)	calcium content (mg)
plain, low-fat yogurt (8 oz)	415
ricotta cheese, part skim (4 oz)	337
sardines, with bones (3 oz)	324
skim milk (8 oz)	302
2% low-fat milk (8 oz)	297
whole milk (8 oz)	291
American cheese (1 oz)	174
molasses, blackstrap (1 tbs)	137
spinach, fresh, cooked (4 oz)	122
cottage cheese, 2% low-fat (4 oz)	78

results so far indicate that cultures that survive in the digestive tract may delay onset or protect against the development of cancer of the colon and breast.

Epidemiological studies of diet and disease in humans have revealed that, in general, individuals who consume yogurt are less susceptible than others to certain cancers. In one study women whose diets were high in dairy fats such as whole milk and cheese had an increased risk of breast cancer; within this group, however, those who ate most of their dairy fat as yogurt had the lowest cancer risk. Possibly, the cancer risk of the women who ate yogurt was influenced by other dietary factors—such as higher intake of fruit, fiber, and vegetables—associated with decreased incidence of cancer. Moreover, one study has actually shown a connection between eating yogurt and developing ovarian cancer. Clearly, it is too early to draw any firm conclusions about yogurt and cancer risk.

Coronary heart disease. The interest in yogurt's possible connection with heart disease prevention began with the early observation that Masai tribesmen of East Africa who consumed large quantities of a yogurt-like food had low blood cholesterol levels despite a high intake of cholesterol. Further studies have both confirmed and refuted the hypothesis that yogurt has cholesterol-lowering properties. More research needs to be done for any health connection between yogurt and heart disease to be fully understood.

Immune function. Scientists have long suspected that the live, active cultures in yogurt enhance immune function. Several studies in experimental animals have found that being fed yogurt cultures or other lactic acid bacteria enhances their immune response either directly or indirectly.

Evidence also shows that when yogurt is heated, killing the bacterial cultures, there is a reduction in its immunologic benefit. This finding suggests that the live, active culture is required for any positive effect on immunity. Further, studies in mice have shown that after they ate yogurt containing live, active bacteria, their defenses against a salmonella pathogen were enhanced. The activity, number, and proliferation of various immune system cells were all increased in mice fed yogurt containing live, active cultures. *L. acidophilus* appears to be the most active of the yogurt cultures on the immune system of mice.

A study of the effects of yogurt on human immune function, conducted at the University of California at Davis, was published in 1992. Sixty-eight healthy adults aged 20–40 were divided into three groups and studied for four months. One group received no yogurt, while the other two ate two cups of yogurt a day. Of the two latter groups, one received yogurt containing live, active cultures, while the other received yogurt in which the cultures had been destroyed by heat treatment. The researchers found that the group

receiving yogurt containing active cultures produced four times more gamma interferon than either the group eating heat-treated yogurt or the non-yogurt-eating group. Gamma interferon is a highly active immune substance that combats and may prevent viral infections. It also reduces the severity of allergic reactions. This important area of research is continuing.

Add some culture to your life

With the constant burgeoning of yogurt types—34 new varieties were added to store shelves in 1992 alone—there should be a product to suit just about any taste. Consumers should keep in mind that yogurt is a milk product and must be refrigerated or kept cool. When buying yogurt, it is imperative to check the "sell by" date stamped on the carton. This date is 30–35 days from the date the yogurt was manufactured, and the product should stay fresh until one week past the indicated date. After that, the flavor may become more tart, and the culture content may diminish. Yogurt should be stored with other milk products on the top shelf of the refrigerator, which is the coolest spot. There is no exact time when yogurt will spoil, but spoilage can be recognized by the "sour" odor, similar to the smell of spoiled milk.

Freezing yogurt is not recommended. Home freezers and refrigerator freezer sections cannot freeze yogurt quickly enough to maintain its creamy consistency; home freezing therefore results in undesirable textural changes, such as the formation of ice crystals. Slow freezing also diminishes the number of active cultures in the yogurt. Yogurt can be frozen properly in a home ice cream freezer, however.

For people who are trying to lower the fat and cholesterol in their diet, plain yogurt or yogurt cheese (made by straining plain yogurt through cheesecloth) can be used as a replacement or partial substitute for sour cream, cream cheese, and mayonnaise in dips, sauces, and spreads. Vanilla- or fruit-flavored yogurt and honey-sweetened plain yogurt make delicious toppings for fresh fruit desserts. Yogurt can also be used to reduce the amount of eggs and oil needed in recipes for some baked goods. And a nutritious, tasty drink can be made in a blender from combinations of fresh fruit, yogurt, and low-fat milk.

People who are watching their calories should be aware of the sugar content of fruit-added yogurts; they may instead want to choose vanilla, coffee, and lemon flavors, which have less added sugar, or add fresh fruit to plain yogurt. Another alternative is to choose a product sweetened with aspartame.

Whether yogurt truly contributes to longevity remains to be seen. Nonetheless, it is clear that yogurt offers many nutritional benefits and is a food that can play an integral part in a healthy diet for people of all ages.

Middle Ear Infections

by Alvin N. Eden, M.D.

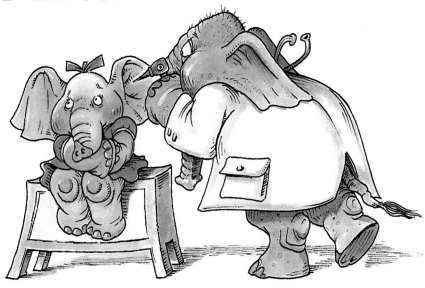

Otitis media, or inflammation of the middle ear, is one of the most common infections in childhood—second only to upper respiratory infections and colds. It can affect children of all ages, including infants. Because middle ear infections occur so frequently in young children and because complications can develop—most notably, hearing loss—it is essential that parents become familiar with the signs and symptoms so that the diagnosis can be made as soon as possible. The treatment of otitis media is a complicated and controversial subject. There is as yet no consensus among physicians as to the optimal treatment or the best way to prevent complications, but all doctors agree that early diagnosis and treatment improve the outcome.

The middle ear and the eustachian tube

Otitis media is defined as an infection or inflammation of the middle ear cavity, the area located just behind the tympanic membrane (better known as the eardrum). In order to understand the mechanisms involved in the development of middle ear infections, it is necessary to know something about the eustachian tube, the bony, cartilaginous tube (sometimes called the auditory tube) that extends from the space in back of the nose to the middle ear cavity. This tube has two main functions. The first is to ventilate the middle ear, replenishing oxygen that has been absorbed and equalizing the air and atmospheric pressures on both sides of the eardrum. With a normally functioning eustachian tube, the lower end of the tube opens during swallowing and yawning, allowing the air that flows up through the tube to balance the air entering through the outer ear canal. This balance of air pressures optimizes the capacity to hear well. The second function

of the eustachian tube is drainage of fluid and mucus out of the middle ear cavity into the nasopharynx. If the tube becomes obstructed or does not function properly and collapses, the fluid becomes trapped in the middle ear cavity and cannot escape. If the fluid remains behind the eardrum for long periods of time, it can cause hearing loss.

Upper respiratory infections and allergies are two common conditions that interfere with eustachian tube function, leading to middle ear inflammation and infection. When a child has an upper respiratory infection, the eustachian tube becomes blocked, thereby trapping fluid inside the middle ear cavity. Middle ear fluid acts as an excellent medium for bacterial growth; bacteria from the back of the nose travel up the eustachian tube directly into the middle ear cavity, where they grow and multiply. This bacterial accumulation causes the fluid to become thick and purulent (filled with pus).

Children with allergies often develop swelling in the back of the nose. This leads to obstruction of the flow of air through the eustachian tube and results in the accumulation of clear fluid in the middle ear cavity. When there is a poorly functioning eustachian tube, the fluid cannot drain out, and the trapped fluid can then become infected with bacteria.

A third condition known to be a cause of obstruction of the eustachian tube is enlarged adenoids. Adenoids are masses of lymphoid gland tissue at the back of the pharynx that, if abnormally enlarged, can obstruct both nasal and ear passages and induce mouth breathing, nasality, and postnasal drip. However, it is unclear exactly what role the adenoids play in the development of middle ear infections.

467

Middle ear infections

Functional obstruction of the eustachian tube can also result in middle ear effusion—*i.e.,* fluid that becomes trapped in the middle ear cavity. In infants and small children the cartilage supporting the eustachian tube is not as stiff as that in older children, which means it can collapse, causing obstruction. In addition, infants and young children have short eustachian tubes, which are quite susceptible to the backup, or reflux, of throat secretions into the middle ear space. This functional eustachian tube obstruction in infants and young children in part explains why middle ear infections are most common between six months and two years of age.

Childhood vulnerability

Two-thirds of all children have had at least one middle ear infection—in one or both ears—by the time they are two years of age. Surveys of practicing pediatricians indicate that except for well-baby and routine child care examinations, otitis media is the most frequent reason for young children's office visits.

Middle ear infections can occur at any age, including the newborn period. As already mentioned, the highest incidence of such infections is between six months and two years. During this period young children are more susceptible to throat infections, both bacterial and viral, and their short eustachian tubes cannot function properly to drain the fluid from the middle ear. After age two the incidence then decreases, but it starts to increase again between ages five and six, the time when children usually enter school and have increased exposure to other children with frequent respiratory infections. Beyond age seven, middle ear infections are comparatively much less frequent in occurrence.

There is no difference in incidence of middle ear infections between boys and girls. American Indians and Eskimos seem to develop more frequent infections; this may be for genetic reasons—because of the shape of their eustachian tubes. Among all children, cases of middle ear infection are reported most often during the winter months, when the incidence of respiratory infections is highest.

Certain conditions make some children more vulnerable to middle ear infections than others. For example, infants under one year of age who spend time in group day-care settings are exposed to more viruses that cause respiratory infection than are those who are cared for at home; they therefore suffer more frequent ear infections. Also, children in day care are often exposed to adults who smoke; children who are exposed to passive, or second-hand, smoke have higher rates of chronic infections (otitis media with effusion) than those who are not so exposed.

There are various ways of classifying otitis media. This discussion will be limited to the two types most frequently seen in children, acute purulent otitis media and otitis media with effusion. The signs and symptoms as well as the complications and treatment are different for each type.

Acute purulent otitis media

In acute purulent otitis media the middle ear cavity is filled with pus, and there is the possibility of abscess formation—*i.e.,* a localized collection of pus that is surrounded by inflamed tissue. Children suffering from this infection are quite ill. The symptoms include severe earache, a feeling of fullness and sometimes ringing in the ear, fever, irritability that is often accompanied by persistent crying, weakness, and headache. Many of these children also have accompanying nausea, vomiting, and complete loss of appetite. In babies the fever may be very high—up to 40.5° C (105° F). The thick purulent material within the middle ear cavity increases the pressure against the eardrum, causing severe pain. A physician examining a child with acute purulent otitis media will find that the eardrum is red and bulging. If the pressure continues to increase, it can result in rupture of the eardrum. Following rupture, the pus then drains out through the ear canal. When this happens, the excruciating pain caused by the pressure on the membrane quickly subsides, and the infection usually clears up in a few days.

Many studies have been conducted to investigate the causes of acute purulent otitis media. Analysis of the thick fluid in the middle ear has shown that the condition is almost always due to a bacterial infection and that *Streptococcus pneumoniae* and *Haemophilus influenzae* are the two most frequently isolated bacteria (but the latter is infrequently seen in children over eight years of age).

A number of antibiotics are effective in treating acute middle ear infections. The child's physician determines the specific antibiotic to be used, the dose to be given, and the duration of the treatment. The consensus among most pediatricians is that a full 10-day course of antibiotic treatment is required for the best results to be achieved. One of the most widely prescribed and effective drugs is amoxicillin. A study reported in the January 1993 issue of *Pediatrics* suggested that a single injection of the antibiotic ceftriaxone, a drug often used to treat pneumonia and meningitis, is as effective as the traditional 10 days of oral treatment with amoxicillin. However, further study of the effectiveness of single-injection therapy is needed.

In almost all cases the child's signs and symptoms will abate dramatically soon after the start of antibiotic treatment. If the organism causing the infection is sensitive to the specific antibiotic chosen, the fluid in the middle ear cavity becomes free of bacteria in over 90% of cases. A small number of children do not improve with antibiotic therapy and continue to suffer pain and fever. In such cases a different antibiotic is then usually given.

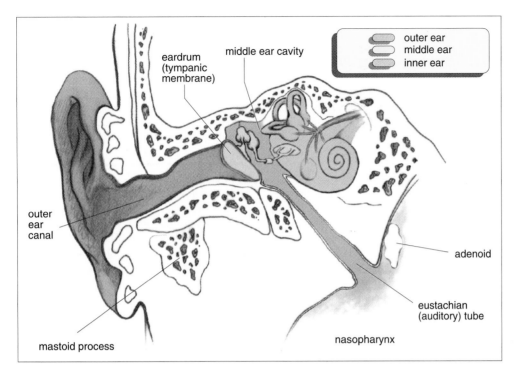

eardrum
(tympanic
membrane)

middle ear cavity

outer ear
middle ear
inner ear

outer
ear
canal

adenoid

eustachian
(auditory) tube

mastoid process

nasopharynx

Many cases of antibiotic treatment failure are due to improper dosage, failure to administer the medication on schedule, or early cessation of the treatment. It is important, therefore, for parents to follow the doctor's prescribed treatment exactly. In rare instances, when pain and fever persist despite a full course of antibiotics, it is necessary to drain the thick pus that remains in the middle ear space in order to relieve the symptoms caused by the increased pressure on the eardrum. (The latter condition is sometimes referred to as glue ear, owing to the sticky consistency of the persisting purulent secretions.)

Many young children are subject to frequent, repeated bouts of acute otitis media. Despite successful treatment of the ear infection, with each new cold or upper respiratory illness there is another episode of acute infection. In such cases some physicians may prescribe prophylactic daily doses of an antibiotic, especially over the winter months, in order to help prevent further infections.

Otitis media with effusion

Despite proper treatment of the acute purulent type of middle ear infection, some children (an estimated one in four) are left with fluid in the middle ear that does not drain out or get absorbed. This chronic condition is called otitis media with effusion, or serous (or secretory) otitis media, and is much more difficult to diagnose than the acute purulent form. Often there are no signs and symptoms, so the diagnosis is delayed or never made. Serous otitis media is characterized by watery, clear fluid in the middle ear cavity that pro-

duces little or no increased pressure on the eardrum and therefore is not associated with pain. The condition most likely to lead to serous otitis media is eustachian tube dysfunction (in conjunction with either allergies or frequent upper respiratory infections).

The most important complication of serous otitis media is the hearing loss that may result if the diagnosis is delayed and the fluid remains in the middle ear cavity for too long a time. In school-age children serous otitis media is considered the most common cause of loss of hearing. There have been a number of reports describing speech problems and behavior and learning deficits resulting from hearing loss associated with prolonged and repeated episodes of serous otitis media during the first three years of life. The problem may not be recognized until a teacher notices that the child is inattentive. Only when it has been determined that this is because the child has trouble hearing is he or she examined by a physician and found to have fluid behind the eardrum.

Even for the skilled clinician, the diagnosis of serous otitis media is not always straightforward. Often the eardrum is difficult to visualize because wax obstructs the physician's view through the otoscope (an instrument that uses a light and magnifying lens to facilitate examination of internal ear structures through the outer ear canal). When the view is blocked, other techniques may be needed for determining whether fluid is present. One such method is tympanometry, the insertion of a probe into the external ear canal that presents a tone and then measures the sound pressure level within the middle ear cavity. In this way the degree of acoustical impedance is determined; when fluid is present behind the eardrum, relatively little sound is absorbed—*i.e.*, acoustical energy is impeded. Another method of determining the presence of middle ear fluid is with the pneumatic otoscope, a device that uses an ear speculum large enough to completely occlude the external ear canal and has a rubber suction bulb to test the reaction of the tympanic membrane to air pressure. If fluid is present, the eardrum's mobility in response to the air flow is impaired.

The child's physician will decide if and when these specialized techniques are needed to diagnose serous otitis media and may refer the patient to a specialist—an otologist or otolaryngologist—to perform the tests. Because the longer fluid remains in the ear, the greater the likelihood that it will cause hearing loss, it is imperative for every child treated for acute purulent otitis media to be reexamined after the treatment has been completed in order to make certain that the middle ear cavity is free of fluid.

The treatment of otitis media with effusion remains both complicated and controversial. When there is no associated or prolonged hearing loss, the consensus of most physicians is that the infection should be treated conservatively and that surgical intervention (discussed below) is not needed.

In the past, many physicians believed that the use of combined decongestant-antihistamine medications for serous otitis media reduced swelling and allowed fluid to drain out of the middle ear cavity through the eustachian tube. Although some doctors still recommend them, many investigations have shown that decongestant-antihistamines are not effective.

Because some studies have concluded that bacteria are still present in the clear fluid in about one-third of the children treated for acute purulent otitis media, some doctors prescribe an additional course of antibiotic therapy. But when there is no hearing loss, the majority of physicians believe that the best method of treatment is no treatment at all. In time, the ear fluid resorbs or drains out of the ear, a process that usually takes from one to three months.

A recent uproar in the medical literature concerning the use of amoxicillin in the treatment of otitis media with effusion was widely covered by the media. A report published in February 1987 in the *New England Journal of Medicine* had concluded that there was some beneficial effect from amoxicillin. One of the investigators who participated in the original study disagreed with the conclusions that were published. In December 1991 a paper in the *Journal of the American Medical Association* reexamined the same data, concluding that amoxicillin had no beneficial effect. This not only added further confusion to the issue of appropriate treatment of middle ear infections but prompted much concern about treatment among physicians and parents alike. While this debate is as yet unresolved, the important point to remember is that the dispute is *not* over the use of amoxicillin in treating acute purulent otitis media, where its effectiveness is well established.

The consensus among both otolaryngologists and pediatricians at present is to intervene surgically when a child with serous otitis media is found to have significant hearing loss over a period of many months or when the child has had a history of frequent, recurrent episodes of serous otitis media with associated hearing loss. The fluid in the middle ear can be drained out either by means of a surgical incision in the eardrum (myringotomy) or by myringotomy and insertion of small ventilation tubes, called tympanotomy tubes, into the eardrum. These tubes, which are left in place for an extended period of time (months or years), are believed to help keep the middle ear cavity free of fluid.

These surgical procedures should not be performed after only one or two episodes of serous otitis media because there are a number of potential complications, such as psychological trauma, risks associated with anesthesia, secondary infection, and eardrum scarring. Some otolaryngologists recommend removal of enlarged adenoids to prevent recurrent episodes of serous otitis media because the inflamed tissue can obstruct the eustachian tube, although the precise role of adenoids in causing middle ear infections, as noted previously, has not been established.

A condition to be taken seriously

The complications of middle ear infections have decreased dramatically in recent years. With the use of appropriate antibiotics, fortunately, many potentially serious or life-threatening complications, including inflammation of the mastoid process and air-filled mastoid cells at the base of the skull, brain abscess, and meningitis, have been almost entirely eliminated. However, owing to the persistence of serous fluid in the middle ear cavity following treatment of acute purulent otitis media, physicians continue to be confronted with the difficult problem of hearing loss in children. Long-standing hearing loss may impair a child's speech, language comprehension, and learning ability. Therefore, all preschool-age children should have their hearing tested, especially those who have had a history of recurrent ear infections, chronic allergies with respiratory symptoms, or frequent upper respiratory infections.

Middle ear infections in children remain among the most poorly understood conditions facing pediatricians and parents. The key to preventing possible complications is maintenance of a high index of suspicion so that an early diagnosis can be made and proper treatment instituted without delay.

How Much Exercise Is Enough?

by Barry A. Franklin, Ph.D.

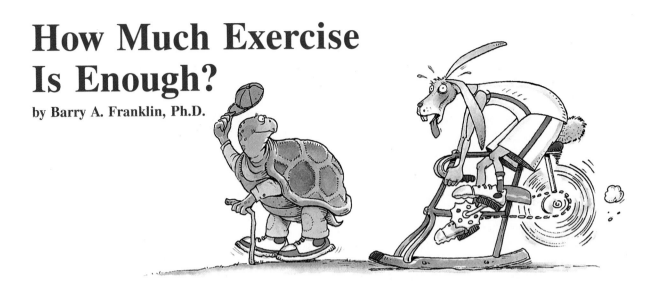

The beneficial effects of regular physical activity are well documented. Aerobic exercise training decreases the heart rate and blood pressure at rest and at any given level of exertion, reducing the workload of the heart. Research has also shown that regular exercise increases one's ability to take in and utilize oxygen. When the body's ability to transport and deliver oxygen improves, individuals have increased energy and do not tire as easily. This index of "cardiorespiratory fitness" is commonly referred to as "maximal oxygen consumption," or "aerobic capacity." Because maximal oxygen consumption normally decreases by about 1% per year after the age of 20, and an exercise program generally increases this variable by about 20%, the physically conditioned 60-year-old can actually achieve the same fitness level as the inactive 40-year-old. In other words, regular exercise can produce a 20-year functional rejuvenation. There are, as well, quite a few general "health" benefits associated with regular exercise participation, including increased bone density, enhanced glucose tolerance, an improved coronary risk factor profile, and reduced cardiovascular-related mortality. Moreover, studies indicate that compared with sedentary people, those who exercise are better able to cope with stress and are less likely to suffer from depression and anxiety.

Experts now agree that the intensity of exercise needed to attain substantial health-related benefits differs from the intensity that is generally prescribed for cardiorespiratory conditioning. In recent years lower levels of physical activity than were previously considered beneficial have been shown to reduce the risk of several chronic degenerative diseases—even though the intensity may be insufficient to improve maximal oxygen consumption. The following will attempt to clarify how much exercise is required for promoting optimal cardiorespiratory fitness, on the one hand, and attaining specific health benefits, on the other.

Attaining cardiorespiratory fitness

The effectiveness of any exercise program is dependent on two basic variables, long-term adherence to the program and appropriateness of the exercise "prescription." The typical exercise session has three phases: a warm-up; a stimulus, or endurance, phase; and a cooldown (*see* Figure, page 473).

Warm-up. The warm-up, which should include both musculoskeletal and cardiorespiratory activities, prepares the body for the transition from rest to vigorous exercise by increasing blood flow, respiration, and body temperature and stretching postural muscles. It also decreases the susceptibility to injury during exercise and lowers the potential for heart rhythm irregularities that may be provoked by sudden strenuous exertion. The warm-up is therefore an important preventive measure; it takes about 5 to 10 minutes and serves to enhance performance capacity.

The warm-up should begin with some light stretching to "warm up" the muscles. The ideal preparation for any endurance activity is then to perform that activity at a low intensity. Hence, people who walk for fitness should conclude their warm-up period with slow walking. Similarly, brisk walking at about 5.6 to 7.2 km/h (3.5 to 4.5 mph) serves as an ideal warm-up for those who jog during the endurance phase of the workout.

Endurance phase. The stimulus, or endurance, phase serves to stimulate the body's oxygen-transport system and maximize caloric expenditure. The exercise prescription should specify the frequency (how often a person exercises), the intensity (how strenuously a person exercises), the duration (the length of each exercise session), and the mode (the type of exercise that is best for the individual).

For persons who wish to develop and maintain cardiorespiratory fitness, most fitness experts recommend exercising at a frequency of three to five days

471

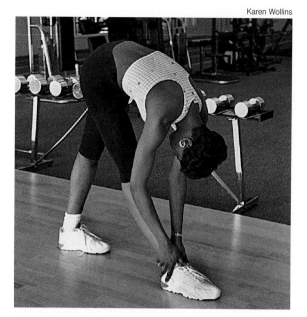

Five to 10 minutes of warming up for a vigorous cardiorespiratory workout are well worth the time spent. The warm-up increases blood flow, respiration, and body temperature; stretching reduces the chance of muscular injury.

a week. The additional benefits provided by a daily workout appear to be minimal, whereas the incidence of musculoskeletal injuries increases markedly, especially with "impact" activities such as jogging and jumping.

The intensity of the exercise can be regulated in several ways: keeping the heart rate within a prescribed training zone; maintaining an assigned pace for walking or jogging or a recommended workload on a stationary bicycle (ergometer); and evaluating perceived exertion by using a standard rating system. This latter method, particularly when used in conjunction with other physiological measurements (*e.g.,* pulse rate), is an especially reliable way to keep exercise within safe and effective limits.

One perceived-exertion scale, which was developed by a Swedish scientist, uses ratings based on the individual's overall feeling of exertion and physical fatigue: rest, very very light, very light, fairly light, somewhat hard, hard, very hard, and very very hard. These ratings correspond well with certain metabolic responses to exercise, such as heart rate and oxygen consumption. This personal assessment of exercise intensity should focus on the overall, or total, feeling of exertion without overemphasizing any one factor, such as leg pain or shortness of breath. Exercise rated as "fairly light" to "hard" is generally appropriate for cardiorespiratory conditioning, corresponding to 70 to 85% of maximal heart rate, which is equivalent to 60 to 80% of the maximal oxygen consumption. For other health benefits (discussed below) it may be enough to exercise at a perceived level of only "very light."

An individual's maximal heart rate may be accurately determined from the results of an exercise stress test; healthy men and women can also estimate it by subtracting their age in years from 220. Thus, for a healthy 40-year-old, maximal heart rate is 180 (beats per minute). However, the variance in maximal heart rate for any given age is considerable—plus or minus 20 beats per minute. The range for 40-year-olds, therefore, is anywhere from 160 to 200.

By taking a 10-second pulse count (and multiplying the result by 6) at several points during the exercise routine, the individual can make sure he or she is exercising within the 70-to-85%-intensity range. It should be emphasized, however, that the training-intensity threshold appears to have a wide variance, and considerable evidence suggests that it increases in direct proportion to the individual's initial level of fitness. Thus, people who are inactive or deconditioned may show improvement in cardiorespiratory fitness at initial training intensities that are below theoretical target levels.

In addition to the warm-up and cooldown, each exercise session should include at least 20 to 30 minutes of sustained activity at the 70-to-85%-intensity level. Sessions longer than 45 to 60 minutes result in little additional cardiorespiratory improvement, while, again, the potential for musculoskeletal and orthopedic injury increases. Although it is widely believed that physical benefits from exercise accrue only from one continuous workout of 30 minutes or longer, recent studies have shown similar improvements in cardiorespiratory fitness in subjects who completed three 10-minute bouts of moderate exercise on a workout day.

The most effective modes of exercise for cardiorespiratory-fitness achievement are those that employ large muscle groups, are maintained continuously, and are rhythmic and aerobic in nature. Examples include: walking, jogging (in place or over a distance), running, stationary or outdoor cycling, swimming, jumping rope, rowing, climbing stairs, and stepping on and off a bench. Conditioning programs for adults who had previously been sedentary may include: calisthenics, particularly those involving sustained total body movement; recreational games such as volleyball, badminton, and tennis; and weight training. The latter may be particularly important, as traditional aerobic conditioning regimens often fail to include activities that improve strength and muscle tone.

Charles Dickens said, "Walk and be happy; walk and be healthy." Walking is undoubtedly the most accessible and easily regulated exercise for almost any goal—to increase cardiorespiratory fitness and particularly to reduce body weight and fat stores. In one recent study of 343 normally sedentary healthy adults (165 men, 178 women), 67% of men and 91% of women achieved a training heart rate (defined as greater than 70% of maximal heart rate) when asked to "walk a mile briskly." Among men over age 50, 83% reached a training heart rate. These findings suggest that most deconditioned adults can improve cardiorespiratory fitness by regular walking. Furthermore, walking is done at an easily tolerated intensity and causes fewer injuries to the legs, knees, and feet than, say, running or jogging would. In addition, it is a "companionable" activity that requires no special equipment other than a pair of well-fitted athletic shoes. Walking in water or with a backpack offers additional benefits for those who wish to substantially improve aerobic capacity.

One who wishes to improve endurance of the upper extremities in addition to achieving cardiorespiratory fitness should choose a training activity that specifically activates these muscles. Equipment suitable for upper-body training includes rowing machines, wall pulleys, simulated cross-country skiing devices, and specially designed arm-crank ergometers or combined arm-leg ergometers.

Cooldown. The cooldown, lasting about 5 to 10 minutes, provides a gradual recovery from the endurance phase. It permits appropriate circulatory adjustments and return of the heart rate and blood pressure to near-resting values. One should never stand still or lie down immediately after exercise; rather, it is important to let the body readjust gradually to the decreased physical demands. Stretching at the end of an exercise session will increase elasticity in muscles and help prevent injury. The cooldown also prevents blood from pooling in the enlarged veins of the exercised muscles, thereby reducing the potential for postexercise hypotension (a sudden drop in blood pressure) that reduces blood circulation to the heart and brain and may result in dizziness or light-headedness, nausea, or even fainting. Additionally, the cooldown facilitates

the dissipation of body heat and helps remove lactic acid, a metabolic product that accumulates in the body during strenuous exercise and can cause fatigue and muscle soreness.

Exercising for health

When it comes to the benefits of regular exercise participation, improved cardiorespiratory fitness is often emphasized more than the potential for disease prevention. Thus, many people have come to think of exercise programs as being synonymous with extremely arduous physical activity. As already noted, however, there are numerous health benefits that can be derived at mild to moderate exercise intensities, provided that the frequency and duration are sufficient. Several of these benefits are detailed as follows:

Effects on bone density. Osteoporosis, in which the bones become excessively porous over time, occurs most commonly in women over the age of 50, owing to a lack of the hormone estrogen after menopause. Symptoms may include a small decrease in height and a rounding of the back. As a result of the gradual loss of bone mass, even minor falls can cause broken bones, especially at the hip and wrist. Indeed, it is estimated that in the United States alone osteoporosis is responsible for 1.2 million fractures each year.

To prevent the problem, attention has generally focused on hormone replacement therapy, adequate calcium intake, and exercise. Weight-bearing activities (such as walking or jogging) are generally better than, say, bicycling or swimming for maintaining bone density. For unfit individuals or those who have suffered previous fractures, however, the latter activities may be preferred. One study done at Washington University, St. Louis, Mo., found that women with osteoporosis who walked for one hour a day three days a week in-

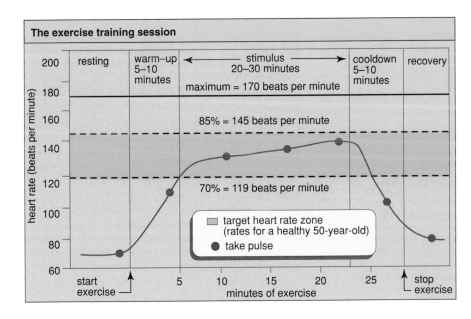

How much exercise is enough?

creased their bone density at the spine (and presumably in other areas) by 6% over nine months. These findings suggest that regular walking can reduce or reverse the bone mineral loss that often occurs in older persons. Moreover, it has been suggested that younger women can help prevent the bone-loss effects that would otherwise occur later if they begin exercising premenopausally.

Effects on glucose tolerance. Diabetes is a disease that is characterized by a chronically elevated blood glucose concentration. It is caused by a lack of insulin (type I, insulin-dependent diabetes) or by a resistance to insulin (type II, non-insulin-dependent diabetes) and, over time, it is associated with retinal damage and possibly blindness, kidney disease, heart disease, stroke, and peripheral vascular disease. By the age of 70 approximately one in four adults is at increased risk of developing adult-onset (type II) diabetes. Studies have shown that the incidence of type II diabetes (which affects as many as 12 million people in the United States) is lower in physically active populations than in predominantly sedentary ones and that its occurrence increases if a population group becomes less active.

In persons with diabetes, glucose levels build up in the blood (top), while relatively little glucose enters the cells to fuel them. The cause can be a lack of insulin, which "unlocks" receptors that allow glucose into the cells, or an insensitivity of the cells to insulin. In normal cells (bottom) insulin admits sufficient glucose to meet energy needs. Studies have shown that for diabetic patients exercise has an insulin-like effect, apparently enhancing glucose movement into cells.

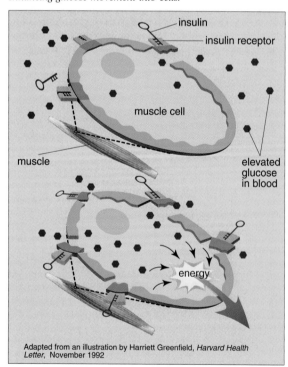

Adapted from an illustration by Harriett Greenfield, *Harvard Health Letter*, November 1992

Dietary changes, weight reduction, and regular exercise are often recommended for both the prevention and treatment of diabetes. Numerous studies have shown that when diabetic patients become less active, their insulin requirements increase, and vice versa. This is presumably because physical activity enhances the transport of glucose into muscle cells and blunts the rise in blood glucose that follows carbohydrate ingestion. In other words, exercise has an insulin-like effect (*see* Figure).

Persons with diabetes can generally participate in the same types of physical activities as their non-diabetic counterparts. Frequent exercise sessions (five or more workouts per week) are recommended for both types of diabetes. Exercise duration for the individual with type I diabetes may be as low as 20 to 30 minutes per session, whereas the person with type II diabetes needs to maximize caloric expenditure and therefore exercise longer (*i.e.,* 40 to 60 minutes) on each workout day. The exercise intensity for type I diabetics is similar to that for healthy adults. In contrast, those with type II diabetes can exercise at more moderate exercise intensities (*e.g.,* 60 to 70% of maximal heart rate) because their prescribed exercise frequency and duration are so high.

When initiating an aerobic training program, it may be important for diabetics to monitor their blood glucose levels before and after exercise. Adjustments in carbohydrate intake or insulin dose may be needed to reduce the risk of hypoglycemic events (symptoms caused by low blood sugar).

Effects on coronary risk factors. Aerobic exercise training programs can result in modest decreases in body weight, fat stores, blood pressure (particularly in hypertensive individuals), total blood cholesterol, serum triglycerides, and low-density lipoprotein (LDL), the "bad" cholesterol. In recent years it has also become quite clear that exercise increases high-density lipoprotein (HDL), the "good" cholesterol. (To differentiate "good" from "bad" cholesterol, one might instead think of HDL as "helpful" and LDL as "lousy.")

Obesity: Exercise programs for the overweight should be performed at least three days per week for 30 minutes or more and include sustained activities involving large muscle groups to promote a caloric expenditure of 300 to 500 kcal (kilocalories) per session. For many persons this may best be accomplished by regular walking for an extended duration. Training regimens lasting less than three months, or those performed only twice a week—regardless of the intensity, duration, or both—are generally ineffective in reducing body weight and fat stores.

Exercise rated between "fairly light" and "somewhat hard" is often recommended for weight-reduction programs, corresponding to 60 to 70% of the maximal heart rate, which is equivalent to 40 to 60% of maximal oxygen consumption. At such an intensity the

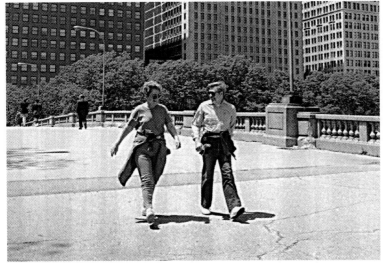

Brisk walking is an ideal form of exercise for meeting almost any fitness goal. It is easily tolerated and unlikely to cause injury; enhances flexibility, strength, and endurance; and is accessible, companionable, and pleasurable. For many people walking is an activity that becomes a lifelong, health-promoting habit.

body preferentially uses free fatty acids as the fuel source, while blood lactate levels generally remain low, allowing the individual to exercise for sustained periods without fatigue or muscle soreness. Most research suggests that it is the total caloric expenditure rather than the exercise intensity that is the most important determinant of weight lost from exercise. Thus, to maximize the caloric cost of exercise, lower-intensity programs need to be compensated for by increased duration of each exercise session, increased frequency of participation, or both.

Hypertension: A recent "meta-analysis"—a compilation and analysis of the findings of 25 relevant studies—demonstrated the efficacy of low-to-moderate-intensity exercise training in the treatment of mild high blood pressure. The studies generally involved men between 15 and 70 years of age, and the physical training programs varied from one to 12 months in length. Approximately two-thirds of the experimental groups in these studies (23 of 33) demonstrated statistically significant decreases in blood pressure, averaging about 10 mm Hg (millimeters of mercury) lower for both systolic and diastolic blood pressure. Interestingly, low-intensity training seemed to be just as effective as high-intensity training and possibly even more so.

Blood lipids and lipoproteins: Similarly, a meta-analysis of the results of 66 training studies demonstrated that in the average exercising subject, total cholesterol, triglycerides, and LDL cholesterol showed small but significant decreases, corresponding to 10, 16, and 5 mg per deciliter, respectively. In contrast, HDL cholesterol increased by only one milligram per deciliter (not significant). None of the changes for the nonexercising control groups was significant. Higher initial levels of total cholesterol and triglycerides and lower initial levels of HDL cholesterol resulted in greater postconditioning decreases and increases, re-

spectively. Cholesterol decreased as the exercise duration and total caloric expenditure increased. Moreover, lower training intensities were associated with more beneficial changes in lipids and lipoproteins.

Although vigorous physical activity like running has most often been associated with an increased "helpful" cholesterol component, recent studies indicate that regular low-intensity, long-duration physical activity may also play an important role in increasing HDL cholesterol. Investigators at Stanford University have reported that approximately 1,000 kcal per week of additional energy expenditure—equivalent to walking or running 13–16 km (8 to 10 mi)—may represent the "threshold" exercise dosage required for increasing HDL. However, other variables, such as age, gender, relative body fatness, heredity, socioeconomic status, smoking, alcohol consumption, and diet, also influence lipid and lipoprotein levels and therefore may partially explain individual differences that are seen in subjects who exercise at the same level.

Effects on "all-cause" mortality. A landmark study conducted at the Cooper Institute for Aerobics Research in Dallas, Texas, revealed that a low level of cardiorespiratory fitness is an independent risk factor for all-cause mortality—in other words, that a lack of exercise reduces longevity. However, this study also demonstrated that only *moderate* exercise is needed to reduce mortality risk.

The investigators prospectively studied 10,224 men and 3,120 women, who were given a preliminary medical examination and a treadmill stress test to assess their aerobic fitness. At the time, none of the individuals showed any evidence of cancer or heart disease. Over an average follow-up of slightly more than eight years, 240 men and 43 women died. The results showed that, in general, the higher the initial level of fitness, the lower the subsequent death rate from cancer and heart disease, even after statistical adjustments were made for age, family history of heart disease, and other coronary risk factors. This relation held up to an "average" fitness level for both men and women. Interestingly, there appeared to be no additional benefit (*i.e.,* lower mortality) associated with higher levels of fitness. Thus, the risk of death for superbly conditioned distance runners was essentially the same as for persons with an average level of fitness. Moreover, the greatest reduction in risk for both men and women occurred among study participants who progressed from the lowest level of fitness (poor) to the next lowest level (below average). As the study's leading investigator, Steven N. Blair, has said, "People who do a little bit of exercise are better off than those . . . who do none. Those who do a little more are better off still."

The study emphasized that the fitness level associated with the lowest mortality rate could be easily achieved by most men and women who walk briskly on a regular basis. Thus, it appears that the protective effects of physical activity can be derived at much more moderate levels of exercise than many had supposed—and far from the fevered pitch some Americans have felt the need to adopt.

Heeding warnings and exercising safely

Although the advantages of regular physical activity are undeniable, there are limitations to the benefits that exercise training offers relative to the prevention of heart disease. Contrary to the speculation of some overzealous enthusiasts, regular exercise training—regardless of the intensity, duration, or both—does not confer "immunity" to heart disease. Furthermore, reports of exercise-related cardiovascular complications have appeared in both the medical literature and the lay press, suggesting that strenuous physical exertion may actually precipitate heart attack or sudden death in some persons.

Fortunately, exercise-related deaths rarely occur in "presumably healthy" adults. Even the vast majority of cardiac patients can exercise safely after a heart attack, coronary artery bypass surgery, or balloon angioplasty. There are, however, a small number of persons who may be predisposed to heart problems during vigorous physical activities like jogging. Almost without exception, these individuals have some form of cardiovascular or structural heart disease.

Can the person "at risk" be accurately identified in advance? Although exercise stress testing is widely recommended and extremely useful in screening for such abnormalities, it is not infallible. Exercise testing has the greatest value in persons with a reasonable likelihood of heart disease—for example, middle-aged or older individuals with a family history of heart disease, major coronary risk factors, or heart disease symptoms (such as angina, or chest pain). On average, the test is accurate in diagnosing certain heart

problems about 70% of the time. In some instances abnormalities that are present go undetected, while in other cases signs or symptoms of heart disease may develop or progress after the test.

Most authorities now agree that it is difficult to predict who may be fatally stricken during exercise. Neither superior fitness nor regular exercise participation nor the absence of cardiac risk factors guarantees protection against an exercise-related death. One clue, however, has emerged. Cardiovascular complications during exercise are often preceded by specific "warnings," including abnormal heart rhythms, chest pain or pressure, and dizziness.

Abnormalities in heart rhythm, called arrhythmias, may include extremely fast, slow, or irregular heartbeats, sometimes perceived as palpitations. Although some arrhythmias are potentially dangerous, most are harmless. Pain or pressure in the center of the chest during or immediately after exercise may suggest a compromised blood supply to the heart muscle. Additional warnings may include arm, back, jaw, throat, or stomach discomfort, which many exercisers fail to recognize as cardiac related. Finally, insufficient blood flow to the brain can cause transient lightheadedness or dizziness. This may be due to serious cardiac rhythm disorders or impaired pumping of the heart muscle. Persons who experience any of these symptoms during activity should stop exercising. They should also consult their physicians to see if a complete workup or further investigation of the problem is warranted.

Not-so-new wisdom

The health and fitness benefits of exercise appear to depend more on the total amount of exercise accomplished—or energy, or calories, expended—than on the specific exercise intensity, frequency, or duration. Low-to-moderate-intensity exercise training can produce beneficial changes in cardiorespiratory fitness, bone density, glucose tolerance, and coronary risk factors and reduce cardiovascular-related and possibly other causes of mortality. These findings may be especially relevant to the inactive adult for whom the perceived discomfort of vigorous physical activity may serve as a deterrent to long-term compliance with an exercise program—or even to beginning such a program.

How much exercise then is enough? Perhaps an earlier observer had the simplest answer and offered the best "exercise prescription" over 2,300 years ago:

All parts of the body which have a function, if used in moderation and exercised in labors in which each is accustomed, become thereby healthy, well-developed and age more slowly, but if unused and left idle they become liable to disease, defective in growth, and age quickly.

That wise doctor was, of course, Hippocrates.

Temper Tantrums

by Elaine A. Blechman, Ph.D.

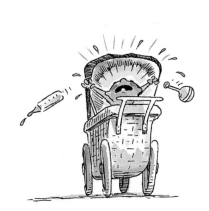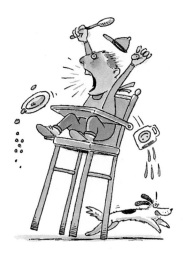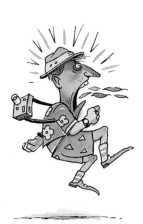

● Betty, a 13-month-old, has a history of ear infections. Painful earaches often kept her awake at night, and she needed to be comforted constantly by her parents. The infections have finally cleared up, but now whenever Betty is left alone in her crib at night, she screams and cries until someone picks her up.

● While waiting in line at the supermarket checkout stand, Rob, aged six, demands that his father buy him a candy bar. When his father refuses, Rob lies down on the floor, kicks his feet, and screams.

● When dropping off four-year-old Jill at the day-care center, her mother tells her they will not be able to go on a picnic that afternoon, as she had previously promised. Jill begins to cry and scream, "You bad mother. I hate you!"

● Tim, an eighth-grader, arrives at math class only to discover that the teacher has decided to spring a surprise quiz. Tim looks at the questions for a few minutes, then stands up, rips up the exam, and throws the pieces at his teacher as he stalks out the classroom door.

● Sally and Harry's first child was born two months ago. Sally has taken maternity leave from her job to stay home with the baby; Harry is working overtime. One night, when Harry finally arrives home much later than usual, his wife greets him, saying, "Glad to see you. You're in charge; I'm on my way to work out at the gym." Harry explodes, throws his briefcase at the kitchen table, scattering and breaking some china, and yells, "This place is a mess. You haven't got dinner ready for me. You're not working. What right do you have to go to the gym?"

To most people, the words *temper tantrum* probably conjure up a vision of a red-faced two-year-old lying on the floor kicking and screaming because he does not want to go to bed. But as the above examples illustrate, people of all ages have tantrums, which take a variety of forms and can occur for a variety of reasons, ranging from serious—Betty's very real fear of pain and being alone at night—to relatively trivial— Rob's dad denying him a candy bar.

A temper tantrum is an irritable outburst that occurs in response to a frustrating, stressful situation. In the very young, the nonverbal, and the unsocialized, such eruptions are an instinctual way of communicating frustration and needs. This was recognized over 2,300 years ago by the Greek philosopher Plato, who suggested that newborns communicate with their caregivers by crying and screaming. In the 18th century the French philosopher Jean-Jacques Rousseau observed, "When children begin to speak, they cry less. This is a natural progression. One language is substituted for another."

It is therefore perfectly normal and healthy for an infant without language—such as Betty—to communicate distress through a noisy outburst. Punishing Betty for such behavior would deprive her of her only way of letting caretakers know of her distress. Young children like Rob and Jill may already have learned how to use language to communicate their everyday needs, but when they are overly tired or confronted with a particularly trying situation, a temper tantrum is normal. During the stressful transition to adolescence, even older children such as Tim, who may not have had a tantrum for years, surprise themselves— and others—by occasionally losing control. For many young people, adolescence is a time for learning how to cope with emotional challenges by talking about feelings with peers rather than exploding in uncontrollable anger at authority figures. Some individuals persist in expressing their displeasure through tantrums during their adult years. By adulthood, however, frequent displays of explosive rage, like Harry's outburst at Sally, are neither normal nor healthy.

A way of communicating

Everybody has a temper tantrum once in a while. Rare exceptions to this rule are people so meek, unassertive, and self-martyred that they do not respond to even legitimate frustrations, such as family members' continually taking advantage of them. Temper tantrums are common because they almost always have some immediate, short-term payoff—coercing someone else into "giving in" or "backing off." Such behaviors tend to be repeated because the capitulation of others provides either positive or negative reinforcement. As an example of the former, in Rob's case the result of his tantrum is a candy bar and a long lecture from his usually remote and emotionally unavailable father. Likewise, Jill gets 10 minutes of cuddling and reassurance from her busy, preoccupied mother. An example of negative reinforcement can be seen in the case of Tim, whose tantrum enables him to escape a test for which he is unprepared. Harry, by exploding at his wife, is able to fend off her questions about why he came home so late. Temper tantrums may be viewed as a necessary survival tool for children who have no other means of getting attention from uninterested parents or of avoiding abuse. Such behavior becomes manipulative, however, when indulged in by someone like Harry, who clearly knows how to use verbal communication to get what he wants and avoid what he does not want. He could, for example, use this opportunity to tell Sally of his mounting dissatisfaction with his demanding job and the changes in his life since the baby was born, as well as to ask about her feelings.

Temper tantrums are never solely an individual's problem; they are always a relationship problem. This is because such outbursts inevitably have an effect on those who are subjected to them. Like Rob's father and Tim's teacher, observers of the tantrum are often startled or frightened; they may also feel guilty or responsible. In order to quell the temper tantrum, observers typically respond by giving in to unreasonable requests or compromising on rules and expectations. In this way they allow themselves to be coerced into supplying the positive and negative reinforcements (a candy bar, a reprieve from a math quiz) that strengthen the future probability and intensity of tantrums. Moreover, each time a temper tantrum is brought to an end by such a reaction (the teacher allows Tim to leave the classroom without taking the quiz), there is a greater chance that the observer too will repeat that same pattern of behavior (the teacher exempts Tim from other obligations in order to avoid his unpleasant outbursts).

Thus, when Sally abandons her plan to go to the gym and begins defending herself against Harry's accusations, she only increases the chances that Harry will continue to have tantrums and that these future outbursts will be more intense and accompanied by greater verbal and physical abuse. In other words, Sally is unintentionally training Harry to be abusive toward her. Worse yet, after Sally spends some time refuting Harry's accusations and placating

him, the tantrum will end, and Harry will turn on his usual charm, becoming apologetic and conciliatory. Through negative reinforcement (end of the tantrum) and positive reinforcement (resumption of endearing behavior), Harry is training Sally to act like a martyr.

Temper tantrums trap family members, teachers, friends, and co-workers into behaving in ways they dislike in order to stop, avoid, or escape the distasteful show of behavior. It is no wonder then that tantrums often make people feel they are being manipulated or used and that the individual having the tantrum is taking unfair advantage. As a result, people tend to dislike, avoid, or reject these consistently explosive individuals. While temper tantrums may at first secure for the individual the attention, support, and nurturance he or she craves, they eventually backfire, depriving the individual of these very same social rewards.

Roots of the problem

Temper tantrums are to be expected among healthy children from birth through early adolescence. In the normal course of development, children use these irritable outbursts to cope with frustrating challenges when they have yet to learn other, more adaptive, socially acceptable methods of coping. Authorities estimate that between the ages of 6 and 12, 80% of children have temper tantrums once a month or more, 48% have tantrums twice a week or more, and 11% have them once a day or more.

And, as was noted above, outbursts of temper often occur in older children and in adults. In some cases they are a manifestation of a mental, behavioral, or physical abnormality. According to the *Diagnostic and Statistical Manual of Mental Disorders,* third edition, revised (*DSM-III-R*), the official manual of the American Psychiatric Association, furious eruptions of anger are a common feature of a wide range of behavior disorders, including intoxication with (and withdrawal from) alcohol, cocaine, and other addictive substances; disorders associated with marked changes in mood (for example, bipolar disorder [manic-depressive psychosis]); childhood behavior problems such as hyperactivity (attention-deficit hyperactivity disorder) and other kinds of disruptive conduct; and posttraumatic stress disorder—to name just a few. Autistic youngsters sometimes have tantrumlike outbursts, as do persons with the neurological condition that is known as Tourette syndrome. None of these disorders is defined solely by the occurrence of occasional temper tantrums, nor are they caused by tantrums; in all of them, however, the occurrence of temper tantrums signals that the individual does not know how to cope with frustration in a constructive fashion. Whenever outbursts of temper are accompanied by many other signs of maladaptive behavior, it is unwise to attempt to do away with the tantrums while ignoring other behavior problems.

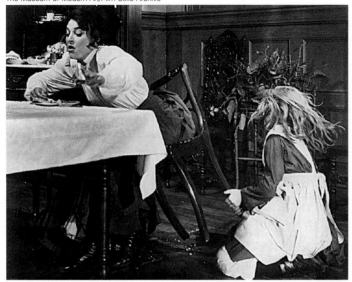

In the 1962 film The Miracle Worker, *teacher Annie Sullivan (played by Anne Bancroft) endures a temper tantrum thrown by Helen Keller (Patty Duke), blind and deaf after a childhood illness. Like many other people with severe physical disabilities, Keller often felt enormous frustration, which frequently erupted in tantrums. After Sullivan was able to get her to understand the connection between sign language and the objects referred to so that she had a means to express herself, Keller's behavior changed dramatically.*

Irritable mood and eruptions of temper are also a typical feature of a wide range of physical disorders that prevent people from functioning as they once did or as most other people do—for example, debilitating injuries, various physical impairments, and certain illnesses. Whenever they accompany such physical limitations, temper tantrums signal that the individual is having difficulty dealing with the frustration of the situation. In some cases the disorder itself—for example, a head injury or stroke—may make it impossible for the individual to articulate this frustration in words; the disorder is then a direct cause of the explosive irritability. Ideally, the rehabilitation process enables the person to express frustration without directing anger at self or others and helps family members and friends to be more tolerant of the recovering individual's expressions of rage. Whenever temper tantrums are accompanied by physical or neuropsychological complaints such as headaches, dizziness, or memory loss, it is unwise to concentrate only on eliminating the tantrums.

While all children have tantrums, they are much more common among youngsters who have a difficult, irritable temperament. From birth, perhaps 10% of infants are "difficult." Even with the most patient, nurturant parenting, children with a difficult temperament have irregular or problematic eating, sleeping, and toilet training. They have a tendency to withdraw from rather than approach new situations, and they are likely to be extremely upset by events that are only mildly distressing to other children. Some of these highly reactive children so intimidate parents and teachers that they are allowed to get away with repeated incidents of bullying and explosive rage. As a result, they are never encouraged to think and talk about their angry, hurt, frightened, or sad feelings. They do not learn to take responsibility for the impact of their rage on other people, nor are they able to soothe their own upset feelings, distract themselves when they are agitated, or solve the problems that give rise to their unhappy state.

Tantrums are not unusual among those adults who did not learn to moderate a difficult childhood temperament. The consequences can be far-reaching: poor personal and professional relationships, failed marriages and repeated divorce, erratic careers, and ill-tempered parenting of their own children. Unfortunately, the explosive behavior may continue throughout life because tantrums channel these individuals into settings that promote continuity of behavior patterns (*e.g.,* menial, low-paying jobs; relationships with volatile, unpredictable partners) and because the outbursts always have some short-term reward. The man who intimidates fellow employees and the woman who bullies her children both get an immediate, if short-lived, payoff: they "let off steam," and other people give in to their demands.

Moreover, tantrums are a form of learned behavior and are therefore more common among people who frequently observe or are subjected to other people's explosive rage. Children, in particular, are likely to become experts at having tantrums when they are constantly exposed to the outbursts of other important people in their lives (*e.g.,* parents, teachers, older siblings, and neighbors). It is unwise and almost always fruitless to try to eliminate outbursts in a child while ignoring the behavior of key figures such as parents and teachers.

Getting help

Temper tantrums are so common that most people cope with them spontaneously, often with good results. For parents who need support in dealing with tantrums that fall into the normal range described above, a good self-help manual may be all that is required. When tantrums exceed the "normal," however, or when they appear to be part of a larger behavioral or physical problem, it is wise to seek expert help.

Since temper tantrums can accompany so many different kinds of behavioral and physical problems, they may fall within the domain of numerous medical and psychological practitioners. One sensible approach is to seek an initial consultation with a Ph.D.-level behavioral psychologist who has specific expertise in the assessment and treatment of tantrums. The Association for Advancement of Behavior Therapy (15 West 36th Street, New York, NY 10018) can provide a list of qualified therapists in each state. After interviewing the individual (or parents, in the case of an infant) and observing family members as they interact, the psychologist may make referrals to other specialists; for example, a neurologist for the purpose of determining whether physical factors are contributing to the behavior problem. Once the medical consultants have done a thorough workup and evaluation and provided their expert opinions, the psychologist can operate as a case manager, supervising the behavior therapy in coordination with any necessary medical treatment.

The behavioral assessment. Whether parents decide to initiate a self-help plan or to consult a professional for guidance, the first step is the same: answering some basic questions about the nature of the tantrum behavior. What exactly does the individual do when he or she has a temper tantrum at home? At school? In a public place? What usually precedes or triggers the outburst? What does the child usually do following the tantrum? How do the parents react? What about teachers? Siblings? Friends? How long do the episodes usually last? How often do they occur? What quells the tantrums? What exacerbates them? Are there certain times of day when these irritable moods are particularly frequent? Do they occur on certain days of the week? Does anyone else in the family have similar outbursts? If so, what is the form and frequency of their tantrums?

Keeping a daily record to answer questions such as those above can help the whole family feel more in control of the situation. The answers to these questions may provide important clues as to why an individual responds to certain situations by having a tantrum and what behavior on the part of others seems to provoke or trigger a tantrum. Sometimes simply keeping a daily record and talking about it in a nonjudgmental fashion reduces the frequency of temper tantrums. If the record keeping alone has a beneficial effect, it is a good idea to continue the procedure until no tantrums have occurred—in any family member—for several months. It may be necessary to reinstate record keeping whenever tantrums recur.

The treatment plan. If the behavioral assessment

and the record-keeping process are not enough to keep the undesirable behavior under control, it is necessary to devise a specific strategy for responding to tantrums on the spot. The details of the plan will vary depending on such factors as the age of the individual who has the tantrums and the time and place they usually occur. The behavior therapist can provide guidance in setting up a treatment plan.

Consider, for example, the case of Betty, the young child who has trouble falling asleep. Betty's parents spend hours in her room each night. They understand that the ear infections contributed to Betty's bedtime tantrums, but they are exhausted and wish she could learn to relax and fall asleep holding her teddy bear after she has been rocked and soothed for 5 or 10 minutes. They have consulted the pediatrician and have been reassured that the child has no signs of continuing pain associated with an ear infection or of sleep apnea (a condition in which breathing ceases during sleep) or any other serious health problems that could interfere with sleep. After consulting a behavioral psychologist, they tried the following regime:

Betty was put to bed as usual. Her mother rocked and sang to her for five minutes, assured herself that Betty was all right, left the room, and stayed out even when the baby began to scream and cry. The first two nights she waited for a full five minutes to pass before she reentered the room and repeated the bedtime procedure. The next two nights she did not reenter the room until 10 minutes had passed. Every two days thereafter, she increased by five minutes the length of the time she refrained from going back into the room, continuing until the crying ceased altogether. From the outset she kept a record of how long she waited to reenter the room and how long Betty cried before stopping and also of her own feelings during the times she stayed out of the room. She continued to keep such a record until nighttime tantrums were no longer a problem. Once, when it seemed that the episodes were beginning again, she reinstated her earlier procedure. And during the daytime, she made a game of teaching Betty to practice putting herself and her teddy bear to sleep; she praised Betty as the child relaxed while having her back rubbed or listening to a story.

Rob and his parents consulted a behavioral psychologist after the boy's violent outburst at the supermarket and numerous tantrums at home. Rob's mother and father lived in dread of his tantrums, and Rob dreaded the anger his behavior provoked in them. The psychologist helped the family to spot a tantrum by defining it—any time when Rob had not been mistreated, was not ill, and for a least one minute continuously screamed, cried, threw things, or struck out at them. The family learned to use a procedure called "time-out" to deal with tantrums at home, and they encouraged Rob's teacher to use a similar pro-

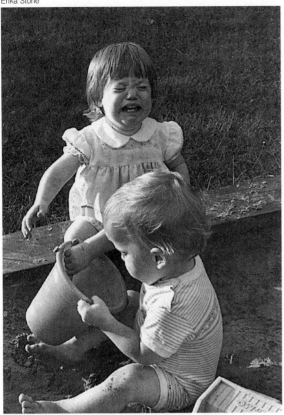
Erika Stone

A temper tantrum can be a normal response of the very young, particularly when they find themselves in a trying situation or when they become tired. Children quickly learn, however, that a tantrum may help them get what they want.

cedure at school. First they picked a "time-out" room for Rob. His bedroom was a good choice; it had a door that closed but had no lock. There was no television in the room, and there was nothing Rob might use to harm himself. (Bathrooms, closets, and other uncomfortable and confining places should never be used for time-out, nor should children ever be physically restrained or locked inside during these periods.) The psychologist recommended that Rob's toys and books be left in his bedroom, since the main purpose was to teach him to eventually go—on his own—to his room to calm himself when he felt he was about to have a tantrum.

At the beginning Rob's parents called time-out at the first sign of an outburst. They did not warn or threaten the youngster; they simply said, "Time-out," and waited for him to go to his room. The psychologist advised Rob's parents that it was not necessary to instruct him to think during time-out about why his behavior had been unacceptable; when children experience time-out consistently, they figure out the reason without being told. Moreover, the purpose of these periods is not to instill guilt—guilty children are not necessarily well behaved.

Rob understood that he was expected to stay in his room quietly (so that no noise could be heard on the other side of his closed door) until a timer set for five minutes went off. If his parents heard any noise from his room, they reset the timer for another five minutes. If they heard no noise, when the timer went off, Rob was free to leave his room. When Rob came out of his room, they praised him for his cooperation and appropriate behavior. Any time Rob ignored the time-out call, they put him to bed 30 minutes earlier than usual. However, on those days when no tantrums occurred and no time-outs were called, they congratulated him and allowed him to stay up an extra hour.

Practices such as that just described not only reduce tantrums but also teach children to cope with their anger by taking themselves out of difficult situations and calming themselves down. Knowing positive ways of dealing with rage not only makes for better behavior but also promotes self-control and enhances a child's self-esteem. The parents are also more effective in their actions and become more confident in their parenting role.

The right strategy

As the above examples illustrate, each case may call for a different strategy, and some may be more resistant to resolution than others. In the long run, however, the time and effort parents put into helping their youngsters control tantrums pay off. Their children will grow into adults who know how to express frustration in an appropriate and constructive way. They are likely to be more successful in their personal and work relationships and to be happier, better adjusted individuals than youngsters whose parents allow them to vent their anger unchecked. While it may seem easier—or sometimes kinder—to give in to the child's demands than to thwart them, parents who do so are not doing the children—or themselves—any favor.

Contributors to HealthWise

Alan L. Bisno, M.D.
Strep Infections (coauthor)
Chief, Medical Service, Miami Veterans Administration Medical Center; Professor, Department of Medicine, University of Miami School of Medicine, Miami, Fla.

Elaine A. Blechman, Ph.D.
Temper Tantrums
Professor, Department of Psychology, University of Colorado, Boulder; Author, *Solving Child Behavior Problems: At Home and at School*

Gladys Block, Ph.D.
Fruits, Vegetables, and Health
Professor, Public Health Nutrition, School of Public Health, University of California at Berkeley

Rafael E. Campo, M.D.
Strep Infections (coauthor)
Fellow, Division of Infectious Diseases, University of Miami School of Medicine, Miami, Fla.

Alvin N. Eden, M.D.
Overweight Children; Middle Ear Infections
Chairman, Department of Pediatrics, Wyckoff Heights Medical Center, Brooklyn, N.Y.; Associate Clinical Professor of Pediatrics, New York Hospital-Cornell Medical Center, New York City

Marc K. Effron, M.D.
Congestive Heart Failure
Senior Cardiologist and Director of Echocardiography, Scripps Memorial Hospital, La Jolla, Calif.; Assistant Clinical Professor, University of California at San Diego School of Medicine, La Jolla

Barry A. Franklin, Ph.D.
Exercise and Weight Loss: The Myths, the Facts; How Much Exercise Is Enough?
Director, Cardiac Rehabilitation and Exercise Laboratory, William Beaumont Hospital, Royal Oak, Mich.; Associate Professor of Physiology, Wayne State University School of Medicine, Detroit, Mich.

Susan M. Kleiner, Ph.D., R.D., L.D.
Yogurt: A Culture in Itself
Nutritionist in private practice, Friedman-Kester and Kleiner, Specialists in Nutrition, Gates Mills, Ohio

Dean Stern, D.P.M.
If the Shoe Fits . . .
Director, Section of Podiatric Medicine and Surgery, Rush-Presbyterian-St. Luke's Medical Center, Chicago, and Rush North Shore Medical Center, Skokie, Ill.

Philip Sanford Zeskind, Ph.D.
Infant Crying
Professor, Department of Psychology, Virginia Polytechnic Institute and State University, Blacksburg

Title cartoons by Richard Laurent

Index

This is a three-year cumulative index. Index entries to World of Medicine articles in this and previous editions of the *Medical and Health Annual* are set in boldface type; *e.g.*, **AIDS**. Entries to other subjects are set in lightface type; *e.g.*, alcohol. Additional information on any of these subjects is identified with a subheading and indented under the entry heading. The numbers following headings and subheadings indicate the year (boldface) of the edition and the page number (lightface) on which the information appears. The abbreviation *il.* indicates an illustration.

All entry headings are alphabetized word by word. Hyphenated words and words separated by dashes or slashes are treated as two words. When one word differs from another only by the presence of additional characters at the end, the shorter precedes the longer. In inverted names, the words following the comma are considered only after the preceding part of the name has been alphabetized. Examples:

      Lake
      Lake, Simon
      Lake Charles
      Lakeland

Names beginning with "Mc" and "Mac" are alphabetized as "Mac"; "St." is alphabetized as "Saint."

Dark type numbers refer to the year of the edition, *e.g.*, **92**–264 for the 1992 edition, page 264.

483

Dark type numbers refer to the year of the edition, *e.g.,* **92**–264 for the 1992 edition, page 264.

Dark type numbers refer to the year of the edition, e.g., **92**–264 for the 1992 edition, page 264.

485

486

Dark type numbers refer to the year of the edition, e.g., 92–264 for the 1992 edition, page 264.

Dark type numbers refer to the year of the edition, e.g., 92–264 for the 1992 edition, page 264.

487

Dark type numbers refer to the year of the edition, *e.g.,* **92**–264 for the 1992 edition, page 264.

Dark type numbers refer to the year of the edition, e.g., 92–264 for the 1992 edition, page 264.

489

Dark type numbers refer to the year of the edition, *e.g.,* **92**–264 for the 1992 edition, page 264.

divorce
temper tantrums **94**–479
Djibouti
child immunization *il.* **94**–38
DL-PLG
child immunization **94**–43
DMPA (drug): *see* Depo-Provera
DMSA (drug): *see* dimercaptosuccinic acid
DNA: *see* deoxyribonucleic acid
DNA fingerprint, *or* genetic fingerprint
gene therapy **93**–307
pathology **94**–70, *il.* 69
do-not-resuscitate order, *or* DNR order
cardiopulmonary arrest **92**–279
dobutamine
heart disease treatment **94**–443
doctor: *see* physician
"Doctor Nicolaes Tulp Demonstrating the
Anatomy of the Arm" (paint.) *il.*
93–10
DOE: *see* Energy, Department of
dog
Depo-Provera research use **94**–393
human disease transmission **93**–463
dog hookworm, *or* Ancylostoma caninum
human infections **93**–464
dog tick, *or* Dermacentor variabilis
human disease transmission **93**–464
Doll, Richard **92**–197
Dome of the Rock (Jerusalem) *il.* **94**–129
dominance
multiple personality disorder **93**–361
domoic acid
nerve-cell death **92**–350
"Don Juan" (Molière)
tobacco (special report) **94**–390
dopamine (drug)
heart disease treatment **94**–443
Parkinson's disease **94**–228
psychoactive drugs and the elderly
(special report) **94**–233
doppelgänger
autoscopy **94**–82
Dorozynski, Alexander
"France: Fuming over a New Antismoking
Law?" (special report) **94**–386
dorsum height **92**–464
Dostoyevsky, Fyodor Mikhaylovich
autoscopy **94**–85
double (psychology)
autoscopy **94**–82
"Double, The" (Dostoyevsky)
autoscopy **94**–85
double depression **92**–80
double dyslexia (special report) **92**–324
double helix
structure of DNA (special report) **94**–305
"Double Secret, Le" (Magritte)
autoscopy *il.* **94**–93
double vision, *or* diplopia
encephalitis lethargica **92**–206
Doucet, Ian Lee
"Persian Gulf War: The Human Tragedy"
93–20
Dow Corning Wright (co., U.S.)
silicone breast implants **93**–411
Down syndrome, *or* Down's syndrome, *or*
DS, *or* mongolism, *or* trisomy 21
Dolly Downs doll **94**–20
Downs, Dolly
Down syndrome **94**–20
doxacurium, *or* Nuromax (drug)
FDA approval **93**–381
doxazosin mesylate, *or* Cardura (drug)
FDA approval **94**–367
DPT vaccine: *see* DTP vaccine
dracunculiasis: *see* guinea worm disease
Dracunculus medinensis: *see* guinea worm
drainage
appendicitis **93**–424, 428
dream
autoscopy **94**–92
DRG: *see* diagnosis-related group
"Drinker, The" (painting) *il.* **92**–157
drinking, alcohol **92**–150
adolescent sexual behavior **93**–209
American Indians **94**–110
Eastern European consumption **92**–372
French dietary paradox **93**–50
health hazards (special report) **93**–170
U.K. attitudes and use **93**–110
U.S. advertising and use **93**–152
see also Alcoholism
drinking water: *see* water
driving
senior citizens **94**–223
dropsy
Withering's research **94**–442
drought
hunger **94**–170
drowning
prevention **93**–334
drug abuse
AIDS association **93**–209
America's children **94**–213
postnatal infant crying **94**–435
professional sports **93**–187
see also Alcoholism

drug-approval process **93**–384
drug interaction
prescription drugs **94**–381
drug testing
National Football League **93**–188
pharmaceuticals **94**–379
Supreme Court decisions **92**–360
drug therapy
asthma **93**–237
women and heart disease **92**–426
Drugs 92–363
see also Pharmaceuticals
"Drugs: Some Do Grow on Trees" (Mason)
93–130
drunk driving
attitudes **92**–153, *il.* 152
traffic fatalities **93**–154
dry commodity, *or* dry food
hunger **94**–177
dry socket
wisdom teeth postoperative pain **92**–436
"DSM-III-R": *see* "Diagnostic and Statistical
Manual of Mental Disorders"
DTP vaccine, *or* diphtheria-tetanus-pertussis
vaccine **93**–382
child immunization **94**–37
dual personality: *see* multiple personality
disorder
dualism
multiple personality disorder (special
report) **93**–360
Duchenne muscular dystrophy **92**–351
duck
French dietary paradox **93**–50
duplex scan
carotid artery blockage **93**–398
Durack, David *il.* **92**–199
Dürer, Albrecht
"Self Portrait" *il.* **93**–11
use of human anatomy knowledge **93**–15
DynaCirc (drug): *see* isradipine
dynamic mutation
stuttering genes **94**–301
dynemicin A
anticancer antibiotic **94**–256
dysgeusia, *or* parageusia
taste disorder **93**–401
dyslexia
adults (special report) **92**–323, *il.*
dysmorphophobia: *see* body dysmorphic
disorder
dysosmia: *see* parosmia
dyspnea
heart failure symptom **94**–440
dysthemia, *or* depressive neurosis **92**–80
dystocia: *see* labor dystocia
dystrophin
Duchenne muscular dystrophy **92**–351

e

ear
allergic reactions *il.* **93**–458
hearing loss noise-induced damage
92–327, *il.* 328
ear infection **94**–467
temper tantrums **94**–480
earache
middle ear infections **94**–468
"Early Arrival—Why Babies Are Born Too
Soon and Too Small" (Luke and
Keith) **94**–134
earphone
dichotic listening use (special report)
94–401
eastern Africa
hunger **94**–160
Eastern Europe
cigarette smoking **92**–396
health care reform (special report)
94–292
medicine and health (special report)
92–370
"Eat, Drink, and Be Healthy!" (Callaway)
93–62
eating habit
obese children, adolescents, and adults
94–453
Ebers Papyrus
guinea worm disease **92**–10
Ebert, Robert H. **93**–346
Ebola virus
hemorrhagic fever outbreak **94**–339
EBV: *see* Epstein-Barr virus
EC: *see* European Community
"Ecclesiastical History of the English
People" (Bede)
near-death experience account **92**–46
ECG: *see* electrocardiography
echocardiography **93**–226
coronary artery disease screening
93–321, 478
congestive heart failure diagnosis **94**–441
economics, health care: *see* health care
economics
ECT: *see* electroconvulsive therapy

ectopic pregnancy
sexual and reproductive health **92**–382
edema
burn injuries **93**–252
congestive heart failure **94**–440
edentulous mouth
wisdom teeth **92**–434
education
adolescent health and sexual behavior
93–211, 451
adult dyslexia (special report) **92**–323
American children's future **94**–219
American Indian health care **94**–106
asthma **93**–240
children's universal access **92**–270
dietary choices **93**–68
hypertension **93**–336
multiple-birth families **92**–69
parental newborn preparation **93**–371
U.K. public health issues **93**–100
Education for All Handicapped Children Act
(1975, U.S.) **93**–286
Educize program
arthritis and exercise (special report)
92–392
EEG: *see* electroencephalograph
EEOC: *see* Equal Employment Opportunity
Commission
effusion
middle ear infections **94**–469
eflornithine hydrochloride, *or* Ornidyl (drug)
FDA approval **92**–364
egg
world diets **93**–47
Egypt
cholera epidemic **93**–77, 88, *il.* 75
Egypt, ancient
dental implants (special report) **94**–265
funerary papyrus *il.* **92**–172
guinea worm disease **92**–10
plant therapy **93**–134
symbolism of bread **93**–445
E.I. du Pont de Nemours & Co. (U.S.)
guinea worm disease **92**–26
Eighth International Congress of Human
Genetics (U.S.)
prenatal diagnosis **93**–306
"Eileen O'Shea After Three Liver
Transplants, Awaiting Her Fourth"
(paint.) *il.* **93**–17
EKG: *see* electrocardiogram
El Tor
cholera treatment **93**–79, 91
elastomer
penile implant use **94**–356
Elavil (drug): *see* amitriptyline
elbow
joint implant (special report) **92**–275
elderly, the: *see* senior citizens
Elders, M. Joycelyn *ils.* **94**–213–220
"America's Children: Our Vision of the
Future" **94**–213
Clinton appointment **94**–8
electric-power-distribution system
environmental health **94**–290
electric shock
muscle stimulating devices **94**–461
electrical impulse
coronary disease **93**–323
taste disorders **93**–403
electrical muscle stimulator, *or* EMS
weight reduction methods **94**–461
electrified blade
surgical use **94**–353
electrocardiogram, *or* EKG
arrhythmia diagnosis **93**–466
heart failure diagnosis **94**–441
stress testing *il.* **93**–475
electrocardiography, *or* ECG
coronary disease testing **93**–320, 473;
92–425
electrocautery
laparoscopic cholecystectomy **92**–406
electroconvulsive therapy, *or* ECT, *or* shock
therapy
body dysmorphic disorder treatment
(special report) **93**–367
depression **92**–93, *il.*
psychoactive drugs and the elderly
(special report) **94**–231
electromagnetic field
environmental health **94**–290
occupational health **94**–371
electron microscopy
pathology **94**–55, 65, *il.* 66
electronic radiology
medical imaging **93**–353
electrophysiological study, *or* EP study, *or*
EPS study
arrhythmias **93**–467, 470
EL530 (drug)
cancer treatment **94**–256
Eliade, Mircea
Jerusalem syndrome **94**–126
Elian, Marta
multiple sclerosis study **94**–365
Ellwood, Paul M., Jr.
U.S. health care system **93**–310

embargo
cholera prevention **93**–94
embolism
strokes **93**–396
embolus
stroke cause **93**–396
embryo
alcohol-related birth defects **94**–122
human development **93**–294
preimplantation genetics **92**–304
X-rays during pregnancy **92**–475, *il.* 476
"Emerging Infections: Microbial Threats to
Health in the United States" (U.S.
publ.) **94**–338
emesis: *see* vomiting
EMG: *see* electromyography
emigration
Eurasian population (special report)
94–295
emission standard
motor vehicles (special report) **92**–255
emmetropia
eye disease treatment **93**–293
emotion
alcohol advertising **93**–156
anatomy and physiology **92**–170
aquatic exercise **93**–430
body dysmorphic disorder (special
report) **93**–363
child and play (special report) **92**–302
depression **92**–74
exercise **92**–143
infant crying **94**–431
memory **92**–126
music and the brain (special report)
94–402
near-death experience **92**–50
only child **92**–444
Employee Retirement Income Security Act,
or ERISA (1974, U.S.)
AIDS patients' rights **94**–315
employment
AIDS issues **94**–315
child care **94**–258
disability act **93**–288
health care costs **94**–320
Japan's aging population **93**–338
occupational health **94**–368
overwork in Japan (special report)
94–373
premature birth **94**–143
senior citizens **94**–223
taste and smell functions **93**–403
U.K. public health efforts **93**–102
U.S. health care system **93**–311
empty calorie **94**–410
EMS (device): *see* electrical muscle
stimulator
EMS (path.): *see* eosinophilia-myalgia
syndrome
enalapril
heart disease treatment **94**–444
encephalitis
encephalitis lethargica **92**–207
epidemiological investigations **92**–99
encephalitis lethargica, *or* sleepy sickness,
or acute epidemic encephalitis, *or*
von Economo's disease **92**–202
"Encounters with Death" (Greyson) **92**–46
endarterectomy
stroke prevention **93**–398
Endo-Clip Applier
laparoscopic cholecystectomy **92**–406
endocrinology
encephalitis lethargica **92**–215
endogenous morphine: *see* endorphin
endometriosis
cancer **93**–259
drug treatment **94**–392; **92**–367
endometrium
estrogen therapy side effects **94**–226
endorphin, *or* endogenous morphine
aquatic exercise **93**–430
endothelial cell
atherosclerotic damage **94**–420
coronary artery **92**–334
endurance phase: *see* stimulus phase
enediyne
cancer treatment **94**–256
Energy, Department of, *or* DOE (U.S.)
radioactive-waste disposal **94**–290
English language
anatomic terms **92**–181
English yew, *or* Taxus baccata (tree)
Taxotere extraction **93**–132
engram **92**–114
Enkaid (drug): *see* encainide
enmeshment
only child **92**–444
enterococcus
strep infections **94**–425
Enthoven, Alain **94**–323, *il.*
entomology **94**–69
environment
Alzheimer's patients' nursing-home care
(special report) **93**–299
multiple sclerosis role **94**–364
Pacific yews controversy **93**–132

Dark type numbers refer to the year of the edition, *e.g.,* **92**–264 for the 1992 edition, page 264.

491

Dark type numbers refer to the year of the edition, e.g., **92**–264 for the 1992 edition, page 264.

Dark type numbers refer to the year of the edition, e.g., **92**–264 for the 1992 edition, page 264.

493

Dark type numbers refer to the year of the edition, e.g., **92**–264 for the 1992 edition, page 264.

Dark type numbers refer to the year of the edition, *e.g.,* **92**–264 for the 1992 edition, page 264.

495

Dark type numbers refer to the year of the edition, *e.g.,* **92**–264 for the 1992 edition, page 264.

Dark type numbers refer to the year of the edition, e.g., **92**–264 for the 1992 edition, page 264.

497

Dark type numbers refer to the year of the edition, *e.g.,* **92**–264 for the 1992 edition, page 264.

Dark type numbers refer to the year of the edition, *e.g.,* **92**–264 for the 1992 edition, page 264.

499

Dark type numbers refer to the year of the edition, *e.g.,* **92**–264 for the 1992 edition, page 264.

Dark type numbers refer to the year of the edition, e.g., 92–264 for the 1992 edition, page 264.

501

Dark type numbers refer to the year of the edition, *e.g.*, **92**–264 for the 1992 edition, page 264.

Dark type numbers refer to the year of the edition, *e.g.*, **92**–264 for the 1992 edition, page 264.

503

Dark type numbers refer to the year of the edition, e.g., **92**–264 for the 1992 edition, page 264.

505

Dark type numbers refer to the year of the edition, e.g., **92**–264 for the 1992 edition, page 264.

Dark type numbers refer to the year of the edition, *e.g.,* **92**–264 for the 1992 edition, page 264.

507

Dark type numbers refer to the year of the edition, *e.g.*, **92**–264 for the 1992 edition, page 264.

Dark type numbers refer to the year of the edition, e.g., **92**–264 for the 1992 edition, page 264.

509

Dark type numbers refer to the year of the edition, e.g., **92**–264 for the 1992 edition, page 264.

Dark type numbers refer to the year of the edition, *e.g.,* **92**–264 for the 1992 edition, page 264.

511